Care of People with Diabetes
A Manual of Nursing Practic

Dedication

This book is dedicated to all people with diabetes who may one day need health care and to all the health professionals who care for them.

Care of People with Diabetes

A Manual of Nursing Practice

Third Edition

Professor Trisha Dunning AM
RN, MEd, PhD, CDE, FRCNA
Inaugural Chair in Nursing
Deakin University and Barwon Health
Geelong, Victoria
Australia

WILEY-BLACKWELL

A John Wiley & Sons, Ltd., Publication

This edition first published 2009
© 2009 Trisha Dunning
© 1994, 2003 Blackwell Publishing Ltd

Blackwell Publishing was acquired by John Wiley & Sons in February 2007. Blackwell's publishing programme has been merged with Wiley's global Scientific, Technical, and Medical business to form Wiley-Blackwell.

Registered office
John Wiley & Sons Ltd, The Atrium, Southern Gate, Chichester, West Sussex, PO19 8SQ, United Kingdom

Editorial offices
9600 Garsington Road, Oxford, OX4 2DQ, United Kingdom
2121 State Avenue, Ames, Iowa 50014-8300, USA

First published 1994
Second edition 2003
Third edition 2009

For details of our global editorial offices, for customer services and for information about how to apply for permission to reuse the copyright material in this book please see our website at www.wiley.com/wiley-blackwell.

Library of Congress Cataloging-in-Publication Data

Dunning, Trisha.
    Care of people with diabetes : a manual of nursing practice / Trisha Dunning—3rd ed.
       p. ; cm.
    Includes bibliographical references and index.
    ISBN 978-1-4051-0111-0 (pbk. : alk. paper) 1. Diabetes—Nursing—Handbooks,
manuals, etc. I. Title.
    [DNLM: 1. Diabetes Mellitus—nursing—Handbooks. WY 49 D924c 2009]
    RC660.D785 2009
    616.4′620231—dc22

                                                                2008047437

A catalogue record for this book is available from the British Library.

Set in 10/12 pt Sabon by Newgen Imaging Systems Pvt Ltd, Chennai, India
Printed and bound in Malaysia by KHL Printing Co Sdn Bhd

1   2009

Contents

List of Figures   xv
List of Tables   xvii
Example Forms and Instruction Sheets   xxi
Foreword   xxiii
Preface   xxv
Acknowledgements   xxvii
List of Abbreviations and Symbols   xxviii

1 Diagnosing and Classifying Diabetes   **1**
   Key points   1
   What is diabetes mellitus?   1
   Prevalence of diabetes   2
   Classification of diabetes   2
   Overview of normal glucose homeostasis   3
   The metabolic syndrome in children and adolescents   6
   Type 1 and Type 2 diabetes   7
   Gestational diabetes   11
   Example Instruction Sheet 1: Preparation for an oral glucose
     tolerance test   18
   Screening for diabetes   19
   Preventing Type 2 diabetes   19
   Managing diabetes mellitus   20
   Aims of management   21
   Exercise/activity   24
   Diabetes education   27
   Complications of diabetes   27
   Cost of diabetes   29
   Aim and objectives of nursing care of people with diabetes   29
   References   32

2 Holistic Assessment, Nursing Diagnosis, and Documentation   **36**
   Key points   36
   Rationale   36
   Holistic nursing   36
   Care models   37

Characteristics of an holistic nursing history   38
Nursing history   40
Example health assessment chart   41
Instruments to measure health status   45
Documenting and charting patient care   47
Nursing care plans   47
Nursing responsibilities   49
Documentation by people with diabetes   49
References   50

3   **Monitoring Diabetes Mellitus**   **52**
Key points   52
Rationale   52
Introduction   52
Monitoring 1: blood glucose   53
Key points   53
Blood glucose testing checklist   63
Monitoring 2: urine glucose   66
Key points   66
Monitoring 3: additional assessment   68
References   73

4   **Nutrition, Obesity and Exercise**   **76**
Key points   76
Rationale   76
The importance of good nutrition   76
Obesity   77
Overview of the pathogenesis of obesity   77
The significance of abdominal obesity   79
Nutrition, obesity and stress   79
Methods of measuring weight   80
Managing obesity and diabetes   82
Method of screening for dietary characteristics and problems   85
Principles of dietary management for people with diabetes   85
The Apple Report   90
Dietary management: obesity   90
Bariatric surgery   91
Complementary weight loss programmes   91
Factors associated with making dietary changes   92
Nursing responsibilities   92
References   97

5   **Medicines Management**   **102**
Key points   102
Introduction   102
Quality Use of Medicines (QUM)   103
Quality Use of Medicines and diabetes   103
Oral hypoglycaemic agents (OHA)   104

The incretin hormones 114
When should insulin be initiated in Type 2 diabetes? 117
Barriers to insulin therapy 119
Some strategies to overcome the barriers 120
Insulin therapy 121
Types of insulin available 122
Injection sites and administration 129
Mixing short- and intermediate-acting insulins 131
Commonly used insulin regimens 131
Interpreting morning hyperglycaemia 133
Continuous subcutaneous insulin infusion (CSII) 133
Continuous blood glucose sensors 135
Subcutaneous insulin sliding scales and top-up regimes 135
Uses of insulin infusions 138
Insulin allergy 141
Transplants 141
Stabilising diabetes 141
Stabilisating diabetes in hospital 142
Community and outpatient stabilisation 143
Lipid lowering agents 146
Monitoring lipid medicines 150
Antihypertensive agents 151
Antiplatelet agents 152
Complementary cardiovascular medicines 154
Medication safety and medication self-management 154
Enhancing medication self-care 155
Example protocol for outpatient stabilisation onto insulin 158
References 160

6 **Hypoglycaemia** 165
Key points 165
Rationale 165
Introduction 165
Definition of hypoglycaemia 168
Recognising hypoglycaemia 169
Counter-regulatory hormonal response to
hypoglycaemia 170
Causes of hypoglycaemia 171
Hypoglycaemic unawareness 172
Nocturnal hypoglycaemia 173
Relative hypoglycaemia 175
Medicine interactions 175
Objectives of care 176
Treatment 176
Prolonged hypoglycaemia 178
Patients most at risk of hypoglycaemia 178
Psychological effects of hypoglycaemia 179
Guidelines for administering glucagon 180

Adverse reactions   181
References   181

7   **Hyperglycaemia, Acute Illness, Diabetic Ketoacidosis (DKA),**
    Hyperosmolar Coma (HONK), and Lactic Acidosis   **184**
    Key points   184
    Rationale   184
    Prevention: proactively managing intercurrent illness   185
    Self-care during illness   186
    Hyperglycaemia   186
    Diabetic ketoacidosis (DKA)   189
    Brittle diabetes and hyperglycaemia   196
    Euglycaemic DKA   197
    Hyperosmolar non-ketotic coma (HONK)   197
    Presenting signs and symptoms   198
    Lactic acidosis   199
    Lactic acidosis associated with metformin   201
    References   202

8   **Long-Term Complications of Diabetes**   **205**
    Introduction   205
    Pathophysiology of diabetes complications   205
    Cardiovascular disease and diabetes   207
    Key points   207
    Rationale   208
    Medicines and cardiovascular disease   209
    Complementary medicines (CAM)   210
    Mental health and cardiovascular disease   212
    Nursing responsibilities   213
    Telephone coaching   217
    Cerebrovascular disease   217
    Signs and symptoms   218
    Diabetes and eye disease   218
    Key points   218
    Rationale   218
    Introduction   218
    Risk factors for retinopathy   219
    Diabetes and renal disease   224
    Key points   224
    Introduction   224
    Risk factors for renal disease   224
    Renal failure   225
    Renal disease and anaemia   227
    Diet and renal disease   227
    Renal disease and older people   228
    Kidney biopsy   229
    Renal dialysis   229
    Objectives of care   230
    Nursing responsibilities   231
    Commencing CAPD in patients on insulin   233
    Educating patient about CAPD   233

Renal disease and herbal medicine (see also Chapter 19)   234
Peripheral and autonomic neuropathy   234
Peripheral   235
Key points   235
Introduction   235
Vascular changes   236
Infection   236
Diabetic peripheral neuropathy   238
Other pain management strategies   239
Stages of peripheral neuropathy   242
Risk factors for the development of foot problems in people with diabetes   242
Objectives of care   243
Nursing responsibilities   243
Classification of foot ulcers   245
Wound management   246
Wound management techniques under study   246
Rehabilitation   246
Autonomic neuropathy   248
Key points   248
Rationale   249
Introduction   249
Diagnosis and management   250
Nursing care   252
References   253

9 **Management During Surgical and Investigative Procedures**   **260**
Key points   260
Rationale   260
Introduction   260
Aims of management   262
Preoperative nursing care   263
Major procedures   266
Postoperative nursing responsibilities   267
Minor procedures   268
Emergency procedures   270
Bariatric surgery   271
Investigative procedures   271
Key points   271
Rationale   272
The objectives of care   272
General nursing management   272
Complementary therapies and surgery and investigative procedures   276
Preoperative phase   276
Postoperative phase   277
Implications for nursing care   278
References   278
Example Instruction Sheet 2(a): Instructions for diabetic patients on oral
   hypoglycaemic agents having procedures as outpatients under sedation
   of general anaesthesia   279

Example Instruction Sheet 2(b): Instructions for diabetic patients on
insulin having procedures as outpatients under sedation or general
anaesthesia   280

10   Managing Common Conditions Associated with Diabetes   281
Key points   281
Introduction   281
Enteral and parenteral nutrition   282
Aims of therapy   282
Routes of administration   283
Choice of formula   284
Nursing responsibilities   285
Diabetes and cancer   286
Objectives of care   288
Nursing responsibilities   289
Managing corticosteroids in people with cancer   290
Complementary therapies and cancer   290
Smoking, alcohol, and illegal drug use   292
Smoking   292
Nicotine addiction   294
Assisting the person to stop smoking   295
Medications to support smoking cessation   296
Alcohol addiction   298
Illegal drug use   299
Effects on diabetes   299
Interactions with medicines   300
Management issues   300
Brittle diabetes   303
Introduction   304
Management   304
Oral health and diabetes   305
Introduction   305
Causal mechanisms   306
Management   306
Diabetes and liver disease   307
Introduction   307
Managing people with diabetes and liver disease   308
CAM medicines   308
Haemochromatosis   309
Iron overload   309
Management   309
Diabetic mastopathy   310
Diagnosis   310
Management   310
Diabetes and coeliac disease   311
Signs and symptoms   311
Management   312
Diabetes and musculoskeletal diseases   312

Management   313
Corticosteroid medications and diabetes   314
Key points   314
Introduction   314
Diabetes and driving   317
Prevalence of and risk factors for driving crashes   317
Diabetes-related effects on driving   322
Hypoglycaemia effects on driving   323
Strategies to enhance driving safety   325
Information for people with diabetes to help them drive safely   326
References   327

11 Diabetes and Sexual Health   **334**
Key points   334
Rationale   334
Sexual health   334
Sexual development   336
Sexual problems   336
Possible causes of sexual difficulties and dysfunction   336
Sexuality and older people   338
Women   338
Men   339
Investigation and management   340
Medication management   340
Non-pharmacological therapy   341
Complementary medicines for sexual problems (CAM)   342
Involving partners in ED management   342
Sexual counselling   343
The PLISSIT model   344
Role of the nurse   345
References   346

12 Diabetes in Older People   **347**
Key points   347
Rationale   347
Introduction   348
Determining functional status   354
Cognitive impairment   355
Depression and older people with diabetes   358
Differentiating depression from dementia   358
Managing diabetes in older people   359
Management aims   359
Factors that affect management decisions   360
Guidelines for administering diabetes medicines with enteral feeds 364
Education approaches   366
Self-care   367
Factors that can affect metabolic control   368
References   377

13   Diabetes in Children and Adolescents   **380**
Key points   380
Rationale   380
Introduction   380
Managing children and adolescents with diabetes   382
Aspects of care that apply to both Type 1 and Type 2 diabetes in
    children and adolescents   383
Managing Type 1 diabetes   384
Managing childhood Type 2 diabetes   388
Medication self-management   388
Complementary therapy use in children   389
Strategies for enhancing adherence during adolescence   390
Ketoacidosis in children   391
References   392

14   Women, Pregnancy, and Gestational Diabetes   **395**
Key points   395
Rationale   395
Polycystic Ovarian Syndrome   395
Pregnancy   398
Complications of pregnancy   403
Effects of diabetes on the baby   404
Longer term effects of maternal hyperglycaemia on the child   404
Gestational diabetes   405
Who is at risk from gestational diabetes?   406
Type 1 diabetes   407
Type 2 diabetes   408
Menopause and diabetes   409
Signs and symptoms of menopause   409
Managing the menopause   410
Contraception options for women with diabetes   410
Complementary approaches to managing the menopause   411
References   414

**15   Psychological and Quality of Life Issues Related to Having
       Diabetes**   **418**
Key points   418
Rationale   418
Introduction   418
Depression   422
Symptoms of depression   423
Maintaining mental health and managing depression   423
Antipsychotic medications and diabetes   425
Type 1 diabetes   426
Type 2 diabetes   427
Compliance/adherence/concordance   428
Psychological distress and cardiovascular disease   428
Quality of life   430
References   432

16   Diabetes Education   436
    Key points   436
    Rationale   436
    Introduction   436
    Learning styles   438
    Education theories   441
    Communication – the central element of effective teaching and learning   443
    Teaching: an art and a process   445
    Health literacy   446
    Survival skills   448
    Sample diabetes education record chart   449
    Empowerment   451
    Special issues   452
    The nurses' role in diabetes education   452
    Insulin administration   454
    Guidelines for instructing patients about insulin delivery systems   455
    Documenting diabetes education   455
    Examples Instruction Sheets   456
    Example Instruction Sheet 3: How to draw up insulin – one bottle only   456
    Example Instruction Sheet 4: How to draw up insulin – two bottles   457
    Example Instruction Sheet 5: How to give an insulin injection using
        syringes or insulin pens   458
    Example Instruction Sheet 6a: Managing your diabetes when you are ill:
        patients with Type 1 diabetes   459
    Example Instruction Sheet 6b: Managing your diabetes when you are ill:
        patients with Type 2 diabetes   462
    References   465

17   Discharge Planning   468
    Key points   468
    On day of discharge   468

18   Community, Practice Nursing, and Home-Based Care   470
    Key points   470
    Introduction   470
    How to obtain advice   471
    General points   471
    Disposing of sharps in the home situation   477
    Storing insulin   478
    Guidelines for premixing and storing insulin doses for home and
        district nursing services   479
    Practice nurses   480
    References   480

19   Complementary and Alternative Therapies and Diabetes   482
    Key points   482
    Rationale   482
    Introduction   483
    CAM philosophy   485

Integrating complementary and conventional care   486
Can complementary therapies benefit people with diabetes?   488
Spirituality   491
CAM and surgery   492
Herb/medicine interactions   495
How can complementary therapies be used safely?   499
Nursing responsibilities   501
Identifying quality health information on the internet   502
References   504

20 **Nursing Care in the Emergency and Outpatient Departments**   507
Rationale   507
The emergency department   507
The outpatient department   509

Appendix A: **Associations Providing Services for People with Diabetes**   511
Diabetes associations   511
Professional diabetes associations   512
International Diabetes Federation (IDF)   512
Other professional associations   513
Pharmaceutical companies   513

Appendix B: **Diabetes Reference Material for Nursing Staff**   514
Guidelines and policy statements   514
Useful reading in addition to the texts listed in the preliminary pages
    and reference list following each chapter   515
Recommended journal   516

Appendix C: **Reading Material for People with Diabetes**   517

Index   519

List of Figures

1.1 Overview of glucose homeostasis showing the key factors operating during the fed and fasting states. Usually the blood glucose is maintained within the normal range by the interplay of the anabolic and catabolic hormones, which are in turn influenced by other hormones and a number of factors such as nutritional status and intake   4

1.2 Schematic representation of the slow progressive loss of beta cell mass following the initial trigger event in Type 1 diabetes   9

1.3 Consequences of the insulin resistance syndrome   10

1.4 Diagrammatic representation of insulin binding, insulin signalling, translocation of GLUT-4 and glucose entry into the cell. GLUT-4 is a glucose transporter contained in vesicles in the cell cytoplasm. Once insulin binds to an insulin receptor GLUT-4 moves to the cell membrane and transports glucose into the cell. During fasting GLUT-4 is low and increases in response to the increase in insulin. Failure of GLUT-4 translocation could explain some of the insulin resistance associated with Type 2 diabetes. The effects of insulin are mediated by two protein pathways: P13-kinase through the insulin receptors (glucose uptake) and MAP-kinase, which stimulates growth and mitogenesis   12

1.5 Example of a screening and preventative model of health care   20

1.6 Suggested diabetes management model. Most diabetes management occurs in primary care settings in collaboration with secondary and tertiary care services   25

1.7 Normal energy sources during exercise. *Note:* At rest free fatty acids are the major energy source. As exercise begins muscle glycogen is utilised as the predominant energy source. As exercise continues the blood glucose is utilised, reverting to free fatty acids as the major energy source if exercise is prolonged. Blood glucose is maintained by hormonal regulation of hepatic glucose output and lipolysis   26

2.1 Example of a combination of a genomap (information inside the circle) and an ecomap (information outside the circle) of a 50-year-old woman with Type 2 diabetes and a history of childhood molestation and sexual abuse. It shows a great deal of conflict within and outside the family and identifies where her support base is   39

2.2 Sample diabetes record charts for (a) 2-hourly testing (e.g. when using an insulin infusion); (b) 4-hourly or less frequent testing   50

3.1   An example of a quality control flow chart for checking blood
      glucose meters   62
5.1   The Quality use of Medicines process applied to diabetes care
      reproduced from The Quality Use of Medicines in Diabetes
      Pharmaceutical Health And Rational use of Medicines (PHARM)
      Committee, Commonwealth Department of Health and Ageing (2005).
      The medication regimen should be reviewed each time a new medicine
      is required, if an adverse event occurs, and at least annually as part
      of routine diabetes complication procedures (September 2005 with
      permission)   105
5.2   Algorithm for achieving blood glucose targets in Type 2 diabetes that
      encompasses a quality use of medicines approach and adopts a
      proactive stepwise approach to initiating insulin   119
5.3   Range of Lilly insulins, their presentation and schematic action profiles.
      Reproduced with permission from Eli Lilly Australia Pty Ltd   125
5.4   (a) Range of NovoNordisk insulins with their time action characteristics
      and insulin profiles and (b) the delivery systems available with each
      insulin. Reproduced with permission from NovoNordisk (Australia)   127
5.5   Diagrammatic representation of insulin action showing different regimes:
      (a) daily, (b) twice daily, (c) basal bolus using short-acting insulins and
      (d) basal bolus using rapid-acting insulins. *Note:* The broken line
      depicts short-acting insulin, the unbroken line intermediate/long-acting
      insulin. The arrows indicate the time of injection   132
5.6   Possible results of a blockage in the IV cannula and three-way adaptor
      during the concurrent administration of insulin and dextrose/saline 140
7.1   An outline of the physiology, signs, and symptoms and biochemical
      changes occurring in the development of diabetic ketoacidosis (DKA) 191
7.2   An outline of the development of hyperosmolar coma   200
8.1   Diagrammatic representation of the factors leading to foot problems
      in people with diabetes   242
14.1 Risk factors for Polycystic Ovarian Syndrome and the possible
      long-term effects. There is still controversy about the diagnostic
      criteria and several degrees of severity exist. There is no single
      diagnostic test: diagnosing PCOS is process of exclusion. Diagnostic
      criteria include National Institute of Health criteria, Rotterdam
      criteria, and International Androgen Excess Society criteria   396
15.1 Model of the diabetic grief cycle   420

List of Tables

1.1 Characteristics of Type 1 and Type 2 diabetes mellitus 13

1.2 Genetic varieties of MODY, the frequency with which they occur and the key features where they are known that account for 85–90% of MODY. Other possible forms are emerging 15

1.3 Diagnostic criteria for diabetes based on the World Health Organisation guidelines. Fasting plasma glucose is the preferred test for diagnosis, but any of the three tests are acceptable 16

1.4 Diabetes management goals (targets) based on the NHMRC Evidence Based Guidelines for the Management of Type 2 Diabetes (2004) and the Australian Alcohol Guidelines (2007) 22

1.5 Guidelines for assessing the patient's blood glucose testing pattern. The results should be considered as part of the overall clinical picture and HbA$_{1c}$. The target HbA$_{1c}$ is <7% (<6.5% in some countries) 23

2.1 Some commonly used assessment instruments. The content of the instruments, the purpose of the assessment, and the particular patient population should be considered when selecting instruments, even when they are valid and reliable. Some are available in languages other than English. Details of most of the diabetes-specific instruments can be found on http://www.musc.edu/dfm/RCMAR/Diabetes Tool.html and Garrett *et al.* (2001) 46

3.1 Blood ketone levels and potential management 65

3.2 Non-glycaemic factors that can affect results of glycosylated haemoglobin assays 72

4.1 Effects of adipokines and changes that occur in the presence of abdominal obesity, which demonstrates their role in the development of insulin resistance, Type 2 diabetes and cardiovascular disease 78

4.2 Dietary fat comes from animal and plant sources and has various effects on blood lipids. Triglycerides are the most abundant dietary fat. Cholesterol and phospholipid dietary fats have a small but significant impact on serum cholesterol 88

4.3 Effect of high carbohydrate, alcohol and fibre on blood fats 89

4.4 Sources of omega-3, -6 and -9 essential fatty acids. And daily intake recommended (RDI) by the National Health and Medical Research Council (2006). A variety of foods high in essential fatty acids should be consumed each day 89

4.5 Drugs whose absorption can be modified by food 93

4.6 Some food-medicine interactions 94

5.1   Oral hypoglycaemic agents, dose range and dose frequency, possible side effects, the duration of action and main site of metabolism   107

5.2   Potential medicine interactions between oral hypoglycaemic agents and other medicines (based on Shenfield 2001)   116

5.3   Some examples of commonly used insulin delivery devices and some of the issues to consider when helping the individual decide which device to use   128

5.4   Some commonly encountered factors that affect insulin absorption   135

5.5   Lipid lowering agents   150

5.6   Antihypertensive medications. Often more than one antihypertensive agent will be required in diabetes to manage the underlying cardiovascular abnormalities. Prescribing information should be followed   153

6.1   Signs and symptoms of hypoglycaemia. These symptoms are so common that they are used in the Edinburgh Hypoglycaemia Scale (Deary *et al.* 1993). Symptoms are different in young children and may vary between episodes in the same individual   169

6.2   The counter-regulatory hormonal response to hypoglycaemia   171

6.3   Commonly prescribed medicines that can increase the hypoglycaemic effect of sulphonylurea medicines   176

7.1   Self-managing blood glucose, ketones and fluid during illness. These recommendations should be tailored to the individual's self-care capabilities, available assistance, and their physical condition. Ketosis can develop rapidly in people using insulin pumps. The underlying cause needs to be ascertained and treated   187

7.2   Early signs, symptoms, and precipitating factors of diabetic ketoacidosis (DKA)   190

7.3   The metabolic consequences of diabetic ketoacidosis and associated risks. Many of these changes increase the risk of falls in older people   192

8.1   Diabetes-specific cardiovascular abnormalities that predispose an individual to heart disease   209

8.2   Risk factors for age-related macular degeneration (Lim 2006). Many of these are similar to the risk factors for diabetic retinopathy and the same risk reduction strategies apply to both conditions. The table shows modifiable and non-modifiable factors. Sun exposure, and iris and hair colour do not appear to be associated with AMD (Khan *et al.* 2006)   220

8.3   Medicines used to manage diabetic peripheral neuropathy. Usually medicines are started at a low dose and titrated up to maximal doses over a few weeks depending on symptoms (Semla *et al.* 2002; Boulton 2005)   240

8.4   Changes in feet due to normal ageing   242

8.5   Management of specific foot problems while the person is in hospital or community settings   247

8.6   Organs commonly affected by diabetic autonomic neuropathy and the resultant clinical features   251

9.1   Hormonal, metabolic, and long-term effects of surgery   261

9.2   Common diabetic complications that can affect surgery and postoperative recovery. Many of these conditions may be documented

in the person's medical record and they may undergo regular
complication assessment but health status can change rapidly especially
older people. Therefore, the current complication status should be
assessed prior to surgery. Hyperglycaemia must be controlled   264

10.1 American Psychiatric Association criteria for drug abuse and drug
addiction. Drug abuse is diagnosed when a person exhibits three
of these criteria for 12 months   292

10.2 Medicines available to assist people to quit smoking. They should be
combined with other counselling and support strategies and good
nutrition and be considered as part of the medication record and their
benefits and risks reviewed regularly while they are being used. The
prescribing information should be consulted for specific information
about each medicine   297

10.3 The effects of the drug or drug combination and duration of action
depends on a number of factors including the dose and frequency of
use and individual factors. Long-term use can contribute to psychiatric
disorders and conversely psychiatric disorders can trigger illegal drug use.
Illegal drugs can interact with conventional and/or complementary
medicines and sometimes alcohol. All can lead to addiction, which has
social, professional and financial implications and increases the risk
of adverse diabetes care, coma, and death   301

10.4 Diabetes-related complications that can affect driving ability and
safety. Frequently more than one factor is present, therefore, the
cumulative effect on driving ability needs to be considered.
MI = myocardial infarction; 'Hypo' = hypoglycaemia   318

12.1 Theories of ageing. Currently there is no general agreement about the
causes of ageing but most experts favour cellular damage theories. These
seem to apply to uncontrolled diabetes where similar theories have been
proposed for the development of diabetes complications. See Chapter 8   349

12.2 Particular problems encountered in the elderly person with diabetes
and the resultant risks associated with the problem. Many of these
conditions affect activities of daily living and extended activities of
daily living. They represent a cumulative health burden and almost
all represent a falls risk and contribute to the risk of driving accidents   350

12.3 Key issues that need to be considered when assessing disability in
older people with diabetes. Repeat measures may be needed especially
during acute illnesses when the physical and mental condition can
change rapidly. These issues should be considered as part of the standard
diabetes complication screening process. Reproduced with permission
from Dunning, T. (2006) *Managing Diabetes in Older People.*
Blackwell Publishing, Oxford   355

12.4 Risk factors for inadequate nutrition and malnutrition in older people   361

12.5 Factors that can affect diabetes control and management
in older people   368

13.1 Self-management expectations according to age and stage.
(a) Metabolic targets need to be appropriate to the age and stage
and revised regularly as the child grows and develops; and
(b) recommended HbA_{1c} targets   386

13.2   Important medicine-related information children need. Information
should be provided using recognised education strategies and quality
use of medicines. Quality use of medicines is discussed in Chapter 5   389

14.1   Medication management during pregnancy. A comprehensive medication
review should be undertaken regularly in all people with diabetes,
when planning a pregnancy and when the woman becomes pregnant.
See also Chapter 5   400

16.1   Learning styles and some teaching strategies that can be used to
facilitate learning. People participating in group education programmes
are likely to learn in different ways. Therefore, a range of teaching
strategies should be used. An individual's preference for one category
may be mild, moderate of strong but generally a balance of styles results
in more effective learning   439

16.2   A simple tool that can be used to estimate an individual's dominant
learning style. It is not comprehensive but can be easily and quickly
incorporated into routine education and care   440

16.3   Some common factors that influence teaching and learning   454

19.1   Commonly used complementary therapies   484

19.2   Medicine-related safety and quality use of CAM and conventional
medicines involves considering all of the inter-related issues outlined
in the table   494

19.3   Commonly used herbs and supplements, their potential interactions,
reported adverse events and some management strategies to use should
an adverse event occur. Many of these interactions are theoretical, others
are well documented. When considering the likelihood of an interaction,
the total individual situation and medication regimen must be
considered. In addition, although 'medicine interactions' is usually used to
denote negative interactions, the term itself is objective and non-judgmental.
Many interactions may actually be beneficial and it is just as important to
document these   496

19.4   Advice health professionals can provide to people with diabetes to
help them use CAM safely   500

19.5   Scale for assessing the likelihood of a CAM-conventional interaction
and information that should be included in the report. One point is
allocated to each of the following criteria   502

Example Forms and Instruction Sheets

Forms

Example of an assessment chart 41
Blood glucose testing checklist 63
Example protocol for outpatient stabilisation onto insulin 158
Sample diabetes education record chart 449

Example Instruction Sheets

1 Preparation for an oral glucose tolerance test 18
2a Instructions for diabetic patients on oral hypoglycaemic agents
having procedures as outpatients under sedation of general anaesthesia 279
2b Instructions for diabetic patients on insulin having procedures as
outpatients under sedation or general anaesthesia 280
3 How to draw up insulin – one bottle only 456
4 How to draw up insulin – two bottles 457
5 How to give an insulin injection using syringes or insulin pens 458
6a Managing your diabetes when you are ill: patients with Type 1 diabetes 459
6b Managing your diabetes when you are ill: patients with Type 2 diabetes 462

Foreword

Worldwide, the prevalence of diabetes is increasing at an alarming rate and much of the care previously considered the domain of the medical practitioner is presently being undertaken by a range of health professionals. Hence, it is essential that health professionals, whatever the context of their working environment, develop a sound clinical understanding of diabetes management.

This remarkably comprehensive book reflects the depth of knowledge and experience of its author and will assist nurses in the process of diabetes management. The text encompasses many areas of diabetic care and bridges the gap between traditional health care texts and diabetes medical textbooks. It will be valuable to health professionals working on the periphery of diabetes in a hospital or community environment as well as to those who have developed a career in diabetes care. The author provides carefully detailed aspects of clinical care such as the caution required when using radio-contrast medium in people with diabetes and renal impairment while also including information about the use of complementary therapies for diabetes management.

The diagnosis of diabetes, whether it is Type 1 or Type 2, has a significant impact on the life of the person and their family. Living with diabetes is not easy and requires considerable dedication and commitment to adapt to the life-long regimen imposed by this chronic disease. While it is inevitable that health professionals will take on an increased clinical role, it is also important that they do not forget the fundamental purpose of health care, which is to care for patients. Health professionals must recognise not only the medical aspects of diabetes but also its psychosocial impact and thus not be judgmental when caring for the person having diabetes. This book emphasises the need for an holistic approach and provides insight into the many physiological and psychological facets of diabetes care.

It is with much delight that I write the foreword to this excellent textbook written by my friend and colleague Dr Trisha Dunning. Her vast experience in diabetes education, clinical management, and research is obvious. I wholeheartedly recommend this text to all health professionals whether working directly in, or on, the fringe of diabetes. This textbook should be considered essential reading for diabetes management.

Marg McGill MSc (Med)
Chair, International Diabetes Federation
Consultative Section on Diabetes Education

Preface

Background to the third edition

Diabetes has come a long way too, since it was first described as *diabetes maigre* (bad prognosis) and *diabetes gros* (big diabetes). Science and technology continue to make major contributions to our understanding of diabetes, and the management options. Qualitative studies highlight the importance of considering the individual's beliefs and attitudes, their explanatory models of diabetes, their social situation and the key central role they play in their care when planning management strategies.

Equally importantly, nurses and other health professionals must reflect on their own beliefs, attitudes, and explanatory models, they affect the care and advice they provide and the example they set for people with diabetes.

However, the accumulating evidence is not always easy to interpret and may not be readily accessible despite the increasing number of databases of systematic reviews such as the Cochrane Collaboration and a bewildering number of management guidelines. Methods of grading the rigor of the evidence have shifted the emphasis to using evidence, preferably from randomised controlled trials, rather than consensus-based guidelines. In other ways we have made very little progress. The incidence of the metabolic syndrome and diabetes is increasing. People are living longer and there is an increasing incidence of Type 2 diabetes in developing countries and depressed populations and worryingly, in children.

Many countries have moved towards managing diabetes in primary care settings with a strong emphasis on multidisciplinary team care delivered in integrated care programmes.

The book has been extensively revised to almost constitute this a new book. New chapters or sections have been included such as smoking cessation, diabetes and driving, coeliac disease and Polycystic Ovarian Syndrome. I have followed the current convention and refer to people/person with diabetes in most places in the text, however, the term 'patient' still occurs prominently in many places. I make no apologies for using that term. To me it signifies caring in a way 'client' and 'customer' will never do. Significantly, The International Alliance of Patient Organisations (IAPO) uses the term 'patient'.

I am constantly indebted to my patients for teaching me so much about living with diabetes. I invite readers to reflect on the following statement made by a young woman with Type 1 diabetes:

Diabetes is a designer disease. It was designed for people with routine lives – and that's NOT me!

Her words eloquently illustrate the enduring truth of Hippocrates (circa 460–370 BC) statement:

> It is more important to know what sort of person has a disease, than to know what sort of disease the person has.

Both statements reflect the imperative to consider the individual in their life context and involve them in planning their care. Hippocrates statement could be regarded as the foundation of diabetes care.

I sincerely hope the revised edition of the Book will continue to contribute to the body of information about diabetes, and that it will help nurses care for people with diabetes in an holistic, caring, and sensitive way and that each person who reads the Book will find something of value.

Using the Book

Health professionals have a responsibility for planning, implementing, and evaluating the care they provide for/with patients under their care. Health professionals function in a variety of settings and the components of their roles vary according to the setting they work in (hospital, community health centres, city or remote areas).

Best practice modern diabetes management relies on team care where health professionals complement each other. Importantly, the person with diabetes is at the centre of care and effective therapeutic relationships with health professionals are necessary to optimal outcomes and patient empowerment. People who have had diabetes for some time are often aware of omissions and poorly performed procedures relating to their care. In the case of people with diabetes, this is particularly true of blood glucose testing, hypoglycaemia, management, and increasingly, medicine management and considerable anxiety and confusion occur if advice and care are not consistent with that of the diabetes specialist team.

This book was designed as a quick reference for the care of people with diabetes mellitus to enable care plans to be formulated in busy situations and to provide references where more information can be found. A list of key points is given at the beginning of most chapters. Important information is referenced throughout the text. In addition, practice points based on research findings, and clinical observations based on personal experience are included.

Chapters are cross-referenced where appropriate. The pathophysiology and medical management of diabetes is discussed only briefly because it is more than adequately covered in other publications, see Appendix B.

The care outlined in this book does support the care that is required to manage the presenting condition, but focuses on the specific and extra needs of people with diabetes. The presence of diabetes will have physiological and psychological effects on the presenting condition if diabetes is not adequately controlled. A careful assessment of individual physical, psychological, and spiritual needs should form the basis of all care.

Practice point

The procedure and policies of the employing institution should be followed. This book does not replace these documents.

Acknowledgements

I would especially like to thank Wiley-Blackwell for promoting the book and for supporting a third edition.

I work in a supportive team of doctors and nurses and say a special thank you to them for their friendship and critical comment on sections of the book: Heather Hart, Patricia Streitberger, Lynn Stack, Leanne Hume, Geoff Nicholson, Mark Kotowicz, and in particular Pam Jones for her comments on managing gestational diabetes and diabetes in pregnancy and Julieanne for commenting on the nutrition chapter.

My sincere thanks also go to Dr Rob MacGinley, Senior Lecturer in Medical Education, at Deakin University and Visiting Nephrologist at The Geelong Hospital for his expert advice in revising the section on renal disease.

Before undertaking the revision I sought critical comment from my diabetes educator colleagues using a structured evaluation framework. I am very grateful to Victoria Stevenson, Fiona Heenan, Margaret Hollis, and especially Michelle Robins for their thoughtful feedback.

My research fellow, Sally Savage, has been an outstanding help chasing references and still smiling!

I particularly acknowledge my colleagues who made helpful suggestions for revising the third edition: Michelle Robins, Victoria Stevenson, Pamela Jones, Heather Hart, and Patricia Strietberger.

My thanks go to Mr Guy Murray, Novo Nordisk Australia, Jehangir Sidhwa, and Peter Giorgis, from Eli Lilly Australia for permission to use their respective insulin charts in Chapter 5, to Sanofi-Aventis for supplying information about Insulin Glargine and Apidra.

I acknowledge the generosity of the Australian Commonwealth Department of Health and Aging for permission to reproduce the figure depicting how the Quality Use of Medicines framework can be applied to diabetes management that appears in Chapter 5.

I continue to learn a great deal about diabetes from the people with diabetes I teach and care for and their families. I thank them for the privilege of caring for them and the information they share about life with diabetes.

I am grateful to Newgen for their careful editing and attention to detail.

Finally I treasure the support and understanding of my family including the furry four legged ones and feathered two legged ones. My special thanks and love go to my husband, John.

List of Abbreviations and Symbols

↑	Increased
↓	Decreased
≤	Equal to, or less than
<	Less than
≥	Equal to, or greater than
>	Greater than
BG	Blood glucose
BMI	Body mass index
BP	Blood pressure
BUN	Blood urea nitrogen
CAPD	Continuous ambulatory peritoneal dialysis
CAM	Complementary and alternative medicine
CCF	Congestive cardiac failure
CCU	Coronary care unit
CSII	Continuous subcutaneous insulin infusion
DA	Diabetes Australia
DKA	Diabetic ketoacidosis
ECG	Electrocardiogram
EN	Enteral nutrition
FFA	Free fatty acids
HbA_{1c}	Glycosylated haemoglobin
HM	Human insulin
HONK	Hyperosmolar non-ketotic coma
IAPO	International Alliance of Patient Organisations
ICU	Intensive care unit
IV	Intravenous therapy lines
LFT	Liver function test
MODY	Maturity onset diabetes in the young
MI	Myocardial infarction
NDSS	National Diabetes Supply Scheme
OGTT	Oral glucose tolerance test
OHA	Oral hypoglycaemic agents
PCOS	Polycystic Ovarian Syndrome
TPN	Total parenteral nutrition
TPR	Temperature, pulse, and respiration
TZD	Thiazolidinediones
WHO	World Health Organisation

The words are used in full the first time they appear in the text. All abbreviations are widely accepted and recognised.

Chapter 1
Diagnosing and Classifying Diabetes

Key points

- Diabetes is the modern pandemic. It represents a considerable global economic and social burden for the person with diabetes and the health system. The prevalence of both Type 1 and Type 2 is increasing.
- Primary prevention and early detection are essential to reduce the personal and community burden associated with the metabolic syndrome and Type 2 diabetes and its complications.
- Type 2 diabetes is a progressive disease and complications are often present at diagnosis. Thus, insulin will eventually be necessary in most people with Type 2 diabetes.
- The prevalence of obesity, the metabolic syndrome and Type 2 diabetes is increasing in children.

What is diabetes mellitus?

Diabetes mellitus is a metabolic disorder in which the body's capacity to utilise glucose, fat and protein is disturbed due to insulin deficiency or insulin resistance. Both states lead to an elevated blood glucose concentration and glycosuria.

The body is unable to utilise glucose in the absence of insulin and draws on fats and proteins in an effort to supply fuel for energy. Insulin is necessary for the complete metabolism of fats, however, and when carbohydrate metabolism is disordered fat metabolism is incomplete and intermediate products (ketone bodies) can accumulate in the blood leading to ketosis, especially in Type 1 diabetes. Protein breakdown leads to weight loss and weakness and contributes to the development of hyperglycaemia and lethargy.

There are different types of diabetes that have different underlying causal mechanisms and clinical presentation. In general, young people are insulin-deficient (Type 1 diabetes), while older people may secrete sufficient insulin and plasma insulin levels may be high (hyperinsulinaemia) but demonstrate resistance to its action (Type 2 diabetes). However, Type 1 occurs in ~10% of older people (see latent autoimmune diabetes (LADA) later in this chapter) and Type 2 is becoming increasingly prevalent in children and adolescents as a result of the global obesity epidemic

(Barr *et al.* 2005; Zimmet *et al.* 2007). Type 2 diabetes is the most common, accounting for ~85% of diagnosed cases; Type 1 accounts for ~15% of diagnosed cases.

Prevalence of diabetes

Diabetes affects approximately 0.5 to >10% of the population depending on the type of diabetes, age group, and ethnic group. The prevalence of diabetes is increasing, particularly in the older age group and in developing countries. The number of individuals with diabetes is projected to reach 215 million by 2010. In western countries the overall prevalence is 4–6% and up to 10–12% among 60–70 year olds. Most countries spend 6–12 of their annual health care budgets on diabetes and its consequences. Most of the morbidity and mortality is associated with Type 2, the prevalence rises to ~20% in developing countries (World Health Organisation (WHO) 2004).

In Australia, AusDiab data show 100 000 people develop diabetes annually (Cameron *et al.* 2003): 7.5% of people over 25 years and 16.8% of people over 65 have diabetes and a further 16.1% >65 have IGT. In addition, >200 000 progress from being overweight to obese, 3% of adults develop hypertension, and 1% reduced kidney function annually, and the average waist circumference increases by 2.1 cm, particularly in women. That is, a significant proportion of the population develop features of the metabolic syndrome with the associated increased risk of Type 2 diabetes and other associated conditions. This is associated with high health costs (Colaguiri *et al.* 2003; Australian Institute of Health and Welfare (AIHW) 2005).

In the UK, an estimated 1.4 million people have diabetes (Audit Commission 2000). In both countries Type 2 is the most common type, accounting for 80–90% of cases. There is wide variation in the incidence rates of newly diagnosed Type 1 diabetes in children in different populations. However, Type 1 in children and adolescents is increasing particularly in developed countries (EURODIAB 2000; The DIAMOND Project Group 2006; Soltesz *et al.* 2006).

Classification of diabetes

The American Diabetes Association (ADA) announced a revised diabetes classification system and diagnostic criteria in 1997. These revised data were a joint activity between the ADA and the WHO. As part of the new classification, the terms insulin-dependent diabetes (IDDM) and non-insulin-dependent diabetes (NIDDM) were replaced with Type 1 and Type 2 diabetes (Expert Committee on the Diagnosis and Classification of Diabetes Mellitus 1997).

- Type 1 diabetes has two forms:
  - Immune-mediated diabetes mellitus, which results from autoimmune destruction of the pancreatic beta cells leading to absolute insulin deficiency.
  - Idiopathic diabetes mellitus refers to forms of the disease that have no known aetiologies.

- Type 2 diabetes mellitus refers to diseases associated with relative insulin deficiency as a result of progressive beta cell failure and insulin resistance.
  - Impaired glucose homeostasis, which is an intermediate metabolic stage between normal glucose homeostasis and diabetes. It is a significant risk factor for cardiovascular disease and Type 2 diabetes. There are two forms:
    (1) Impaired fasting glucose (IFG) where the fasting plasma glucose is higher than normal but lower than the diagnostic criteria.
    (2) Impaired glucose tolerance (IGT) where the plasma glucose is higher than normal and lower than the diagnostic criteria after a 75 g glucose tolerance test. IFG and FPG often occur together and are associated with the metabolic syndrome.
- Gestational diabetes mellitus, which occurs during pregnancy.
  - Other specific types, which include diabetes caused by other identifiable disease processes:
  - Genetic defects of beta cell function such as MODY.
  - Genetic defects of insulin action.
  - Diseases of the exocrine pancreas such as cancer and pancreatitis.
  - Endocrine disorders such as Cushing's disease and acromegaly.
  - Medicines, such as glucocorticoids and atypical antipsychotics have been associated with weight gain but the newest second-generation antipsychotic medications such as aripiprazole is weight neutral (Citrome *et al.* 2005). Possible causes of weight gain associated with medicines include food cravings and eating more, changed resting metabolic rate, changes in neurotransmitters and neuropeptides such as leptin, which regulate appetite, and weight loss before medicines are commenced (Zimmermann *et al.* 2003). Individuals with schizophrenia are generally more overweight than those without.
- Chemical induced diabetes.

Overview of normal glucose homeostasis

Blood glucose regulation (glucose homeostasis) relies on a delicate balance between the fed and fasting states and is dependent on several simultaneously operating variables including hormones, nutritional status, especially liver and muscle glucose stores, exercise, tissue sensitivity to insulin, and the type of food consumed. Figure 1.1 shows the key features of the fed and fasting states. Note that insulin release occurs in two phases. The first phase is important to control the post prandial blood glucose rise and is lost early in the progression to Type 2 diabetes. Insulin action is mediated via two protein pathways: Protein 13-kinase through insulin receptors and influences glucose uptake into the cells and MAP-kinase, which stimulates growth and mitogenesis.

The metabolic syndrome

The metabolic syndrome consists of a cluster of risk factors for cardiovascular disease and Type 2 diabetes. Several researchers have explored the factors that predict diabetes risk including the Paris Prospective Study, Diabetes Epidemiology Collaborative Analysis of Diagnostic Criteria in Europe (DECODE), Epidemiology Study on the Insulin Resistance Syndrome (DESIR), and the European Group for the Study of Insulin

Anabolism (fed state)	Catabolism (fasting state)
• Driven by insulin • Insulin release stimulated by the rise in blood glucose • Two phase response • Facilitates glucose uptake • Reduces hepatic glucose output	• Driven by a variety of hormones, e.g. catecholamines, cortisol, growth hormone, glucagon • Increases endogenous glucose output: 80% liver, 20% kidney • Induces insulin resistance • Reduces glucose utilisation • Insulin output reduced • Protective during hypoglycaemia

– Fasting state 12–16 hours after an overnight fast and is an important determinant of day long glycaemia
– Postprandial (fed) state – dynamic regulated by insulin and glucagon especially in the first 30–60 minutes
– insulin is secreted in two phases and regulates the rate of glucose entry into cells and removal from the circulation:

  • Post prandial blood glucose rise is usually transient
  • Peaks 60–90 minutes
  • Usually returns to normal within 3 hours
  • Usually there is very little diurnal variation in the blood glucose level
  • Isolated post prandial hyperglycaemia occurs in IGT

Figure 1.1   Overview of glucose homeostasis showing the key factors operating during the fed and fasting states. Usually the blood glucose is maintained within the normal range by the interplay of the anabolic and catabolic hormones, which are in turn influenced by other hormones and a number of factors such as nutritional status and intake.

Resistance: Relationship Between Insulin Sensitivity and Cardiovascular Disease Risk (EGIR-RISC).

The metabolic syndrome has been known as syndrome X, the deadly quartet, the awesome foursome, diabesity, and metabolic syndrome X. Currently, no agreed definition of the metabolic syndrome exists, particularly with respect to assessing risk or outcomes in children and adolescents. Four main definitions for adults have been described. They disagree about the predictive ability of the various metabolic features for cardiovascular disease and Type 2 diabetes due to ethnic, gender and age differences, which affect the syndrome components and may not identify groups at risk at lower waist circumference such as Asian people:

• World Health Organisation (1999).
• European Group for the Study of Insulin Resistance (2002).
• National Cholesterol Education Program – Adult Treatment Panel 111 (2001).
• International Diabetes Federation (IDF) (2005).
• The IDF Consensus Report on the Metabolic Syndrome in Children and Adolescents (2005).

Key features of the metabolic syndrome

• The metabolic syndrome appears to be a result of genetic predisposition and environmental factors, which include high saturated fat diets, inactivity, smoking, hormone imbalances contributing to metabolic stress, age and some medicines. These factors represent a cumulative risk and are largely modifiable.
• Central obesity – waist circumference: Europoids >94 cm in men and >80 cm in women. South Asian and South-East Asian men >90 cm, women >80 cm:

(WHO 2004; Zimmet 2005) and childhood/adolescent Body Mass Index (BMI) 25–29 overweight, >30 obese.

- Raised serum triglycerides >1.7 mmol/L.
- Low serum HDL-c: <1.03 mmol/L males, <1.29 mmol/L women.
- Hypertension: systolic > 130 mmHg or diastolic >85 mmHg in women.
- IFG: >5.6 mmol/L or previously diagnosed diabetes (e.g. gestational diabetes (GDM). IFG is associated with a 20–30% chance of developing Type 2 diabetes within 5–10 years. The chance increases if FPG is also present.

Other key features include:

- Insulin resistance
- Hyperinsulinaemia, which occurs in the presence of insulin resistance and exaggerates the proliferative effects of the MAP-kinase pathway.
- Procoagulent state: elevated plasma fibrinogen and plasminogen activator inhibitor-1 (PAI-1).
- Vascular abnormalities: increased urinary albumin excretion and endothelial dysfunction, which affect vascular permeability and tone.
- Inflammatory markers such as cytokines, Interleukin, adhesion molecules, and TNF-alpha, which alter endothelial function. C-reactive protein is a significant predictor of cardiovascular disease and possibly depression, and there is an association among diabetes, cardiovascular diseases and depression. In fact some experts suggest depression could be an independent risk factor for Type 2 diabetes (Loyd *et al.* 1997) and accelerates the progression of coronary artery disease (Rubin 2002). Depression is associated with behaviours such as smoking, unhealthy eating, lack of exercise and high alcohol intake, which pre-disposes the individual to obesity and Type 2 diabetes. Peripheral cytokines induce cytokine production in the brain, which activates the hypothalamic–pituitary–adrenal axis and the stress response, which inhibits serotonin and leads to depression. Inflammation appears to be the common mediator among diabetes, cardiovascular disease and depression (Lesperance & Frasure-Smith 2007).
- Hyperuricaemia: More recently, liver enzymes such as sustained elevations of alanine aminotransferase (ALT) and gamma-glutamyl transferase (GGT), which are associated with non-alcoholc fatty liver disease and low adiponectin, have been associated with diabetes and cardiovascular disease. Therefore, the relationship is complex. Conversely, higher testosterone levels appear to be protective against diabetes in men but indicate greater risk in women and high oestradiol levels confer increased diabetes risk in both men and women (American Diabetes Association 2007 Preventing Diabetes).

Consequences of the metabolic syndrome include:

- A five-fold increased risk of Type 2 diabetes.
- A two to three fold increased risk of cardiovascular disease (myocardial events, stroke and peripheral vascular disease).
- Increased mortality, which is greater in men but women with Type 2 diabetes have a greater risk than non-diabetic women.

- Increased susceptibility to conditions such as:
  - Gestational diabetes (GDM)
  - Fetal malnutrition
  - Polycystic Ovarian Syndrome
  - Fatty liver
  - Gallstones
  - Asthma
  - Sleep problems
  - Some forms of cancer.

The risk of developing cardiovascular disease and Type 2 diabetes increases significantly if three or more risk factors are present (Eckel *et al.* 2005).

The metabolic syndrome in children and adolescents

The prevalence of metabolic syndrome in children and adolescents is usually extrapolated from adult definitions and may not be accurate. However, it is vital that children and adolescents at risk of developing the metabolic syndrome be identified early. Future risk appears to be influenced *in utero* and early childhood by factors such as GDM, low birth weight, feeding habits in childhood, genetic predisposition and socio-economic factors (Burke *et al.* 2005). The IDF proposed that the metabolic syndrome should not be diagnosed before age 10 but children at risk should be closely monitored especially if there is a family history of metabolic syndrome, diabetes, dyslipidaemia, cardiovascular disease, hypertension and obesity, and preventative strategies implemented (Weiss *et al.* 2005; Zimmet *et al.* 2007).

In the 10–16-year-old age range diagnostic features are waist circumference >90th percentile, triglycerides >1.7 mmol/L, HDL-c >1.03 mmol/L, glucose >5.6 mmol/L (OGGT recommended), systolic blood pressure >130 mmHg and diastolic >85 mmHg. Adult criteria are recommended for adolescents over 16 years. The long-term impact on morbidity and mortality will emerge as young people with the metabolic syndrome become adults. However, heart disease may be apparent in children as young as 10 (Sinaiko 2006) and early onset of Type 2 diabetes in adolescents is associated with more rapid progression of complications than occurs in Type 1.

Management of the metabolic syndrome in children and adults consists of primary prevention through population-based strategies aimed at early detection, regular follow-up of at-risk individuals and personalised education. Secondary prevention concentrates on preventing the progression to diabetes and cardiovascular disease. Lasting effects demonstrating reduced cardiovascular and Type 2 diabetes risk has been demonstrated in studies such as the Diabetes Prevention Program (DPP), the Finnish Diabetes Prevention Study and the Da Quing IGT and Diabetes Study. These studies showed the importance of multidisciplinary team care, modifying lifestyle factors that contribute to obesity by improving diet and activity levels to reduce weight (10% body weight in the long term), and stop smoking. Some programmes include health coaching but the cost–benefit has not been demonstrated (Twigg *et al.* 2007). The transformational Model of Change is frequently used to implement preventative strategies.

Medicines might be required for secondary prevention for example, to control blood glucose and lipid lowering, antihypertensive, and weight management medicines in addition to lifestyle modification. Several medicines have been shown to reduce the incidence of diabetes in people with the metabolic syndrome. These include Metformin 850 mg BD, which showed a 31% risk reduction in the DPP; 100 mg of acarbose TDS by 25% after three years (STOP-NIDDM); and women with a history of GDM in the TRIPOD trial were less likely to develop diabetes when they were treated with troglitazone. Troglitazone was withdrawn from the market because of the tendency to cause liver disease. Other thiazolidinediones such as pioglitazone and rosiglitazone do not have the same adverse effects on the liver. Rosiglitazone reduced the risk of prediabetes progressing to diabetes by 60% over three years in the DREAM study. Orlistat, an intestinal lipase inhibitor taken TDS, reduced the risk of progression to diabetes in obese adults with metabolic syndrome by 37% over four years (XENDOS study). However, compliance with orlistat is low due to the side effects, see Chapter 5.

The macrovascular risk factors need to be managed proactively and screening programmer are imperative so abnormalities treated early, see Chapter 8. A 75 g OGGT may be performed initially to diagnose the metabolic syndrome and repeated after 12 months to determine whether glucose tolerance has changed, then the test interval can be increased to every two to three years (WHO 1999). However, if an individual demonstrates significant changes in weight gain, then OGGT may be performed earlier.

The Consensus Development Conference on Antipsychotic Drugs and Obesity and Diabetes (2004) recommend monitoring people on antipsychotic medicines including:

- BMI at baseline and every visit for 6 months then quarterly and treat if weight increases by one BMI unit.
- Blood glucose and lipids at baseline and if weight increases by 7% and then annually; HbA$_{1c}$ 4 months after starting antipsychotic medicines and then annually in people with metabolic syndrome or diabetes risk factors.

Type 1 and Type 2 diabetes

Type 1 diabetes

Type 1 diabetes is a disease of absolute insulin deficiency that usually affects children and young adults but can occur in older people where it is known as latent autoimmune diabetes (LADA), see the following section.

The symptoms usually occur over a short space of time (two to three weeks) following a subclinical prodromal period of varying duration where the beta cells are destroyed. The precipitating event may have occurred many years prior to the development of the symptoms. Type 1 diabetes can be due to an autoimmune or idiopathic process. Various researchers have demonstrated that exogenous factors play a role in the development of Type 1 diabetes on the basis that <10% of susceptible people develop diabetes and <40% of monozygotic twins both develop diabetes, the >10-fold increase in the incidence of Type 1 diabetes in European Caucasians in the last 50 years, and migration studies that show the incidence of Type 1 has risen in people who migrated from low to high incidence regions (Knip *et al.* 2005). This is known as the trigger-bolster hypothesis. Seasonal variations in incidence of new diagnosis occur.

The EURODIAB substudy 2 Study Group researchers (1999) suggested low plasma 25-hydroxyvitamin D may be implicated in the development of Type 1 diabetes (1999). Later, Stene & Jones (2003) suggested there was no link between vitamin D supplementation and lower rates of Type 1 diabetes. More recently, a systematic review and meta-analysis of observational studies and a meta-analysis of cohort studies suggest vitamin D supplementation in early childhood might reduce the risk of Type 1 diabetes by 30% (Zipitis & Akoberng 2008). However, randomised controlled trials are required to clarify whether there is a causal link and the optimal dose, duration of treatment, and the best time to begin using vitamin D supplements.

A range of other environmental triggers has been implicated in the development of Type 1 such as potatoes, cow's milk, and various viruses. Thus, the cause of Type 1 diabetes appears to be multifactorial due to a combination of genetic predisposition and a diabetogenic trigger that induces an immune response, which selectively destroys pancreatic beta cells. Islet cell antibodies (ICA), glutamic acid carboxylase (GAD), or tyrosine phosphatase (IA-2A) antibodies are present in 85% of cases.

Type 1 diabetes in children usually presents with the so-called classic symptoms of diabetes mellitus:

- Polyuria
- Polydipsia
- Lethargy
- Weight loss
- Hyperglycaemia
- Glycosuria
- Blood and urinary ketones.

In severe cases the patient will present with diabetic ketoacidosis (DKA) (see Chapter 7). Bed-wetting may be a consequence of hyperglycaemia in children. Classically, insulin secretion does not improve after treatment but tissue sensitivity to insulin usually does.

Figure 1.2 is a schematic representation of the progression of Type 1 diabetes. It shows the progressive relentless destruction of the beta cells from the time of the initial triggering event. Five to ten per cent of first-degree relatives of people with Type 1 diabetes have beta cell antibodies, usually with normal glucose tolerance, and some progress to diabetes.

Immunosuppression with Azathioprine or Cyclosporin, and immunomodulation using Nicotinamide to prevent further beta cell destruction has been used in newly diagnosed or pre-Type 1 diabetes but these treatments are uncommon. These medicines are potent immunosuppressive agents and their use cannot be warranted in the long term. Insulin has also been used in an attempt to stimulate immune tolerance, but not successfully.

Latent autoimmune diabetes (LADA)

LADA is a genetically linked autoimmune disorder that occurs in ~10% of people initially diagnosed with Type 2 diabetes. The prevalence varies among ethnic groups (www.actionlada.org). LADA has some features of both Types 1 and 2 diabetes. The UKPDS (1998) identified that one in 10 adults aged between 25 and 65 presumed to have Type 2 diabetes were GAD antibody positive, and these findings have been evident

Figure 1.2 Schematic representation of the slow progressive loss of beta cell mass following the initial trigger event in Type 1 diabetes.

in other studies (Zinman *et al.* 2004). LADA often presents as Type 2 but has many of the genetic and immune features of Type 1 (see the previous section and Table 1.2).

The progression to insulin dependency is usually rapid when GAD and IA-2A antibodies are present. The clinical features also resemble Type 1 in that people with LADA are not usually obese, are often symptomatic, and do not have a family history of Type 2 diabetes. A number of LADA trials are currently underway such as ACTIONLADA in Europe and the INIT 11 (LADA Trial) in Australia. LADA is also known as latent autoimmune diabetes of adulthood, late-onset autoimmune diabetes of adulthood, slow onset Type 1, and Type 1.5 (type one-and-a-half) diabetes.

Management includes:

- Testing non-obese people presenting with Type 2 diabetes for autoantibodies especially GAD, which has higher sensitivity to prevent episodes of ketoacidosis (Niskanen *et al.* 1995).
- Testing C-peptide levels in the blood to assess beta cell function. C-peptide is usually low in LADA indicating deficient insulin secretion, which predicts the need for insulin.
- Diet and exercise changes relevant to the individual.
- Avoiding metformin because of the potential risk of lactic acidosis in the presence of insulin deficiency.
- Introducing insulin early to support insulin secretion. Insulin is usually required within 4–6 years of diagnosis.
- Stress management and regular complication screening and mental health assessment (as per Types 1 and 2 diabetes).
- Appropriate education and support.

Type 2 diabetes

Type 2 diabetes is not 'just a touch of sugar' or 'mild diabetes'. It is an insidious progressive disease that is often diagnosed late when complications are present. Therefore, population screening and education programs are essential. Type 2 diabetes often presents with an established long-term complication of diabetes such as neuropathy, cardiovascular disease, or retinopathy. Alternatively, diabetes may be diagnosed during another illness or on routine screening. The classic symptoms associated with Type 1 diabetes are often less obvious in Type 2 diabetes, however, once diabetes is diagnosed and treatment instituted, people often state they have more energy and are less thirsty. Other subtle signs of Type 2 diabetes especially in older people include recurrent candida infections, incontinence, constipation, symptoms of dehydration and cognitive changes. As indicated, insulin resistance often precedes Type 2 diabetes.

Insulin resistance is the term given to an impaired biological response to both endogenous and exogenous insulin that can be improved with weight loss and exercise. Insulin resistance is a stage in the development of impaired glucose tolerance. When insulin resistance is present, insulin production is increased (hyperinsulinaemia) to sustain normal glucose tolerance; however, the hepatic glucose output is not suppressed and fasting hyperglycaemia and decreased postprandial glucose utilisation results.

Insulin resistance is a result of a primary genetic defect and secondary environmental factors (Turner & Clapham 1998). When intracellular glucose is high, free fatty acids (FFAs) are stored. When it is low FFAs enter the circulation as substrates for glucose production. Insulin normally promotes tryglyceride synthesis and inhibits postprandial lipolysis. Glucose uptake into adipocytes is impaired in the metabolic syndrome and Type 2 diabetes and circulating FFAs as well as hyperglycaemia have a harmful effect on hepatic glucose production and insulin sensitivity. Eventually the beta cells do not respond to glucose and this is referred to as glucose toxicity. Loss of beta cell function is present in over 50% of people with Type 2 diabetes at diagnosis (United Kingdom Prospective Study (UKPDS) 1998) (Figure 1.2). Figure 1.3 depicts the consequences of insulin resistance.

Insulin is secreted in two phases: the first phase plays a role in limiting the post prandial rise in blood glucose. The first phase is diminished or lost in Type 2 diabetes leading to elevated post prandial blood glucose levels (Dornhorst 2001). Postprandial hyperglycaemia contributes to the development of atherosclerosis, hypertriglyceridaemia and coagulant activity, endothelial dysfunction, and hypertension, which

Figure 1.3 Consequences of the insulin resistance syndrome.

add to the effects of chronic hyperglycaemia and contribute to long-term diabetes complications (Ceriello 2003).

Interestingly, the beta cells do respond to other secretagogues, in particular sulphonylurea medicines.

The net effects of these abnormalities is sustained hyperglycaemia as a result of:

- impaired glucose utilisation (IGT)
- reduced glucose storage as glycogen
- impaired suppression of glucose-mediated hepatic glucose production
- high fasting glucose (FPG)
- reduced postprandial glucose utilisation.

People most at risk of developing Type 2 diabetes:

- have the metabolic syndrome,
- are overweight: abdominal obesity, increased body mass index (BMI), and high waist-hip ratio (>1.0 in men and >0.7 in women). The limitations of the waist circumference in some ethnic groups are outlined later in the chapter. Elevated FFAs inhibit insulin signalling and glucose transport (see Figure 1.4) and are a source of metabolic fuel for the heart and liver. Binge eating precedes Type 2 diabetes in many people and could be one of the causes of obesity; however, the prevalence of eating disorders is similar in Type 1 and Type 2 diabetes (Herpertz *et al.* 1998):
- are over 40 years of age, but note the increasing prevalence in younger people (see also Chapter 13)
- are closely related to people with diabetes,
- are women who had gestational diabetes or who had large babies in previous pregnancies.

Other associated risk factors have already been described. In addition, active and former smoking and acanthosis nigricans are associated with hyperinsulinaemia (Kong *et al.* 2007). Baseline and hypertension progression are independent predictors (Conen *et al.* 2007). Recent research suggests insulin lack might be partly due to the enzyme PK Cepsilon (PKCe), which is activated by fat and reduces the production of insulin. Future medicines may target this deficiency and restore normal insulin function (Biden 2007). The characteristics of Type 1 and Type 2 diabetes are shown in Table 1.1.

The majority of people with Type 2 diabetes require multiple therapies to achieve and maintain acceptable blood glucose and lipid targets over the first nine years after diagnosis (UKPDS 1998). Between 50% and 70% require insulin, which is often used in combination with OHAs. This means diabetes management progressively becomes more complicated for people with Type 2 diabetes, often coinciding with increasing age when their ability to manage may be compromised, which increases the likelihood of non-compliance and the costs of managing the disease for both the patient and the health system.

Gestational diabetes

Gestational diabetes is the most common medical complication of diabetes accounting for 0–95% (Menato *et al.* 2008). Diabetes occurring during pregnancy is referred to

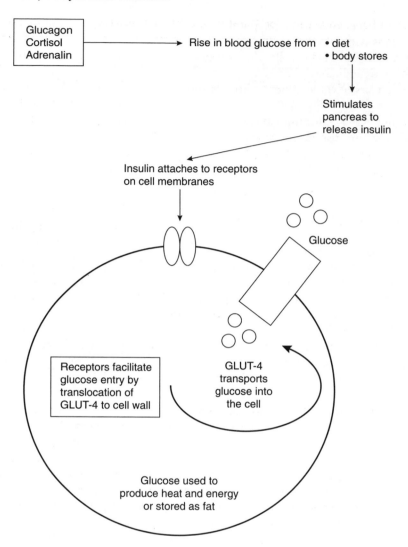

Figure 1.4 Diagrammatic representation of insulin binding, insulin signalling, translocation of GLUT-4 and glucose entry into the cell. GLUT-4 is a glucose transporter contained in vesicles in the cell cytoplasm. Once insulin binds to an insulin receptor GLUT-4 moves to the cell membrane and transports glucose into the cell. During fasting GLUT-4 is low and increases in response to the increase in insulin. Failure of GLUT-4 translocation could explain some of the insulin resistance associated with Type 2 diabetes. The effects of insulin are mediated by two protein pathways: P13-kinase through the insulin receptors (glucose uptake) and MAP-kinase, which stimulates growth and mitogenesis.

as gestational diabetes (GDM). GDM describes carbohydrate intolerance of varying degrees that first occurs or is first recognised during pregnancy, generally indicated by fasting blood glucose >6 mmol/L. GDM occurs in 1–14% of pregnancies. The exact cause of gestational diabetes is unknown, but several factors have been implicated including diet and lifestyle, smoking, some medicines, older age, genetic background, ethnicity, number of previous pregnancies and recently, short stature (Langer 2006). For more information on GDM refer to Chapter 14.

Table 1.1 Characteristics of Type 1 and Type 2 diabetes mellitus.

	Type 1	Type 2
Age at onset	Usually <30 years[a]	Usually >40 years[b]
Speed of onset	Usually rapid	Usually gradual and insidious
Body weight	Normal or underweight; often recent weight loss	80% are overweight
Heredity	Associated with specific human leukocyte antigen (HLA-DR3 or 4)	No HLA association Genetic predisposition
	Autoimmune disease and environmental triggers	Environmental and lifestyle factors contribute
Insulin	Early insulin secretion Impaired later; may be totally absent Insulin resistance is reversible if appropriate diet and exercise regimens are instituted	Often preceded by the metabolic syndrome (see section on 'The metabolic syndrome'). Type 2 is associated with slow, progressive loss of beta cell function
Ketosis	Common	Rare
Symptoms	Usually present	Often absent, especially in the early stages Acanthosis nigricans is common
Frequency	~15% of diagnosed cases	~85% of diagnosed cases
Complications	Common but not usually present at diagnosis	Common, often present at diagnosis
Treatment	Insulin, diet, exercise, stress management, regular health and complication assessment	Diet, OHA, exercise, insulin, stress management, regular health and complication assessment

[a] Increasing incidence of the metabolic syndrome and Type 2 diabetes in children and adolescents.
[b] Occurs in older people; see LADA.

Malnutrition-related (tropical) diabetes

Childhood malnutrition, genetic predisposition and environmental factors are implicated in the development of diabetes in people living in tropical countries. It is not included as a specific category in the revised classification but could fit into the 'other' category. 'Tropical diabetes' or malnutrition-related diabetes differs from Type 1 diabetes because ketoacidosis is rare, and from Type 2 diabetes because it often occurs in young, thin people with no family history of diabetes. However, researchers have not yet agreed about the underlying causal mechanisms.

Maturity onset diabetes of the young (MODY)

Maturity onset diabetes of the young is a rare group of diabetes disorders, formerly also called Mason-type diabetes and non-insulin-dependent diabetes of the young (NIDDY). MODY can develop at any age up to 55 in 2–2% of people with non-Type 1 diabetes.

It has a genetic basis and there are at least six varieties in many ethnic groups (Dean & McEntyre 2004). MODY can be distinguished from Type 1 diabetes by the absence of GAD antibodies and ketosis and from Type 2 because MODY is caused by a single gene and Type 2 is caused by minor problems in several genes that occur simultaneously (Froguel & Velho 1999). Likewise, MODY people often do not have insulin resistance. The age at onset in at least one genetic type depends on which parent carries the mutant gene: it occurs at a younger age if the mother passed it on especially if she had GDM. Women with MODY are often diagnosed during pregnancy. The varieties of MODY are shown in Table 1.2.

Treatment is with oral hypoglycaemic agents, diet and exercise, although insulin may eventually be required. Interestingly, Ehilishan *et al.* (2004) suggested diabetes diagnosed in children younger than six years is likely to be a genetic defect rather than Type 1 diabetes. If that is the case, there are implications for diabetes education and management.

Recognition can be difficult and the diagnosis is often missed (Appleton & Hattersley 1996). This can have implications for the individual and their family in commencing appropriate treatment for the specific type of MODY and genetic counselling.

Practice points

(1) MODY is a different disease process from Type 2 diabetes that occurs in young people and has a different genetic and inheritance pattern from Type 2. The prevalence of Type 2 diabetes in children is increasing and is associated with obesity and insulin resistance (Sinha *et al.* 2002).
(2) MODY has been misdiagnosed as Type 1 diabetes and insulin commenced unnecessarily. MODY has also been diagnosed instead of Type 1 diabetes in the UK (Health Service Ombudsman 2000).

These points demonstrate the importance of taking a careful clinical history and undertaking appropriate diagnostic investigations.

Diagnosing diabetes

Urine glucose tests should not be used to diagnose diabetes; if glycosuria is detected, the blood glucose should be tested. When symptoms of diabetes are present, an elevated blood glucose alone will usually confirm the diagnosis. See Table 1.3 for diagnostic criteria.

If the person is asymptomatic, abnormal fasting blood glucose values of >7 mmol/L should be demonstrated on at least two occasions before the diagnosis is made (note that some guidelines suggest >6.5 mmol/L). A random plasma glucose >11.1 mmol/L and symptoms are diagnostic of Type 2 diabetes. An oral glucose tolerance test (OGTT) using a 75 g glucose load may be indicated to determine the presence of glucose intolerance if results are borderline. The criteria for diagnosing diabetes according to the World Health Organisation are shown in Table 1.3. A protocol for preparing the patient and performing an OGTT are outlined later in the chapter. However, some experts suggest 75 g may be too high a load for some ethnic groups such as Vietnamese.

Table 1.2 Genetic varieties of MODY, the frequency with which they occur and the key features where they are known that account for 85–90% of MODY. Other possible forms are emerging.

Genetic variety	Prevalence	Features[a]
MODY 1 HNF-4?	Rare	Adequate insulin produced in infancy then declines progressively Diabetes develops in early adulthood Treated with sulphonylureas and eventually insulin Similar to MODY 3
MODY 2 (Glucokinase)	Causes 10–65% of cases	Often diagnosed in childhood or pregnancy Complications are rare Can be managed with diet and exercise Autosomal dominant mother will pass on to 50% of children
MODY 3 HNF-1 alpha	Causes 20–75% of cases Most common type in Europeans	Reduced beta cell mass or impaired function, which is progressive Chronic mild hyperglycaemia usually asymptomatic Often detected through screening during pregnancy Can be controlled using sulphonylureas but eventually insulin is required Often misdiagnosed as Type 1 Can develop complications
MODY 4 IPF-1	Rare Only a single family has been studied	
MODY 5 HNF-1 beta	Rare	Associated with kidney disease, often cystic kidney disease, which is often diagnosed before MODY Various genitourinary malformations Elevated liver enzymes are common Hyperuricaemia may occur Develops from infancy to middle age
MODY 6 Neuro-D1	Very rare Only three kindreds have been identified to date	Most diagnosed after 40 Some required insulin

[a] General characteristics: mild-to-moderate hyperglycaemia, first-degree relative with a similar presentation, absence of autoantibodies, low/not requiring insulin, not obese and no other features of the metabolic syndrome and diabetes occurring in the neonatal period or apparent Type 1 before the age of 6 months. The diagnosis is confirmed by genetic testing.

Practice point

Hyperglycaemia often occurs as a stress response to serious intercurrent illness such as cardiovascular disease and it may be difficult to diagnose diabetes in such circumstances. However, controlling the blood glucose during the illness is important and leads to better outcomes including in non-diabetics.

Table 1.3 Diagnostic criteria for diabetes based on the World Health Organisation guidelines. Fasting plasma glucose is the preferred test for diagnosis, but any of the three tests are acceptable.

Stage	Fasting plasma glucose	Random plasma glucose	Oral glucose tolerance test (OGTT)
Normal	<6.1 mmol/L		2 hour plasma glucose <7.8 mmol/L
Impaired glucose tolerance	Impaired fasting glucose – fasting glucose ≥6.1 and <7.0 mmol/L		Impaired glucose tolerance – 2 hour plasma glucose ≥7.8 and <11.1 mmol/L
Diabetes	≥7.0 mmol/L	≥11.1 mmol/L and symptoms	2 hour plasma glucose >11.1 mmol/L

Note: In this table venous plasma glucose values are shown. Glucose in capillary blood is about 10–15% higher than venous blood.

Abnormal plasma glucose identifies a subgroup of people at risk of diabetes-related complications. The risk data for these complications is based on the 2-hour OGTT plasma glucose level. However, the fasting glucose of >7.8 mmol/L does not equate with the 2-hour level used to diagnose diabetes. Recently, the ADA and the WHO lowered the fasting level to 7.0 mmol/L to more closely align it to the 2-hour level.

The WHO continues to advocate routine OGTT screening in at-risk individuals to identify people at risk of complications early, in order for early treatment to be instituted. The ADA does not advocate routine OGTT use because it believes that the revised fasting level is sensitive enough to detect most people at risk. Therefore, there could be differences internationally about the routine use of the OGTT. The ADA and the WHO do agree on how the test should be performed. Australia supports the continued use of the OGTT when the diagnosis is equivocal and to detect GDM (Hilton *et al.* 2002; Twigg *et al.* 2007).

Other screening and prevention measures include providing the public with information about screening programmes, health maintenance programmes, and self-risk assessment lists, for example checklists from the Agency for Healthcare Research and Quality (AHRQ). Checklists can be downloaded from the Internet (http://www.ahrq.gov/ppip/helthywom.htm or http://www.ahrq.gov/ppip/helthymen.htm). The information is based on the US Preventative Services Task Force recommendations.

Although HbA_{1c} is a useful measure of blood glucose control its utility as a screening tool is still debated. It is not clear whether it can be used to diagnose Type 2 diabetes and cardiovascular disease, although elevated HbA_{1c} was shown to be a strong predictor of diabetes but not cardiovascular disease after multivariate analysis and after excluding people diagnosed with diabetes within 2–5 years of follow-up (Pradhan *et al.* 2007). Despite these findings the researchers did not recommend using HbA_{1c} as a single measure of diabetes risk.

Spectroscopic measurement of dermal advanced glycation end products (SAGE), a non-invasive procedure, has been compared with FPG and HbA_{1c} as a screening test for diabetes (Maynard *et al.* 2007). Advanced glycated end products (AGE) are biomarkers of diabetes and are implicated in diabetes complications especially retinopathy and nephropathy. AGE accumulate faster in the presence of hyperglycaemia. SAGE provides a quantitative diabetes risk score. SAGE does not require the person to fast and provides an immediate result. Compared to PFG and HbA_{1c} SAGE was statistically more sensitive than the two comparator measures detecting 28.8% more cases of diabetes using the OGGT criteria than FPG and HbA_{1c}. If further research confirms these findings SAGE could be a useful non-invasive screening tool.

Oral glucose tolerance test (OGTT)

An OGTT is used to diagnose diabetes:

- When fasting and random blood glucose results are equivocal.
- When there is a strong family history of diabetes, especially during pregnancy.
- If the suspicion of diabetes is high but blood and urine glucose tests are normal.

An OGTT should not be performed when the patient:

- Is febrile.
- Is acutely ill, for example postoperatively, or if uraemic.
- Has been immobilised for more than 48 hours.
- Has symptoms of diabetes or an elevated blood glucose before commencing of the test.

Rationale for OGTT

Early diagnosis and treatment of diabetes reduces the morbidity and mortality associated with the disease.

Preparing the patient for an OGTT

(1) Give specific oral and written instructions to the patient. A sample is given in Example Instruction Sheet 1 overleaf.
(2) Ensure the diet contains at least 200 g/day carbohydrate for at least 3–5 days before the test.
(3) If possible stop medicines that can influence the blood glucose levels 3 days before the test: some of these will need to be reduced gradually, for example steroids. People should be informed about the consequences of stopping their medicines and when to resume taking them after the test:
  - thiazide diuretics
  - antihypertensive medicines
  - analgesic and anti-inflammatory medicines
  - antineoplastic medicines
  - steroids.
(4) Fast from 12 midnight, the night before the test.
(5) Avoid physical/psychological stress for 1 hour prior to, and during, the test.
(6) Avoid smoking for at least 1 hour prior to the test.
(7) Allow the patient to relax for 30 minutes before beginning the test.

Example Instruction Sheet 1: Preparation for an oral glucose tolerance test

---

PATIENT INSTRUCTIONS FOR ORAL GLUCOSE TOLERANCE TEST

Date of test: **Name:**

Time: **I.D. label**

Location where test will take place:

(1)   Please ensure that you eat high carbohydrate meals each day for 3 days before the test. Carbohydrate foods are: breads, cereals, spaghetti, noodles, rice, dried beans and pulses, vegetables, fruit. These foods should constitute the major part of your diet for the 3 days.

(2)   Have nothing to eat or drink after 12 midnight on the night prior to the test day, except water.

(3)   Specific information about managing medicines: ....

(4)   Bring a list of all the tablets you are taking with you when you come for the test.

(5)   Do not smoke for at least one hour before the test.

The test

The test is performed in the morning. You are required to rest during the test, which will take approximately 3 hours to complete. A small needle will be inserted into an arm vein for blood sampling. The needle will stay in place until the test is completed. You will be given 300 mL of glucose to drink. This is very sweet but it is important to drink it all over the 5 minutes, so that the results of the test can be interpreted correctly. Water is permitted.

   You will be given a drink and something to eat when the test is finished. The doctor will discuss the results with you.

Test protocol

(1) The person should rest during the test to avoid dislodging the cannula.

(2) A cannula is inserted into a suitable vein for blood sampling.

(3) The blood glucose should be tested before commencing the test. If elevated, clarify with the doctor ordering the test before proceeding. Two millimetres of blood are collected in fluoride oxalate tubes for laboratory analysis.

(4) The cannula is flushed with saline between samples to prevent clots forming in the sample. One to two milliletres of blood should be withdrawn and discarded before collecting each sample to avoid contaminating the sample with saline left in the tubing.

(5) Blood samples are collected at the following times. However, sometimes only baseline (0) and a two-hour sample are collected:

   minutes: −10

                        0

                        ⇨   75 g glucose, consumed over 5 minutes Water can be given after the glucose. It is very sweet and some people find it difficult to drink.

                  +30

                  +60

                  +120

The glucose used for an OGTT is prepacked in 300 mL bottles containing exactly 75 g of glucose.

(6) Ensure the person has a follow-up appointment with the referring doctor whose responsibility it is to explain the test results and commence appropriate management and education.

Screening for diabetes

Because of the insidious nature and increasing incidence and prevalence of Type 2 diabetes, many countries have instituted population-based education and screening and/or case detection programmes in at-risk populations. Fasting plasma glucose tests are preferred to capillary (fingerpick) tests to diagnose diabetes, see Table 1.3 for the diagnostic criteria. Some programmes also involve checking for obesity and cardiovascular risk factors. At-risk groups include:

- age >55 years;
- high-risk ethnic groups;
- women with Polycystic Ovarian Syndrome (PCOS)
- previous GDM;
- family history of diabetes;
- people with symptoms – often absent in Type 2 diabetes;
- older people >65 years;
- those with known diabetes complications such as cardiovascular, erectile dysfunction, and renal disease
- active smokers (Willi *et al.* 2007).

Screening for Type 1 diabetes is not usually necessary because it presents differently and has a more rapid onset and symptoms are usually present. First-degree relatives of people with Type 1 diabetes can be tested for risk markers (autoantibodies) for diabetes but the preventative strategies applicable to Type 2 diabetes do not apply.

An example of a screening and preventative model of care is shown in Figure 1.5.

Preventing Type 2 diabetes

A number of clinical trials have demonstrated that it is possible to prevent Type 2 diabetes and may in turn prevent the associated morbidity from long-term complications. Most prevention trials were conducted among people with IGT because it is a strong predictor of Type 2 diabetes. These programmes include the DaQuing Study (1997), the Diabetes Prevention Program (DPP) (2002), and the Finnish Diabetes Prevention Study (DPS) (2003), which showed a 58% reduction in the progression to diabetes in people who followed a healthy lifestyle and the effects were still present at the four year follow up. (Tuomilehto *et al.* 2001). The DPS was stopped early because the intervention was so successful but the researchers continued to follow people who did not develop diabetes for up to 10 years. The intervention group achieved a reduction of ~40% compared to controls. The DPS has been adapted and implemented in many

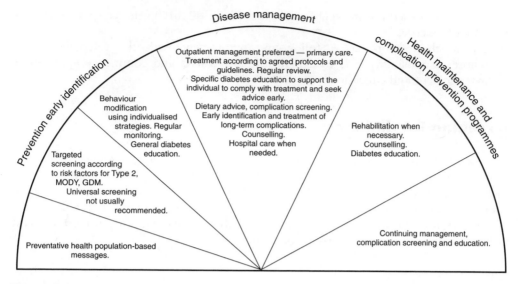

Figure 1.5   Example of a screening and preventative model of health care.

countries since the findings were first published for example *Go For Your Life* and the Life Programme in Australia.

Key features of the DPS are weight reduction (~5%), reducing fat intake to <30% with <10% coming for saturated fats, fibre intake of >15 g per 1000 calories and >30 minutes of moderate exercise per day. In the DPS, weight loss and exercise appeared to be more important than dietary goals in preventing diabetes. Achieving weight loss and making dietary changes is difficult and only 2% of participants in the DPS achieved four or five targets but no participant who did so developed diabetes compared to 50% of the control group. Weight management strategies are discussed in Chapter 4.

Studies concentrating on increasing fibre and magnesium to prevent Type 2 diabetes show inconsistent results despite current guidelines to increase the total fibre intake. The type of fibre consumed may be important in that soluble fibre may enhance gastric emptying and reduce the post prandial glucose rise. A meta-analysis revealed lower diabetes risk with increased intake of cereal fibre but no significant association with fruit and vegetable fibre, thus, including whole grain foods is important in diabetes prevention diets (Krishnan *et al.* 2007). An example of a screening, prevention model is shown in Figure 1.5.

Managing diabetes mellitus

The diabetes team

Effective diabetes management depends on having a collaborative multidisciplinary health care team. The person with diabetes is the central player in the team. Good communication among team members is vital and information given to the patient must be consistent between, and within, hospital departments and health services to ensure smooth transition among services and avoid confusing the patient with inconsistent information. The team usually consists of some or all of the following:

- Diabetologist
- Diabetes nurse specialist/diabetes educator and/or diabetes nurse practitioner
- Dietitian
- Podiatrist
- Social worker
- Psychologist
- General practitioner.

Other professionals who contribute regularly to the management of the patient are:

- Opthalmologist
- Optometrist
- Pharmacist
- Specialists such as vascular and orthopaedic surgeons, neurologists, and urologists
- Cultural health workers, for example, aboriginal health workers in Australia and traditional healers in Africa
- Exercise physiologists
- Physiotherapists.

The ward staff who care for the patient in hospital and the community also become team members during presentations to hospital and emergency rooms including:

- Doctors
- Nurses
- Dietitians
- Physiotherapists
- Occupational therapists.

The management of diabetes consists of dietary modification, regular exercise/activity and in some cases insulin or OHAs. Diabetes education and regular medical assessment of diabetic control and complication status is essential. In addition, general health care is very important and includes dental checks, mammograms, prostate checks and preventative vaccination, for example, fluvax and pneumovax.

Aims of management

Diabetes management should be determined within the quality use of medicine framework, see Chapter 4. Management aims for Australia are defined in the National Diabetes Strategy and a number of other specific guidelines such as those described in the Australian Diabetes Society Position Statements, Clinical Management Guidelines for Diabetes in General Practice, and a range of self-management guidelines produced by various countries some of which are listed in Chapter 16 and Appendix B. The UK also has a number of specific guidelines including the newly released *Diabetes National Service Framework: Standards*, a ten-year implementation

(2001). Likewise Diabetes Australia published a *Plan for a Better Life for People with Diabetes* in 2004.

The aim of diabetes management is to maintain quality of life and keep the person free from the symptoms of diabetes, and the blood glucose and blood lipids in an acceptable range. The range is determined on an individual basis, usually between 3- and 6.5 mmol/L for 90% of tests, especially during acute illness and surgery, young people and during pregnancy. The aim is to obtain results as near as possible to normal blood glucose but there must be a balance between the food plan, medication (insulin/OHAs) and exercise/activity. Maintaining emotional well being is essential, see Chapter 15. General management goals (targets) are shown in Table 1.4.

The regimen should affect the person's lifestyle as little as possible, although some modification is usually necessary. Type 1 people require insulin in order to survive. Type 2 obese patients can sometimes be treated effectively with a combination of diet and exercise but research suggests that people managed with diet are not as rigorously monitored and have more hyperglycaemia and hypertension than those on medicines (Hippisley-Cox & Pringle 2004). Many people with Type 2 diabetes require OHAs and often eventually insulin.

Practice point

The recommendations in the previous section are general. Individual needs must be taken into consideration. For example, aiming for normoglycaemia in an older person could put them at risk of adverse events such as falls by causing hypoglycaemia see Chapters 6 and 12.

In the current person-centred empowerment model of diabetes care, the person with diabetes is the pivotal person in the management team. Forming a therapeutic partnership with the individual and accepting their choices is essential to achieving

Table 1.4 Diabetes management goals (targets) based on the NHMRC Evidence Based Guidelines for the Management of Type 2 Diabetes (2004) and the Australian Alcohol Guidelines (2007).

Glucose: Fasting blood glucose 4–6 mmol/L; HbA$_{1c}$ <7%
Lipids: LDL-c <2.5 mmol/L; triglycerides <1.5 mmol/L; HDL-c >1.0 mmol/L
Blood pressure: 130/80 mmHg; 125/75 mmHg if proteinuiria exceeds 1 g/day: 140/90 if over 65 years.
BMI <25 kg/m^2 (ideal); waist circumference women <80 cm, men <94 cm.
Renal function: Urine albumin excretion 20 μm/min in timed overnight collection; <20 μm/min spot collection; albumin–creatinine ratio <3.5 mg/mmol in women, <2.5 mg/mmol men eGFR.
Alcohol intake: Women, 1 standard drink/day, men, 2 standard drinks/day.
No smoking
Exercise/activity: >150 minutes/week; at least 30 minutes brisk walking or equivalent/day or on at least five days/week

optimal outcomes and is important when the individual elects not to follow advice after receiving adequate information (informed decision).

Clinical observation

Diabetes is a balancing act. The individual's physical, psychological, spiritual and social and relationship needs must be balanced to enable people to undertake the necessary self-management to achieve management targets (optimal physical health). In fact, the emphasis should be on balance rather than control. Spirituality, in particular, is an important but neglected aspect of current diabetes management strategies and is key to self-empowerment and self-determination (Parsian & Dunning 2008).

Management involves educating the person with diabetes and other family members in order to help them:

- Understand diabetes, be involved in deciding their care plan and adopt relevant self-care strategies necessary to maintain optimal health and meet glycaemic targets.
- Manage the impact of diabetes on their physical, psychological and spiritual functioning to maintain an acceptable quality of life.
- Obtain and maintain an acceptable weight.
- Achieve acceptable blood glucose levels.
- Achieve a normal blood lipid profile.
- Relieve symptoms of diabetes (polyuria, polydipsia and lethargy). This involves helping the person recognise and manage relevant signs and symptoms associated with diabetes and any concomitant condition/s.
- Prevent complications of diabetes and of treatment.
- Maintain a healthy, independent lifestyle where the person is able to manage the necessary self-care tasks to achieve acceptable glycaemic control and have a good quality of life.

Some guidelines for assessing metabolic control are shown in Table 1.5.

Table 1.5 Guidelines for assessing the patient's blood glucose testing pattern. The results should be considered as part of the overall clinical picture and HbA_{1c}. The target HbA_{1c} is <7% (<6.5% in some countries).

% haemoglobin A1c	Glucose (mmol/L)		Control
	Fasting	2 hours after food	
4.0–6.0	4	<7	Excellent or 'too good'[a]
6.0–7.4	7	9	Upper limit of normal
7.5–9.4	10	14.5	Unacceptable
>9.5	14	20	Unacceptable

[a] Risk of hypoglycaemia, especially in older people and young children.

A suggested model for managing diabetes is shown in Figure 1.6. The model is divided into phases and indicates that management, education and counselling are required for life.

Exercise/activity

Exercise plays a key role in the management of Type 1, Type 2 diabetes, and GDM. It increases tissue sensitivity to insulin aiding in the uptake and utilisation of glucose during exercise and for several hours afterwards. The energy sources during exercise are depicted in Figure 1.7.

In addition, regular exercise may have beneficial effects on the risk factors that contribute to the development of diabetes complications especially cardiovascular disease (Boule *et al.* 2001). Exercise:

- Increases cardiovascular efficiency.
- Reduces blood pressure.
- Reduces stress.
- Aids in weight reduction and appetite control.
- Promotes a sense of wellbeing.
- Aids in blood glucose control.
- Improves strength and reduces the risk of falls in older people, which helps them remain independent (anaerobic exercise).

All of these factors also reduce the risk of developing the long-term complications of diabetes. People are advised to have a thorough physical check-up before commencing an exercise programme; in particular, the cardiovascular system, eyes, nerves and feet should be examined. Food, fluid and clothing should be suitable for the type of exercise and the weather.

Insulin/OHA doses might need to be adjusted. Where the duration of the exercise is <30 minutes adjustments are generally not required. Adjustments are often necessary where the duration of the exercise exceeds 30 minutes (Perlstein *et al.* 1997). Exercise should be decided in consultation with the individual and suited to their preferences and physical capabilities. It is advisable that they test their blood glucose before and after exercising and to have some carbohydrate available during exercise in case of hypoglycaemia. Infrequent exercise is not advisable; the aim should be to begin with 10–15 minutes exercise and progress to 30–60 minutes of moderate intensity three to five times per week, daily if possible.

Footwear and clothing should be appropriate to the type of exercise and the feet inspected after exercising. Exercise is not recommended in extremes of temperatures, or at periods of hyperglycaemia, especially if ketones are present in the urine or blood. People should discuss their exercise plans with the diabetes team in order to plan an appropriate routine, adequate carbohydrate intake, and appropriate medication doses. Ensure adequate fluid intake to replace water loss especially in hot weather.

Figure 1.6 Suggested diabetes management model. Most diabetes management occurs in primary care settings in collaboration with secondary and tertiary care services.

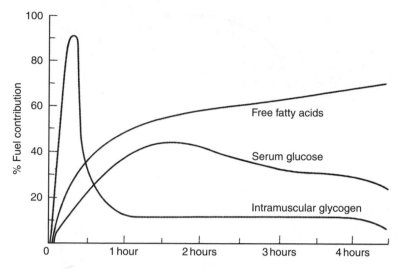

Figure 1.7 Normal energy sources during exercise. *Note:* At rest free fatty acids are the major energy source. As exercise begins muscle glycogen is utilised as the predominant energy source. As exercise continues the blood glucose is utilised, reverting to free fatty acids as the major energy source if exercise is prolonged. Blood glucose is maintained by hormonal regulation of hepatic glucose output and lipolysis.

Practice point

Hypoglycaemia can occur several hours after vigorous or prolonged aerobic exercise due to continuing glucose uptake by muscles. People need to be informed about adequate carbohydrate intake and medication dose adjustment as well as recognising and treating hypoglycaemia before and after exercise see Chapter 5.

In general, anaerobic exercise (e.g. weight lifting) does not significantly enhance glucose utilisation. It does build muscle mass and improve strength but does not improve cardiovascular fitness. Anaerobic exercise is unlikely to cause an increase in blood glucose. Aerobic exercise (e.g. running, cycling, swimming) uses glucose as the major fuel source and hypoglycaemia can occur. It also confers cardiovascular benefits.

Specific advice about medications and food intake needs to be tailored to the individual. The relationship between hypoglycaemia and exercise is generally well recognised. Hyperglycaemia can also occur if insulin levels are low when exercising. In this situation the counter-regulatory hormones predominate and increase the blood glucose.

Exercise for the patient in hospital

(1) Encourage as much mobility/activity as the person's condition allows.
(2) Increase movement and activity gradually after a period of being confined to bed.
(3) Consider postural hypotension and differentiate it from hypoglycaemia to ensure correct management is instituted.

(4) Consult the physiotherapy department for assistance with mobility, chair or hydro-therapy exercises.
(5) Consider having the occupational therapist undertake a home assessment to ensure safety at home, for example, following a stroke.

Practice point

Be aware that resuming normal activity after a period of prolonged inactivity, for example in rehabilitation settings, constitutes unaccustomed exercise and can result in hypoglycaemia, especially if the person is on insulin/OHAs and is not eating well or is malnourished. Exercise/activity increases the basal energy requirement by ~20%.

Diabetes education

Diabetes education is an integral part of diabetes management. Regular support and contact with the diabetes care team assists people to self-manage their diabetes by providing advice and support when necessary. For more details see Chapter 16.

Practice points

(1) People with Type 2 diabetes do not become Type 1 when insulin is needed to control blood glucose. The correct term is insulin-treated or insulin-requiring diabetes. The basic underlying pathophysiology does not change and usually enough endogenous insulin is produced to prevent ketosis occurring except during severe intercurrent illness.
(2) Type 2 diabetes is characterised by progressive beta cell destruction and insulin is eventually required by >50% of people (UKPDS 1998). People with LADA require insulin within 4–6 years; therefore, people need to be informed at diagnosis that they are likely to need insulin in the future.

Complications of diabetes

Many people with diabetes are admitted to hospital because they have an active diabetes complication. The presence of a diabetic complication can affect the duration of the admission and the patient's ability to care for him or herself. Hence diabetic complications contribute to the overall cost of health care for these patients. In addition, they represent significant physical and mental lifestyle costs to the person with diabetes and their family.

Complications can be classified as acute or long term. Acute complications can occur during temporary excursions in blood glucose levels. Long-term complications occur with long duration of diabetes and persistent hyperglycaemia, especially in the presence of other risk factors. In Type 2 diabetes long-term complications are frequently present at diagnosis. Often there are few symptoms and both the diagnosis of diabetes and the coexisting complication/s can be overlooked.

Acute complications

(1) Hypoglycaemia (refer to Chapter 6).
(2) Hyperglycaemia:
   • diabetic ketoacidosis (refer to Chapter 6)
   • hyperosmolar coma (refer to Chapter 7).
(3) Infections can occur if blood glucose control is not optimal. Common infections include dental disease, candidiasis and urinary tract infections.
(4) Fat atrophy/hypertrophy and insulin allergy occur very rarely with modern highly purified insulins and correct injection site rotation.

Long-term complications

Two important studies, the DCCT in 1993 and the UKPDS in 1998, demonstrated the relationship between the development and progression of the long-term complications of Type 1 and Type 2 diabetes, respectively. In addition, the UKPDS demonstrated the importance of controlling blood pressure to reduce the risk of cardiovascular disease. Diabetes management guidelines and metabolic targets are regularly revised as new evidence emerges.

Current management targets are shown in Table 1.4.

(1) Macrovascular disease or disease of the major blood vessels, for example:
   • myocardial infarction
   • cerebrovascular accident
   • intermittent claudication.
(2) Microvascular disease or disease of the small blood vessels associated with thickening of the basement membranes of the small blood vessels, for example:
   • retinopathy
   • nephropathy.
(3) Neuropathy: diabetes can also cause damage to the central and peripheral nerves:
   • *peripheral*: decreased sensation in hands and particularly the feet, which can lead to ulcers, Charcot's arthropathy and amputation.
   • *autonomic*: erectile dysfunction, atonic bladder, gastroparesis, mononeuropathies.
(4) Complications of pregnancy: diabetes during pregnancy carries risks for both mother and baby:
   • *mother*: toxaemia, polyhydramnous intrauterine death, and Caesarian section
   • *baby*: congenital malformations, prematurity, respiratory distress, hypoglycaemia at birth.

A number of other factors might play a role in the development of diabetic complications. For example, studies are under way to determine the role of free radicals (ROS), advanced glycated end products (AGE), changes in cellular signalling and endothelial humoral components that determine coagulation status and the tendency to form microthrombi. A list of recommended reading that deals with this subject is included in Appendix B and they are discussed in detail in Chapter 8.

It is the responsibility of all health professionals involved in providing care to comprehensively assess the patient including the presence of complications to determine their self-care potential and devise an appropriate achievable management plan, and to be involved in preventative teaching about reducing risk factors for the development of diabetic complications. Health professionals need to be proactive about identifying opportunities for health screening and education.

Cost of diabetes

The Australian Institute of Health in 1991 and 2005 estimated the cost of diabetes in Australia to be >$7000 million per year. The cost of diabetes in the UK was recently estimated to be 10% of health service resources, nearly £5 billion per annum. These costs are increasing, especially for older people. In addition, the length of stay in hospital is longer for people with diabetes. Many of the hospitalisations are a result of diabetic complications, which should be largely preventable.

Sixty per cent of the costs associated with diabetes are direct costs of providing service and medical supplies. The indirect costs (40%) are more difficult to assess; they include psychological costs to the person with diabetes, life years lost and loss of quality of life. There are also costs to the caregivers (relatives and family), which are difficult to estimate and which probably reduce direct health costs.

Diabetes is the fourth major cause of death after cardiovascular disease, cancer and musculo-skeletal disease, distributed across all age groups. Cardiovascular disease is a major complication of diabetes. Therefore it is not unreasonable to conclude that a person with diabetes will require at least one hospital contact/admission during their lifetime. It is documented that the need for hospital admission and the length of stay in hospital can be improved by diabetes education, and appropriate medical and nursing care. It is envisaged that this Manual will contribute to the provision of that care.

Practice points

(1) Hyperglycaemia and insulin resistance commonly occur in critically ill patients, even those who do not have diabetes (Van den Berghe *et al.* 2001).

(2) It is important to control these states in people with diabetes during illness because of the extra stress of the illness and/or surgery, and their compromised insulin response. Elevated blood glucose in these situations in people without diabetes will require decisions to be made about the diagnosis of diabetes after the acute episode resolves.

Aim and objectives of nursing care of people with diabetes

In hospital

Being hospitalised is more common for people with diabetes than those without, and they are more like to stay longer. Current diabetes management guidelines are heavily weighted towards screening and primary care management. Good evidence for acute care is more difficult to locate. The care suggested in this Manual is extrapolated from the research quoted, discussion with nurse experts in particular areas, and the extensive clinical and nursing experience of the author.

Factors that complicate diabetes management during illness

- Age
- Gender
- Type and duration of diabetes
- Nutritional status
- Potentially erratic insulin absorption, especially in Type 1.
- Haemodynamic changes in blood flow.
- Counter-regulatory stress response to illness, hospitalisation, treatment, pain, psychological stress and fear.
- Timing of meals and snacks as well as during TPN, fasting and renal dialysis.
- Duration of time between insulin administration and meals.
- Effect of medications on the gut, especially narcotics for pain relief. Glucose requirements may need to be increased to compensate for slow transit times, to supply sufficient energy and prevent hypoglycaemia.
- Increased white cell count and impaired leukocyte function as a result of hyperglycaemia.
- Delayed wound healing and strength of healing tissue.
- Increased risk of thrombosis.
- Presence of ketoacidosis and/or hyperosmolar states if hyperglycaemia is not reversed, see Chapter 7.
- Impaired cognitive function and lowered mood can make problem-solving, self-care, and learning difficult.
- Depression.

Clinical observations – patients' stories

(1) People with diabetes worry that hospital staff will make mistakes, especially with their medication doses and administration times and management of hypoglycaemia.
(2) They dislike being made to feel incompetent and not trusted by staff who take over the self-care tasks they usually perform for themselves, and who do not believe what they say.
(3) Conversely, some people prefer the nurses to take on these tasks because it is an opportunity to 'let go of' the responsibility for a short time.
(4) They find judgmental attitudes about eating sweet things demeaning, especially when they are accused of dietary indiscretions when their blood glucose is high.
(5) They dislike being labelled non-compliant, or uncooperative, if they have difficulty learning and remembering information.

Aims and objectives of nursing care

Aims

To formulate an individual nursing management plan so that the person recovers by primary intention, maintains their independence and quality of life as far as possible and does not develop any complications of treatment. In some cases helping them prepare for a peaceful death.

Recognise the importance of support from the family and other key individuals to the individual's well being, self-care capacity and ability to take responsibility for their disease.

Rationale

Early diagnosis of diabetes and monitoring for short- and long-term complications enables early treatment and improved outcomes. The nurse's understanding of the pathophysiology and classification of diabetes will improve the care they provide.

Objectives

(1) To assess the person's:
- physical, mental and social status
- usual diabetic control
- ability to care for themselves
- knowledge about diabetes and its management
- the presence of any diabetes-related complications including lowered mood and depression
- acceptance of the diagnosis of diabetes
- presence of concomitant disease processes.

(2) To encourage independence as far as the physical condition allows in hospital (test own blood glucose, administer own insulin, select own meals).

(3) To obtain and maintain an acceptable blood glucose range, thereby preventing hypoglycaemia or hyperglycaemia so that the person is free from distressing symptoms and fluctuating blood glucose levels.

(4) To prevent complications occurring as a result of hospitalisation (e.g. falls associated with hypoglycaemia).

(5) To observe an appropriate management plan in order to achieve these objectives.

(6) To inform appropriate health professionals promptly of the patient's admission, for example, diabetes nurse specialist/diabetes educator, dietitian, or podiatrist.

(7) To ensure the patient has the opportunity to learn about diabetes and its management, particularly self-management.

(8) To plan appropriately for discharge including managing medicines and undertaking or referring the person for a home medicine review if they meet the criteria.

(9) To prevent further hospitalisations as a result of diabetes.

In the longer term, especially for diabetes nurse specialist/diabetes educators who often see the patient regularly over many years, establishing a therapeutic relationship based on respect, equality and trust. The value of a therapeutic relationship has been recognised from the time of Hippocrates as being essential to healing.

References

American Diabetes Association, American Psychiatric Association, American Association of Clinical Endocrinologists, North American Association for the Study of Obesity (2004) Consensus Development Conference on Antipsychotic Drugs and Obesity and Diabetes. *Diabetes Care*, **27**, 596–601.

American Diabetes Association (ADA) (2003) Evidence based nutrition principles and recommendations for the treatment and prevention of diabetes and related complications. *Diabetes Care*, **26** (Suppl. 1), S51–S61.

Appleton, M. & Hattersley, A. (1996) Maturity onset diabetes of the young: a missed diagnosis. *Diabetic Medicine*, (Suppl. 2), AP3.

Audit Commission (2000) *Testing Times: a Review of Diabetes Mellitus Services in England and Wales*. Audit Commission, London.

Australian Diabetes Society (1990–1996) *Position Statements*. Australian Diabetes Society, Canberra.

Australian Institute of Health and Welfare (2005) Costs of diabetes in Australia, 2000–01. (AIHW) Cat. No. CVD 26). Canberra.

Barr, E.L., Magliano, D.J., Zimmet, P.Z., Poilkinghorne, K.R., Atkins, R.C., Dunstan, D.W. et al. (2005). *The Australian Diabetes, Obesity and Lifestyle Study (AusDiab). Tracking the Accelerating Epidemic: Its Causes and Outcomes*. International Diabetes Institute, Melbourne.

Biden, T. (2007) Major breakthrough in understanding type 2 diabetes. Interview in *Nursing Review*, November 2007, 10.

Boule, N., Haddard, E., Kenny, G., Wells, G. & Sigal, R. (2001) Effects of exercise on glycaemic control and body mass index in Type 2 diabetes mellitus: a metaanalysis of controlled clinical trials. *Journal of the American Medical Association*, **286**, 1218–1227.

Burke, V., Beilin, U. & Simmer, K. (2005) Predictors of body mass index and associations with cardiovascular risk factors in Australian children: a prospective cohort study. *International Journal of Obesity*, **29**, 15–23.

Ceriello, A. (2000) The postprandial state and cardiovascular disease: relevance to diabetes mellitus. *Diabetes Metabolism Research Reviews*, **16**, 125–132.

Chiasson, J., Josse, R., Gomis, R. et al. (2002) Acarbose for prevention of type 2 diabetes mellitus: the STOP-NIDDM randomized trial. *Lancet*, **359**, 2072–2077.

Citrome, L., Blonde, L. & Damatarca, C. (2005) Metabolic issues in patients with severe mental illness. *South Medical Journal*, **98** (7), 714–720.

Conen, D. (2007) Blood pressure may predict incident type 2 diabetes in healthy women. *European Heart Journal* (published online 9–10-2007).

Conen, D., Ridker, P., Mora, S., Buring, J. & Glynn, R. (2007) Blood pressure and risk of developing type 2 diabetes mellitus: the Women's Health Study. *European Heart Journal*, **28** (23), 2937–2943.

Dean, L. & McEntyre, J. (2004) The genetic landscape of diabetes (http>//www.ncbi.nlm.nih.gov/books/bv.fegi?call=bv.View.ShowTOC&rid=diabetes. TOC accessed January 2008).

DECODE Study Group (2001) Glucose tolerance and cardiovascular mortality: comparison of fasting and two hour diagnostic criteria. *Archives of Internal Medicine*, **161**, 397–405.

Diabetes and Control and Complications Trial Research Group (1993) The effect of intensive insulin treatment on the development and progression of long term complications of insulin dependant diabetes. *New England Journal of Medicine*, **329**, 977–986.

Dornhorst, A. (2001) Insulinotrophic meglitinide analogues. *Lancet*, **358** (9294), 1709–1716.

Dunstan, D., Zimmet, P. & Welborn, T. (2000) On behalf of the AusDiab Steering Committee, Diabesity and associated disorders in Australia 2000: the accelerating epidemic. *Australian Diabetes, Obesity and Lifestyle Report*. International Diabetes Institute, Melbourne.

Dunstan, D., Zimmet, P., Welborn, T. *et al.* (2002) The rising prevalence of diabetes and impaired glucose tolerance: the Australian obesity and lifestyle study. *Diabetes Care*, **25**, 829–834.

EUROBIAB Substudy 2 Study Group (1999) Vitamin D supplement in early childhood and risk for Type 1 (insulin-dependent) diabetes mellitus. *Diabetologia*, **42** (1), 51–54.

EURODIAB ACE Study Group (2000) Variation and trends in incidence of childhood diabetes in Europe. *Lancet*, **355**, 873–876.

Ehtisham, S., Hattersley, A., Dunger, A. & Barrett, T. (2004) First UK survey of paediatric type 2 diabetes and MODY *Archives Diseases in Child*, **89**, 526–529.

Expert Committee on the Diagnosis and Classification of Diabetes Mellitus (1997) Report of the expert committee on the diagnosis and classification of diabetes *Diabetes Care*, **20**, 1183–1197.

Froguel, P. & Velho, G. (1999) Molecular genetics of maturity-onset diabetes of the young. *Trends in Endocrinology and Metabolism*, **10** (4), 142–146.

Gerstein, H., Yusuf, S., Bosch, J. *et al.* (2006) DREAM (Diabetes Reduction Assessment with ramipril and rosiglitazone Medication) trial Investigators. Effect of rosiglitazone on the frequency of diabetes patients with impaired glucose tolerance or impaired fasting glucose: a randomized controlled trial. *Lancet*, **368** (9541), 1096–1105.

Health Service Ombudsman (2000) *Errors in the Care and Treatment of a Young Woman with Diabetes*. The Stationary Office, London.

Herpertz, S., Albus, C. & Wagener, R. (1998) Cormorbidity of eating disorders. Does diabetes control reflect disturbed eating behaviour? *Diabetes Care*, **21** (7), 1110–1116.

Hilton, D., O'Rourke, P., Welbourn, T. & Reid, C. (2002) Diabetes detection in Australian general practice: a comparison of diagnostic criteria. *Medical Journal of Australia*, **176**, 104–107.

Hippisley-Cox, J. & Pringle, M. (2004) Diabetics treated with diet only have more complications. *Lancet* (http://www.medscape.com/viewarticle/484479 5.8.2004).

International Diabetes Federation (IDF) (2006) *The IDF Consensus Worldwide Definition of the Metabolic Syndrome*. IDF, Brussels (accessed December 2007).

Knip, M., Veijola, R., Virtanen, S., Hyoty, H., Vaarala, O. & Akerblom, H. (2005) Environmental triggers and determinants in type 1 diabetes. *Diabetes*, **54** (Suppl. 2), s125–s126.

Knowler, W., Barrett-Connor, E., Fowler, S. *et al.* (2002) Diabetes Prevention Program Research Group. Reduction in incidence of type 2 diabetes with lifestyle intervention of metformin. *New England Journal of Medicine*, **346**, 393–403.

Krishnan, S., Rosenberg, L., Singer, M., Hu, F. Djoussé, L., Cupples, A. & Palmer, J. (2007) Glycaemic index, glycaemic load and cereal fiber intake and risk of Type 2 diabetes in US Black Women *Archives Internal Medicine*, **167** (21), 2304–2309.

Kong, A., Williams, R., Smith, M., Sussman, A., Skipper, B., Hsi, A., Rhyne, R., RIOS Net Clinicians (2007) Acanthosis nigricans and diabetes risk factors: prevalence in young persons seen in southwestern US primary care practices. *Annals of Family Medicine*, **5** (3), 202–208.

Langer, O. (2006) Management of gestational diabetes: pharmacological treatment options and glycaemic control. *Endocrinology Metabolic Clinics of North America*, **35**, 53–78.

Lesperance, F. & Frasure-Smith, N. (2007) Depression and heart disease. *Cleveland Clinic Journal of Medicine*, **74** (Suppl. 1), S63–S66.

Lindstrom, J., Louheranta, A., Mannelin, M. *et al.* (2003) The Finnish Diabetes Prevention Study (DPS): lifestyle intervention and 3-year results on diet and physical activity. *Diabetes Care*, **26**, 3230–3236.

Lindstrom, J., Ilanne-Parikka, P. & Peltonen, M. (2006) Sustained reduction in incidence of type 2 diabetes by lifestyle intervention: follow-up of the Finnish Diabetes Prevention Study. *Lancet*, **368**, 1673.

Loyd, C., Wilson, R. & Forrest, K. (1997) Prior depressive symptoms and onset of coronary heart disease. *Diabetes*, **46**, 3A.

MacKinnon, M. (1998) *Providing Diabetes Care in General Practice. A Practical Guide for the Primary Care Team*. Class Publishing, London.

Maynard, J., Rohrscheib, M., Way, J., Nguyen, C. & Ediger, M. (2007) Non-invasive Type 2 diabetes screening: supervision substudy to fasting plasma glucose and A_{1c}. *Diabetes Care*, 30 (5), 1120–1126.

National Divisions Diabetes Programs (1998) Commonwealth Department of Health and Family Services, Canberra.

Nichols, G. (2007) Preventing and predicting diabetes. *Medscape Diabetes and Endocrinology* (posted 8.10.2000).

Nilsson, C., Ursing, D., Torn, C., Aberg, A. & Landin-Olsson, M. (2007) Presence of GAD-antibodies during gestational diabetes predicts type 1 diabetes. *Diabetes Care*, DOI: 10. 2337/dc07–0157.

Niskanen, L., Tuomi, T., Groop, L. & Uusitupa, M. (1995) GAD antibodies in NIDDM. Ten-year follow-up from diagnosis. *Diabetes Care*, 18 (12), 1557–1565.

Oomichi, T., Emoto, M., Tabata, E., Morioka, T. Tsujimoto, Y., Tahara, H., Shoji, T. & Nishizawa, Y. (2007) Impact of glycemic control on survival of diabetic patients on chronic regular hemodialysis: a 7-year observational study. *Diabetes Care*, 29, 1496–1500.

Pan, X., Li, G., Hu, Y. *et al*. (1997) Effects of diet and exercise in preventing NIDDM in people with impaired glucose tolerance. The Da Quing IGT and Diabetes Study. *Diabetes Care*, 20, 537–544.

Perlstein, R., McConnell, K. & Hagger, V. (1997) *Off to a Flying Start*. International Diabetes Institute, Melbourne.

Pradhan, A., Rifai, N., Buring, J. & Ridker, P. (2007) Hemoglobin A1c predicts diabetes but not cardiovascular disease in nondiabetic women. *The American Journal of Medicine*, 120 (8), 720–727.

Rubin, R. (2002) Was Willis right? Thoughts on the interaction of depression and diabetes. *Diabetes Metabolism Research Reviews*, 18, 173–175.

Schultz, M. (2007) Fiber and magnesium intake protects against developing type 2 diabetes. *Archives of Internal Medicine*, 167, 956–965.

Sinha, R., Fisch, G., Teague, B. *et al*. (2002) Prevalence of inpaired glucose tolerance among children and adolescents with marked obesity. *New England Journal of Medicine*, 346 (11), 802–810.

Snitker, S., Watanabe, R., Avi, L. *et al*. (2004) Changes in insulin sensitivity in response to troglitazone do not differ between subjects with and without the common functional pro12Ala perixisome proliferator-activated receptor gamma2 gene variant: results form the Troglitazone in Prevention of Diabetes (TRIPOD) study. *Diabetes Care*, 27, 1365–1368.

Smith, M. (2001) Pathogenesis of Type 2 diabetes and effect of lifestyle changes. *Journal of Diabetes Nursing*, 5 (4), 123–127.

Soltesz, G., Patterson, C. & Dahlquist, G. (2006) Global trends in childhood obesity. International Diabetes Federation (IDF) *Diabetes Atlas*, 3rd edn. IDF, Brussels, pp. 154–190.

Stene, L. & Joner, G. (2003) Use of cod liver oil during the first year of life is associated with lower risk of childhood-onset type 1 diabetes: a large, population-based, case-control study. *The American Journal of Clinical Nutrition*, 78 (6), 1128–1134.

The Agency for Healthcare Research and Quality www.ahrq.gov/ppip (accessed 12–1-2008).

Torgerson, J., Hauptman, J., Boldrin, M. & Sjostrom, L. (2004) XENical in the prevention of diabetes in obese subjects (XENDOS) study: a randomized study of orlistat as an adjunct to lifestyle changes for the prevention of type 2 diabetes in obese patients. *Diabetes Care*, 27,155–161 (erratum in 2004; 27: 856).

The DIAMOND Project Group (2006) Incidence and trends of childhood type 1 diabetes worldwide 1990–1999. *Diabetic Medicine*, 23, 857–866.

Tuomilehto, J., Eriksson, J. & Valle, T. (2001) Prevention of type 2 diabetes mellitus by changes in lifestyle among subjects with impaired glucose tolerance. *New England Journal of Medicine*, 344, 1343–1350.

Turner, N. & Clapham, C. (1998) Insulin resistance, impaired glucose tolerance and non-insulin-dependant diabetes pathologic mechanisms and treatment: current status and therapeutic possibilities. *Progress in Drug Research*, **51**, 33–94.

Twigg, S., Kamp, M., Davis, T., Neylon, E. & Flack, J. (2007) Prediabetes: a position statement from the Australian Diabetes Society and Australian Diabetes Educators Association. *Medical Journal of Australia*, **186** (9), 461–465.

UKPDS (United Kingdom Prospective Diabetes Study) (1998) Intensive blood glucose control with sulphonylureas or insulin compared with conventional treatment and risk of complications in patients with Type 2 diabetes (UKPDS 33). *Lancet*, **352**, 837–853.

Van den Berghe, G., Wouters, P., Weekers, F. *et al.* (2001) Intensive insulin therapy in critically ill patients. *New England Journal of Medicine*, **345** (19), 1359–1367.

Van der Laar, F., Lucassen, P., Akkermans, R. *et al.* (2006) Alpha-glucosidase inhibitors for people with impaired glucose tolerance or impaired fasting blood glucose. *Cochrane Database of Systematic Reviews*, **4**, CD005061.

Weiss, R. & Caprio, S. (2005) The metabolic consequences of childhood obesity. *Best Practice & Research Clinical Endocrinology & Metabolism*, **19** (3), 405–419.

Wild, S. Roglic, G., Green, A., Sicree, R. & King, H. (2004) Global prevalence of diabetes estimates for the year 2000 and projections for 2030. *Diabetes Care*, **27** (5), 1047–1057.

Willi, C., Bodenmann, P., Ghali, W., Faris, P. & Cornuz, J. (2007) Active smoking and the risk of Type 2 diabetes: a systematic review and meta-analysis. *Journal of the American Medical Association*, **298**, 2654–2664.

World Health Organization (WHO) (1999) *Definition, Diagnosis and Classification of Diabetes Mellitus and Its Complications: Report of a WHO Consultation. Part 1: Diagnosis and Classification of Diabetes Mellitus*. WHO, Geneva.

Zimmermann, U. & Himmerich, H. (2003) Epidemiology, implications and mechanisms underlying drug-induced weight gain in psychiatric patients. *Journal of Psychiatric Research*, **37**, 193–220.

Zinman, B., Kahn, S., Haffner, S., O'Neill, C., Heise, M. & Freed, M. (2004) Phenotypic characteristics of GAD antibody-positive recently diagnosed patients with type 2 diabetes in North America and Europe. *Diabetes*, **53** (12), 3193–3200.

Zimmet, P., Alberti, G. & Shaw, J. (2005) Mainstreaming the metabolic syndrome: a definitive definition. *Medical Journal of Australia*, **183** (4), 175–176.

Zipitis, C. & Akoberng, A. (2008) Vitamin D supplementation in early childhood and risk of Type 1 diabetes: a systematic review and meta-analysis. *Archives of Disease in Childhood*, March 13 [Epub ahead of print].

Zimmet, P., Alberti, G., Kaufman, F., Tajima, N., Silink, M., Arslanian, S., Wong, G., Bennett, P., Shaw, J., Caprio, S. & IDF Consensus Group (2007) The metabolic syndrome in children and adolescents – an IDF consensus report. *Paediatric Diabetes*, **8**, 299–306.

Zoungas, S. & Kerr, P. (2008) The impact of glycaemic control on outcomes in patients with end-stage renal disease and type 2 diabetes. *Nephrology*, **13** (2), 124–127.

Chapter 2
Holistic Assessment, Nursing Diagnosis, and Documentation

Key points

- An holistic diabetes education and management plan must encompass:
  - The physical, emotional, spiritual, social, and environmental factors relevant to the individual and be developed in collaboration with them and significant family members and carers.
  - General nursing and health care needs as well as diabetes.
- Incorporate diabetes-specific factors likely to affect self-care, health professional care and outcomes.
- Develop and document individual care plans based on the best available evidence and communicate them to other relevant health professionals, family and carers keeping in mind the individual's right to privacy.
- Evaluate outcomes relevant to the overall management goals, agreed metabolic targets as well as short-term goals formulated within the overall plan for a specific episode of care such as an admission to hospital.
- Discharge planning and transitional care among health services should be part of the care plan.

Rationale

Best practice diabetes education and care relies on a combination of the best available evidence, intuition, and clinical judgement, effective communication skills and the informed participation of the person with diabetes. Careful assessment enables physical, psychological, spiritual and social issues that impact on care to be identified and incorporated into nursing management and discharge/transition plans. Life balance and emotional well being are essential to achieving metabolic targets.

Holistic nursing

Holistic care aims to heal the whole person using art and science to support the individual to mobilise their innate healing potential: that is, to become empowered.

Healing occurs when the individual embraces and transforms traumatic life events and is open to and/or recognises his or her potential (Dossey *et al.* 1995, p. 40). Transcending traumatic life events such as the diagnosis of diabetes or a diabetes complication is part of the spiritual journey to self-awareness, self-empowerment, and wholeness. Significantly, spirituality is not the same as religion, although it may encompass religion (Dossey *et al.* 1995, p. 6; Parsian & Dunning 2008).

Thus, in order to achieve holistic care, nurses must consider the individual's beliefs and attitudes because the meaning people attach to their health, diabetes, and treatment, including medicines, affects their self-care behaviour and health outcomes. At least eight broad interpretations of illness have been identified: challenge, enemy, punishment, weakness, relief, irreparable loss/damage, value adding, and denial (Lipowski 1970; Dunning 1994; Dunning & Martin 1998). In addition, the author has identified other explanatory models as part of routine clinical care: diabetes as an opportunity for positive change; diabetes is a visitation from God.

Care models

Wagner *et al.* (2002) suggested many care models have limited effectiveness and reach because they rely on traditional education methods and do not support self-management, and transition among services. The essential elements needed to improve outcomes encompass:

- Evidence-based planned care including management guidelines and policies.
- Appropriate service and practice design that encompasses prevention and expedites referral and communication among services.
- Systems to support self-management.
- Process to ensure practitioners are knowledgeable and competent, collaborate and communicate effectively, have sufficient time to provide individual care and are supported to do so and where health professional roles are clearly defined and complementary.
- Clinical information systems that enable disease registries to be maintained, outcomes to be monitored, relevant reminders to be sent to patients and performance to be evaluated (Wagner *et al.* 1996).

Many current diabetes management models such as the Lorig and Flinders Models, the Group Health Cooperative Diabetes Roadmap, Kaiser-Permanente in Colorado, nurse-led case management, and various shared care models including computer programs (Interactive Health Communication Applications (IHCA)) encompass these elements and improve patient adherence to management strategies and satisfaction. However, their application is still limited by time and resource constraints, including timely patient access to health professionals.

Preliminary research suggests Internet-based support can improve patient–practitioner communication and collaboration, and enhance patient's sense of being valued and secure (Ralston *et al.* 2004). However, more research is needed to determine the best way to use these programmes and their effects in specific patient groups (Murray *et al.* 2005). Generally, patients have a better understanding of what is expected of them if they receive both written and verbal information (Johnson *et al.* 2003).

The font size, colour and language level of any written material provided including instructions for procedures and appointments and health professional contact details needs to be appropriate to the age, education level, and culture of the individual concerned (see Chapter 16).

In addition, health professionals must clearly promote a patient-centred approach care (National Managed Care Congress 1996) that is evident within the service. For example, patients are involved in decisions about their care and see the same doctor each time they attend an appointment. Although patient-centred care is difficult to define and achieve, often because of time constraints, it encompasses ways to:

- achieve personalised care
- ensure care is culturally sensitive and relevant
- increase patient trust in health professionals (Wagner *et al.* 1996a)
- help patients acquire the information they need to make informed decisions (McCulloch *et al.* 1998)
- improve patient adherence to management recommendations (Wagner *et al.* 1996b): also see Chapters 15 and 16.
- make collaborative decisions.

Specific programs that train health professionals how to deliver patient-centred care improve patient trust in doctors (Lewin *et al.* 2001; McKinstry *et al.* 2006), and the delivery of patient information (Kinnersley *et al.* 2007). In addition, patients may need specific education about how to ask relevant questions during consultations, and how to participate in making management decisions. Both parties may need education about how to negotiate the complex nature of shared decision-making to balance the imperative for evidence-based care with the need to incorporate the individual's values and preferences (Kilmartin 1997). In order to assist the process, the Foundation for Informed Decision-Making in the USA (2007) developed a series of interactive videos and written materials for patients about a range of common medical conditions.

In order to meet these requirements it is necessary to undertake a thorough assessment, use clinical reasoning to identify the patient's needs and management guidelines to determine whether the recommended treatment is likely to benefit the individual, whether the benefits outweigh the risks, and whether the individual can/will adhere to the recommendations including their self-care capacity, and then select the most appropriate treatment option.

Characteristics of an holistic nursing history

The nursing history

- Includes demographic data (age, gender, social situation).
- Collects units of information about past and current individual and family health and family and social relationships (see Figure 2.1) to permit individual care plans to be formulated considering the person's goals and expectations.
  - Obtains baseline information about the person's physical and mental status before and after and the presenting complaint.

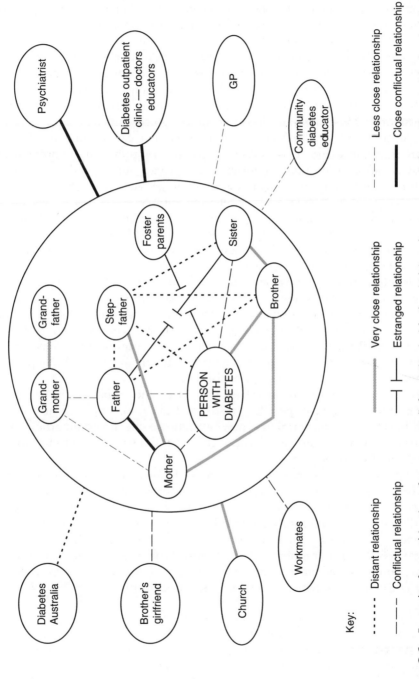

Key:

· · · · · Distant relationship   Very close relationship   – – – – Less close relationship

– – – Conflictual relationship   ─┤├─ Estranged relationship   Close conflictual relationship

Figure 2.1 Example of a combination of a genomap (information inside the circle) and an ecomap (information outside the circle) of a 50-year-old woman with Type 2 diabetes and a history of childhood molestation and sexual abuse. It shows a great deal of conflict within and outside the family and identifies where her support base is.

o Collects information about the person's general health and diabetes-related beliefs and attitudes and the meaning they attach to, and the importance they place on symptoms.
- Should be concise to enable information to be collected in a short time.
- Should focus on maintaining the person's independence while they are in hospital (e.g. allowing them to perform their own blood glucose tests).

The findings should be documented in the patient record and communicated to the appropriate caregivers. There is an increasing trend towards electronic data collection and management process that enable information to be easily and rapidly transferred among health professionals. Some systems enable patients to access their health information. Most modern electronic blood glucose meters have a facility for marinating a record of blood glucose test result that can be downloaded into computer programs. These systems have the capacity to significantly improve health care, however, consideration must be given to the privacy and confidentiality of all personal information and appropriate access and storage security mechanisms should be maintained according to the laws of the relevant country

Note: A guideline for obtaining a comprehensive nursing history follows. However, it is important, to listen to the patient and not be locked into 'ticking boxes', so assumptions can be checked and non-verbal messages and body language noted and clarified, so that vital and valuable information is not overlooked.

Most of the information is general in nature, but some will be specifically relevant to diabetes (e.g. blood glucose testing and eating patterns). The clinical assessment in this example is particularly aimed at obtaining information about metabolic status.

Assessment of the person with diabetes does not differ from the assessment performed for any other disease process. Assessment should take into account social, physical and psychological factors in order to prepare an appropriate nursing care plan, including a plan for diabetes education and discharge/transition.

Any physical disability the patient has will affect their ability to self-manage their diabetes (inject insulin, inspect feet, test blood glucose). Impaired hearing and psychological distress and mental illness may preclude people attending group education programmes. Management and educational expectations may need to be modified to take any disability into account.

If the person has diabetes, however, metabolic derangements may be present at admission, or could develop as a consequence of hospitalisation. Therefore, careful assessment enables potential problems to be identified, a coordinated collaborative care plan to be developed and appropriate referral to other health professionals (medical specialist, podiatrist, diabetes nurse specialist/diabetes educator, dietitian, psychologist) to take place. A health 'problem list', that ranks problems in order of priority can also assist in planning individualised care that addresses immediate and future management goals. The first step in patient assessment is to document a comprehensive health history.

Nursing history

A nursing history is a written record of specific information about a patient. The data collected enables the nurse to plan appropriate nursing actions considering individual patient's worldviews and needs. A good patient care plan will enable consistent care to be delivered within, and among, service departments. An example patient assessment chart follows. It was formulated to collect relevant diabetes-specific data, which could be used in conjunction with other relevant tools such as those shown in Table 2.1. Some electronic data management systems enable some information to be collected electronically from existing records when the patient has attended the service before.

Example health assessment chart

Formulated for people with diabetes in hospital but most issues are relevant in any health care setting. Other systems-based assessment may also be necessary for example respiratory, renal, nervous, and gastrointestinal systems.

A. Demographic data

Name: ....

Age: ....   Gender: ☐ Male   ☐ Female

Type of diabetes: ☐ Type 1   ☐ Type 2   ☐ Other ....

Duration of diabetes .... years

Known allergies ....

Social

Language spoken: ....

Command of English/language of relevant country: ☐ Written   ☐ Spoken

Important cultural practices, e.g. fasting, dietary requirements, practices related to dying and death

Marital status: ....

Living arrangements: ☐ With partner   ☐ Alone   ☐ Other

Support systems: ....

Age and health status of significant other/carer ....

Work type: ....

Responsibility in the home ....

Hobbies ....

Education level ....

Religion ....

Important religious practices, e.g. prayer ....

Meals

Regular meals: ☐ Yes   ☐ No

Food allergies ....

Usual diet ....

Appetite generally .... currently ....

Who does the cooking: ....

Who does the shopping ....

Eating out: ....

Current nasogastric tube .... TPN .... IV ....

Alcohol consumption: ☐ Yes   ☐ No   How much: ....

How often: ....

Smoking

☐ Yes   ☐ No   Cigarettes/pipe:..

How many per day: .... Marijuana: ....

Current medications

Record dose and dose frequency for each medicine, when they administer it in relation to food and exercise, whether they miss doses, if so how often and why, whether they alter doses, if so how often and why.

Check insulin injection sites, and blood glucose test sites if relevant.

General: ....

Diabetic: ....

Self-prescribed: ....

Insulin delivery system used ....

Insulin administration technique/accuracy: ....

Preparing injection using usual system: ....

Patient can name type/s of insulin: ☐ Yes   ☐ No. Do they adjust their insulin dose?

Why? ....What criteria do they use to adjust doses? ....

Complementary therapies: name of the product/therapy, why they are using it and what they are using it for.

If on insulin or oral hypoglycaemic agents: ask whether they have hypoglycaemia.

How often?

Do they ever lose consciousness during a hypoglycaemic episode?

Do they recognise the signs and symptoms of hypoglycaemia?

What signs/symptoms do they experience?

When does it usually occur?

What is the blood glucose level before they treat the hypo?

How do they treat the hypo?

Do they always have some form of glucose with them? ....

Usual activity level

Sports: ....

Gardening: ....

Walking: ....

Other: ....

Sleep pattern

Approximately how long do they sleep for?

Do they have trouble getting to sleep?

Do they have trouble staying asleep?

Do they need to get up at night to go to the toilet? .... How often?

Can they go back to sleep after going to the toilet?

What prevents them from sleeping?

Do they use anything to help them sleep? .... What? ....

Disabilities

What activities are limited: ....

To what degree: ....

(1)   General: ....

(2)   Hearing: ....

(3)   Related to diabetic complications: ....

Reduced vision: ☐ glasses   ☐ contact lenses   ☐ registered blind

Neuropathy: (a)   Peripheral: ....

                (b)   Autonomic: ....

Vascular: (a)   Cardiac: ....

                (b)   Legs and feet: ....

Kidney function: ....

Sexuality: (a)   Erectile dysfunction: ....

                (b)   Sexual difficulties ....

(4)   Mobility and flexibility:

(5)   Dexterity (fine motor skills):

Self-monitoring of diabetes status (testing methods)

....

Tests own blood glucose: ☐ Yes   ☐ No

Tests blood ketones during illness: Yes ☐   No ☐

Testing frequency: ....

System used:

Blood glucose meter type: ....

Testing accuracy: ....

Psychological status

Anxiety
Depression

Adjustment to diabetes

☐ Anxious ☐ Denial ☐ Depression ☐ Well adjusted
Usual mental state: .... Current mental state: ....
Current stressors: ....
Coping mechanisms: ....

Diabetes knowledge

Previous diabetes education: ☐ Yes   ☐ No   How long ago: ....
Attendance at education support groups: ☐ Yes   ☐ No
Name of group: ....

Patient's stated reason for being in hospital

....
....

B. Clinical and laboratory examination

A detailed physical examination is essential. Particular attention should be paid to the following areas.

(1) General inspection

- Conscious state
- Temperature, pulse and respiration
- Blood pressure lying and standing; note any postural drop
- Height
- Weight and history of weight gain/loss; BMI, ...Waist circumference
- Hydration status, skin turgor
- Presence of diabetic symptoms, thirst, polyuria, polydipsia, lethargy
- Full urinalysis
- Blood glucose
- Presence of ketones in blood ☐   urine ☐

(2) Skin

- Pigmentation (Acanthosis nigricans)
- Skin tone/turgor, colour

- Presence of lesions, rashes, wounds, ulcers
- Inspect injection sites, including abdomen; note any thickening, lumps, bruises

(3)   Mouth

- Mucous membranes (dry/moist)
- Lips
- Infection, halitosis
- Teeth: evidence of dental caries, loose teeth, red gums, incorrectly fitting dentures

(4) Feet and legs

- Temperature of feet and legs, noting any differences between two legs and parts of the feet and legs.
- The skin of the feet and legs may be hairless and shiny due to poor circulation
- Muscle wasting
- Ulcers or pressure areas on soles of feet and toes, including old scars
- Loss of pain sensation that may be due to nerve damage; estimate the size and depth of any ulcers using a template filed in the medical record, note their location and how long they have been present
- Presence of oedema
- Infection including fungal infection; inspect between the toes
- Condition of nails and general cleanliness of feet
- Type of footwear
- Record podiatry contact or referral, if any

Laboratory tests

Full blood count
Glucose
HbA_{ic}
Lipid profile
Kidney function
Liver function
Urea and electrolyte
Other relevant tests

Instruments to measure health status

Other specific instruments can be very helpful to determine health status, quality of life (QOL), beliefs and attitudes, and satisfaction. QOL is a complex, multifactioral, and individual construct encompassing the individual's physical, social and mental functioning, satisfaction with life and whether/how these factors are affected by illness and its management (Salek 1998). Significantly, social well being is strongly correlated

Table 2.1 Some commonly used assessment instruments. The content of the instruments, the purpose of the assessment, and the particular patient population should be considered when selecting instruments, even when they are valid and reliable. Some are available in languages other than English. Details of most of the diabetes-specific instruments can be found on http://www.musc.edu/dfm/RCMAR/Diabetes Tool.html and Garrett *et al.* (2001).

Generic instruments	Diabetes-specific instruments
Sickness Impact Profile (Bergner *et al.* 1976)	Audit of Diabetes-dependent Quality of Life (ADDQoL) (Bradley *et al.* 1999)
Nottingham Health Profile (Hunt & McKenna 1985)	Appraisal of Diabetes Scale (ADS) (Carey *et al.* 1991)
Short Form Health Survey (SF-36) (Ware *et al.* 1992)	Diabetes Health Profile (DHP-1, DHP-18) (Meadows *et al.* 1996)
Quality of Life After Acute Myocardial Infarction (Oldridge *et al.* 1991)	The Diabetes Impact Measurement Scale (DIMS) (Hammond & Aoki 1992)
K10+ depression scale, which is sometimes used as part of the psychosocial profile developed by the Department of Human Services Victoria in Australia	Diabetes Quality of Life (DQOL) (Jacobson *et al.* 1988)
Perceived Therapeutic Efficacy Scale (PTES)	Diabetes Specific Quality of Life Scale (DSQOLS) for Type 1 diabetes (Mulhauser *et al.* 1998)
Spiritual Assessment Tool (Dossey *et al.* (1995)	Questionnaire on Stress in Diabetic Patients (QSD-R) (Duran *et al.* 1995)
Hospital Anxiety and Depression Scale (HADS)	Well-being Enquiry for Diabetics (WED) (Mannucci *et al.* 1996)
Self Assessment Health Status (EQ-5D)	Problem Areas in Diabetes (PAID) (Polonsky *et al.* 1995)
Center for Epidemiological Studies Depression Scale (CESD) (Radloff 1997)	Diabetes Treatment Satisfaction Questionnaire (DTSQ) (Bradley 1994)
Patient Health Questionnaire (PHQ-9) (Pfizer Inc 2003)	Diabetes Care Profile (DCP) (Fitzgerald *et al.* 1996)
	Diabetes-39 Questionnaire (D-39) (Boyer & Earp 1997)
	Spirituality Questionnaire for young adults with diabetes (Parsian & Dunning 1997 not listed on the RCMAR website)

with emotional well being. A range of instruments generally designated as generic and disease-specific is available. Generic instruments were designed for use in a wide range of patients and populations. Disease-specific instruments have a narrower focus on particular illnesses, in this case, diabetes.

Table 2.1 presents an overview of generic and diabetes specific instruments commonly used to collect important subjective information from individuals about their health status and beliefs. The instruments have all been extensively validated.

Note: permission from the authors may be needed before the tools can be used and specific training in interpreting the data is needed with some instruments. Other useful instruments include pain scales, falls risk tools, activities of daily living and mental assessment such as Folstein's Minni Mental.

The Victorian Department of Human Services (DHS) (2006) produced a range of profiles such as the Psychosocial Profile, which encompasses mental health and well-being, and the Health Behaviours Profile that are used in many Australian DHS funded projects.

Documenting and charting patient care

Documenting in the health record

Documentation is an essential part of health management. Alternative methods of documenting care are emerging, for example charting by exception, where only events outside the normal expected progress are recorded. This form of charting requires supportive documentation in the form of guidelines, flow charts, care plans and care maps. They can avoid duplication and streamline documentation. The use of care pathways is becoming increasingly common in Australia and in the UK (O'Brien 2000).

Other ways of documenting holistic care incorporate genomaps and ecomaps (see Figure 2.1), which can effectively convey a great deal of information about the social relationship and support base aspects of an individual's life (Cluning 1997). They are particularly useful for long-term chronic diseases such as diabetes where these factors affect management outcomes, see Chapters 15 and 16. They also record information that is often passed on anecdotally during handover or in the 'corridor', which means vital information that could assist in planning care is not available or is misinterpreted.

Genograms illustrate how an individual relates to other people in the family and ecomaps place the family in the context of the wider social situation in which they live. Ecograms and ecomaps can be simple or convey complex and detailed information. Together they give a great deal of information about:

- the individual's environment
- their relationships with people in their environment
- family structure
- family and extended support
- family health history
- family functioning
- health service utilisation
- social orientation.

This information helps determine how social support and other networks influence the person's self-management and the assistance they can rely on, for example to manage serious hypoglycaemia and intercurrent illness.

Nursing care plans

The employing institution's policy regarding the method of documentation should be followed. Good nursing documentation enables the required care to be communicated to all staff. In the future, changes will occur to the methods of documenting care; for example, focus charting and flow charts may replace narrative notes. Flow charts are designed to enable all healthcare providers to document care on a single care plan, which reduces duplication and enhances communication

Standardised care plans of common medical and nursing diagnosis are being developed to serve as blueprints and may reduce the time spent on documentation. There is a move towards computerised or 'paperless' documentation. Where this form of documentation is used, due consideration of the security of the information is essential. Confidential information should be labelled as such in the record. Extra care is required with mobile technology such as laptops and palm pilots to ensure patient confidentiality is protected.

Nursing notes

Due consideration needs to be given to standard policies for good documentation and the laws governing privacy and confidentiality and people's right to access their medical records. Nursing notes are a record of the patient's hospital admission, healthcare and response to treatment, and act as a guide for discharge planning. They should be written legibly and objectively. They are not legal documents but may be subpoenaed for a court hearing.

Documentation should contain the following:

- The condition of the patient recorded objectively; for example, describe wounds in terms of size and depth.
- Quantification of the patient's condition, recording swelling, oedema, temperature, pulse, and respiration (TPR) and blood pressure (BP) using objective measures.
- All teaching the patient receives and that still required.
- The patient's response to treatment.
- All medications received.
- Removal of all invasive medical devices (e.g. packs, drains, IV lines).
- Psychological, spiritual, and social factors.

Clinical observation

In some cases it is possible to refer to standard protocols in medical records if there is a set procedure documented and regularly revised, for example there is a standard procedure for performing an oral glucose tolerance test. The documentation could note relevant details such as the time, date and person's name and then state 'OGGT performed according to the standard protocol'. Where any deviation from the protocol occurred it should be recorded. If required, the standard protocol could be produced.

Diabetes documentation

The purposes of the chart are:

- To provide a record of blood glucose measurements so the blood glucose pattern can be identified and used to adjust insulin/oral hypoglycaemic agent dose forms, doses, and/or dose intervals.
- To record blood ketone measurements to detect risk of ketoacidosis especially in Type 1 diabetes.
- To provide a record of the dose and time of administering insulin/oral hypoglycaemic agents.
- To record episodes of hyper or hypoglycaemia.

Frequency of blood testing depends on the patient's status and the management plan (see Chapter 3).

Practice point

A common error is that medication doses are not recorded and it can be difficult to interpret the blood glucose pattern without the medication information.

Nursing responsibilities

(1) Write legibly. Avoid using unauthorised abbreviations. Insulin doses should be documented as 'units' not u/s.
(2) Accurately record all medication doses and dose intervals.
(3) Record hypoglycaemic episodes (symptoms, treatment, time, activity and food omission) in the appropriate column. Hypoglycaemia should also be documented in the patient's unit record.
(4) Do not add unnecessary details.
(5) Sign and include the date and time of all entries.

Figure 2.2 depicts example charts for (a) frequent testing and (b) testing 4-hourly or less often.

Documentation by people with diabetes

People with diabetes also document a great deal of information about their disease. They use a variety of written and electronic record-keeping methods including blood glucose monitoring diaries, complication screening records and other management information such as medication doses and the results of investigative procedures. These records are a vital part of the documentation process. They not only supply written information, they also contain a great deal of information about an individual's self-care ability, for example a blood glucose diary covered with blood smears could mean the person is having difficulty placing the blood on the strip.

(a)

DIABETIC FREQUENT MONITORING							
						IDENTIFICATION	

		INSULIN		BLOOD GLUCOSE	BLOOD KETONES	URINALYSIS	NURSING COMMENTS E.g. Adverse reactions or food omission
DATE	TIME	TYPE	DOSE				

(b)

INSTRUCTION TYPE OF INSULIN BLOOD GLUCOSE AND URINE TESTS MUST BE RECORDED IN FULL						
					IDENTIFICATION	
DATE		0700	1100	1600	2100	COMMENTS
	Insulin type Dose					
	Blood glucose mmol/L					
	Urine ketones Ketones					
	Insulin type Dose					
	Blood glucose mmol/L					
	Urine ketones Ketones					

Figure 2.2   Sample diabetes record charts for (a) 2-hourly testing (e.g. when using an insulin infusion); (b) 4-hourly or less frequent testing.

Discussion with the patient might reveal that they often get the shakes and their vision is blurred due to hypoglycaemia. It is important, however, that all such assumptions are checked.

References

Cluning, T. (1997) Social assessment documentation: genomaps and ecomaps. In: *Nursing Documentation: Writing What We Do* (ed. J. Richmond), Chapter 7. Ausmed Publications, Melbourne.

Culloch, D. *et al.* (1998) A population based approach to diabetes management in a primary care setting: early results and lessons learned. *Effective Clinical Practice*, 1, 1222.

Dossey, B., Keegen, L., Guzzetta, C. & Kolkmeier, L. (1995) *Holistic Nursing: A Handbook for Practice*. Aspen Publishers, Maryland, pp. 20–21.

Dunning, P. (1994) Having diabetes: young adult perspectives. *The Diabetes Educator*, 21 (1), 58–65.

Dunning, P. & Martin, M. (1998) Beliefs about diabetes and diabetes complications. *Professional Nurse*, 13 (7), 429–434.

Foundation for Informed Medical Decision Making (2007) http:// www.fmdm.org/decision_ sdms.php (accessed December 2007).

Garratt, A., Schmidt, L. & Fitzpatrick, R. (2002) Patient-assessed health outcome measures for diabetes: a structured review. *Diabetic Medicine*, 19, 111.

Hunt, S. & McKenna, J. (1985) Nottingham Health Profile. http://.www.eygnus-group.com/ cidm/risk/html (accessed January 2008).

Johnson, A., Sandford, J. & Tyndall, J. (2003) Written and verbal information versus verbal information only for patients being discharged from acute hospital settings to home. *Cochrane Database of Scientific Reviews*. Issue 4 Art No Cd003716. DOI; 10. 1002/14651858. CD 003716.

Kilmartin, M. (1997) Evidence is lacking on shared decisions. *Journal of Health Services Research and Policy*, 2 (2), 112–121.

Kinnersley, P., Edwards, A., Hood, K., Cadbury, N., Ryan, R., Prout, H., Owen, D., McBeth, F., Butow, P. & Butler, C. (2007) Interventions before consultations for helping patients address their information needs. *Cochrane Database of Scientific Reviews*, Issue 3, Art. No. CD 004565. DOI 10. 1002/14651858. CDOO4565.pub2.

Lewin, S., Skea, Z., Entwistle, V., Zwarenstein, M. & Dick, J. (2001) Interventions for providers to promote a patient-centred approach in clinical consultations. *Cochrane Database of Systematic Reviews*, Issue 4, Art. No. CDOO 3267. DOI 10. 1002/14651858.CDOO3267.

McKinstry, B., Ashcroft, R., Car, J., Freeman, G. & Sheik, A. (2006) Interventions for improving patients' trust in doctors and groups of doctors. *Cochrane Database for Systematic Reviews*, Issue 3, Art. No. CDOO4134. DOI: 10. 1002/14651858.CDOO4134.pub2.

Murray, E., Burns, J., See Tai, S., Lai, R. & Nazareth, I. (2004) Interactive health communication applications for people with chronic illness. *Cochrane Database of Systematic Reviews*, Issue 4, Art. No. CDOO4274. DOI: 10. 1002/4651858.CDOO4274.pub4.

National Managed Health Care Congress. Inc (NHCG) (1996) *The Disease Management Strategic Research Study and Resource Guide*. NHCG, Washington.

O'Brien, S. & Hardy, K. (2000) Impact of a care pathway driven diabetes education programme. *Journal of Diabetes Nursing*, 4 (5), 147–150.

Parsian, N. & Dunning, T. (2008) spirituality and coping in young adults with diabetes. *Diabetes Research and Clinical Practice*, 79 (182), S82–S121.

Ralston, J., Revere, D. & Robins, L. (2004) Patients' experience with a diabetes support program based on an interactive electronic medical record: qualitative survey. *British Medical Journal*, 328, 115–162.

Salek, S. (1998) *Compendium of Quality of Life Instruments*. John Wiley & Sons, Chichester.

Wagner, E. *et al.* (1996a) Improving outcomes in chronic illness. *Managed Care Quarterly*, 4 (2), 1225.

Wagner, E. *et al.* (1996b) Organising care for patients with chronic illness. *The Millbank Quarterly*, 74 (4), 51–54.

Chapter 3
Monitoring Diabetes Mellitus

Key points

- Regular assessment of the individual's physical, emotional, social, spiritual, relationship status, and their capability to perform their usual activities of daily living and self-care is essential to enable proactive management strategies to be implemented.
- Structured regular complication screening programmes that encompass mental health, self-care, driving safety, and a structured medication review should be undertaken at least annually. In some cases the health and well being of spouses need to be considered especially older spouses who provide care and support.
- Diabetes education and management programmes should be evaluated and revised regularly to ensure they remain current. Patients should be involved in the evaluation processes.
- The patient has a responsibility to undertake appropriate self-care to manage their disease.

Rationale

Proactive monitoring programmes enable blood glucose and lipid patterns, complication status, and self-care ability to be identified and the management regimen appropriately tailored to the individual. The accuracy of the self-testing technique and appropriate maintenance of equipment is an important aspect of the individual's ability to manage their diabetes and helps ensure management decisions are based on the best available data when used in conjunction with laboratory investigations and physical and mental assessment Self-monitoring enables people with diabetes to identify the effects of diet, exercise and other factors on their blood glucose levels, and gives them greater insight into and control over their disease.

Introduction

Monitoring blood glucose is an important part of diabetes management. The results obtained form the basis for adjusting medication, food intake, and activity levels.

Urine glucose is not a reliable method of assessing metabolic control, but *might* still be useful for some people and in some countries where no other method is available provided the renal threshold for glucose has been established. Most glucose circulating in the blood is reabsorbed in the renal tubules, however, the capacity to reabsorb glucose is exceeded during hyperglycaemia and glucose appears in the urine. The renal threshold for glucose is fairly constant, about 10 mmol/L, but may be higher in older people and during pregnancy (Sonksen *et al.* 1998). Glucose in the urine represents the amount of glucose that collects in the urine since the bladder was last emptied and is therefore, a retrospective value.

People with diabetes are expected to manage their diabetes at home. They should be encouraged to continue to self-monitor in hospital if they are well enough to do so. If health professionals perform the test they should always inform the patient of the result of their blood glucose test unless they are too ill to understand the information. Blood glucose testing time can be used as teaching time.

The results of blood and urine tests are useful only if tests are accurately performed. The following section explores monitoring blood glucose.

Monitoring 1: blood glucose

Key points

- Follow correct procedure when performing tests. 7
- Perform meter control and calibration tests regularly.
- Clean and maintain equipment regularly.
- Record and interpret results according to the clinical situation.

The role of blood glucose monitoring in the care of diabetes

Blood glucose monitoring provides insight into the effectiveness of the diabetes management plan. It enables direct feedback to the patient about their blood glucose.

Some experts suggest the cost and time associated with self-blood glucose monitoring is not cost effective, even when patients are taught to adjust their management regimen. For example, the DiGEM investigators undertook a randomised control trial involving people with treated Type 2 diabetes over age 25 treated with diet or OHAs and showed no statistically significant difference in HbA_{1c} at 12 months but there was a significant change in total cholesterol (Farmer 2007). Subjective parameters such as quality of life and sense of control were not measured. Other researchers also show that people who monitor their blood glucose are younger at diagnosis and present with a higher HbA_{1c} than people who do not test (Franciosi *et al.* 2005; Davis *et al.* 2006).

In contrast, the ROSSO study (Schneider *et al.* 2006) showed metabolic control improved in people with Type 2 diabetes who performed frequent blood glucose tests, and demonstrated a 51% lower risk of death and a 32% lower risk of micro and macrovascular complications. In addition, people who monitored were more aware of their blood glucose levels and sought advice from health professionals sooner. Likewise, Karter *et al.* (2006) demonstrated improved HbA$_{1c}$ after home blood glucose testing was instituted in the Kaiser Permanente study.

Other researchers have shown lower rates of self-blood glucose monitoring in men and those with low education level, those who do not have health insurance, in countries where equipment is not subsidised, as well as those not on insulin, those taking OHAs, having less than two consultations with the doctor annually, and not attending diabetes education programmes (Centers for Disease Control and Prevention (CDC) 2007).

These studies suggest there may be gender and age differences in the rates of self-blood glucose monitoring but the rates are similar in different countries. Nevertheless, most management guidelines continue to recommend self-blood glucose testing as an integral part of the management plan. Testing frequency should be individualised depending on glycaemic control and health status in Type 2 diabetes but at least daily when insulin and/or OHAs are used. People with Type 1 should monitor at least TDS (Canadian Diabetes Association).

Blood glucose testing is performed to:

- Monitor the effectiveness of diabetes therapy and guide adjustments to the food plan, OHAs/insulin dose, exercise/activity, mental well being and quality of life, see Chapter 2.
- Detect hyperglycaemia, which can be confirmed by laboratory blood glucose tests and elevated HbA$_{1c}$ levels, a marker of the average blood glucose over the preceding three months, and more recently, A$_{1c}$-derived average glucose.
- Achieve blood glucose targets, which has a role in preventing or delaying the onset of diabetes-related complications and maintaining independence and quality of life.
- Diagnose hypoglycaemia, including nocturnal hypoglycaemia, which can present as sleep disturbances, snoring, restlessness or bad dreams.
- Establish the renal threshold for glucose to determine the reliability of urine testing in those rare cases where people still test their urine glucose.
- Achieve 'tight' control in pregnancy and thereby reduce the risks to both mother and baby.
- Provide continuity of care following hospitalisation.

Blood glucose monitoring is of particular use in:

- Frequent hypoglycaemic episodes and hypoglycaemic unawareness.
- Unstable or 'brittle' diabetes.
- Managing illnesses at home and when recovering from an illness.
- GDM, pregnancy and in neonates born to women with GDM and diabetes.
- Establishing a new treatment regimen.
- Stabilising OHA and/or insulin doses.
  - Patients with renal failure, autonomic neuropathy, cardiovascular or cerebrovascular insufficiency where hypoglycaemia signs can be masked or not recognised.
  - During investigations such as angiograms and surgical procedures.
  - Detecting actual or potential medicine/medicine or medicine/herb interactions.
  - During travel.

Clinical observation

In the home situation, blood glucose testing enables the person with diabetes to take more responsibility for and control over their disease and is a tool they can use to maintain their quality of life. It is not a means by which health professionals control people with diabetes. It is only one aspect of an holistic, individualised assessment, see Chapter 2.

The target blood glucose range and frequency of testing should be assessed individually when people with diabetes are in hospital. The aim is to achieve a blood glucose pattern as close to normal as possible. Generally accepted blood glucose targets are: premeal ≤5.5 mmol/L and two-hour post prandial <7.8 mmol/L (IDF 2007). However, the management regimen must target both fasting and post prandial blood glucose to achieve optimal control and reduce the risks associated with hyperglycaemia see Chapters 1, 7, and 8.

Increasing emphasis is being placed on reducing post prandial hyperglycaemia because it is associated with increased risk of retinopathy, cardiovascular disease, increased risk of cancer and impaired cognitive function in older people (IDF 2007). Significantly, elevated post prandial hyperglycaemia is present before Type 2 diabetes is diagnosed and partly accounts for why cardiovascular complications are frequently present at diagnosis. Management of post prandial hyperglycaemia is discussed in Chapters 5 and 8.

Although the focus is on achieving optimal blood glucose control to prevent or delay the onset of diabetes complications, optimal control is often not achieved. The person is usually blamed for not 'complying' with recommendations. However, the progressive nature of Type 2 diabetes and clinician inertia also play a part (Grant *et al.* 2004). Clinical inertia refers to health professionals recognising a problem but failing to act. Like 'non-compliance', clinical inertia is a derogatory term for a complex phenomenon where behaviours are influenced by factors such as competing demands in the clinical setting including time constraints and patients presenting with multiple problems that cannot all be addressed at the same time (Parchman *et al.* 2007). However, clinician inertia combined with patient non-adherence might increase the risk of poor control and may be mutually causative.

Factors that influence blood glucose levels

(1) Food: times of last food intake, quantity and type of carbohydrate/fibre consumed in relation to meals and activity.
(2) Exercise: timing with respect to food, medication and insulin doses, injection site, type of exercise and blood glucose level when commencing exercise.
(3) Intercurrent illness, for example, influenza, urinary tract infection.
(4) Medications used for diabetes control blood glucose: oral agents, insulin.
(5) Other medicines, for example, corticosteroids, oral contraceptives, beta blockers, and non-prescription medications that contain glucose, ephedrine, pseudoephedrine

or alcohol, for example, cold remedies and glucose lowering complementary medicines see Chapters 5 and 19.

(6) Alcohol: type, relationship to food intake, amount consumed.
(7) Insulin type, injection site, injection technique.
(8) Complementary medicines/therapies, for example, glucose lowering herbs, stress management techniques, see Chapter 19.
(9) Emotional (emotional dwelling) and physical stress – not only stress itself but medications used to treat stress.
(10) Accuracy of monitoring technique, including not hand washing before testing if sweet substances have been handled.
(11) Pregnancy in people with diabetes and gestational diabetes.
(12) Childhood: erratic swings in blood glucose levels are common.
(13) Adolescence: hormonal factors during adolescence can make control difficult.
(14) Renal, liver, and pancreatic disease.
(15) Other endocrine disorders, for example, thyroid disease, Cushing's disease, and acromegaly.
(16) Parenteral nutrition.
(17) Obtaining the blood sample from unwashed fingers, for example, after the patient or health professional treated a hypoglycaemic event with oral glucose.

Clinical observation

Insulin absorption can be delayed if insulin is injected into an oedemateous or ascitic abdomen. The delayed absorption can affect the blood glucose level. The thigh or upper arm may be preferable sites in this instance.

Guidelines for the frequency of blood glucose monitoring
(1) In care settings, capillary blood glucose tests should be performed only by adequately qualified health professionals.
(2) Medical staff and sometimes diabetes educators are usually responsible for interpreting the results and adjusting the diabetes management plan. Over time, many people with diabetes become expert at adjusting their insulin doses to account for carbohydrate intake (Dose Adjustment for Normal Eating (DAFNE)) and during illness and exercise.

The following recommendations are guidelines only; the policies and procedures of the employing institution should be followed.

Suggested protocol in hospital settings.   Blood glucose tests performed before meals and before bed (e.g. 7 AM, 11 AM, 4 PM, and 9 PM) in order to obtain a profile of the effectiveness of diabetes therapy. Occasionally, urine glucose will be measured at these times for 24 hours to establish the renal threshold. As indicated, testing 2 hours after food, especially in Type 2 diabetes, may be preferable to provide information about glucose clearance from the blood stream after a meal as an indicator of cardiovascular risk. Blood glucose tests may be performed at 2 AM or 3 AM for two to three days if the blood glucose is high before breakfast and there is a possibility of nocturnal hypoglycaemia, see Chapter 6.

Blood ketones should be monitored in all patients with Type 1 diabetes and in Type 2 people during severe stress, for example, surgery, infection, and myocardial infarction if blood glucose tests are elevated. Urine ketone tests might still be used in some places but are a less reliable indicator of ketosis than blood ketones. Each person's needs should be assessed individually and the testing schedule tailored to individual requirements where work routines and staffing levels allow. One way to achieve an individualised monitoring regime is to allow the patient to perform their own blood glucose tests where their condition permits them to do so.

Regimen for patients on insulin.   Initially, for 48 hours, monitor at 7 AM, 11 AM, 4 PM, and 9 PM to assess the effectiveness of the prescribed insulin therapy. Review after 48 hours and alter testing frequency if indicated. If the insulin regimen is altered, review again after 48 hours.

Note: The timing of blood glucose monitoring depends on the insulin regimen and the action profile of the prescribed insulin see Chapter 5.

Patients using insulin pumps and those on IV insulin infusions require more frequent monitoring.

Patients on oral hypoglycaemic agents.   Initial monitoring as for insulin-treated patients. Review after 48 hours and reduce monitoring frequency to twice daily, daily or once every second or third day, alternating the times of testing, as indicated by the level of control and the general medical condition of the patient.

Patients using diet and exercise.   Initially, twice daily monitoring, decreasing to daily or once every second or third day, unless the patient is having total parenteral nutrition (TPN), diagnostic procedures, is undergoing surgery or is actually ill.

In the acute care setting, patients are usually ill and require at least 4-hourly monitoring. The frequency can often be reduced in rehabilitation, mental health and care facilities for the elderly, and in the end stages of life.

Special circumstances.   These might require a prescription from the medical staff. They include:

(1) Insulin infusion: tests are usually performed every 1–2 hours during the infusion and reviewed every 2 hours. Reduce to 3–4 hourly when blood glucose levels are stable (see Chapter 5).

(2) People on glucocorticoid therapy because these medicines induce insulin resistance and increase hepatic glucose output, which might be greater in people who already have insulin resistance and hyperglycaemia and may be a risk factor for hyperosmolar states see Chapters 7 and 10. Ketones should also be monitored in Type 1 diabetes because some corticosteroids also induce lipolysis and increase the risk of ketoacidosis.

(a) Non-diabetic patients: regularly screen for hyperglycaemia. The effects on blood glucose depend on the formulation, dose, dose frequency, and duration of action, and the response of the individual to the particular preparation used. Often the blood glucose increases during the day and is higher in the afternoon (Dunning 1996). Oral preparations have a greater impact on blood glucose than IV preparations, which usually do not cause a great rise in the blood glucose.

    (b)   People with diabetes: see protocols in sections Regime for patients on insulin, Patients on oral hypoglycaemic agents or Patients using diet and exercise.

(3) TPN guidelines suggest:

    (a)   Routine blood glucose testing for the first 48 hours, 7 AM, 11 AM, 4 PM, and 9 PM, until the patient is stable on TPN, then revert to protocol in section Regime for patients on insulin or Patients on oral hypoglycaemic agents.

    (b)   Monitor blood for ketones, 7 AM, 11 AM, 4 PM, and 9 PM.

Practice point

Never prick the feet of an adult because it causes trauma and increases the risk of infection. Heel pricks can be performed on babies.

Blood glucose meters

Blood glucose meters are devices used to monitor blood glucose in the home or at the bedside in hospital. The first capillary blood glucose meter was introduced in 1974. Over the following decades the technology of both meters and test strips has changed rapidly. Modern meters are small, light, only require small quantities of blood, and are accurate if the factors that influence the results are taken into account. Staff should become familiar with the system used in their place of employment. Consult the diabetes educator/specialist team or manufacturer for specific advice.

Where meters are used, a blood glucose meter quality management programme with a centralised coordinator is desirable. As part of such a programme it is recommended that:

- Individual nurses and other users demonstrate competence to use the system in operation.
- Meters are subject to regular control testing and calibration according to the manufacturer's recommendations and are calibrated as required, usually when a new pack of strips is opened, and are appropriately cleaned and maintained and that these processes are documented.
- A procedure for dealing with inaccurate results and meter malfunction is in place.

Two main types of meter are available, reflectance photometers and biosensors. The former measures the colour change that occurs when chemical reagents in the test strip react with glucose in the blood. A light in the test chamber of the meter illuminates the test strip and the amount of reflected light is measured electronically and converted into a blood glucose concentration, which is displayed as a number in the test result window.

Biosensors measure an electrical current that is generated when glucose in the blood reacts with chemical reagents in the strip (known as a sensor). The current is generated in proportion to the concentration of glucose in the blood and is displayed in the result window as a number. Most meters can be programmed to read in mmol/L or mg/dL, which is used in the United States. Most meters also store a record of blood glucose tests that can be downloaded into computer software programmes that enable the data to be displayed in a range of ways.

Modern meters are small and light, easy to operate, and only require a very small amount of blood. Particular meters are designed specifically for particular target audiences such as children and older people, who have different requirements. For example, large result display screens and 'talking' meters for vision impaired people. Test strips require a minimal amount of blood. Therefore, many of the systems errors associated with early meters have been eliminated. However, inaccuracies still occur and are mostly due to technique errors.

Meter technology changes rapidly and health professionals need to be aware that the system in use in the hospital may be different from the system the person uses at home and note the following points.

Although blood glucose readings obtained from the fingertip most closely correlate with arterial glucose, alternative site testing (from sites other than the fingertip such as the forearm, abdomen and thigh) are available and cause less discomfort but only yield small quantity of blood ~3 µL. However, blood glucose levels vary among different sites. For example, there is a lag in increases and reductions in blood glucose by up to 30 minutes at the forearm compared with the fingertip, which can lead to delay in detecting and treating hypoglycaemia (Jungheim *et al.* 2002). Less variation occurs between the palm and ball of the thumb.

Practice point

'Glucometer' is not a generic term for blood glucose meters. It was the name of a specific meter no longer available. A more appropriate term is 'blood glucose meter' or use the name of the particular meter.

Continuous glucose monitoring systems

The technology to enable continuous glucose monitoring is developing rapidly towards the ultimate 'closed loop system'. Fingerprick blood glucose tests may miss many hypo and hyperglycaemic levels: continuous blood glucose monitoring systems enable 'real-time' continuous blood glucose levels to be identified. Sampling generally occurs from interstitial and tissue sites. Interstitial glucose concentrations are often lower than capillary concentrations during the night compared with capillary glucose (Monsod *et al.* 2002. However, continuous monitoring enables the trend toward hyper or hypoglycaemia (trend analysis) to be monitored and preventative action to be taken.

Glucowatch® G2 Biographer

The Glucowatch® G2 Biographer Glucose Monitoring System is a non-invasive blood glucose monitoring method that works by iontophoresis to extract tissue liquid and monitor blood glucose approximately every 20 minutes. It shows a good correlation with capillary glucose but has a lag time similar to alternative site testing and may underestimate the actual level (Garg *et al.* 1999).

The device works by reverse iontophoreses and uses an electric current that stimulates sweat production. Glucose is absorbed from the sweat by an autosensor, a small disposable pad, on the back of the device. The autosensor transforms the electrical signal to a glucose reading that can be displayed by pressing a button. The autosensor must be changed every 24 hours. An alarm sounds if the blood glucose goes too low or too high. The Glucowatch® holds up to 4000 tests in the memory and is only approved for adult use at present. The manufacturer, The Animas Corporation, announced they would discontinue selling the current model in the US because new products are being developed. The sensors will be available until July 2008 (http://www.glucowatch.com, accessed February 2008).

Continuous glucose monitoring system (CGMS)

The CGMS system consists of a pager-sized glucose monitor, disposable subcutaneous glucose sensor, a cable connecting these two components to a communication system that stores data, which is downloaded into a computer software program that enables the results to be displayed in graph form. Glucose concentrations are measured every 10 seconds; 1440/day. Glucose sensors need to be changed after 72 hours. At least four capillary blood glucose measurements are required each day to calibrate the CGMS and when there is likely to be a variation such as following severe hypoglycaemia or a glucose load (Guerci 2003).

Glucose targets can be assigned, the duration and frequency of hypo and hyperglycaemic episodes, and modal time determined using modern software. This provides important information that can help health professionals and patients understand the differences between their home blood glucose testing results and HbA$_{1c}$ and detect unrecognised hypoglycaemia. It is primarily used to determine blood glucose profiles before using insulin pumps, during GDM, in paediatrics, and to detect unrecognised hypoglycaemia rather than for routine home monitoring because of the cost. Other CGMS systems include the Pendragon Medical Company impedance spectroscopy system (Caduff *et al.* 2003) and the Freestyle Navigator Continuous Glucose Monitoring System (Weinstein *et al.* 2007).

Interpreting different results

Patients often comment that their blood glucose results are different from the results obtained using the meter in the outpatient clinic and doctor's rooms or at when they retest their blood glucose after a few minutes. Blood glucose meter tests only reflect individual points in time and may not detect fluctuations in blood glucose especially post prandially and overnight. CGMS is useful to detect such fluctuations.

Different meters give different results even when the tests are performed correctly and close together in time but generally should not differ by more than ~5%. Squeezing the finger to obtain a drop of blood can dilute the sample with tissue fluids and affect the accuracy of the test result.

Likewise, capillary glucose values are likely to differ from laboratory values reported on venous blood. Capillary glucose is ~5% higher than venous glucose. Laboratory values can be affected by glycolysis. Glucose in whole blood decreases by ~5–7% per hour because of the glycolytic enzyme activity in red blood cells. Thus venous samples should be sent to the laboratory promptly or kept at 4°C for short periods if it is not possible to transport the sample immediately. Preservatives such as fluoride in blood tubes slow but do not stop glycolysis in blood samples.

People are often confused by the different ways of reporting blood glucose (mmol/L or mg/dL) and HbA$_{1c}$ (%). Meter blood glucose results may not give an accurate indication of the average blood glucose level or of the minute fluctuations that occur minute-by-minute, see continuous blood glucose monitoring on the previous page. Discrepancies between blood glucose meter readings and HbA$_{1c}$ could be used as an opportunity to explore testing technique, other factors that affect the results of both testing methods and the individual's feelings about diabetes and its management. The differences may be a sign of underlying stress, especially in adolescents (Rose *et al.* 2002) see Chapter 13.

Practice point

Incorrect operator technique, inadequate quality control testing, incorrect meter calibration, and using out-of-date test strips are the major causes of inaccurate results using blood glucose meters.

Reasons for inaccurate blood glucose results

Inaccurate blood glucose readings can occur for the following reasons:

(1) Meters and test strips
  • using the incorrect strip for the meter
  • using the incorrect calibration or code
  • using an unclean meter
  • low or flat battery
  • inserting the strip incorrectly or facing the wrong way
  • insufficient blood on the strip will give a false low reading
  • quality control tests/calibration are not performed.
  • strips used after the expiry date
  • failure to wash hands before testing, especially if sweet substances have been handled
  • humidity and high temperatures affect some meters and/or strips.

If in doubt, repeat the test or confirm biochemically.

Figure 3.1 outlines the steps to be taken when performing quality control testing of blood glucose monitoring equipment.

Practice points

(1) It is not necessary to swab the finger with alcohol prior to testing because it can dry the skin. Alcohol swabbing does not alter the blood glucose results (Dunning *et al.* 1994).

(2) The hands should be washed in soap and water and dried carefully before testing, especially if the person has been handling glucose, for example, in an accident and emergency department/casualty when the person presents with hypoglycaemia.

Monitoring blood ketones

A 10-second capillary blood ketone testing meter is a useful adjunct to blood glucose testing for people with Type 1 diabetes during illness by enabling them to detect ketosis and institute treatment early to prevent ketoacidosis, see Chapter 7. It is increasingly

Figure 3.1   An example of a quality control flow chart for checking blood glucose meters.

being used in the clinical setting for the same reasons as well as giving an indication of the adequacy of the treatment during illness (Wallace *et al.* 2001).

Blood ketones are raised after fasting, in the morning, during starvation, may indicate a UTI in non-diabetic patients, after hypoglycaemia not due to excess insulin, some inborn errors of metabolism and ketoacidosis, which is most commonly due to diabetes. It is characteristic of untreated Type 1 diabetes and can occur in LADA and Type 2 diabetes. The main ketone bodies are:

- Acetoacetate, which is an end product of fatty acid metabolism.
- Acetone, which is formed from spontaneous decarboxylation of acetoacetate. Acetone is volatile and is expelled in expired air. It is the ketone responsible for the acetone smell of ketoacidosis.
- Beta-hydroxybutyrate (B-OHB), which is a reduced form of acetoacetate and the major ketone formed in acidosis.

Acetoacetate and beta-hydroxybutyrate are important energy substrates for many tissues especially the brain particularly during fasting and inadequate food intake. Blood ketone testing for B-OHB is more reliable than urine ketone testing (Fineberg *et al.* 2000). Currently available urine ketone test strips do not measure B-OHB and laboratory ketone testing often does not do so either, unless it is specifically requested.

The meter measures capillary B-OHB, which is the most abundant ketone body and the best guide to the patient's metabolic status: Levels >1 mmol/L require further action, for example, extra insulin, levels >3 mmol/L require medical assessment.

Blood glucose testing checklist

> **Nursing actions**
>
> (1) Assemble materials and prepare environment according to hospital policy and testing system used:
>   - test strip removed from vial and cap replaced immediately or open foil package;
>   - dry cotton or rayon ball or tissue to blot the test site if required;
>   - disposable fingerpricking device or a device with disposable end cap to avoid the possibility of cross-infection from blood left on the device.
> (2) Explain procedure to patient.
>
> **Obtaining a drop of blood**
>
> (1) Wash patient's hands with soap and warm water, dry carefully.
> (2) Choose a site on any finger, near the side or tip. Avoid using the pad of the finger where nerves and arteries are concentrated: it is more painful.
> (3) Prick finger firmly, using a fingerprick device.

(4) 'Milk' along the length of the finger to well up blood at the puncture site. Avoid squeezing too hard.

(5) Allow the drop of blood to fall onto the strip or be drawn up by capillary action depending on the type of meter and strips in use.

(6) Dispose off sharps into appropriate sharps container.

Documenting the results

(1) Record test results on diabetes chart and in any other pertinent record.

(2) Communicate results to appropriate person, for example, doctor and the patient.

Tips

(a) Warm hands bleed more readily.

(b) If peripheral circulation is deficient, obtaining blood can be difficult. Trap blood in fingertip with one hand, by milking the length of the finger and applying pressure with finger before pricking.

(c) Excess squeezing can dilute the red cells with plasma and lead to inaccurate results.

(d) Check with biochemistry result if the result does not match the clinical picture.

People with Type 1 diabetes are advised to test for ketones during illness, hyperglycaemia, pregnancy, if polyuria, polydipsia, and lethargy are present and if they have abdominal pain. Abdominal pain is common in ketoacidosis and usually resolves as the ketosis clears. If it persists it could indicate an abdominal emergency, see Chapter 7. Type 1 patients with hyperglycaemia and HbA_{1c} >8.5%, in association with B-OHB, are insulin deficient and at risk of ketosis. Normal blood B-OHB is 0–0.5 mmol/L. Table 3.1 depicts normal and abnormal ketone levels and suggests the management required.

Table 3.1   Blood ketone levels and potential management.

Blood ketone level (B-OHB)	Potential management
Normal <0.5 mmol/L	
Elevated 0.5–1.5 mmol/L and blood glucose ≥16 mmol/L	Ketosis risk/impending ketosis
	Insulin dose may need to be increased
	Food intake might be low due to fasting, poor intake or anorexia
Acidosis >1.5 mmol/L and blood glucose >16 mmol	Ketones established and ketoacidosis risk
	Medical review required
	Insulin required, possibly as an IV infusion
	Infection could be present

It should be noted that these levels are an indication and are not evidence based (Laffel & Kettyle 2000).

Testing for ketones is important during illness in.

- All people with Type 1 diabetes.
- People with Type 2 who are severely ill.
- During fasting.
- After-severe hypoglycaemia.
  - Severe stress.
  - TPN feeds high in glucose or lipids.
  - In the operative period.

Clinical observation

Lower than actual capillary blood glucose levels can be recorded using some blood glucose meters in the presence of moderate-to-heavy ketosis. The reason for this finding is not clear. As a consequence, health professionals and patients can underestimate the severity of the hyperglycaemia, miss developing ketoacidosis, and delay appropriate treatment.

Practice points

(1) Ketones are present in non-diabetic individuals during fasting and can be detected in 30% of first voided morning urine specimens of pregnant women.

(2) Ketone test strips using nitroprusside reagents (used on urine test strips) give false-positive ketone results in the presence of sulphydryl drugs such as captopril.

(3) Insulin replacement corrects the acidosis by facilitating the conversion of B-OHB into acetoacetate and indicates the ketosis is resolving. However, urine ketone tests can indicate the ketones are still high. That is, urine ketone clearance lags behind actual blood ketone levels.

(4) Urine ketone test strips give false-negative results when they have been exposed to the air for some time, have passed their expiry date and if the urine is highly acidic such as in a person taking large doses of vitamin C.

The rate of fall of B-OHB using blood ketone strips can potentially avoid these situations and improve self-care and enable preventative action to be taken early to avoid ketoacidosis.

Blood ketone strips can be used as an indicator of the adequacy of the treatment in acute care settings.

Monitoring 2: urine glucose

Key points

Urine glucose testing is not recommended. If it is used:

- Establish renal threshold to determine the reliability of urine tests.
- Fluid intake, hydration status, and urine concentration affect results.
  - Renal status affects the results.
  - The time since last voiding influences the result.
- Double voiding is unnecessary.
- However, a full urinalysis can provide important clinical information such as presence of infection, which is often silent in people with diabetes, haematuria, and indicate jaundice.

In the presence of normal kidney function glycosuria is correlated to the blood glucose concentration. Glycosuria occurs when the tubular maximum reabsorption is exceeded, usually around 8–10 mmol/L blood glucose. The test reflects the average glucose during the interval since the person last voided, rather than the level at the time the test is performed. This is called the renal threshold for glucose and varies within and between individuals. The renal threshold may be changed by:

- Increasing age
- Renal disease
- Long-standing diabetes.

Therefore:

- The blood glucose can be elevated without glycosuria being present.
- Traces of glucose in the urine can indicate loss of control.
- The renal threshold can be low in children and glycosuria present when blood glucose is normal.

It is important to establish the renal threshold during a period of good control (normoglycaemia) by simultaneously testing blood and urine glucose.

Practice point

Urine glucose monitoring is not recommended. It is not an accurate reflection of the blood glucose. In addition, it does not give warning of impending hypoglycaemia and a negative urine glucose finding does not indicate hypoglycaemia.

Indications for urine glucose tests

(1) If a person refuses to monitor their blood glucose.
(2) When the aim is to avoid glycosuria.

Double voiding prior to testing is not necessary.

Monitoring kidney function

Diabetic nephropathy is the leading cause of end-stage renal disease thus early identification of declining renal function is imperative see Chapter 8. Twelve- and 24-hour urine collections are used to monitor kidney function and detect early kidney damage by monitoring creatinine clearance rates and microalbumin excretion rates. Microalbuminuria reflects abnormally elevated albumin level not detectable on urine dipsticks. It is the earliest marker of the onset of kidney and cardiovascular damage and predicts deteriorating renal function (Krolewski *et al.* 1995). Up to 30% of newly diagnosed people with Type 1 diabetes already have high urine albumin levels, of these ~75% have microalbuminuria and 25% have overt nephropathy. People with Type 2 in the MICRO-Hope study (2000) had a 20% risk of progression from normal to microalbuminuria to nephropathy over 5 years, which is similar to Type 1.

Early diagnosis and treatment can delay the onset by 24 years and decrease the need for dialysis and increase life expectancy (Borch-Johnsen *et al.* 1993). Seventeen per cent of people with essential hypertension develop proteinuria despite satisfactory treatment (Ruilope *et al.* 1990).

Methods of screening for microalbuminuria

Several methods are available and include:

* Timed 12- or 24-hour urine collections.
* Spot urine tests. The first voided morning specimen is often used for initial screening (Jerums *et al.* 1994).
* Random urine tests using dipsticks or automated urine analysers to measure microalbumin and calculate the microalbumin–creatinine ratio (normal level in males is <2 mg:mmol and <2.8 mg:mmol in women). These tests should be negative for protein (Sheldon *et al.* 2002).
* Micral-Test dipstick tests (Boehringer Mannheim, GmbH Mannheim, Germany) is an immunochemiclly based urinary dipstick used to test for microalbuminuria and can be used in the ward situation. Compared to radioimmunoassays Micral-Test has a sensitivity of 92.2% and specificity of 92.3% and a positive predictive value of 37.8% in predicting an albumin excretion rate >20 µ/minute (Jerums *et al.* 1994).
* Glomerular filtration rate (GFR). The degree of reduction in the GFR is linked to the development of renal disease. GFR is used as the index to classify the severity of renal disease, see Chapter 8.
* Serum creatinine, which is used as a surrogate marker of GFR is relatively inaccurate (Chadban *et al.* 2003). Significantly, serum creatinine is not reliable in older people; especially those with lean muscle mass who can have creatinine in the normal range despite severely compromised renal disease (Mathew 2003).

- Estimated GFR (e-GFR) is calculated using a predictive equation that uses serum creatinine, age, and gender. It is less accurate in Chinese people and possibly other Asian peoples and Indigenous Australians (Zuo 2005). In the US, the Modification of Diet in Renal Disease (MDRD) is a valid method of determining e-GFR and classifying renal disease (National Kidney Foundation 2002). e-GFR may be unreliable in the following situations:
  ○ Acute changes in kidney function.
  ○ People on dialysis.
  ○ High protein and high vegetable diets and those who take creatine supplements.
  ○ Skeletal muscle diseases such as paraplegia and amputees.
  ○ Those with high muscle mass.
  ○ In the presence of severe liver disease.
  ○ When the e-GFR is >60 mL/min/1.73 m^2.
  ○ Children <18 years.
  ○ Asian peoples.
  ○ Maori and Pacific Islander peoples.
  ○ Aboriginal and Torres Strait Islander peoples.

Microalbuminuria is diagnosed when the urine albumin level is >30 mg/dL and is expressed as the quantity of albumin excreted in a given time (>20 μ/minute) or as a concentration (>20 μ/L urine). Most experts prefer the albumin–creatinine ratio because the other tests can be affected by the concentration of the urine.

Nurses have a role in screening and detecting declining renal function and educating the person about appropriate preventative measures. If timed urine collections are needed the procedure for collecting the urine should be explained to the patient carefully. Written instructions should be supplied if the collection is to be performed at home. Collections are best obtained at a period of good control and normal activity, not during illness or menstruation; therefore, the urine is often collected on an outpatient basis. The opportunity can be taken during a hospital admission to collect 12- or 24-hour timed urine collections when people repeatedly fail to collect them as outpatients. In some cases the first early morning voided specimen will be collected ~50 mL.

Ensure the correct containers are used for the collection and the specimen is correctly labelled.

Monitoring 3: additional assessment

In addition to blood and urine testing, diabetic status is assessed by:

(1) Regular weight checks. Height is also required to calculate BMI. Waist circumference is preferred.
(2) Regular physical examination, especially:
  - blood pressure (lying and standing to detect any postural drop that could indicate the presence of autonomic neuropathy)
  - eyes (retina) and visual acuity
  - cardiac status
  - feet

- kidney function
- Driving safety especially in older people.
(3) Regular education about:
  - diet
  - self-monitoring techniques
  - injection sites
  - general diabetes information especially new technology and research findings that need to be discussed in the context of the individual, see Chapter 16.
  - changes to diabetes care as a result of research.

Practice point

Normal ranges for the tests described differ among laboratories depending on the assay methods used. It is helpful if people attend the same pathology service to have blood and urine tests performed.

Nursing responsibilities

(1) To have a basic knowledge of the tests in order to be able to explain them to the patient.
(2) Ensure patients who are required to fast are given appropriate *written* instructions before the test about their medications and any other preparation required.
(3) To ensure the correct collection technique, appropriate amount of blood and correct tubes are used.
(4) Mix the sample by inverting the tube two or three times if an anticoagulant tube is required. Vigorous shaking causes haemolysis of red blood cells, which affects the results.
(5) To ensure the specimen reaches the laboratory within 30 minutes of collection or be refrigerated to prevent glycolysis occurring and consequent inaccurate results.
(6) To ensure results are available for medical evaluation.
(7) To know the effects of illness and stress on the results of the test.
(8) To ensure appropriate sterile blood collection technique is used.
(9) To ensure appropriate disposal of used equipment and to protect themselves from needlestick injury.
(10) To ensure patients are given their medication and something to eat after completing tests when fasting is required and that they are informed about when to recommence any medications that were temporarily stopped and the doses to take.

Blood glucose
Venous glucose is measured to:

- Screen for and diagnose diabetes.
- Monitor effectiveness of and determine the need for glucose lowering medicines and the dose and dose frequency required.

- Evaluate diabetic control.
- Confirm high/low capillary glucose result.

Glycosylated or glycated haemoglobin (HbA$_{1c}$)

It is most useful to have the HbA$_{1c}$ result at the time the person is assessed by the doctor/diabetes educator. Blood can be drawn from a vein and measured in the laboratory before the clinic/doctor visit so the result is available at the time of the consultation. Alternatively, blood can be drawn from a fingerprick sample at the time of the visit using devices such as the DCA 2000 (Bayer) analyser.

Circulating blood glucose attaches to the haemoglobin in the red blood cells and undergoes an irreversible non-enzymatic interaction with amino groups of lysine and valine residues in haemoglobin (Amadori reaction) whereby the glucose becomes permanently fixed to the haemoglobin (glycosylation). The glycosylated haemoglobin, HbA$_{1c}$ (A$_{1c}$ in the US) can be measured and quantified to give an indication of the average blood glucose concentration over the preceding 3 months (normal 4–5.9%) and to predict risk of long-term diabetes complications (Bloomgarden 2007; Kilpatrick *et al.* 2007). Currently, four main assays and ~20 different measurement methods are used that measure different glycated products and report different units (% HbA$_{1c}$, % HbA1, and total GHb) (Colman *et al.* 2008). The four assay methods are: ion-exchange chromatography, electrophoresis, affinity chromatography, and immunoassay.

Fasting prior to obtaining the blood sample for HbA$_{1c}$ is not necessary.

Tests are usually performed at least three months apart but can be done sooner to gauge the effect of a treatment modification and in research.

Kirkpatrick *et al.* (2007) point out that HbA$_{1c}$ is a proxy measure of average blood glucose and can be misleading because individuals are higher or lower glycosylators at specific mean blood glucose levels, which emphasises the importance of considering the individual and the overall clinical picture.

Current assay methods use a mixture of glycated haemoglobins to determine the HbA$_{1c}$. Representatives from the American Diabetes Association, The European Association for the Study of Diabetes, the International Diabetes Federation and the International Federation of Clinical Chemistry and Laboratory Medicine (IFCC) have been discussing methods of standardising HbA$_{1c}$ measurement for a number of years and released a consensus statement in Milan in 2007 (Consensus Committee 2007). Key recommendations were:

- Standardising the method of measuring HbA$_{1c}$ and the reference system used to report results.
- The IFCC reference system is the only currently valid method of measuring HbA$_{1c}$ and should be used as the basis to standardise HbA$_{1c}$ measurements.
- The results should be reported in IFCC units (mmol/mol) and derived national Glycohaemoglobin Standardisation Program Units (NGSP) (%) should be calculated using the IFCC-NGSP master equation.
- Laboratories should be able to maintain a CV <3% at HbA$_{1c}$ between 6 and 9% and manufacturer's assays should have a CV <5% (Colman *et al.* 2008).
- If the ongoing 'average plasma glucose study' using frequent capillary glucose measurements and continuous glucose monitoring due to be published in early 2008 fulfills its priori-specified criteria, an A$_{1c}$-derived average glucose value

(ADAG) should also be reported (Nathan 2007). The ADAG value is calculated from the individual's A_{1c} result to deduce an estimate of their average blood glucose (O'Riordan 2007).
- That clinical guidelines be revised and glycaemic targets be expressed as IFCC units, derived NGSP units, and ADAG.

If these recommendations are adopted, education programmes for health professionals and people with diabetes will need to be developed and existing teaching material including health professional texts will need to be revised. Glycaemic targets should not be considered independently of other risk factors for complications such as hyperlipidaemia, hypertension and smoking, age and comorbidities. A_{1c} targets differ slightly among various guidelines. It is generally accepted that targets should be:

- As low as possible to reduce the likelihood of microvascular complications. Most recommend <6.5% or <7% for most people with Type 2 diabetes.
- Individualised for specific patients after discussing the risks and benefits with them. For example, children, older and frail people, and those with limited life expectancy might require higher targets and those at very high risk of microvascular complications may need lower targets (range 7–7.5%).
- Avoid adverse events such as frequent hypoglycaemia.

Practice points

(1) People who experience frequent hypoglycaemic episodes may have a low HbA_{1c} that might not reflect their complication risk.
(2) HbA_{1c} results should be evaluated as part of the total clinical picture and not viewed in isolation.
(3) HbA_{1c} does not represent the blood glucose profile, but gives an average level. It is considered to be the 'gold standard' for monitoring metabolic control.

Table 3.2 lists some factors that might affect HbA_{1c} results.

Fructosamines
The fructosamines are a group of glycosylated blood and tissue proteins that reflect the average blood glucose levels within the preceding 3 weeks. Fructosamine results can be lower in patients with low serum albumin, cirrhosis of the liver or haemoglobinopathies. Fructosamine estimations are not performed very often but they are useful for monitoring:

- diabetes during pregnancy
- initial response to diabetes medication
- patients with chronic anaemia
- patients with haemoglobinopathies.

Table 3.2 Non-glycaemic factors that can affect results of glycosylated haemoglobin assays.

False high	False low
Chronic alcohol abuse	Anaemia
Fetal haemoglobin	Abnormal haemoglobins such as HbS,
Hyperlipidaemia	HbC, HbD found in some ethnic groups
Hyperbilirubinaemia	Chronic blood loss
Renal failure	Haemolysis
Splenectomy	Haemorrhage

Serum lipids

Serum lipids are usually elevated if the blood glucose is elevated. Three classes of lipids are measured as shown with the target range in brackets:

(1) Cholesterol (<4.0)
(2) Triglycerides (<1.5)
(3) Lipoproteins:
    • very low-density lipoprotein (VLDL)
    • low-density lipoprotein (LDL) (<2.5)
    • high-density lipoprotein (HDL) (>1.0).

Although it is generally accepted that fasting blood lipid levels are most useful, recent research suggests non-fasting levels correlate more closely with cardiovascular risk (Bansal *et al.* 2007; Nordestgaard *et al.* 2007). However, there are many forms of hypertriglyceridaemia and more research is needed to determine the exact relationship to atherosclerosis. High lipids, especially elevated triglycerides and LDL, and low HDL is a common lipid profile in people with poorly controlled Type 2 diabetes and may be secondary to hyperglycaemia and is a clinical useful measure of the need for lipid-lowering medications such as fibrates, fish oil concentrates or nicotinic acid depending on the type of lipid abnormality present, see Chapter 5.

Alcohol should not be consumed for 24 hours before the blood sample for serum lipid measurements is taken.

C-peptide

C-peptide is the connecting peptide, which determines the folding of the two insulin chains during insulin production and storage in the pancreas. It splits off in the final stages and can be measured in the blood. It is used to measure endogenous insulin production, to determine the type of diabetes (along with various antibodies, see Chapter 1) if it is not clear in the clinical presentation. C-peptide is present in normal or elevated amounts in Type 2 diabetes, indicating that insulin is being produced and that diet and/or OHAs with exercise could achieve acceptable control. However, progressive beta cell loss occurs in Type 2 diabetes and C-peptide levels fall proportionally.

• C-peptide is absent or low in people with Type 1 diabetes and can be a useful indicator in slow onset Type 1 diabetes (LADA) occurring in adults (Cohen 1996) see Chapter 1.

- It is not changed by injecting exogenous insulin.
- Fasting results are most useful.

Islet cell antibodies

Islet cell antibodies (ICA) are found in most newly diagnosed people with Type 1 diabetes, indicating that diabetes is an autoimmune disease. The beta cells of the pancreas are the specific target in diabetes and other pancreatic functions are not affected. In the laboratory, impaired insulin release can be demonstrated when ICA are present but the clinical implication is still unclear.

ICA are present in the prediabetic state before the disease is clinically obvious. They can also be present in close relatives who are at high risk of developing diabetes if they have ICA.

GAD antibodies are also present in 80% of people with Type 1 diabetes and enable it to be distinguished from Type 2 diabetes (Cohen 1996).

Creatinine clearance and urea

As indicated, creatinine clearance is used to estimate renal function. It is also used to determine nutritional status in relation to protein especially during TPN and continuous ambulatory peritoneal dialysis (CAPD). An increase in the blood urea nitrogen (BUN) may indicate impaired renal function, however, the BUN can also be increased if the patient is dehydrated, has internal bleeding or is on steroids. Anorexia, a low protein diet and fasting can lead to a decrease in urea.

References

Bansal, S. (2007) Fasting compared with nonfasting triglycerides and risk of cardiovascular events in women. *Journal of the American Medical Association*, 18 (298), 309–316.

Bloomgarden, Z. (2007) Glucose variability. Comment on sessions presented during the 67th *American Diabetes Association, Scientific Sessions* June 22–26, Chicago, Illinois. http://www.medscape.com/viewarticle/560754 (accessed January 2008).

Borch-Johnsen, K., Wenzel, H., Vibert, G. & Mogensen, C. (1993) Is screening and intervention for microalbuminuria worthwhile in patients with IDDM? *British Medical Journal*, 306, 1722–1725.

Canadian Diabetes Association (2008) Reduce your risk of serious complications associated with diabetes. www.canadiandiabetes association.ca accessed on 9 January 2008).

Chadban, S., Briganti, E. & Kerr, P. (2003) Prevalence of kidney disease in Australian adults: the AusDiabe kidney study. *Journal of the American Society of Nephrologists*, 14 (7) (Suppl. 2), S121–S138.

Cohen, M. (1996) *Diabetes: A Handbook of Management*. International Diabetes Institute, Melbourne.

Colman, P., Goodall, I., Garcia-Webb, P., Williams, P. & Dunlop, M. (2008) Glycohaemoglobin: a crucial measurement in modern diabetes management. Progress towards standardization and improved precision of measurement. *EMJA* http://www.mja.com.au/public/issues/jul21/colan/colman.html (acessed February 2008).

Consensus Committee (2007) Consensus Statement on the Worldwide Standardisation of the Haemoglobin A$_{1c}$ Measurement. The American Diabetes Association, European Association for the Study of Diabetes, International Federation of Clinical Chemistry and Laboratory Medicine, International Diabetes Federation. *Diabetes Care*, 30, 2399–2400.

Davis, T., Bruce, D. & Davis, T. (2006) Is self-monitoring of blood glucose appropriate for all type 2 diabetic patients? The Freemantle Diabetes Study. *Diabetes Care*, **29**, 1764–1770.

Dunning, T., Rantzau, C. & Ward, G. (1994) Effect of alcohol swabbing on capillary blood glucose. *Practical Diabetes*, **11** (4), 251–254.

Dunning, T. (1996) Corticosteroid medications and diabetes mellitus. *Practical Diabetes International*, **13** (6), 186–188.

Farmer, A. (2007) Self-monitoring of blood glucose does not improve HbA_{1c} levels in patients with non-insulin treated diabetes the DIGEM study. Presented during the 67th *American Diabetes Association, Scientific Sessions* June 22–26, Chicago, Illinois. Also published in the *British Medical Journal Online* June 6, 2007.

Fineberg, S. (2000) Comparison of blood beta-hydroxybutyrate and urine ketones in 4 weeks of home monitoring by insulin-requiring children and adults. American Diabetes Association Scientific Meeting, USA, June.

Garg, S., Potts, R., Ackerman, N., Fermi, S., Tamada, J. & Chase, H. (1999) Correlation of fingerstick blood glucose measurements with Glucowatch biographer glucose results in young subjects with type 1 diabetes. *Diabetes Care*, **22**, 1708–1714.

International Diabetes Federation (IDF) (2007) *Guideline for Management of Postmeal Glucose.* IDF, Brussels.

Jerums, G., Cooper, M., O'Brien, R. & Taft, J. (1994) ADS Position Statement 1993: microalbuminuria and diabetes. *Medical Journal of Australia*, **161**, 265–268.

Jungheim, K. & Koschinsky, T. (2002) Glucose monitoring at the arm: evaluation of upper dermal blood glucose kinetics during rapid systemic blood glucose changes. *Hormone Metabolism Research*, **34**, 325–329.

Kilpatrick, E., Rigby, A. & Atkin, S. (2007) Variability in the relationship between mean plasma glucose and HbA_{1c}: implications for the assessment of glycaemic control. *Clinical Chemistry*, **53**, 897–901.

Kolb, H., Schneider, B., Heinemann, L., Lodwig, V. & Martin, S. (2007) Is self-monitoring of blood glucose appropriate for all type 2 diabetic patients? Comment on the The Freemantle Diabetes Study. *Diabetes Care*, **30**, 183–184.

Krolewski, A., Laffel, L., Krolewski, M., Quinn, M. & Warram, J. (1995) Glycosylated haemoglobin and risk of microalbuminia in patients with insulin dependent diabetes mellitus. *New England Journal of Medicine*, **332**, 1251–1255.

Laffel, L. & Kettyle, W. (2000) Frequency of elevations in blood b-hydroxybutyrate (B-OHB) during home monitoring and association with glycaemia in insulin-treated children and adults. *Proceedings, ADA Scientific Meeting*, USA.

McGowan, K., Thomas, W. & Moran, A. (2002) Spurious reporting of nocturnal hypoglycaemia by CGMS in patients with tightly controlled type 1 diabetes. *Diabetes Care*, **25**, 1499–1503.

Monsod, T., Flanagan, D. & Rife, F. (2002) Do sensor glucose levels accurately predict plasma glucose concentrations during hypoglycaemia and hyperinsulinaemia? *Diabetes Care*, **15**, 899–893.

Nathan, D. (2007) The problem with ADAGE (A1c-derived average glucose equivalent). 67th *American Diabetes Association, Scientific Sessions* June 22–26, Chicago, Illinois.

Nordestgaard, B. (2007) Nonfasting triglycerides and risk of myocardial infarction, ischemic heart disease, and death in men and women. *Journal of the American Medical Association*, **18** (298), 299–308.

Outcomes Prevention Evaluation Study Investigators (2000) Effects of ramipril on cardiovascular and microvascular outcomes in people with diabetes. Results of HOPE and MICRO-HOPE substudy. *Lancet*, **355**, 253–259.

O'Riordan, M. (2007) Average blood glucose instead of HbA_{1c}? Change appears to be coming for diabetes care. *Heartwire*, July 3. http://www.medscape.com.viewarticle/559262 (accessed December 2007).

Parchman, M., Pugh, J., Romero, R. & Bowers, K. (1997) Competing demands or clinical inertia: the case of elevated glycosylated hemoglobin. *Annals of Family Medicine*, 5 (3), 196–201.

Rose, M., Fliege, H., Hildebrandt, M., Schirop, T. & Klapp, B. (2002) The network of psychological variables in patients with diabetes and their importance for quality of life and metabolic control. *Diabetes Care*, 25, 35–42.

Ruilope, L., Alcazar, J., Hernandez, E. & Rodico, J. (1990) Does an adequate control of blood pressure protect the kidney in essential hypertension? *Journal of Hypertension*, 8, 525–531.

Schneider, M., Heinemann, B., Lodwig, L., Kurth, H.-J., Kolb, H. & Scherbaum, W. (2006) The ROSSO Study group: self-monitoring of blood glucose in type 2 diabetes and long term outcome: an epidemiological study. *Diabetelogia*, 49, 271–278.

Sonksen, P., Fox, C. & Judd, C. (1998) *Diabetes at Your Fingertips*. Class Publishing, London, pp. 105.

Wallace, T., Meston, N., Gardnert, S. & Matthews, D. (2001) The hospital and home use of a 30-second hand-held blood ketone meter: guidelines for clinical practice. *Diabetic Medicine*, 18 (8), 640–645.

Weinstein, R., Schwartz, S., Brazg, R., Bugler, J., Peyser, T. & McGarraugh, G. (2007) Accuracy of the 5-day Freestyle navigator Continuous Glucose Monitoring system: comparison with frequent laboratory reference measurements. *Diabetes Care*, 30, 1125–1130.

Zuo, L., Ma, Y. & Zhou, Y. (2005) Application of GFR – estimating equations in Chinese patients with chronic kidney disease. *American Journal of Kidney Diseases*, 45, 463–472.

Chapter 4
Nutrition, Obesity and Exercise

Key points

- Obesity is an increasing global health issue.
- Obesity is associated with more than 30 medical conditions and impacts on many other conditions. Weight loss can improve some obesity-related conditions including the metabolic syndrome, Type 2 diabetes, and hypertension and reduce cardiovascular risk.
- The relationship between weight, health outcomes and life expectancy is complex and affected by gender and age.
- Genetic and environmental factors play a role in obesity.
- Population based and targeted screening and prevention programs are required to address the problem.
- Dietary advice for people with diabetes is applicable to the whole population.
- Diet and exercise continue to be the cornerstone of diabetes management even when medicines are required.
- Regular dietary assessment is advisable.

Rationale

Good nutrition is vital to health and well being and is an essential basis of diabetes management. Obesity is a significant health problem and a major risk factor for serious disease including Type 2 diabetes. Managing obesity is difficult. Regular nutritional assessment is important to maintain the optimal health of people with diabetes as their general health, age and diabetes-related circumstances changes.

The importance of good nutrition

Good nutrition is essential to health. Inadequate nutrition leads to many diseases and affects the primary condition and response to treatment (Sydney-Smith 2000). Sixty per cent of deaths are related to nutritional factors, for example, diabetes-associated cardiovascular disease (Middleton *et al.* 2001). In particular, micronutrients and protein intake are often inadequate and mineral deficiencies are common in Australia, especially in people living in poverty.

Diets low in vitamins and minerals are also deficient in antioxidants that modulate oxidative tissue damage. Oxidative tissue damage is implicated in the development of long-term diabetic complications and is compounded by smoking, alcohol and chronic inflammatory diseases, see Chapter 8. Vitamins C, E, and A and some plant chemicals (phytochemicals) are naturally occurring antioxidants derived from a well balanced diet.

Obesity

Obesity is defined as excess body fat and is now recognised as a disease in its own right (Marks 2000). Obesity is emerging as a complex phenomena caused by a number of inter-related factors including a high fat energy-dense diet, inadequate amounts of exercise, and genetic, hormonal and environmental factors (Brunner & McCarthy 2001; Bouchard *et al.* 2004). The estimated risk of becoming obese using data from the Framingham Study suggests a normal weight person has a 50% long-term risk of becoming overweight and 25% risk of becoming obese (Reynolds *et al.* 2005). Significantly, a number of studies suggest underweight might confer greater health risks in older people (Diehr *et al.* 1998, 2008).

Some medicines such as corticosteroids, antipsychotics, birth control medicines, insulin, sulphonylureas, and thiazolidinediones (TZDs) also contribute to weight gain, see Chapter 5. There is increasing evidence that ethnicity, difficult social environments, social isolation, being teased about weight, low self-esteem and low global self-worth contribute to obesity in children (Goodman & Whitaker 2002; Eisenberg *et al.* 2003). Contributing environmental factors include excess television viewing, insufficient physical activity, which might be influenced by living in unsafe areas, and high consumption of fast foods (Burdett & Whitaker 2005).

The prevalence of overweight and obesity are increasing globally but there are differences among populations and among ethnic groups within populations. Rates of overweight and obesity are also increasing in children and adolescents. A child with one overweight parent has a 40% chance of becoming overweight and the risk increases to 80% when both parents are overweight. Significantly, obesity makes it difficult for health professionals to perform some preventative health care interventions such as Papinocolou smears and mammograms and overweight women are more likely to have false-positive results than non-obese women (Elmore *et al.* 2004).

Overview of the pathogenesis of obesity

Abdominal fat is not inert. It produces signalling molecules, adipokines, which exacerbate endothelial dysfunction. A number of adipokines are produced, see Table 4.1. In addition, the endocannabinoid (CRB) neuroregulatory system influences the activity of other neurotransmitter systems including hormone secretion and modulates immune and inflammatory responses. Likewise, understanding of the role of white adipose tissue in regulating body metabolism, insulin sensitivity, and food intake has increased rapidly over the past few years.

The CRB consists of many CRBs including CB_1 and CB_2. CB_I occurs through the body including the brain, adipose tissue, vascular endothelium and sympathetic nerve

Table 4.1 Effects of adipokines and changes that occur in the presence of abdominal obesity, which demonstrates their role in the development of insulin resistance, Type 2 diabetes and cardiovascular disease.

Name of adipokine	Effects in the body	Effect of increasing abdominal obesity on adipokine levels
Tumour necrosis factor-alpha	Disrupts insulin signalling processes in the cell membranes. Reduces endothelial vasodilatation by reducing nitric oxide	Higher
Interleukin -6	Stimulates rate of C-reactive protein release from the liver. Induces insulin resistance. Damages endothelial function	Higher
Plasminogen Activator Inhibitor-1	Enhances prothrombotic state	Higher
Leptin	Regulates: • Appetite • Energy expenditure • Insulin sensitivity Stimulates the sympathetic nervous system Acts as a signalling factor in hypertension	Higher
Adiponectin	Improves tissue sensitivity. Anti-inflammatory. Reduces atherogenesis	Lower
Angiotensinogen	Contributes to hypertension	Higher

terminals. CB_2 mostly occur in lymph tissue and macrophages. In addition, a number of subtypes exist whose function is yet to be determined. They regulate metabolism in a number of ways. Blocking CB_1 reduces food intake, abdominal fat, triglycerides, LDL, C-reactive protein (CRP), and insulin resistance; it increases HDL. Activating CB_1 has the opposite effect. Data from the RIO-Europe trial showed significant weight reductions and reduction in cardiometabolic risk factors such as waist circumference, triglyceride levels and elevated HDL using the CB_1 blocker, Rimonabant, compared to controls (Van Gaal 2005). The latter effects occurred independently of weight loss. People taking Rimonabant averaged 4.7 kg weight loss after a year and were more likely to achieve a 10% weight loss than controls.

White adipose tissue has many functions including acting as a storage depot for triglycerides. It is regarded as an endocrine organ that secretes a range of adipokines, which influence weight, inflammation, coagulation, fibrinolysis, tissue response to insulin, and contribute to the development of metabolic syndrome and Type 2 diabetes. Energy balance is impaired and obesity results if white adipose tissue function is disrupted (Iqbal 2007), see Table 4.1. Ghrelin is produced in the stomach and mediates hunger. Ghrelin levels are increased by restricting calories and exercising (Leidy *et al.* 2007).

Adipose tissue has a major role in hormone metabolism such as synthesising oestrogen in postmenopausal women, which is protective against osteoporosis (Moyad 2004). Likewise, replacing testosterone preserves skeletal muscle and reduces abdominal obesity in non-obese men over 50 years whose testosterone level is <15 nM (Allan 2009).

The significance of abdominal obesity

People with central or abdominal obesity are at increased risk of obesity-related diseases such as metabolic syndrome, Type 2 diabetes, dyslipidaemia, fatty liver, and therefore are at significant risk of cardiovascular disease. Obesity is a risk factor for shortened life expectancy in younger but not older people (Heiat *et al.* 2001) and the importance of overweight and obesity as predictors of health status decline in people >65 years. In fact, some research indicates being overweight is associated with better quality of life and health status in this age group (Stevens 2000).

Weight circumference is significantly correlated with triglycerides, CRP, cholesterol and glucose but not HbA_{1c} in healthy women (Behan & Mbizo 2007). Likewise, the INTERHEART Study Group (2005) demonstrated that waist circumference is strongly related to myocardial infarction but the level of risk is still debated. Physical fitness may reduce the inflammation associated with abdominal obesity and lower cardiovascular risk (Zoeller 2007).

Various cardiovascular risk scores have been developed based on parameters such as age, gender, total cholesterol, LDL, systolic blood pressure, being treated for hypertension and smoking, for example, The Framingham Risk Score (Expert Panel on Detection, Evaluation, and Treatment of High Blood Cholesterol in Adults (2002) and the Systemic Coronary Risk Evaluation (SCORE) (Third Joint Taskforce of European and Other Societies on Cardiovascular Disease Prevention in Clinical Practice (2003). However, a 12-year US study of people in their 60s suggests obese people live as long as people of normal weight and are less likely to develop diabetes or lipid abnormalities if they are fit. However, at BMI >30 people experience difficulty performing usual activities of daily living and develop other obesity-related disorders such as musculoskeletal disease that cause pain and have lower muscle strength and reduced cardiovascular fitness (ABC Health and Well Being 2007). Thus, the focus of weight management must also include reducing disability.

Other obesity-related diseases include osteoarthritis, rheumatoid arthritis, and other musculoskeletal diseases, some forms of cancer, for example, breast, oesophagus, colorectal, endometrial and renal cell, sleep apnoea and daytime sleepiness, gout, urinary stress incontinence, surgical complications, and maternal obesity has been associated with a higher incidence of birth defects.

Nutrition, obesity and stress

There is a complex association between nutrition and stress and overweight/obesity. Stress affects eating behaviour: most people eat more and gain weight; 30% reduce weight (Stone *et al.* 1994) but the reasons for the increased intake are unclear. Likewise, Fiegal *et al.* 2002) found people are concerned about life stress and 50% eat more calorie dense food when they are stressed, and undertake less activity. A suggested mechanism for the effect of stress on weight is that cortisol levels are increased during stress, which stimulates appetite: managing stress reduces stress-related intake. In addition, chronic low level stress reduces insulin sensitivity and contributes to abdominal obesity and metabolic syndrome.

Significantly, 45% of women and 23% of men think they are overweight and 20% of underweight women think they are overweight and are dieting to lose weight (Better Health Channel, January 2008). People use a range of self-initiated strategies to lose weight, which are often successful initially, but regain half to two thirds of the weight lost in the first 12 months and nearly all within 5 years. In contrast, the NHANES 1999–2002 showed 58% of people who lost >5% of their bodyweight maintained the weight loss for up to 5 years. Factors associated with weight gain included:

- Mexican-American peoples.
- Significant weight loss.
- Fewer years since reaching their maximum weight.
- Long time spent watching TV including children.
- Attempting to control weight.
- Sedentary lifestyle.
- Frequent attempts to diet were associated with increased risk of developing an eating disorder.

Ethnic differences could partly explain the different findings. In addition, people who are supported are more likely to stay motivated than those who 'go it alone.' Self-perception and body image influence quality of life and mood and there is a pervasive association between perception of being overweight and depression and disordered body image.

Methods of measuring weight

Measuring obesity is difficult. A number of methods are used. Each has advantages and disadvantages.

Crude weight

Weighing people is the simplest way to estimate obesity using height/weight standards. It does not take into account muscular builds at different heights or that lean body mass weighs more than fat tissue. Mild obesity = 20– 40% overweight; moderate obesity = 41–100%, and severe obesity = twice the actual weight for height.

Body Mass Index

The Body Mass Index (BMI), sometimes referred to as Quetelet's Index, is a simple method of assessing obesity but, like crude weight, it does not take into account muscular builds at different heights. However, despite the limitations BMI >30 generally indicates excess adipose tissue. BMI should be interpreted according to growth charts in children. BMI is calculated using the following formula: Weight in kilograms divided by height in metres squared.

Waist-hip ratio

The waist-hip ratio (WHR) is measured with the person standing and specifically measure abdominal obesity. The waist is defined as the largest abdominal circumference midway between the costal margin and the iliac crest. A WHR >90 in men and >80 in women is generally regarded as an accurate predictor of obesity-related disorders, independently of the BMI. WHR can be affected by postprandial status, time of day, and depth of inspiration to an unknown degree. It includes both intra-abdominal fat (the area of interest) and subcutaneous fat, but it is not clear how to adjust the WHR for subcutaneous fat. There are also differences among ethnic groups that need to be considered. It is useful to record the WHR on a regular basis.

Other ways of measuring body fat include:

- Dual energy X-ray absorptiometry (DEXA), which is often used in research and to determine risk of osteoporosis. Lean body mass, skin fold thickness, densitometry hydrostatic weighing and bioelectrical impedence analysis are other ways to measure obesity.

Strategies used to measure food consumption:
A number of tools are used to estimate food intake over various time periods. These include:

- Food records: the individual keeps a detailed record of their intake for varying periods from 3 to 7 days. Maintaining a food record can be burdensome and requires the person to be literate. In addition, actually recording intake often influences the person to consider what they eat and change their usual eating pattern.
- Food frequency questionnaires (FFQ) to retrospectively estimate usual dietary intake over time, usually 6–12 months. Information is collected about specific types of food and the quantities and frequency with which they are consumed. Short (60 foods) and long (100 foods) FFQs are used. FFQs must be culturally relevant and a number of culturally relevant forms exist. Modified FFQs identify dietary fat, fibre, fruit, and vegetable intake.
- Dietary recall, often over 24-hours to estimate current intake. Accuracy is influenced by the individual's ability to recall the type and quantity of food consumed. Most people underestimate their intake.
- Visual estimation, where trained observers monitor an individual's food choices, classifies foods using a rating scale and estimates serving sizes. This is intimidating and may influence the individual's food selection. Nurses can undertake this type of monitoring process.
- Plate waste methodology, which has been used extensively in studies of food intake in school children but is not practical in clinical practice.
- Screening tools such as;
  - Malnutrition Universal Screening Tool (MUST) for adults (Malnutrition Advisory Group (MAG) 2000).
  - Nutritional Risk Screening (NRS-2002) for hospital settings.

○ Mini Nutritional Assessment (MNA©) for the elderly (Vellas *et al.* 1999).
○ The Healthy Eating Index (HEI) and Modified HEI for children and adolescents (Feskanich *et al.* 2004).
○ Biomarkers to identify specific food components in body fluids or tissue, which independently reflect intake of the particular food.

Managing obesity and diabetes

Obesity and Type 2 diabetes are chronic conditions and long-term management strategies are needed. Usually a combination of strategies is most effective especially when they are developed in consultation with the individual. In the first instance, energy-dense food intake such as simple carbohydrates and saturated and *trans* fats should be reduced, exercise increased, and possibly more sleep (Lamberg 2006). Exercise needs to be enough to increase total energy expenditure to 160–180% of the resting metabolic rate (Erlichman *et al.* 2002). Increasing exercise with or without a weight loss diet induces a modest weight loss. People with diabetes should have a thorough physical assessment before undertaking exercise and weight loss programs that need to be individualised for best effect. Along with diet, exercise prescriptions (Elfhag *et al.* 2005) and wearing a pedometer (Richardson *et al.* 2008) can help the individual achieve weight loss.

Counselling and behavioural strategies that encompass support, exercise and dietary counselling are effective and in Australia are supported through some health benefit funds. For example, commercial diet oriented weight loss programmes such as *Step into Life, Mass Attack Weight Loss Program, Lite n' Easy, ClubOptiSlim*. Some of these programs deliver nutritionally balanced portion controlled low fat meals to the individual's home.

Prepared low-energy meals or meal replacements that replace some or all of the individual's diet can be useful as an initial weight loss strategy or to avoid refeeding syndrome after severe calorie restriction or bariatric surgery. However, they can be expensive in the long term.

Self-help programmes often combine lifestyle change, computer-assisted interventions, packaged programmes such as Internet correspondence courses, and take home weight loss kits. Self-help programmes are difficult to measure but Latner (2001) claimed 45% of people using such programmes lose weight and keep it off. Knowledgeable clinicians can support individuals likely to benefit from a self-help approach (Tan *et al.* 2006).

Significantly, public health programmes that involve health providers, legislators, the food industry, and health insurers are needed and must include children and adolescents. Weigh loss strategies may need include strategies to keep people physically active in the longer term and recent research suggests it could be important to minimise exercise variation because maintaining exercise at a consistent level moderates age-related weight gain in proportion to the amount of exercise performed (Williams 2008). Even fit people tend to gain weight with increasing age, thus the amount of exercise may need to be increased to reduce age-related weight gain (Williams 2008). Significantly, stopping exercise leads to weight gain.

Dietary management: diabetes

Diet is the mainstay and first line of treatment of Type 2 diabetes to control blood glucose and manage cardiovascular and other health risks. The aim is to achieve a healthy weight range for the individual. The aim is to achieve an appropriate weight within the healthy weight range for the individual, but focusing on weight might mean the under nutrition is not considered, which as indicated, might confer more health risks than overweight especially in older people.

Expert dietary advice is essential but the changing role of the nurse and the focus on the preventative aspects of healthcare mean that nurses have a responsibility to develop a knowledge of nutrition and its role in preventing disability and disease. A number of basic screening tools can be used to identify dietary intake and nutritional characteristics and can be incorporated into usual nursing assessment and patient care plans and enable useful information to be communicated to the dietitian.

The general dietary principles apply to the whole population as well as all people with diabetes. Precise advice depends on the individual's age, gender, lifestyle, eating habits, cultural preferences and nutritional requirements. It is important that realistic targets are negotiated with the patient, particularly if weight control is necessary. The goal is to achieve gradual progressive weight loss to reduce weight by 5–10%, which is usually achievable and improves the health profile (Pi-Sunyer 2006).

The effect of medications, fasting for procedures, and gastrointestinal disturbances such as diarrhoea and vomiting, on food absorption and consequently blood glucose levels is an important consideration especially during illness.

Optimal nutritional care is best achieved by collaboration among nurses, other health professionals and the dietitian to decide the most appropriate management regimen. Nurses have the greatest continuous contact with the patient in hospital; consequently they have an invaluable role in nutritional management by:

(1) Identifying patients at high risk of nutritional deficiencies. Approximately 30% of all patients in hospital are undernourished (Kondrup *et al.* 2003).
(2) Screening patients' nutritional characteristics to identify actual and/or potential problems, for example:
   • inappropriate, erratic, and over eaters, and those with eating disorders. Screening processes should be connected to relevant actions. For example, if the person is eating appropriately, arrange for regular screening at specified intervals. If the person is at risk of an eating disorder, an appropriate nutrition plan needs to be determined. If functional, metabolic, or diabetes-related complications are present, standard nutrition plans may not be appropriate and dietitian advice will be needed (Kondrup *et al.* 2003). The following factors need to be considered when deciding the level of risk: the current condition, whether the condition is stable (weight loss/gain can be assessed from the health history), the significance of the condition and whether it is likely to deteriorate or improve, and any disease processes that affect nutritional status such as appetite, diabetes complications, and hyperglycaemia. Managing eating disorders is challenging because people often do not consider their eating behaviour as a problem, or deny they have an eating problem. Repeated episodes of ketoacidosis (DKA) could indicate an eating disorder and needs to be investigated. Young people with diabetes often run their blood glucose levels high to loose weight, which puts them at risk of DKA (see Chapters 7 and 13). Cognitive behaviour therapy may be a useful strategy when the eating disorder is mild-moderate. The complex underlying issues need to be ascertained and managed.
   • those with domestic, financial, and/or employment problems.
(3) Providing ongoing patient monitoring on a meal-to-meal basis.

Example questions to ask when taking a diet history. The questions should be asked sensitively as part of a nutritional assessment.

(1) Do you have regular meals?
- It is important to clarify what the individual means by 'regular' and whether they skip meals and if they do when and why. For example, a nurse with diabetes working in the operating theatre might find it difficult to always predict when the operation will finish.

(2) Do you have a good breakfast?
- Poor morning appetite can indicate nocturnal hypoglycaemia and catecholamine production to maintain the falling blood glucose.
- People who do not eat breakfast often snack later in the day on energy-dense foods and can be protein deficient.
- Missing breakfast interferes with work performance.

(3) How often do you eat takeaway foods?
- Takeaway foods tend to be high in fat, salt and sugar and low in fibre, protein and essential vitamins and minerals.

(4) Do you eat cream biscuits, chocolates or lollies?
- This question is a way of checking the individual's intake of sugar and fat.

(5) Can you tell me some of the foods you eat that contain carbohydrate?

This information provides the basis from which nursing staff can quickly and effectively refer patients to the dietitian who can support nursing staff by:

- Setting dietary management goals for the individual consistent with their health status, lifestyle and healthcare goals.
- Identifying possible nutritional problems. Estimating caloric intake is difficult because people generally underestimate their caloric intake by as much as 50% despite trying to keep accurate food records (Fabricatore 2004) but 3-day food records can be helpful to health professionals and the person with diabetes.
- Identifying causes of possible nutritional problems and suggesting strategies to overcome them.
- Counselling and educating the patient about how to reduce the risks associated with these problems.
- Supporting nursing and medical staff on an ongoing basis to ensure most effective nutritional management is achieved and maintained (Dunning & Hoy 1994).

Practice points

Dietitians are essential members of the multidisciplinary team.
   Dietary requirements change with increasing age, activity level, health status, pregnancy, and lactation, and during specific disease processes, for example, renal and cardiac disease.

Method of screening for dietary characteristics and problems

Nutritional status

(1) Identify whether the person is overweight or underweight and whether the person's health is affected by their weight status. For example, calculate BMI and/or waist-hip ratio.

(2) Review any current haematological and biochemical measurements, which reflect the person's nutritional status such as haemoglobin and serum albumin levels, creatinine, folate and cholesterol. Clinical signs such as tiredness, fatigue and obesity can indicate inadequate protein intake and can be confirmed by blood urea nitrogen (BUN) and serum creatinine levels. Low creatinine suggests protein intake is low. Low BUN and creatinine suggests a catabolic state such as hyperglycaemia. Consider coeliac disease in Type 1 diabetes, see Chapter 10.

Recent research indicates malnourished patients have a longer length-of-stay, are older and have increased mortality rates compared with well-nourished patients. Most malnourished patients are not identified as being at risk (Middleton *et al.* 2001). Clues to nutritional deficiency are:

- Weight loss.
- Low lymphocyte count.
- An illness lasting longer than three weeks.
- Serum albumin <3.5 g/dL.

If a patient is identified as being malnourished their nutritional status should be monitored by being weighed regularly, using the same scales and with the person wearing similar clothing, and by monitoring nitrogen balance. Nutritional supplements may be needed.

Dietary characteristics

The tools and questions described earlier in the chapter can be used to determine:

- The regularity/irregularity of meals and/or snacks.
- Whether the person consumes foods and fluids containing refined sugar.
- Whether the person omits any of the major food groups.

If one or more problems are identified the person should be referred to the dietitian for further dietary analysis and advice.

Principles of dietary management for people with diabetes

A number of dietary guidelines have been developed such as the American Diabetes Association, the Diabetes and Nutrition Group of the European Association for the

Study of Diabetes, The Canadian Diabetes Association, Diabetes UK, The Indian Council of Medical Research and Diabetes Australia. The macronutrient content of these guidelines varies despite the fact they are all evidence based and largely draw on the same evidence. Socio-economic factors and food availability appear to influence the dietary advice health professionals provide (Kapur & Dunning 2007).

Diets such as the traditional Mediterranean, Okinawan, Dietary Approaches to Stop Hypertension (DASH) antihypertensive, anti-inflammatory diet, South Beach diet, Atkins type diet, Omniheart, Onish, and Onish Zone (A to Z) diets all appear to improve metabolic risk factors by reducing lipids and weight to various degrees (Carey *et al.* 2005; Gardner *et al.* 2007; Fung 2007; Tay *et al.* 2008). They include different combinations of macronutrients.

There are various methods of counting carbohydrate, for example, exchanges and portions. They help to ensure an even distribution of carbohydrate when planning meals for individual patients. The difference between the two terms relates to the amount of carbohydrate measured. An exchange is equal to 15 g and a portion 10 g. Exchanges are often used in the UK while Australia often uses glycaemic index (GI) and glycaemic load. More recently, portions are making a comeback in programs such as The German Diabetes Training and Treatment Program (DTTP) and its counterpart the Dose Adjustment for Normal Eating Program (DAFNE). These programs are being widely adopted and adapted, for example, OzDAFNE in Australia.

Using these programs people with diabetes estimate their carbohydrate intake based on 10 g portions and calculate their short-acting insulin doses as a ratio to carbohydrate consumption. Basal insulin doses are adjusted to address preprandial and bedtime blood glucose targets, see Chapter 1. HBA$_{1c}$ reductions of ~1% and improved quality of life have been demonstrated without increasing hypoglycaemia or weight (Muhlhauser *et al.* 2002; DAFNE Study Group 2002).

In general, people with diabetes should:

- Eat foods high in complex carbohydrate with low GI (50–60% of total intake), high fibre unprocessed foods. Rapidly digested carbohydrates cause a rapid rise in blood glucose and a greater demand on the pancreas to release insulin to maintain the normal blood glucose range. Low GI foods are associated with a lower risk of diabetes and the related complications (Brand-Miller 2003). GI is a method of ranking foods based on their immediate effect on the blood glucose level. Foods that enter the blood stream quickly have a high GI, for example, sugars. Foods that enter more slowly are known as low GI, for example, cereals. The GI is the area under the glucose response curve measured after ingestion of a test food and multiplied by 100. Foods with a GI <55 are classified as low GI, 56–69 as moderate GI, and >70 are high GI foods. In general, the lower the GI, the smaller the impact on the blood glucose level.

However, many factors affect the rate at which carbohydrate is absorbed including the types of sugar and starch in food, the degree of processing, cooking methods and the presence of other nutrients such as fat and fibre and the particular combination of foods. Foods high in fat have a low GI because the fat delays their digestion and they are absorbed slowly but high fat foods are not recommended.

Low GI foods are the preferred basis of a well-balanced diet. They slow food absorption from the gut so the post prandial glucose load is reduced, cause satiety and help control weight, reduce HBA$_{1c}$, improve insulin sensitivity and help control lipids (Brand-Miller 1994).

People with diabetes are advised to include low GI foods in at least one meal each day. Simple sugars do not have to be excluded using the GI food plan. The move to GI-based diets is not universal and GI can be difficult for some people to understand. Generally, if people are accustomed to working in portions or exchanges and have reasonable metabolic control they should not be expected to change, particularly if they are elderly. Scientists are currently undertaking research to reduce the GI of some foods such as rice by altering their amylopectin structure to improve consumer acceptability (Rahman *et al.* 2007).

GI is not related to the quantity (portion size) of carbohydrate, which is measured by glycaemic load (GL). GI is taken into account when determining GL. That is GI indicates how rapidly the food enters the blood as glucose and the GL indicates how much carbohydrate is in a portion/serving; both are important to understanding the effect of a particular carbohydrate on blood glucose. The type of dietary fibre influences GI, water-soluble fibres such as hemicellulose, mucilages, gums and pectins have low GI because they slow digestion and absorption of carbohydrate.

- Be low in fat (<10% of total energy value), especially saturated fat and *trans* fatty acids; see Tables 4.2 and 4.3 which depict the main types of dietary fats and their effects on blood lipids, respectively. Some fat is necessary to supply essential fatty acids and fat-soluble vitamins A, D, E, and K. Despite an overall reduction in dietary fat, the mean Australian serum cholesterol has not fallen since 1980 (National Heart Foundation 2008). Omega 3 and 6 fatty acids are crucial to healthy brain function, normal growth and development and skin and hair growth, bone health, regulating metabolism, and maintaining reproductive function. Omega 6 fatty acids have an important role in modulating the inflammatory response by generating eicosanoids (prostaglandins and leukotrienes) and cytokines (interleukins). For example, gamma-linolenic acid (omega 6) is synthesised from linolenic acid reduces inflammation. There is strong evidence that replacing saturated fatty acids with omega 3 and 6 reduces cardiovascular disease in people with diabetes and non-diabetics (Eddy 2008). Dietary sources are not high in gamma-linolenic acid. Some are found in green leafy vegetables and nuts. The richest sources are borage oil, blackcurrant and evening primrose oil and breast milk. The conversion of linolenic acid into gamma-linolenic acid is inefficient in older age, diabetes, high alcohol consumption, eczema, viral infections, excess fat intake, hypercholestrolaemia and deficiency of vitamin B6, zinc, magnesium, calcium and biotin. Deutsch (2007) suggested *Euphasia superba* (krill) is a better source of omega-3 than plant sources and rapidly reduces C-reactive protein, a marker of inflammatory disease. Sources of omega 3, 6, and 9 are shown in Table 4.4.
- Contain adequate protein (15% of total intake).
- Be low in simple sugar, less than 25 g/day.
- Ensure a variety of food is eaten daily from each of the five food groups.
- Ensure that complex carbohydrate is consumed at each meal to reduce the postprandial blood glucose rise and the likelihood of hypoglycaemia in patients on insulin or diabetes medication.
- Limit salt. A typical western diet contains about ~10 g of salt per day and 75% of salt consumed is added salt. The National Health and Medical Research Council

Table 4.2 Dietary fat comes from animal and plant sources and has various effects on blood lipids. Triglycerides are the most abundant dietary fat.[a] Cholesterol and phospholipid dietary fats have a small but significant impact on serum cholesterol.

Saturated fatty acids (SFA)	Monounsaturated fatty acids (MUFA)	Polyunsaturated fatty acids (PUFA)	Trans fatty acids (TFA)
Not essential fatty acids[b]	Not essential fatty acids[b]	Omega-3 (Eicosapentaenoic acid (EPA and Docosahexaenoic acid (DHA)) and omega-6 (Gamma- Linolenic acid GLA) are essential fatty acids (EFA)[c]	Can be MUFAs or PUFAs TFA are formed when hydrogen is added to vegetable oils but small amounts are found in animal fats. Some dietary supplements contain TFA Amounts >0.5 must be listed on the label in the US.
With cholesterol contributes to hypercholesterolaemia	Small beneficial effect on lipoproteins	Has a beneficial effect on cholesterol Increasing omega-3 intake lowers LDL and triglycerides but not as much as reducing dietary SFA. Different omega-3 may have different effects on serum cholesterol. Reduce platelet aggregation and risk of myocardial infarction Retard deposition of atherosclerotic plaque and have anti-inflammatory effects. May help reduce abdominal fat in insulin-resistant people. Improves morning stiffness in rheumatoid arthritis and has additive effects with anti-inflammatory medicines. High doses may increase the risk of bleeding. Omega-9 might reduce cancer risk and reduces abdominal fat but increases HDL but it also increases LDL, cholesterol and triglycerides so it may not be cardioprotective (Jepersen 2001)	Increase LDL reduce HDL and lipoprotein (a)

[a] Provides SFAs, MUFAs and PUFAs.
[b] Can be obtained from protein and carbohydrate if necessary.
Serum cholesterol is more responsive to changes in dietary SFAs than PUFAs or cholesterol.
TFAs are found in foods containing hydrogenated vegetable oils and fat from ruminant animals.
[c] Omega-6 is derived from linoleic acid; omega-3 is derived from alpha-linolenic acid. All other longer chain PUFAs can be synthesised in the body from these precursors. Omega-3, -6, and -9 compete for the same desaturase enzymes. The desaturase enzymes show preference for the omega-3, -6, and -9 in that order so that synthesis of some EFAs might only occur when the intake of omega-3 and -6 EFAs is low.

Table 4.3 Effect of high carbohydrate, alcohol and fibre on blood fats.

Carbohydrate	Fibre[a]	Alcohol	Non-nutrient components[b]
Increases VLDL and triglycerides	Reduces cholesterol	Increases triglycerides and VLDL and possibly cholesterol	HMG-CoA-like activity
Lowers HDL		Small increase in HDL	Reduces cholesterol and LDL

[a] Effects depend on the type of fibre. Insoluble fibres only have a small effect on lipoproteins; soluble fibre has a favourable effect.
[b] For example allicin, saponins, isoflavonoids, phyto-oestrogens, and anthocyanins. Individually they only have a small LDL lowering effect but combining several components may produce a cumulative effect.

Table 4.4 Sources of omega-3, -6 and -9 essential fatty acids. And daily intake recommended (RDI) by the National Health and Medical Research Council (2006). A variety of foods high in essential fatty acids should be consumed each day.

Omega-3 (EPA) RDI 50–200 mg/day	Omega-6 RDI 150–1500 mg/day	Omega-9 <50 g/day
Fresh tuna	Safflower	Olive oil
Halibut	Evening primrose	Avocado
Sardines	Sunflower	Almond
Mackerel	Corn and maize	Apricot
Herring	Hempseed	Canola
Trout	Walnut	Peanut
Krill	Pumkin seed	Butter
Cod liver oil[a]	Borage	Lard
	Blackcurrant	Eggs
	Soya bean	Milk
	Flax and linseed	Coconut

RDI = recommended daily intake. The RDI varies among publications. Consider the quantity of EPA and DHA in omega-3 supplements rather than the total quantity of fish oil in the product. Different types of fish contain different quantities of omega-3.
Consider the risk of bleeding before recommending supplements if the person is on anticoagulant medicines or has bleeding conditions.

[a] Cod liver oil may be contraindicated in pregnancy without medical advice.

(NHMRC) (2003) and The Heart Foundation recommend an upper level of 6 g of salt per day. High salt diets are leading causes of cardiovascular disease and hypertension (WHO 2002) and reducing salt intake reduces blood pressure.
- Reduce alcohol. Small amounts of alcohol (0.5–1 drink/day) can reduce cardiovascular risk and post prandial blood glucose levels if consumed with the evening meal containing carbohydrate. Greater quantities impairs glucose metabolism and contributes to hyperlipidaemia, In Australia, the current recommendation is 2 standard drinks per day for men and 1 standard drink per day for women.

The Apple Report

The Apple Report (2008) suggests there may be a grain of truth in the old adage, An apple a day keeps the doctor away. The Apple Report suggests:

- A 100 g apple has the equivalent antioxidant effect of 1740 mg of vitamin C. Apples contain vitamins C and B, phytochemicals especially flavonoids quercetin and quercetin conjugates, fibre, potassium and other minerals, and has a low GI (38).
- Several studies suggest an association between eating one apple per day and lower risk of cancer, particularly lung cancer, possibly due to their high flavonoid content. Different varieties of apples have different effects on liver cancer cells *in vitro*.
- Apple consumption is linked to a ~22% lower risk of cardiovascular disease and reduced mortality associated with coronary heart disease and cardiovascular disease.
- Apples appear to reduce cholesterol and increase HDL in animal studies
- An association between apple consumption and improved lung function in people with asthma including lower risk of children of mothers who ate apples during pregnancy having asthma at age 5.
- Apple peel demonstrates antiproliferative properties, which reduce inflammation and cell apoptosis.
- An apple before each meal helps weight loss and overall health profile.

It is not clear whether these findings translate to people with diabetes but there is no reason to suspect they do not.

The goals of dietary management are to:

- Improve the person's overall health.
- Attain optimal body weight.
- Attain lipid and blood glucose levels as close to normal as practical considering hypoglycaemia risk and its consequences, see Chapter 6.
- Ensure normal growth and development in children.
- Decrease the risk of diabetes- and obesity-related complications and comorbidities.
- Identify nutrition-related disorders that can affect diabetes management and interpreting investigative procedures, for example, anaemia.

Dietary management: obesity

Public health strategies are required, see Chapter 1. These should be age, gender and culturally specific, and address environmental issues such as safe, accessible areas to exercise and understandable food labels.

As well as diet and exercise, a combination of behaviour change strategies tailored to the individual, and support are required. Diets high in fruit, vegetables, whole grains, legumes, and low in fat are generally safe and effective and promote fullness and satiety (National Institute of Health 2000). However <20% of people trying to lose weight consume these foods.

As indicated, commercial weight loss programmes such as Weight Watchers, The slim-fast plan, Dr Atkin's New Diet and the Rosemary Conley Program result in significant weight loss and lower WHR after six months compared to controls who gained an average of 0.6 kg. However, the improvements were not sustained after the trial was completed. More sustained benefit was noted in programs that included a support group (Truby *et al.* 2006).

Other popular diets include the following, which all have advantages and disadvantages. People with diabetes should be advised to discuss these diets with a dietitian and/or their doctor before they try them:

- High protein-low carbohydrate (ketogenic) diets.
- Meal replacement plans where 1–2 meals per day are replaced with meal supplements.
- Dairy diet. Preliminary data suggest 3 servings/day of calcium rich food enhances weight loss through a variety of mechanisms but more research is needed to confirm these preliminary results (Zemel 2003).

Fish oil supplements (3 g fish oil containing 1.8 g polyunsaturated fatty acids) have been shown to reduce adiposity and atherogenic risk factors in a randomised controlled trial of women with Type 2 diabetes (Rizkalla 2007). However, fish oil may affect the INR in patients taking anticoagulants.

If the BMI is >30 or BMI >27 and diabetes or cardiovascular risk factors are present and diet and exercise is ineffective, medicines such as lipase inhibitors (Xenical) or serotonin reuptake inhibitors such as Sibutramine can be used but they only reduce weight by ~10%. Sibutramine can increase blood pressure (Donohoe 2008). Research into future weight loss medicines is likely to focus on the hormones involved in regulating satiety (leptin, ghrelin and CRBs). Fucoxanthin, an antioxidant obtained from brown seaweed, which is commonly used in Asian cuisine, has been shown to induce weight loss and increase omega-3 fatty acid levels in rats (Miyashita 2006) but its application in humans is unknown.

Bariatric surgery

Gastric bypass surgery effectively reduces weight and improves quality of life and lowers the risk of comorbidities after two years compared to controls (Adams 2006). Improved mood has been demonstrated using the Beck Depression Inventory (Mitka 2003). Several procedures are used such as Roux-en-Y gastric bypass, stapled gastroplasty, and adjustable gastric banding all of which reduce the stomach size and control caloric intake. Although the risks are high people lose weight and blood glucose levels normalise (Encinose *et al.* 2006).

Complementary weight loss programmes

Many complementary weight (CAM) loss strategies are similar to conventional programmes and these are beneficial and effective. However, many of the CAM medicines have limited evidence of any benefits (Egger 2005). Some are dangerous, for example, weight loss products that contain ephedra should be avoided and have been banned in some countries. Likewise, creams, soaps, and body wraps are unlikely to lead to weight loss but they may improve body image and self-concept and help the individual mentally. Hypnosis may be a useful adjunct to other strategies.

People also use topical creams and 'anticellulite' preparations to improve their body image and research is continuing on such medicines. Caruso *et al.* (2007) reported 11% reduction in waist circumference compared to 5% after 12 weeks in controls with equal reductions in women and men using a 1200 calorie balanced diet, a walking programme and 0.5% topical aminophylline cream applied to the waist BD. The diet and exercise could confound the results. Likewise, the study was not blinded. Thus, there is no compelling evidence to recommend using currently available anticellulite preparations and some that contain aminophylline could affect heart rhythm, which might be undesirable in people with diabetes.

In Australia, weight control products (complementary and conventional) must conform to the Weight Management Industry Code of Practice (htt://www.weightcontrol. org/browse.asp?page=349. People can be advised to check whether products conform to this Code before they purchase the product.

Factors associated with making dietary changes

Kapur *et al.* (2008) described a number of factors associated with positive dietary changes in India. These included:

- being older
- a shorter time since being fit and acceptable weight
- having strong family support
- having a less busy work life
- being conscious of their health
- having received dietitian advice and frequent visits to a dietitian
- being interested in overall health not just diabetes.

Motivational interviewing in addition to diet and exercise leads to weight loss in African-American in a randomised prospective trial in women. HbA_{1c} was correlated with weight loss at 6 months but was not sustained at 18 months (Smith-West 2007). Galuska *et al.* (1999) demonstrated cost savings in people being counselled and suggested frequent reminders and support were essential.

These findings suggest important issues for health professionals to consider when developing weight management strategies and delivering dietary advice. They might also indicate health professionals also need to make some behaviour changes and become better educated about nutrition and how to deliver dietary and weight loss advice.

Nursing responsibilities

(1) To assess dietary and nutritional characteristics and problems and refer to a dietitian as required, for example at a change from tablets to insulin, if there are frequent high or low blood glucose levels, the diagnosis of a complication such as renal disease, if the patient displays inadequate knowledge, or when the person requests a referral.

Table 4.5 Drugs whose absorption can be modified by food.

Reduced absorption	Delayed absorption	Increased absorption
Aspirin	Aspirin	Diazepam
Cephalexin	Cefaclor	Dicoumarol
Erythromycin	Cephalexin	hydrochlorothiazide
Penicillin V and G	Cimetidine	Hydrochlorothiazide
Phenacetin	Digoxin	Metoprolol
Tetracycline	Indoprofen	Nitrofurantoin
Theophylline	Metronidazole	Propranolol

(2) To observe and, if necessary, record food intake, with particular reference to carbohydrate intake of patients on glucose lowering medication.

(3) To promote general dietary principles to patients in accordance with accepted policies and procedures.

(4) To ensure the meals and carbohydrate content are evenly spaced throughout the day.

(5) To ensure adequate carbohydrate intake for fasting patients and those with diminished intake to avoid hypoglycaemia.

(6) Administer medicines at an appropriate time in relation to food.

(7) To know that the absorption of some medicines can be modified by food especially antibiotics and their effectiveness may be diminished or increased, see Table 4.5. The pharmacological response to medicines is influenced by the individual's nutritional status. In turn, medicines can affect the nutritional status. The sense of smell and taste play a significant role in adequate dietary intake. Both these senses diminish with age and can be changed by disease processes and some medicines. Gastrointestinal (GIT) disorders can lead to malabsorption, pH changes alter the bioavailability of nutrients and medicines, inhibit medicine binding and chelation and impair the metabolism and excretion of medicines (NHMRC 1999). Interactions can also occur with commonly used dietary supplements, see Chapter 19 and the International Bibliographic Information on Dietary Supplements (National Institute of Health).

(8) To observe for signs and symptoms of hyper- and hypoglycaemia, and correct the blood glucose level by appropriate nutritional management as part of the management plan.

Inadequate nutrition and low protein stores can delay the healing process.

Some foods that interact with medicines are shown in Table 4.6.

'Sugar-free' foods

'Sugar-free' usually refers to the sucrose content of foods. Other sugars are often used to sweeten foods labelled sugar-free (e.g. dextrose, fructose, maltose, lactose, galactose).

Recent evidence suggests fructose, which is used to sweeten most soft drinks, causes a greater increase in triglycerides and LDL than glucose (American Dietetic Association

Table 4.6   Some food-medicine interactions.

Food	Medicine	Possible effects
Black liquorice in large doses	Digoxin Diuretics Calcium channel blockers	Irregular heart rhythm Hypertension High serum sodium Muscle pain Weakness
Aged cheese such as brie, parmesan, Roquefort Sauerkraut Over ripe avocadoes Pepperoni	MAO antidepressants	Hypertension
Grapefruit juice	Calcium channel blockers Lipid lowering medicines Some oral contraceptives Some psychiatric medicines	Modifies medicine metabolism
Orange juice	Aluminium-containing antacids Antibiotics	Increases aluminium
Milk and other dairy products	Tetracycline digitalis Laxatives containing bisacodyl	Enhanced effects
Oatmeal and high fibre cereals	Many oral medicines including antihypertensive agents	Can affect absorption
Leafy and green vegetables high in vitamin K	Warfarin and other anticlotting medicines	Interferes with blood clotting
Caffeinated foods such as tea, coffee, chocolate	Asthma medications Quinolone antibiotics Some oral contraceptives	Excessive excitability
Alcohol	Medicines containing pseudoephedrine Antidepressant medicines Antipsychotics Muscle relaxants Sedatives Glucose lowering medicines	Excitability Sedation Hypoglycaemia
High salt foods	Steroids	Fluid retention
Iodine-rich food	Thyroid medicines	Reduced efficacy Might affect blood glucose through its effect on the thyroid

Note: Alcohol interacts with almost all medicines. Some medicines increase the risk of nutritional deficiencies. For example, metformin leads to vitamin B-12 deficiency; cholestyramine increases excretion of folate and vitamins A, D, E, and K; and antacids interfere with the absorption of many essential minerals. Thus, the person being prescribed medicines should be advised about when to take them in relation to food. People at high risk of a food–medicine interaction are older, taking medicines for chronic diseases such as diabetes, have hypertension, depression hypercholesterolaemia, renal disease, or congestive heart failure.

2004; Havel 2007). The study was undertaken in overweight and obese individuals but the findings are likely to apply to non-obese people because fructose is more likely to pass into the lipogenic pathway than glucose after being metabolised in the liver. More research is needed to confirm these findings to determine the percentage of total energy consumption at which fructose has an atherogenic effect. These foods may not be appropriate for people with diabetes. Low calorie and artificially sweetened foods are generally recommended.

Alternative sweeteners

Alternative sweeteners elicit a pleasurable sensation without affecting the blood glucose and are generally safe if used at the recommended doses. They may also play a role in reducing dental caries (American Dietetic Association 2004). They are an acceptable alternative to sugar for people with diabetes. However, a small amount of sugar included in a balanced diet does not adversely affect the blood glucose. There are two types of alternative sweeteners: non-nutritive (or artificial) and nutritive. Non-nutritive sweeteners are kilojoule free, for example:

• Saccharin
• Acesulphame-K
• Aspartame (Equal)
• Cyclamate
• Isomalt
• Neotame
• Sucralose (Splenda)
• Alitame
• Neotame

These products are safe to use. If used in cooking they are best added after cooking because heat can change the taste. The best choices for pregnant women are Acesulphame-K, Alitame, Aspartame, and Sucralose.

Nutritive sweeteners are usually derived from different types of carbohydrate and products containing these sweeteners are often labelled 'carbohydrate modified'. Nutritive sweeteners include:

• Sorbitol
• Fructose (Sweetaddin)
• Mannitol
• Xylitol
• Maltilol
• Isomalt
• Polydextrose (Litesse)
• Maltodextrin (hydrolysed corn syrup)
• Thaumatin

Many nutritive sweeteners are sugar alcohols, for example, sorbitol. These sweeteners can cause diarrhoea in high doses. Likewise, 'diet' products containing alternative sweeteners can be high in fat.

Stevia (*Stevia rebaudiana*), a herb much sweeter than sugar, is being promoted as a suitable sugar alternative for people with diabetes and may have glucose lowering effects but it has not been extensively evaluated in clinical practice. Only very small quantities are required. Larger doses may cause diarrhoea.

Food additives

Many people are allergic to food additives, which can result in sensitivities or in severe cases, analphylaxis. Different additives are used for different classes of foods. A list of food additives and their code numbers can be obtained from www.foodstandards. gov.au. Types of additives include acidity regulators, antioxidants, bulking agents, colourings, flavourings, emulsifiers, gelling agents, humectants, preservatives, and thickeners. Some of these additives are also used in some medicines.

It is important to learn to read labels and to get to know the alternative names for foods and additives that commonly cause allergies such as cow's milk, soy, nuts, and gluten as well as alternative names for fat and sugar. Key information on a food label people need to look for includes:

- The nutrition claims, for example, fat free, high fibre, low fat, reduced fat, cholesterol free, low in salt, low in sugar and sugar free.
- How to interpret the list of ingredients.
- How to interpret the allergy information.
- The country of origin.
- Use by dates and storage recommendations.
- Understand the nutrition information.
- How to interpret information about recommended daily intake.
- Understanding the figures and symbols such as the GI symbol, genetically modified foods, and the Heart foundation tick.

These key aspects should be part of routine dietary advice or the person can be referred to Reid (2007) www.healthyfoodguide.com.au.

Alcohol

Alcohol reduces hepatic glucose output but does not have a direct affect on insulin secretion or glucose disposal (Shai 2007). It is recommended that alcohol consumption be limited because of its potential to affect blood glucose and contribute to or mask, hypoglycaemia (see Chapter 6). Sweet alcoholic drinks can lead to *hyper*glycaemia, while the alcohol itself leads to *hypo*glycaemia. The hypoglycaemic effect may depend on the nutritional state and glucose stores. Alcohol should *never* be consumed on an empty stomach.

Alcohol supplies considerable calories and provides little or no nutritional value. In addition, alcohol clouds judgment and can lead to inappropriate decision-making. Drunkenness can resemble hypoglycaemia and treatment of hypoglycaemia may be delayed. Appropriate education about hypoglycaemia risk with alcohol consumption is essential. Alcohol has a range of other physical effects including liver cirrhosis, malnutrition and peripheral neuropathy.

Although, moderate amounts of alcohol may reduce cardiovascular risk current recommended intake still applies. In Australia 2 standard drinks per day for men and 1 standard drink per day for women. See also Chapter 10.

Exercise/activity

Exercise has an important role in controlling the blood glucose and increasing overall fitness. It should be combined with a suitable diet. People commencing an exercise programme should first have a medical assessment.

Structured aerobic and resistance training programmes improve blood glucose levels and lower HbA_{1c} by ~0.6% and reduce cardiovascular risk in Type 2 diabetes (Krause & Levine 2007). A 1% reduction was associated with 15–20% reduction in major macrovascular events and 37% reduction in microvascular events. In addition, exercise has mental health benefits such as improved body image and feelings of self-worth (Goldfield *et al.* 2007).

Exercise capacity is an independent predictor of non-fatal cardiac events and mortality of patients referred for treadmill testing (ETT) (Peterson *et al.* 2008). For example, low exercise capacity is associated with increased risk of MI on ETT but it is not clear whether low exercise capacity indicates the presence of underlying disease is a marker of cardiovascular events.

Exercise can result in hypo or hyperglycaemia. Under normal circumstances exercise stimulates hepatic glucose output and glucose utilisation to maintain glucose in the normal range. However, if exercise occurs in times of metabolic stress the sympathetic drive can be stimulated, which leads to reduced glucose utilisation (Van de Veire *et al.* 2006).

Before exercising people should check their blood glucose levels. It is important to make a gradual start to the exercise. Strenuous activity can cause hypoglycaemia; extra carbohydrate may be needed.

Various strategies are suggested to help people begin, maintain an exercise/activity regimen. The beneficial effects of exercise are less evident if exercise is the sole focus of the intervention (Conn *et al.* 2007). Effective strategies include:

- Providing exercise education.
- Setting achievable goals and focusing on achieving one goal at a time.
- Providing individual supervision is as effective as group programmes and is more acceptable to some people.
- Suggesting written 'exercise prescriptions' that take account of the individual's interests, gender, age and capabilities.
- Wearing a pedometer, especially when combined with a step goal diary. Reduction in BMI of 0.38 kg/m^2 and reductions in blood pressure by 3.8 mmHg have been described (Bravata *et al.* 2007). A recent meta-analysis suggests people lose an average of 0.05 kg representing 2–3% of body weight over 12 months and continues if the individual continues to wear the pedometer (Richardson *et al.* 2008). People often hope to lose much more weight than this so it is important that they realise even small weight loss is beneficial and to set reasonable goals. Steps walked increased from ~2000 to ~4000 per day on average in Richardson *et al.*'s meta-analysis. Pedometers provide feedback on the number of steps a person takes per day but exercise duration, intensity and frequency and the long-term benefits are unknown.

- Combining exercise with rehabilitation programmes.
- Tai Chi, particularly in older people and those in wheelchairs has a range of benefits such as improved: muscle strength, flexibility, balance, range of movement, lower risk of: falls, cardiovascular fitness, cholesterol and abdominal fat and younger vital age (ICCMR 2008), see Chapter 19.

References

Adams, T., Walker, J., Litwin, S. & Pendelton, R. (2006) Two-year improvement in morbidity following gastric bypass surgey. *NAASO: The Obesity Society Annual Scientific Meeting*, Dallas, Texas. Abstract 16-0R October.

Allan, C. (2008) Testosterone reduces visceral fat gain in non-obese older men. *Journal of Clinical Endocrinology and Metabolism*. pp. 139–146.

American Dietetic Association (ADA) (2004) Use of nutritive and non-nutritive sweeteners. *ADA*, **104** (2), 255–275.

Australian Dietary Guidelines (1991) Australian Government Publications, Canberra.

Behan, K. & Mbizo, J. (2007) The relationship between waist circumference and biomarkers for disease in health non-obese women. *American Society for Clinical Pathology*, **38** (7), 422–427.

Better Health Channel Fact Sheet: Weight Loss – Common Myths. Htpp://www.betterhealth.vic.gov.au/bhcv2/bhcarticles.nsf/pages/Weight_loss_common (accessed January 2008).

Brand-Miller, J. (1994) Importance of glycaemic index in diabetes. *American Journal of Clinical Nutrition*, **59** (Suppl.), 7475–7525.

Block, G. (1982) A review of validations of dietary assessment methods. *American Journal of Epidemiology*, **115**, 492–505.

Bravata, D., Smith-Sprangler, C. & Sundaram, V. (2007) Using pedometers to increase physical activity and health. A systematic review. *JAMA*, **298**, 2296–2304.

Bouchard, L., Drapeau, V., Provencher, V. & Lemieux, S. (2004) Neuromedin beta: a strong candidate gene linking eating behaviours and susceptibility to obesity. *American Journal of Clinical Nutrition*, **80** (6), 1478–1486.

British Diabetic Association Report (1992) Dietary recommendations for people with diabetes. *Diabetic Medicine*, **9**, 189–202.

Burdette, H. & Whitaker, R. (2005) A national study of neighbourhood safety, outdoor play, television viewing, and obesity in preschool children. *Pediatrics*, **116** (3), 657–662.

Donohoe, M. (2007) Weighty matters: public health aspects of the obesity epidemic. *Medscape Obstetrics and Gynaecology and Women's Health*. Available at http://www.medscape.com.viewarticle/566056 (acccessed January 2008).

Carey, V., Bishop, L. & Charleston, J. (2005) Rationale and design of the optimal macronutrient intake heart (Omni-Heart) trial. *Clinical Trials* **2** (6), 529–537.

Caruso, M., Pekarovic, S., Raum, W. & Greenway, F. (2007) Topical treatments for fat reduction do they work? A best evidence review. *Diabetes Obesity and Metabolism*, **9**, 300–303.

Deutsch, L. (2007) Evaluation of the effect of Neptune krill oil on chronic inflammation and arthritis symptoms. *Journal of American College of Nutrition*, **26** (1), 39–48.

Conn, V. & Hafdahl, A. (2007) Metabolic effects of interventions to increase exercise in adults with type 2 diabetes. *Diabetologia*, **50**, 913–921.

DAFNE Study Group (2002) Training in flexible, intensive insulin management to enable dietary freedom in people with type 1 diabetes: dose adjustment for normal eating (DAFNE) randomized controlled trial. *British Medical Journal*, **325**, 746.

Diehr, P., Bild, D. & Harris, T. (1998) Body mass index and mortality in non-smoking older adults. The cardiovascular effects. *Journal of Public Health*, **88**, 623–629.

Diehr, P., O'Meara, E., Fitzpatrick, A. & Newman, A. (2008) Weight, mortality, years of healthy life and active life expectancy. *Journal American Geriatric Society*, **56** (1), 76–83.

Dunning, T. & Hoy, S. (1994) *What to Do till the Dietitian Gets There*. Servier Australia, Melbourne.

Eddy, S. (2008) Omega-6 and 9 fatty acids. *Journal of Complementary Medicine*, **7** (2), 34–39.

Egger, G. & Thorburn, A. (2005) Environmental policy approaches: methods of dealing with obesity . In: *Clinical Obesity in Adults and Children* eds Kopleson, P., Caterson, I. & Deitz, W., 2nd edition. Blackwell Publishing, Oxford.

Erlichman, J., Kerbey, A. & James, W. (2002) Physical activity and its impact on health outcomes. Paper 2: prevention of unhealthy weight gain and obesity by physical activity: an analysis of the evidence. *Obesity Review*, 3, 273–287.

Elmore, J., Carney, P. & Abraham, L. (2004) The association between obesity and screening mammography accuracy. *Archives of Internal Medicine*, **164**, 1140–1147.

Encinosa, W., Bernard, D., Steiner, C. & Chen, C. (2006) Healthcare utilization and outcomes after bariatric surgery. *Medical Care*, **44**, 706–712.

Fegal, K., Carroll, M., Ogden, C. & Johnston, C. (1999) Prevalence and trends in obesity among US adults 297: 969–977.1999–2000. *JAMA*, **288**, 1723–1727.

Feskanich, D., Rockett, H. & Colditz, G. (2004) Modifying the healthy eating index to assess diet quality in children and adolescents. *Journal of the American Dietetic Association*, **104** (9), 1375–1383.

Fung, T. (2007) DASH-style diet may reduce risk of CHD and stroke. *American Heart Association Scientific Sessions*, Abstract 2369. November 5th.

Galuska, D., Will, J., Serdula, M. & Ford, E. (1999) Are health care professionals advising obese patients to loose weight? *JAMA*, **282**, 1576–1578.

Gardner, C., Kiazand, A. & Alhassan, S. (2007) Comparison of the Atkins, Zone, Ornish and LEARN diets for change in weight and related risk factors among overweight premenopausal women: the A to Z Weight Loss Study: a randomized trial. *JAMA*, **297**, 969–977.

Goldfield, G., Mallory, R., Parker, T., Cunningham, T. & Legg, C. (2007) Effects of modifying physical activity and sedentary behaviour on psychosocial adjustment in overweight/obese children. *Journal Pediatric Psychology*, **32** (7), 783–793.

Havel, P. (2007) Fructose but not glucose consumption linked to atherogenic lipid profile. *American Diabetes Association 67th Scientific Sessions*, Abstract 0062-0R June.

Iqbal, O. (2007) Endocannabinoid system and pathophysiology of adipogenesis: current management of obesity. *Personalised Medicine*, **4** (3), 307–319.

Jespersen, I. (2001) The effect of dietary oils on blood lipids and the risk of ischemic heart disease with special emphasis on olive oil. A Literature review. *Ugeskr Laeger*, **163** (35), 4736–4740.

Kapur, K., Kupur, A., Ramachandran, S., Mohan, V., Aravind, S., Bagandi, M. & Srishyla, M. (2008) Barriers to changing dietary behaviour. *JAPI*, **56**, 27–32.

Kapur, K. & Dunning, T. (2007) Global nutritional recommendations: a combination of evidence and food availability. *Practical Diabetes International*, **24** (9), 1–8.

Katan, W. (1990) Biochemical indicators of dietary intake. *European Journal of Clinical Nutrition*, **52**, S5.

Kraus, E. & Levine, B. (2007) Aerobic and resistance training improve glycaemic control in type 2 diabetes. *Annals of Internal Medicine*, **147**, 357–369; 423–425.

Kondrup, S., Allison, S., Elia, M., Vallas, B. & Plauth, M. (2003) EPSEN guidelines for nutrition screening 2002. *Clinical Nutrition*, **22** (4), 415–421.

Kondrup, J., Rasmussen, H. & Hamberg, O. (2003) Nutritional risk screening (NRS 2002): a new method based on an analysis of controlled clinical trials. *Clinical Nutrition*, **22**, 321–336.

Lamberg, L. (2006) R$_x$ for obesity: eat less, exercise more, and – maybe get more sleep. *JAMA* http:// www.medscape.com/viewarticle/566056 (accessed February 2008).

Latner, J. (2001) Staff help in the treatment of obesity. *Obesity Review*, **2**, 87–97.

Malnutrition Advisory Group (MAG) (2000) *MAG – Guidelines for Detection and Management of Malnutrition.* British Association for Parenteral and Enteral Nutrition, Redditch, UK.

Marks, S. (2000) Obesity management. *Current Therapeutics*, **41**, 6.

Middleton, M., Nazarenko, G., Nivison-Smith, I. & Smerdely, P. (2001) Prevalence of malnutrition and 12-month incidence of mortality in two Sydney teaching hospitals. *Medical Journal of Australia*, **31**, 455–461.

Mitka, M. (2003) Surgery for obesity: demand soars amid scientific, ethical questions. *JAMA*, **289**, 1761–1762.

Miyashita, K. (2006) Brown seaweed may burn away brown fat. *American Chemical Society 232nd National Meeting and Exposition*, San Francisco, 10–14th Sept.

Moyad, M. (2004) Fad diets and obesity-Part 1: measuring weight in a clinical setting. *Urology Nurse*, **24** (2), 114–119.

Muhlhauser, I. & Berger, M. (2002) Patient education-evaluation of a complex intervention. *Diabetologia*, **45**, 1723–1733.

National Institutes of Health (NIH) Office of Dietary Supplements IBIDS database. Available at: http://grande.nal.usda.gov/index.php (accessed January 2008).

National Health and Medical Research Council (NHMRC) (1999) *Diet for Older Australians.* Commonwealth of Australia, Canberra.

National Health and Medical Research Council (NHMRC) (2003) Dietary Guidelines for Australian Adults. NHMRC Ref. No. N29-N34.

NHMRC (2006) Healthy eating Club Fact Sheets: fat & cholesterol. www.healthyeatingclub. org/info/articles/fats-chol/index.htm (accessed January 2008).

Peterson, P.N., Magid, D.J. & Ross, C. (2008) Association of exercise capacity on treadmill with future cardiac events in patients referred for exercise testing. *Archives of Internal Medicine*, **168**, 174–179.

Pi-Sunyer, F. (2006) Use of lifestyle changes treatment plans and drug therapy in controlling cardiovascular disease and obesity. *Obesity*, **14** (Suppl 3), 135S–142S.

Rahman, S., Morell, M., Topping, D., Bired, A., Zhongyi, Li, Dennis, E. & Peacock, J. (2007) Low glycaemic response cereals for enhanced human health. *International Diabetes Monitor*, **19** (3), 21–25.

Reynolds, S., Yasuhkio, S. & Crimmins, E. (2005) The impact of obesity on active life expectancy in older Americans. *Gerontologist*, **45**, 438–444.

Richardson, C., Newton, T., Abraham, J., Sen, A. & Swartz, M. (2008) A meta-analysis of pedometer-based walking interventions and weight. *Annals of Family Medicine*, **6** (1), 69–77.

Reid, C. (2007) www.healthyfoodguide.com.au.

Rizkalla, S. (2007) Fish oils supplements cut adiposity in type 2 diabetes. *American Journal of Clinical Nutrition*, **86**, 1670–1679.

Stevens, J. (2000) Impact of age on associations between weight and mortality. *Nutrition Review*, **58**, 129–137.

Smith-West, D. (2007) Motivational interviewing improves weight loss in women with type 1 diabetes. *Diabetes Care*, **30**, 1018–1087.

Stone, A. & Brownell, K. (1994) The stress eating paradox: multiple daily measurements in adult males and females. *Psychological Health*, **9**, 425–436.

Sydney-Smith, M. (2000) Nutritional assessment in general practice. *Current Therapeutics*, **41** (9), 13–24.

Tay, J., Brinkworth, G. & Noakes, M. (2008) Metabolic effects of weight loss on a very-low-carbohydrate diet compared with an isocaloric high-carbohydrate diet in abdominally obese subjects. *American Journal of Cardiology*, **51**, 59–67.

Truby, H. & Baic, S. (2006) Randomised controlled trial of four weight loss programmes in the UK: initial findings from the BBC "diet trials". *British Medical Journal*, **332**, 1309–1314.

Tsai, A. & Wadden, T. (2005) Sytematic review: an evaluation of major commercial weight loss programs in the United States. *Annals of Internal Medicine*, **142**, 56–66.

Third report of the National Cholesterol Education Program (NCEP) Expert Panel on Detection, Evaluation and Treatment of High Blood Cholesterol in Adults (2002) (Adult Treatment Panel 111) Final Report. *Circulation*, **106** (25), 3143–3421.

Third Joint Taskforce of European and Other Societies on Cardiovascular Disease Prevention in Clinical Practice (2003) European guidelines on cardiovascular disease prevention in clinical practice. *European Journal of Cardiovascular Prevention Rehabilitation*, **10** (Suppl. 1), S1–S78.

Van de Veure, N., De Winter, O., Gir, M., De Buyzere, M., van de Wiele, C. & Sutter, J. (2006) Fasting blood glucose levels are related to exercise capacity in patients with coronary artery disease. *American Heart Journal*, **152** (3), 486–492.

Van Gaal, L., Rissanen, A. & Scheen, A. (2005) RIO-Europe Study group. Effects of the cannabinoid-1 receptor blocker rimonabant on weight reduction and cardiovascular risk factors in overweight patients: 1-year experience from the RIO-Europe Study. *Lancet*, **365**, 1389–1397.

Vellas, B., Guigoz, Y. & Garry, P. (1999) The Mini Nutritional Assessment (MNA) and its use in grading nutritional state of elderly patients. *Nutrition*, **15**, 116–122.

Weiss, E. (2007) Certain factors associated with weight regain after weight loss. *American Journal of Preventative Medicine Online June 5th 2007*.

Williams, P. (2008) Asymmetric weight gain and loss from increasing and decreasing exercise. *Medicine Society Sports Exercise*, **40** (2), 296–302.

World Health Organisation (WHO) (2000) *The World Health Report – Reducing Risk, Promoting Healthy Life*. WHO, Switzerland.

Zemel, M. (2003) Role of dietary calcium and diary products in modulating adiposity. *Lipids*, **38**, 139–146.

Chapter 5
Medicines Management

Key points

- Medications should be managed within the principles of the Quality Use of Medicines.
- Understanding the pharmacology of the different oral hypoglycaemic agents, insulins and other medicines enables meals, activity, and medicine administration times to be planned appropriately.
- Medicine-related outcomes need to be proactively monitored according to management targets, the indications for their use, and individual benefits and risks.
- Type 2 diabetes is a progressive disease of beta cell decline and insulin will eventually be needed by >50% of people with Type 2 diabetes.
- Polypharmacy is common in diabetes, especially Type 2, and could be considered best practice.
- Medicine-related non-adherence is common, complex and multifactorial. It has its basis in patient and health professional-related issues as well as system-related issues.
- People with diabetes frequently use complementary medicines/therapies (CAM), which needs to be considered when selecting management options.

Introduction

The main 'diabetes medicines' listed below are discussed in this chapter. Other medicines are described in the relevant chapters:

(1) Oral hypoglycaemic agents
(2) Insulin
(3) Lipid lowering agents
(4) Cardiovascular agents
(5) Antiplatelet agents

The author prefers to use the term 'medicines' rather than 'drugs', which is reserved for describing illegal drugs. Medicines should be managed within a quality use of medicine framework (QUM), which is an holistic risk management approach that encompasses all types of medicines and recommends using non-medicine options first. People with diabetes also frequently use complementary medicines (CAM) and these are discussed throughout the book but principally in Chapter 19. Medicines are also mentioned in other chapters throughout the book where relevant.

Quality Use of Medicines (QUM)

The information in this section was adapted from *The Quality Use of Medicines in Diabetes* (2005) a paper developed by the Pharmaceutical Health and Rational use of Medicines (PHARM) Committee, a Committee of the Australian Commonwealth Department of Health and Ageing. It is reproduced with permission. QUM is a key aspect of the National Medicines Policy. QUM aims to help health professionals and consumers make the best possible use of medicines to improve their health outcomes. QUM recognises the central role of the consumer in medicines use and that many people maintain their health without using medicines, while for others medicines are important to their health and wellbeing. It also recognises that medicines may be needed for prevention as well as treatment.

'QUM means:

• Selecting management options wisely.
• Choosing suitable medicines if a medicine is considered necessary.
• Using medicines safely and effectively' (Commonwealth Department of Health and Ageing, 2002).

Quality Use of Medicines and diabetes

Medicines are central to effective diabetes management to control metabolic abnormalities and manage the complications of diabetes and other concomitant conditions. However, even when medicines are required, lifestyle factors, diet, exercise and smoking cessation, are necessary to achieve optimal outcomes. Prevention programmes such as SNAP have a central, primary and ongoing role (Commonwealth Department of Health and Aging 2001).

Medicines are used in four main areas in diabetes:

(1) *Primary prevention* focuses on lifestyle factors to prevent or delay the need for medicines in those at risk of diabetes and its complications. However, medicines may be needed for prevention, for example, lipid lowering and antihypertensive medicines, and flu vaccine to prevent intercurrent illness in at-risk individuals.

(2) *Secondary prevention* where medicines are usually necessary to reduce the risk of diabetes complications diabetes such as renal disease, atherosclerosis, and retinopathy.

(3) *Clinical care*, which involves using medicines to achieve optimal metabolic, psychological and quality of life targets by appropriately selecting management options including choosing suitable medicines if medicines are required, obtaining informed consent, ensuring patients have the information and skills to participate in medication management, and monitoring the outcomes to ensure medicines are used safely and effectively. Educating the person with diabetes and their carers and supporting them to manage their diabetes generally, and medicines in particular, are key aspects of QUM. Medicines prescribed for other conditions, self-initiated non-prescription medicines and CAM use need to be considered as part of holistic assessment and care. Significantly, polypharmacy is usually necessary to achieve optimal outcomes in people with diabetes and may be considered best practice. However, polypharmacy increases the complexity, risks and costs of the

management regimen. Therefore, as few medicines as possible should be used. Insulin and sometimes other medicines are needed at diagnosis in Type 1 diabetes and many people with Type 2. Type 2 diabetes is a progressive disease and, consequently the medication regimen becomes progressively complex with increasing duration of diabetes.

(4) *Clinical trials* commonly investigate new medicines and other interventions before they are licensed for use to ensure they are safe, efficacious, and determine cost benefit. Information from trials is also used to develop clinical practice guidelines and consumer and health professional information. Health professionals are often asked to help recruit participants for clinical trials. The fact that an individual is participating in a clinical trial should be clearly documented in the person's medical record.

QUM is a useful framework for reducing polypharmacy and duplicate prescribing because it encompasses prevention using non-medicine options, regular medication reviews, and effective communication among health professionals and with people with diabetes (National Prescribing Service 2000).
Medicines are selected taking into account:

- The individual's physical and mental health status.
- Whether there is a suitable non-medicine option.
- The risks and benefits of using medicines for the individual.
- Dosage, dose interval, and duration of treatment.
- Other medicines, CAM and therapies that the individual may be using.
- The process required to monitor the outcomes of medicine use including adverse events, medication self-management and other relevant self-care such as blood glucose monitoring, processes for communicating the medication plan among the relevant health professionals when the individual makes transitions among health providers and services, and strategies for regularly reviewing the continued benefits and risks of the medication regimen and the individual's self-care capacity.
- The costs to the individual, the community, and the health system. A process for integrating QUM into existing care is shown in Figure 5.1.

Oral hypoglycaemic agents (OHA)

Different OHAs target the various underlying abnormalities of glucose homeostasis in Type 2 diabetes. They are not appropriate for Type 1 diabetes. Type 2 diabetes is a progressive disease of beta cell decline, thus the medication regimen needs to be constantly monitored and adjusted and medicines included as necessary. The UKPDS study (Turner *et al.*1999) showed monotherapy was ineffective in 75% of people with Type 2 diabetes. An appropriate diet and exercise regimen remain essential regardless of whether medicines are required.

Sulphonylureas were the first OHAs to become available in the 1940s. The Biguanides followed in the 1950s. The value of these medicines has been established and they have been consistently improved over time with new generations of the original sulphonylureas. In addition, new classes of OHAs have been introduced, which might extend the life of the beta cells and delay the need for insulin (Dornhorst 2001).

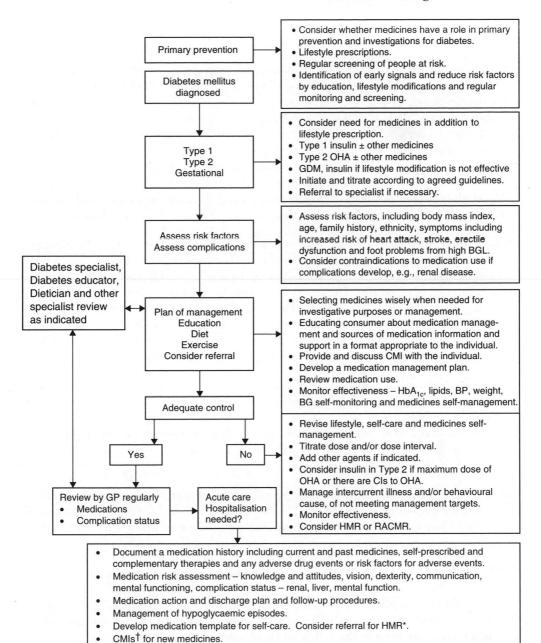

Figure 5.1 The Quality use of Medicines process applied to diabetes care reproduced from The Quality Use of Medicines in Diabetes Pharmaceutical Health And Rational use of Medicines (PHARM) Committee, Commonwealth Department of Health and Ageing (2005). The medication regimen should be reviewed each time a new medicine is required, if an adverse event occurs, and at least annually as part of routine diabetes complication procedures (September 2005 with permission). *HMR = home medicines reviews, †CMI = consumer medicines information.

OHAs target the different underlying abnormalities of glucose homeostasis associated with Type 2 diabetes. These OHAs are:

- Biguanides, which reduce insulin resistance and fasting glucose and are the medicine of first choice in overweight people with Type 2 diabetes (UKPDS 1998). Biguanides are insulin sensitisers.
- Sulphonylureas and Glitinides, which are secretagogues that stimulate insulin production. Therefore, the beta cells must be capable of responding by producing insulin. Sulphonylureas are insulin secretagogues.
- Thiazolidinediones (TZD), which reduce insulin resistance, reduce daytime preprandial hyperglycaemia, and have some effect on the fasting blood glucose.
- Alpha-glucosidase inhibitors, which slow carbohydrate digestion and glucose absorption and reduce postprandial glucose levels (Phillips 2000; Braddon 2001).

Each of these medicines can be used alone or in combination, which is common practice because they individually target different metabolic abnormalities. Biguanides and sulphonylureas reduce HbA_{1c} by 1–2% (Kuritzky 2006). OHAs can also be effectively combined with insulin. The commonly available OHAs are listed in Table 5.1.

Blood glucose and HbA_{1c} monitoring are essential to assess, whether, when, and which OHA should be commenced and when insulin is required. When OHAs are started it is necessary to monitor the blood glucose in order to appropriately adjust the dose and dose interval. Normal endogenous insulin secretion consists of two components:

(1) Basal secretion, a constant low secretion rate to suppress hepatic glucose production between meals and overnight (fasting).
(2) Bolus secretion, which occurs in response to increasing glucose levels after meals (postprandial). These insulin boluses also consist of two phases: first phase, an initial high spike, which is lost early in the development of Type 2 diabetes, and a lower more prolonged second phase.

The different OHAs and insulins target these components. Testing the blood glucose is a key to determining their effectiveness. HbA_{1c} only provides an overall average blood glucose level (see Chapter 3). Thus both measures provide important information. Key testing times are:

(1) Before breakfast to assess the fasting blood glucose, an indicator of overnight hepatic glucose output.
(2) Postprandial, usually two hours after food, to assess glucose disposal. Postprandial hyperglycaemia is common in Type 2 diabetes because of the loss of first phase insulin response early in the course of the disease.

Sometimes testing at both of these times will be required and sometimes overnight (2–3 AM) to detect nocturnal hypoglycaemia, see Chapter 6.

Biguanides

Biguanides are the medicine of first choice for overweight people with Type 2 diabetics when the HbA_{1c} is >7%. Metformin effectively lowers all-cause mortality and diabetes complications among overweight people with diabetes (UKPDS 1998). It is also used to manage insulin resistance associated with PCOS, where it may delay the progression to

Table 5.1 Oral hypoglycaemic agents, dose range and dose frequency, possible side effects, the duration of action and main site of metabolism.

Medicine	Usual daily dose	Frequency	Possible side effects	Duration of action (DA)	Site of metabolism
(1) *Sulphonylureas: these are sulphonamides, urea derivatives*					
Glibenclamide Daonil 5 mg	2.5–20 mg	Up to 10 mg as a single dose	Side effects rarely encountered include:	DA: 6–12 h Peak: 6–8 h	Liver
Euglucon 5 mg		>10 mg in divided doses	Nausea, anorexia, skin rashes		
Glimel 5 mg		Taken with, or immediately before food	Severe hypoglycaemia especially in elderly and those with renal dysfunction		
Glipizide Minidiab 5 mg	2.6–40 mg	Up to 15 mg as a single dose >15 mg in a twice daily dosage Taken immediately before meals	GIT disturbances Skin reactions Hypoglycaemia (rare)	DA: Up to 24 h Peak: 1–3 h	Liver
Gliclazide Diamicron MR (a sustained release preparation)	30–120 mg Dose increments should be two weeks apart Should not be crushed	Daily	Hypoglycaemia	Released over 24 hours	Liver
Glimepiride (Amaryl)	1–4 mg	2–3 per day	Hypoglycaemia	DA: 5–8 h	Liver

(Continued)

Table 5.1 Continued.

Medicine	Usual daily dose	Frequency	Possible side effects	Duration of action (DA)	Site of metabolism
(2) Biguanides Metformin					
Diaformin 500 mg	0.5–1.5 g	1–3 times/day	GIT disturbances	DA: 5–6 h	Unchanged in urine
Diabex 500 mg	May be increased to 3–0 g	Taken with or immediately after food	Lactic acidosis		
Glucophage 500 mg			Hypoglycaemia with other OHAs		
			Decrease B$_{12}$ absorption		
Combination sulphonylurea and biguanide					
Glucovance: metformin (M) and glibenclamide (G): M 250 mg G 1.25 mg M 500 mg, G 2.5 mg M 500 mg G 5 mg			Hypoglycaemia especially in older people Side effects associated with each medicine		Liver
(3) Glitinides Repaglinide, Nataglitinide	0.5–16 mg	2–3 per day	Hypoglycaemia with other OHAs Weight gain GIT disturbance		Liver

	Dose	Frequency	Side effects / comments	DA: 24 h	
(4) *Thiazolidinediones* Rosiglitazone;: 4, 8 mg Pioglitazone: 15, 30, 45 mg	4–8 mg	Daily	Oedema, weight gain, CCF, heart failure Raised liver enzymes, pregnancy risk in women with polycystic ovarian disease (rosiglitazone)	DA: 24 h	Liver
(5) *Alpha-glucosidase inhibitors* Acarbose: 50, 100 mg	50–100 mg	TDS with food	GIT problems, for example, flatulence, diarrhoea Hypoglycaemia		Faeces and urine
DPP-4 inhibitors (Incretin mimetics) Sitagliptin (Januvia) Vildagliptin	100 mg per day in BD regimen in combination with metformin, or a sulphonylurea (experience is with glimepride) or a TZD (experience is with pioglitazone) Moderate renal failure 50 mg Severe renal disease 25 mg	With or without food	Hypoglycaemia – reduce dose of sulphonylurea if used as dual therapy to reduce hypoglycaemia risk Safety with insulin has not been established More research is needed in older people		Unchanged in urine

Note: Only some of the many trade named formulations are listed. Formulations in each class have similar actions although there are minor differences among them. The table is a guide only. Specific prescribing information for each medicine should be consulted as well as relevant regulatory authority licensing and approvals. Combination medicines such as Glucovance (metformin and glibenclamide) may be useful in reducing the overall number of medicines an individual needs to take.

Type 2 diabetes and is being trialed in the treatment of GDM (Hamilton *et al.* 2003), see Chapter 14. Metformin is the most commonly used Biguanide. It acts by:

- Impairing the absorption of glucose from the gut.
- Inhibiting hepatic glucose output.
- Increasing glucose uptake in peripheral tissues (muscle and fat).
- Increasing the effects of insulin at receptor sites.
- Suppressing the appetite (mild effect).

Practice points

(1) Biguanides do not stimulate the production or release of insulin and therefore, are unlikely to cause hypoglycaemia.
(2) They have favourable effects on the lipid profile and slow glucose absorption from the intestine.
(3) They do not stimulate the appetite and are unlikely to cause weight gain.

Possible side effects

(1) Nausea and/or diarrhoea occurs in 10–15% of patients. Most patients tolerate Biguanides if they are started at a low dose, the tablets are taken with or immediately after food, and the dosage is increased gradually.
(2) Lactic acidosis is the most significant side effect, see Chapter 7. Although lactic acidosis is rare, 48 cases were reported to the Australian Adverse Drug Reactions Advisory Committee (ADRAC) between 1985 and 2001. Of these, known risk factors were present in 35 of the 48 cases (Jerrell 2002). However, the true incidence is unknown and could be higher because not all adverse events are reported. Nisbet *et al.* (2004) identified 13 cases of lactic acidosis possibly related to metformin since 2000. Of these, two died, three required dialysis for renal failure, and one had severe neurological deficits and required nursing home care. The average age was 67 and average serum creatinine was 0.31 mmol/L (normal 0.05–0.11 women; 0.06–0.12 men mmol/L). Nisbet *et al.*'s study highlights the importance of appropriate clinical assessment before prescribing or represcribing medicines, especially in older people. The risk of lactic acidosis is increased in people with diseases likely to cause hypoxia such as alcohol abuse and liver, renal, and cardiac disease. Early signs of lactic acidosis include:
    - anorexia
    - nausea and vomiting
    - abdominal pain
    - cramps
    - weight loss
    - lethargy
    - respiratory distress.
(3) Biguanides should not be prescribed:
    - during pregnancy
    - for patients with chronic renal failure

- Type 1 diabetes
- any disease likely to cause hypoxia such as severe respiratory diseases and hepatic or cardiovascular disease.

There is some evidence that at higher doses and longer duration of use metformin inhibits absorption of vitamin B_{12}. The metformin dose is the strongest predictor of vitamin B_{12} deficiency (Ting *et al.* 2006). However, Ting *et al.* did not assess calcium intake or measure vitamin B_{12} metabolites (homocysteine and methylmalonic acid), which could have affected the results. Nevertheless, Vitamin B_{12} deficiency should be considered in people at high risk of malnourishment, for example, older people and those with eating disorders, people who have been on metformin for long periods of time especially at high doses, and those with malabsorption syndromes.

Biguanides should be ceased for two days before IVP, CAT scans and investigations that require IV-iodinated contrast media to be used (Calabrese *et al.* 2002).

Sulphonylureas

Sulphonylureas can be used alone or combined with metformin. They are usually well tolerated but there is a tendency for people to gain weight, especially with older OHAs. Weight gain occurs to a less extent with newer OHAs (Inzucchi 2002). They generally have a rapid onset of action except for long-acting formulations. Hypoglycaemia is a risk especially in older people on long-acting agents, although these are rarely used and are no longer available in some countries. However, glibenclamide is available in combination with metformin (Glucovance). People with renal impairment and those who are malnourished are also at risk of hypoglycaemia.

Sulphonylureas act by:

- Stimulating insulin secretion from the pancreatic beta cells.
- Increasing the effects of insulin at its receptor sites.
- Sensitising hepatic glucose production to inhibition by insulin.

Possible side effects

(1) Hypoglycaemia may result due to oversecretion of insulin if the dose of the OHA is increased, food is delayed, meals are missed, or activity is increased see Chapter 6
(2) Liver dysfunction
(3) Nausea, vomiting
(4) Various skin rashes
(5) Increased appetite
(6) *Rarely*, agranulocytosis and red cell aplasia may also occur.

Note: (2)–(6) are very uncommon. Sulphonylureas are contraindicated in pregnancy although they are used during pregnancy in some countries. They are mostly metabolised in the liver and severe liver disease is a contraindication to their use. Caution should be taken in people who are allergic to 'sulphur medicines' because the sulphonylureas have a similar chemical makeup.

Glitinides

These medicines increase insulin secretion at meal times and they should only be taken with meals, usually 2–3 times per day. They are short acting and have a low hypoglycaemic risk.

They target early phase insulin secretion, which is essential for postprandial glucose and control the postprandial glucose load (Dornhorst 2001). In this way they initiate an insulin response pattern close to normal. They can be used in combination with Biguanides and possibly Thiazolidinediones (TZD). The two main formulations are repaglinide and nataglinide. These medicines are rarely used in Australia because they are not listed on the PBS. However, because of their short duration of action and the requirement to take them with meals they could be very useful in older people at high risk of hypoglycaemia.

Thiazolidinediones

The Thiazolidinediones (TZD) are also known as peroxisome-proliferator-activated receptor-γ (PPAR-γ). They are given as a daily dose. It takes several days before they show an effect. In Australia, authority is required to prescribe TZDs and they are not subsidised for use as monotherapy (Schedule of Pharmaceutical Benefits (PBS) 2006). There are two forms Pioglitazone and Rosiglitazone. Pioglitazone can be used as dual therapy in combination with metformin OR a sulphonylurea in Type 2 diabetes when the HbA_{1c} is >7% when combining metformin and a sulphonylurea is contraindicated. It can be combined with insulin in Type 2 diabetes if the HbA_{1c} is >7% despite treatment with OHAs and insulin, OR insulin alone OR if metformin is contraindicated. Rosiglitazone can be combined with metformin AND a sulphonylurea in Type 2 diabetes when the HbA_{1c} is >7% despite maximum tolerated doses of these medicines.

TZDs reduce HbA_{1c} by ~1–2% (Ko *et al.* 2006) with similar improvements to adding insulin. However, long-term data is not yet available for TZDs. If adding a TZD does not adequately reduce HbA_{1c} to <8 5% in 3 months, insulin should be commenced (Nathan *et al.* 2006).

Practice points

(1) Pioglitazone is not listed for use as monotherapy or triple therapy in Australia. It can only be prescribed as dual therapy with metformin OR a sulphonylurea OR insulin.
(2) Rosiglitazone can be used as triple therapy with metformin and a sulphonylurea.
(3) It is usual to start at low dose and monitor the person closely for signs of heart failure especially those with pre-existing cardiovascular disease. Significant cardiovascular disease is a contraindication to TZDs.
(4) Rosigitazone might prevent/delay the transition to Type 2 diabetes in at-risk individuals (DREAM 2006). However, subsequent modelling of the DREAM data suggests people taking rosiglitazone to prevent diabetes would end up taking more medicines than those who start medicines after diabetes is diagnosed and are at risk of TZD side effects (Montori *et al.* 2007).

TZDs lower fasting and postprandial blood glucose by increasing insulin sensitivity in muscle, fat, and liver cells. Some improve lipid profiles, enhance insulin sensitivity and may restore the beta cell mass.

An early form of the medicine was responsible for causing liver failure and was withdrawn from the market. This effect is unlikely with currently available TZDs but it is recommended that liver function be monitored and caution be exercised in people with liver damage or whose albumin excretion rate is elevated.

Hypoglycaemia is possible because TZDs reduce insulin resistance and enhance the effectiveness of endogenous insulin.

Side effects

- Localised oedema, which can be significant and may occur to a greater extent in people treated with TZD and insulin (product prescribing information: Actos 2004; Avandia 2005).
- Congestive cardiac failure and heart failure. People with diabetes are 2.5 times more likely to develop heart failure than non-diabetics (Nichols *et al.* 2004) and TZDs increase the risk of heart failure. Rosiglitazone doubles the risk among those with pre-existing cardiovascular disease (Home *et al.* 2007). TZDs are contraindicated in people with New York Heart Association Class III or IV heart failure. The person should be closely monitored for signs of heart failure such as oedema and rapid weight gain.
- Myocardial infarction and death associated with rosiglitazone (Nissen & Wolski 2007). This report caused significant debate among diabetes experts and stress for patients prescribed rosiglitazone. The risk appears to be small (DREAM 2006). The information should be used in the context of individual risk. For example, rosiglitazone might increase the risk of MI in people with ischaemic heart disease, those on insulin or nitrates, those with an atherogenic lipid profile, and those at high risk of MI (ADRAC 2007). Pioglitazone does not appear to carry the same risk because it has fewer adverse effects on lipids (Dormandy *et al.* 2005). Diabetes Australia recommended patients not to stop rosiglitazone without consulting their doctor. The Australian Diabetes Society (2007) issued a position statement recommending patient's concerns be acknowledged, rosiglitazone continued to be used until further evidence arises, or discontinuing rosiglitazone and maintaining glycaemic control using other OHAs or commencing insulin. Regulatory authorities such as the FDA and NPS issued advisories but did not withdraw or limit the prescribing indications for rosiglitazone at the time,
- Reduced red and white cell counts.
- Weight gain, especially deposition of subcutaneous fat, while visceral obesity is reduced. Weight gain appears to continue as long as TZDs are continued. Gains between 2 and 5 kg are reported (Dormandy *et al.* 2005). However, insulin also causes weight gain (~3 kg), as do sulphonylureas (~4 kg). Weight gain is lower when patients are taking metformin before a TZD is added (Strowig 2004).
- Hypercholesterolaemia.
- Liver damage although it is uncommon. TZDs are contraindicated if liver disease is present or serum transiminase is >2.5 times the upper limit of the normal. Liver function tests should be performed before starting a TZD and then monitored regularly while the patient remains on TZDs. Signs of liver toxicity include nausea, vomiting, jaundice, dark urine, and right upper abdominal discomfort.

- Macular oedema (European Medicine Agency Press 2005). Macular oedema is a known complication of diabetes and there some reports the condition worsens with TZD.
- Fractures occurring in the arms and lower leg usually in women (Khan *et al.* 2006), however the risk is small. Fracture risk may be significant in older women at risk of osteoporosis and increase the risk of falls if the fractures occur in the feet or legs.
- Women with Polycystic Ovarian Disease should be counselled about contraception because TZDs may improve fertility in these women.
- They are contraindicated in pregnancy and during breast feeding.
- Care should be taken in lactose intolerant people because TZDs contain a small amount of lactose.

These data suggest a thorough assessment including a medication review is warranted before commencing TZDs. Health professionals and people with diabetes should be alert to the possibility of silent MI.

Alpha-glucosidase inhibitors

These medicines are usually taken in a TDS regimen.

They act by slowing glucose uptake of many carbohydrates by inhibiting alpha-glucosidase, which slows the breakdown of complex and simple carbohydrates in the brush border of the proximal small intestine so the glucose load is spread over a longer time frame. They reduce fasting and postprandial glucose.

Their major side effects are due to the arrival of undigested carbohydrate in the lower bowel – bloating, flatulence, and diarrhoea. These symptoms can be distressing and embarrassing and people often stop their medications because of these side effects.

Taking the medicines with meals, starting with a low dose and increasing slowly to tolerance levels, and careful explanation to the patient can reduce these problems.

Hypoglycaemia is possible if they are combined with other OHAs. They may be contraindicated or need to be used with caution in people with gastrointestinal disease such as gastroparesis, coeliac disease, and irritable bowel syndrome.

Practice point

Oral glucose may not be an effective treatment for hypoglycaemia occurring in people on alpha-glucosidase inhibitors because absorption from the gut will be delayed. IM Glucagon is an alternative.

The incretin hormones

The incretins enhance glucose-mediated insulin secretion by the beta cells. Approximately 60% of insulin secreted in response to food is due to the activity of incretins (Eli Lilly 2005). The incretin effect is due to peptide hormones released by K and L cells in the intestine directly into the blood stream. The incretins include:

(1) Glucose-dependent insulinotropic peptide (GIP) secreted by the K-intestinal cells. Postprandially, GIP levels are ~10 times higher than GLP-1 and have similar insulinotrophic actions when the glucose level is ≤6 mmol/L, but its effects are limited at blood glucose levels >7.8 mmol/L. GIP does not inhibit glucagon secretion. It is not clear whether it has any effect on eating behaviour.

(2) Glucagon-like peptide (GLP-1) is secreted by the L-cells in the intestine. It primarily regulates postprandial glucose. GLP-1 binds to its specific receptor but has a very short half-life (60–90 seconds) because it is rapidly broken down by dipeptidyl peptidase-1V (DPP-1V). The active metabolites may act as GLP-1 receptor antagonists. GLP-1:
   (a) stimulates insulin in a glucose-dependent way
   (b) suppresses postprandial glucagon secretion, thus reducing hepatic glucose output
   (c) maintains an appropriate ratio of gastric acid secretion to food solids in the stomach
   (d) regulates gastric emptying, which reduces food intake
   (e) has a central effect on the brain in regulating food intake
   (f) there is some evidence that GLP-1 may stimulate beta cell proliferation (Abraham *et al.* 2002).

The incretin hormones are either incretin mimetics or incretin enhancers. GLP-1 is a mimetic (receptor agonist) injectable synthetic agent, for example, Exanatide (Byetta); sometimes referred to as 'lizard spit'. It lowers HbA_{1c} by 0.5–1% (Nathan *et al.* 2006). Incretin enhancers are oral agents known as DPP-1V inhibitors, for example, Sitagliptin (Januvia) and Vildagliptin, see Table 5.1.

Medicine interactions

Possible interactions between OHAs and other commonly prescribed medicines are shown in Table 5.2.

Medicine and OHA interactions are possible and can lead to hypo- or hyperglycaemia. A number of mechanisms for the interactions are known and they include:

- Displacing the medicine from binding sites;
- Inhibiting or decreasing hepatic metabolism;
- Delaying excretion;
- Reducing insulin release;
- Antagonising insulin action.

Consideration should also be given to potential medicine and herb or herb/herb interactions, see Chapter 19.

Table 5.2 Potential medicine interactions between oral hypoglycaemic agents and other medicines (based on Shenfield 2001).

Medicine	Possible mechanism
Medicines that increase blood glucose	
Clonidine	Adrenergic response
Clozapine	Impaired insulin secretion
Corticosteroids	Oppose insulin action
Diuretics, especially Thiazides	Oppose insulin action
Nicotinic acid	Unknown
Nifedipine	Delays insulin action
Oral contraceptives	Unknown
Phenytoin	Impairs insulin secretion
Sugar-containing medicines, for example, cough syrup	Increase blood glucose
Medicines that lower blood glucose	
ACE inhibitors	Enhance insulin action
Alcohol	Reduce hepatic glucose production
Fibrates	Unknown
MOA inhibitors	Unknown
Salicylates	Unknown

Practice points

(1) The clinical relevance of some postulated medicine interactions is uncertain.
(2) Other miscellaneous interactions that should also be considered are:
  • beta blockers can mask tachycardia and other signs of hypoglycaemia resulting in delayed recognition and treatment increasing the risk of hypoglycaemic coma.
  • chronic alcohol consumption can stimulate the metabolism of sulphonylureas and delay their effectiveness, cause hypoglycaemia, mask signs of hypoglycaemia, and with metformin, predispose the individual to lactic acidosis. It may also increase the bioavailability of ACE-1.

Potential interactions have not yet emerged for TZIs and the glitinides. Medicines that alter hepatic enzymes have the potential to cause interactions with these OHAs because they are metabolised in the liver.

Medicines that interfere with access to the gut by alpha-glucosidase inhibitors can inhibit their action, for example, charcoal, digestive enzymes, cholestyramine, neomycin, and some CAM medicines such as slippery elm.

Combining OHAs and insulin

Any combination of currently available OHAs only lowers HbA_{1c} by ~3% (Endocrinologists Medical Guidelines for the Management of Type 2 Diabetes 2002), thus people with HbA$_{1c}$ >10% are unlikely to achieve management targets using OHA alone. Therefore, insulin is assuming an increasingly important role in Type 2 diabetes. As indicated, most people with Type 2 diabetes have progressive beta cell dysfunction and a decline in beta cell mass. Proposed mechanisms for these defects include the interplay among a range of factors that reduce beta cell mass and secretory function such as hyperglycaemia, elevated free fatty acids, and inflammatory processes

Practice point

Medication administration times should be planned so that OHAs are administered with, or before, meals to reduce the risk of hypoglycaemia.

associated with adipocyte-derived cytokines. Apoptosis appears to be a key underlying mechanism (Leiter 2006). In addition, lifestyle factors, concomitant diseases, and often medicines, compound the metabolic abnormalities. In some cases medication non-adherence may be a factor and should be assessed in a non-judgmental manner.

When should insulin be initiated in Type 2 diabetes?

Commencing insulin should be a proactive decision and should not be delayed. Some experts refer to 'tablet failure'. The choice of words should be considered carefully when conveying the need for insulin to a patient: they may interpret 'tablet failure' to mean *they* have failed.

The time to commence insulin in Type 2 diabetes depends on the individual's blood glucose pattern, HbA$_{1c}$, adherence to medicines, and complication status especially cardiovascular and renal status and willingness to use insulin. Indications for insulin include:

- Women with Type 2 diabetes who become pregnant and sometimes women with gestational diabetes, see Chapter 14.
- When the person actually has LADA (see Chapter 1).
- As rescue therapy in DKA, HONK, during other acute illnesses, and surgical procedures, see Chapters 7 and 9.
- Persisting hyperglycaemia indicated by elevated fasting blood glucose and/or random postprandial blood glucose.
- Symptomatic especially polyuria, polydipsia and weight loss.
- OHA intolerance or contraindication, for example, metformin if creatinine is high.
- People on two OHAs and not achieving targets where insulin may be preferable to adding a third OHA given that most people with Type 2 diabetes eventually need insulin especially if the OHAs are at maximal doses. However, there is no consensus about whether the second agent added to metformin should be another OHA or insulin. Insulin might be preferable if the HbA$_{1c}$ is >8.5% or the person is very symptomatic (Nathan *et al.* 2006). In these cases it might be appropriate to consider LADA especially if the individual is thin. The National Prescribing Service advised health professionals to be '... more aggressive in their management of patients with Type 2 diabetes' (NPS media release, 26 March 2008).

- Recent research suggests insulin may have anti-inflammatory properties in addition to its other actions (Dandona *et al.* 2008).

The goals are to achieve optimal control without causing hypoglycaemia or excessive weight gain and with minimal impact on lifestyle. Thus, understanding the individual's perspective is essential. For some peoples commencing insulin and ceasing OHAs may represent a simpler more manageable medication regime.

Insulin is often added to the OHA regimen at bedtime to reduce fasting glucose levels (Riddle *et al.* 2003; Janka *et al.* 2005). The dose is titrated according to the fasting blood glucose pattern including self-adjustment by the patient to achieve targets with minimal hypoglycaemia according to a simple algorithm (Yki-Jarvinen *et al.* 2007). Yki-Jarvinen *et al.* (2007) showed insulin could be successfully initiated in groups and achieve glycaemic targets. In addition, group insulin initiation was acceptable to patients.

The specific initiation process depends on the policies and guidelines of individual health services. Over recent years, research has demonstrated the efficacy of several processes for initiating and titrating insulin in Type 2 diabetes using various insulins and usually starting with small doses. They all used a stepwise approach and include:

- The Treat-To-Target study used basal Glargine at bedtime and titrated the dose weekly in 10 weeks (Riddle *et al.* 2003). This regimen is suitable for older people because it is associated with fewer hypoglycaemic events and is well tolerated (Janka *et al.* 2005). Isophane insulin can also be used as the basal insulin but has a higher risk of hypoglycaemia.
- The 1-2-3 study, which used daily bedtime doses of NovoMix 30 initially and subsequently added doses pre-breakfast then pre-lunch if necessary to achieve targets (Raskin *et al.* 2005).
- The INITIATE study that used BD doses of NovoMix 30 (Jain *et al.* 2005).

The advantage of using basal bolus insulin dose regimens is that they usually achieve better postprandial control but eating after injecting is important. BD Lispro/isophane mix and Metformin also improves pre and postprandial blood glucose with few episodes of nocturnal hypoglycaemia (Malone *et al.* 2005).

Many researchers have compared different brands of insulin and dose regimens. Overall, the findings suggest the pharmacokinetic differences among insulin brands may not be clinically relevant and there are likely to be variations in individual patient's response to the different formulations (Zeolla 2007). In reality, the choice of insulin may actually be made according to prescriber preference and local availability. Despite the similarities, indiscriminate switching between different insulin brands or using them simultaneously is not generally recommended.

Except in specific circumstances, outpatient or community-based initiation is preferable.

A proforma initiation process is outlined in this chapter that can be adapted as necessary and a simple algorithm for commencing insulin in Type 2 diabetes is shown in Figure 5.2. Usually, OHAs are continued with basal insulin regimens if there are no contraindications to their use. When bolus insulin doses are added secretagogue doses are usually reduced or the medicines discontinued.

Figure 5.2   Algorithm for achieving blood glucose targets in Type 2 diabetes that encompasses a quality use of medicines approach and adopts a proactive stepwise approach to initiating insulin.

The algorithm is based on the premise that the individual undertakes blood glucose monitoring, relevant monitoring and assessments are undertaken, relevant education is provided and the response to therapy is monitored at each step. Consider LADA if the person is not overweight, loses weight, has significant hyperglycaemia, and is very symptomatic because insulin should not be delayed in these people, see Chapter 1.

Management aims:

(1) Proactively initiate insulin. Insulin should not be delayed
(2) Control fasting and postprandial hyperglycaemia without causing serious hyperglycaemia
(3) Achieve HbA_{1c} target relevant to the age of the individual generally <7% but maybe higher in older people
(4) Normalise lipids to reduce cardiovascular risk
(5) Control symptoms

OHA = oral hypoglycaemic agents; TZD = Thiazolidinediones.

Barriers to insulin therapy

There are many barriers to initiating insulin therapy in Type 2 diabetes: most relate to either the individual with diabetes or health professional factors. Although patients often view insulin negatively, early explanations about the nature of Type 2 diabetes (from diagnosis), with support and encouragement most people usually accept they need insulin. However, their fears and concerns must be acknowledged and respected. People often regard insulin as 'the last resort', fear hypoglycaemia, and weight gain (Dunning & Martin 1999). The DAWN study (Rutherford *et al.* 2004) showed people on insulin worried about hypoglycaemia more than non-insulin users and insulin was associated with worse quality of life in people with Type 2 diabetes.

Type 2 diabetes is a silent disease with few symptoms; thus, it is often difficult for people to accept they have a serious, progressive disease. They are often reluctant to test their blood glucose frequently and feel blood glucose monitoring and insulin interferes with their lifestyle. For some people, the stigma associated with needles is an issue.

Many doctors are reluctant to use insulin in Type 2 diabetes and often compound the patient's concerns, albeit usually unintentionally, by delaying insulin initiation. This has been referred to as 'clinical inertia' (Riedel *et al.* 2006), and, like non-adherence is a complex, multifactorial issue. Other health professional-related barriers include inadequate knowledge, lack of time, support and resources, worry about causing hypoglycaemia and complicating the management regimen. For example, UK practice nurses felt commencing insulin in primary care was beneficial for patients but lack of time, support, and confidence, and concerns about medico-legal implications and personal accountability made it difficult to achieve (Greaves *et al.* 2003).

Some strategies to overcome the barriers

The therapeutic relationship between the patient and the health professional has a significant effect on health outcomes and patient behaviours including adherence to medicines and improved safety (Worthington 2003). Thus, a first step is to establish a non-judgmental, trusting relationship. Specific approaches depend on the individual and the circumstances in which insulin is required. Health professionals need to acknowledge that:

- Managing insulin is a complex process and is only one self-care and life task the person is expected to fulfil.
- 'Things might get worse before they get better'. For example vision often deteriorates temporarily.
- The ability to self-care changes over time due to physical and mental functional changes often associated with diabetes complications.
- There are usually added costs involved.

The transformational model of change can be a useful framework for addressing the need to commence insulin, especially if it is integrated with aspects of the health belief model and holistic care, where insulin is discussed as one aspect to be addressed not an isolated event in a person's life. Research suggests timing is important when trying to initiate change. That is it needs to be linked to an individual's stage in the change process (Prochaska & Velicer 1997) and significant life transitions, which are often also accompanied by changes in identity and behaviour (George 1993).

Providing personalised and customised advice and written information is most useful when it is delivered in a caring relationship where the individual's concerns are acknowledged and they are invited to suggest ways they could address the issues they identity. Thus, listening, clarifying, and following up by asking about progress are essential. However, despite the focus on patient-centred care, the patient's views are often not sought and they are inadvertently placed in a passive rather than an active role particularly when communication barriers such as language, culture, or disabilities are present.

Identifying and discussing the person's concerns is essential. For example, 'needle phobia', weight gain, and hypoglycaemia. Demonstrating the various insulin delivery devices often helps reduce some concerns about needles. People on insulin gain more weight than those on diet over 10 years (Mayfield & White 2004) due to better glycaemic control and losing less glucose in the urine, the fact that insulin is an anabolic hormone, lower metabolic rate and people may eat more to prevent hypoglycaemia (Birkeland *et al.* 1994). Weight gain appears to be less on Levemir in both Type 1 and Type 2 diabetes (Dornhurst *et al.* 2007).

Strategies to avoid weight gain include selecting insulin formulations and other medicines least likely to contribute to weight gain if possible, regular exercise perhaps using a pedometer, and individualised nutrition advice. Once symptoms are controlled people often feel more active and exercise helps control weight and blood glucose.

Understanding and exploring the person's concerns about hypoglycaemia and helping them identify strategies to reduce the incidence. Explain that the frequency and severity of hypoglycaemia is lower in people with Type 2 diabetes than Type 1 diabetes (UKPDS 1999). The risk increases when the HbA_{1c} is <7.4%. Carefully explaining the likely risk factors and helping the person develop strategies to minimise their individual risk is important.

Vision can deteriorate when insulin is commenced. Sight is not usually threatened but it is very distressing for the person with diabetes and they need a careful explanation and reassurance to help them understand. Activities of daily living such as reading and driving can be affected. Visual changes occur because the lens absorbs excess glucose in much the same way as sponge soaks up water. Changes in the amount of glucose in the lens can lead to blurred vision and can occur with high and low blood glucose levels. This phenomenon is quite different from diabetic retinopathy, which can threaten the sight.

The starting dose may not be the 'right' dose and the 'right' dose changes according to specific circumstances and individual need.

Insulin therapy

Overview of insulin action

Insulin is a hormone secreted by the beta cells of the pancreas. Normal requirements are between 0.5 and 1.0 units/kg/day. Insulin synthesis and secretion are stimulated by an increase in the blood glucose level after meals. Insulin attaches to insulin receptors on cell membranes to facilitate the passage of glucose into the cell for utilisation as fuel or storage, and reduces hepatic glucose production. Insulin also stimulates the storage of fatty acids and amino acids, facilitates glycogen formation and storage in the liver and skeletal muscle, and limits lipolysis and proteolysis. Therefore, insulin deficiency results in altered protein, fat and carbohydrate metabolism (also refer to Chapter 1).

Insulin is vital to survival for people with Type 1 diabetes and is eventually required by most people with Type 2 diabetes.

Objectives of insulin therapy

(1) To achieve blood glucose and lipid levels within an acceptable individual range by replacing absent insulin secretion in Type 1 and supplementing insulin production in Type 2 diabetes (see previous section).
(2) To approximate physiological insulin secretion and action.
(3) To avoid the consequences of too much insulin (hypoglycaemia) or too little insulin (hyperglycaemia).
(4) Improve quality of life and reduce the risk of long-term diabetes complications.

Types of insulin available

Insulin cannot be given orally at this stage. It is a polypeptide. Polypeptides are digested by gastric enzymes and do not reach the circulation. Research is currently underway to coat insulin in a substance that can withstand gastric juices and enable it to pass unchanged into the intestine before breaking down. Inhaled insulin is also the subject of research but is not generally used in clinical practice. Likewise, some trials have been abandoned.

A number of different brands of insulins are available, for example, Novo Nordisk, Eli Lilly, and SanofiAventis.

Animal insulins (bovine and porcine) are rarely used nowadays but still available in some countries often under special access schemes. 'Human' insulin (HM) is manufactured by recombinant DNA technology . The amino acid sequence of HM insulin is the same as that of insulin secreted by the beta cells of the human pancreas. In the past few years rapid acting insulin analogues have been developed that give a more physiologic response after injection and improve the blood glucose profile, for example, Humalog, Aspart, and Apidra. The advantages of these insulins are reduced postprandial hyperglycaemia and reduced risk of hypoglycaemia.

Long-acting analogues are Glargine and Levemir. Glargine has a slower onset than Isophane insulins and a smooth peakless action profile for up to 24 hours (Buse 2001). Levimir may be shorter acting than Glargine and has its maximal effect between 3 and 14 hours. It was only registered for use in Type 1 diabetes in Australia at the time of writing. These insulins enable greater management flexibility and lower risk of hypoglycaemia.

Rapid acting insulin

Rapid acting insulin should be clear and colourless. Examples are:

- Lispro (Humalog)
- Novorapid (Aspart)
- Glulisine (Apidra)

They have a rapid onset of action, within 10–15 minutes, peak at 60 minutes and act for 2–4 hours.

They need to be given *immediately* before meals and are used in basal bolus regimes, in combination with intermediate acting insulin and long–acting analogues, or used in combination with OHAs or in insulin pumps.

Combining them with alpha-glucosidase inhibitors, which reduce glucose absorption from the gut, can increase the risk of hypoglycaemia.

The first hour after injection and 2–3 hours after exercise are other peak times for hypoglycaemia.

Short-acting insulin

This should be clear and colourless. Examples are:

- Actrapid
- Humulin R
- Hypurin neutral (beef)

They begin to take effect in 20–30 minutes, and act between 4 and 8 hours. They can be used:

- Alone two to four times per day.
- In combination with intermediate or long-acting insulins.
- As IV insulin infusions

Intermediate-acting insulin

This must be mixed gently before use and should be milky after mixing. Examples are:

- Protophane
- Humulin NPH
- Hypurin (isophane)

They begin to act in 2–3 hours. The duration of action is between 12 and 18 hours. They can be used:

- In combination with short-acting insulin – this is the usual method.
- Alone for patients who are sensitive to short-acting insulin, or in combination with oral hypoglycaemic agents.

Long-acting insulin

- Glargine (Lantus)
- Detemir (Levemir) as described in the preceding section.

Biphasic insulins

Biphasic insulins are often prescribed for people with Type 2 diabetes.

These contain both short- and intermediate-acting insulins in various combinations. They must be mixed before using. They do not enable independent adjustment of the short or intermediate components. Examples are:

- Mixtard 30/70   Humalin 30/70
- Mixtard 50/50   Humulin Mix 50
- NovoMix 30   Humalog Mix 25

The range of Lilly insulins is shown in Figure 5.3 and the Novo Nordisk range in Figure 5.4. They also depict the insulin delivery devices available for each product. Apidra is dispensed in a prefilled disposable injection device (Apidra SoloStar) and is blue to distinguish it from the Lantus SoloStar, which is white and mauve and is also disposable. Lantus is also dispensed in 3 mL cartridges and 10 mL glass vials. Each insulin administration device has advantages and disadvantages and patient preference should be considered (see Table 5.3). The diabetes educator can help individuals decide which device (and therefore, to some extent which insulin) suits them best.

Storing insulin

The temperature at which insulin is stored is important to maintaining its efficacy. Insulin should be stored according to the manufacturer's directions. Unopened vials should be stored in the refrigerator at 2–8°C. Insulin vials in use can be stored out of the refrigerator, for example, in the patient's medication drawer, provided they are not stored near a source of heat or light (Campbell *et al.* 1993; individual product prescribing information).

People with diabetes need to be educated about correct storage and handling of insulin as well as sharps disposal as part of their education about insulin therapy.

Clinical observation

Hyperglycaemia associated with using incorrectly stored insulin and insulin that has passed the expiry date does occur.

Practice points

(1) Long-acting analogues cannot be mixed with other insulins. Nor can they be injected in the same site.
(2) They are clear and great care must be taken to ensure they are not mistaken for rapid or short-acting insulins. Look alike medicine alert policies should be initiated. For example, consider storing them in a different part of the refrigerator and clearly flagging them with a 'look alike' medication alert label.
(3) Carefully check the dose to be administered of NovoMix 30 and Humalog Mix 25 or 50 and do not mistake the numbers in the name of the insulin for the insulin dose, which has occurred and led to an adverse medicine event.

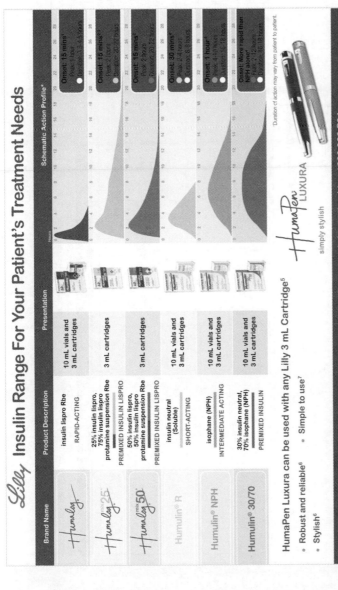

Figure 5.3 Range of Lilly insulins, their presentation and schematic action profiles. Reproduced with permission from Eli Lilly Australia Pty Ltc. PBS information refers to Australian prescribing information.

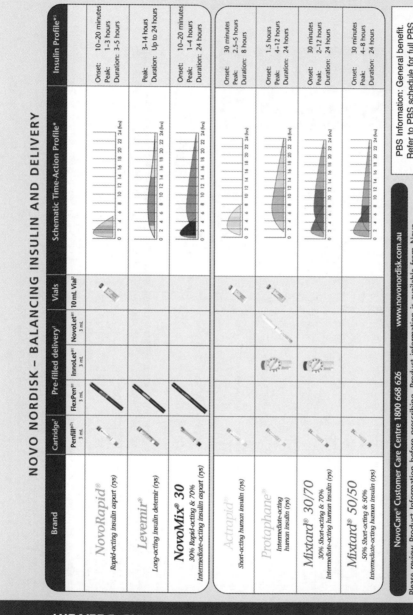

NOVO NORDISK – BALANCING INSULIN AND DELIVERY

Brand	Cartridge	Pre-filled delivery			Vials	Schematic Time-Action Profile*	Insulin Profile*
	Penfill 3 mL	FlexPen 3 mL	InnoLet 3 mL	NovoLet 3 mL	10 mL Vial		
NovoRapid® Rapid-acting insulin aspart (rys)							Onset: 10–20 minutes Peak: 1–3 hours Duration: 3–5 hours
Levemir® Long-acting insulin detemir (rys)							Peak: 3–14 hours Duration: Up to 24 hours
NovoMix® 30 30% Rapid-acting & 70% Intermediate-acting insulin aspart (rys)							Onset: 10–20 minutes Peak: 1–4 hours Duration: 24 hours
Actrapid® Short-acting human insulin (rys)							Onset: 30 minutes Peak: 2.5–5 hours Duration: 8 hours
Protaphane® Intermediate-acting human insulin (rys)							Onset: 1.5 hours Peak: 4–12 hours Duration: 24 hours
Mixtard® 30/70 30% Short-acting & 70% Intermediate-acting human insulin (rys)							Onset: 30 minutes Peak: 2–12 hours Duration: 24 hours
Mixtard® 50/50 50% Short-acting & 50% Intermediate-acting human insulin (rys)							Onset: 30 minutes Peak: 4–8 hours Duration: 24 hours

NovoCare® Customer Care Centre 1800 668 626   www.novonordisk.com.au

Please review Product Information before prescribing. Product information is available from Novo Nordisk Customer Care Centre 1800 668 626. Novo Nordisk Pharmaceuticals Pty Ltd. ABN 40 002 879 996. Level 3, 21 Solent Circuit, Baulkham Hills, NSW 2153. ® Registered trademark of Novo Nordisk A/S

PBS Information: General benefit.
Refer to PBS schedule for full PBS listing information for each product.
Levemir: Restricted benefit.
Type 1 diabetes.

novo nordisk

NOVO NORDISK – BALANCING INSULIN AND DELIVERY

(a)

(b)

MINIMUM PRODUCT INFORMATION*
NovoMix® 30 (insulin aspart) (rys)
Indications: Treatment of diabetes mellitus. **Contraindications:** Hypoglycaemia. Hypersensitivity to insulin aspart or excipients. **Precautions:** Inadequate dosing or discontinuation of treatment, especially in type 1 diabetes, may lead to hyperglycaemia and diabetic ketoacidosis. Where blood glucose is greatly improved, e.g. by intensified insulin therapy, patients may experience a change in usual warning symptoms of hypoglycaemia, and should be advised accordingly. The impact of the rapid onset of action should be considered in patients where a delayed absorption of food might be expected. Do not use in insulin infusion pumps. No studies in children and adolescents under the age of 18. No clinical experience in pregnancy. **Adverse Effects:** hypoglycaemia. **Dosage and Administration:** Dosage as determined by physician. NovoMix®30 should be administered immediately before a meal, or when necessary after the start of a meal. Resuspend immediately before use. Discard the needle after each injection. Subcutaneous injection only. NovoMix®30 must not be administered intravenously. Refer to full PI before prescribing, available on request (June 2007).

*Note changes in Product Information

Novo Nordisk Pharmaceuticals Pty Ltd
A.B.N. 40 002 879 996
Level 3, 21 Solent Circuit
Baulkham Hills NSW 2153

MINIMUM PRODUCT INFORMATION*
NovoRapid® (insulin aspart) (rys)
Indication: Treatment of diabetes mellitus. **Contraindications:** Hypoglycaemia. Hypersensitivity to insulin aspart or excipients. **Precautions:** Inadequate dosing or discontinuation of treatment may lead to hyperglycaemia and diabetic ketoacidosis. Where blood glucose is greatly improved, e.g. by intensified insulin therapy, patients may experience a change in usual warning symptoms of hypoglycaemia, and should be advised accordingly. The impact of the rapid onset of action should be considered in patients where a delayed absorption of food might be expected. *Pregnancy Category: A.* NovoRapid (insulin aspart) can be used in pregnancy. Data from two

randomised controlled clinical trials (157 + 14 insulin aspart-exposed pregnancies, respectively) did not indicate any adverse effect of insulin aspart on pregnancy or on the health of the foetus/newborn when compared to human insulin (see 'Clinical Trials' in full PI). Intensified blood glucose control and monitoring treatment of pregnant women with diabetes (type 1 diabetes, type 2 diabetes or gestational diabetes) are recommended throughout pregnancy and when contemplating pregnancy. **Adverse Effects:** hypoglycaemia. **Dosage and Administration:** Dosage as determined by physician. NovoRapid® should be administered immediately before a meal, or when necessary after the start of a meal. Discard the needle after each injection. *NovoRapid can be used in children. Clinical experience is available in children aged 2 years and over (see 'Clinical Trials' in full PI). NovoRapid® can be used during pregnancy (see 'Use in Pregnancy' and 'Clinical Trials' in full PI). NovoRapid® can be used subcutaneously, intravenously or (10 mL vial only) via continuous subcutaneous insulin infusion ('CSII'). Refer to full PI before prescribing, available on request (December 2007).

*Note changes in Product Information

Novo Nordisk Pharmaceuticals Pty Ltd
A.B.N. 40 002 879 996
Level 3, 21 Solent Circuit
Baulkham Hills NSW 2153

ABRIDGED PRODUCT INFORMATION
Human Insulin

Actrapid® (Neutral Insulin Injection, short-acting solution)

Protaphane® (Isophane Insulin Injection, intermediate-acting suspension)

Mixtard® 30/70, Mixtard® 50/50 (Biphasic Isophane Insulin Injection, intermediate-acting suspension)

Composition: Human insulin (rys). **Indications:** Treatment of insulin-requiring diabetes. **Contraindications:** Hypoglycaemia. Hypersensitivity to human insulin or excipients. Insulin suspensions should not be administered intravenously or for treatment of diabetic ketoacidotic coma. **Precautions:** Inadequate dosing or discontinuation of treatment may lead to hyperglycaemia and diabetic ketoacidosis.

Insulin requirements may increase during illness and decrease with renal or hepatic impairment, insufficient food intake or increased physical activity. Avoid hypoglycaemia whilst driving or operating machinery. Transfer of patients between insulin types should be done under strict medical supervision and may require a change in dose. On transfer from animal-source insulin to human insulin, a few patients have reported the early warning symptoms for hypoglycaemia were less pronounced than with animal-source insulins. Patients whose blood glucose control is greatly improved may experience a change in their usual warning symptoms of hypoglycaemia. *Pregnancy and Lactation* Intensified treatment is recommended throughout pregnancy and when contemplating pregnancy. Insulin requirements vary during pregnancy and in nursing mothers and dose adjustments may be necessary. **Interactions:** Oral hypoglycaemic agents, octreotide, ACE inhibitors, salicylates, anabolic steroids, quinine, quinidine, sulphonamides, glucocorticoids, diuretics, oral contraceptives, thyroid hormones, sympathomimetics, growth hormone, diazoxide, asparaginase, nicotinic acid, monoamine oxidase inhibitors, alpha and betablockers, alcohol. In general, insulin should only be added to compounds with which it has known compatibility. **Adverse Effects:** Hypoglycaemia, lipodystrophy, insulin resistance, hypersensitivity, oedema, refraction abnormalities. **Dosage and Administration:** Dosage as determined by physician. Rotate injection sites. Insulin suspensions should not be used in infusion pumps or given intravenously. Eat within 30 minutes after injection of Actrapid® or Mixtard®. **Actrapid®** Subcutaneous. In an emergency, Actrapid® is suitable for intramuscular administration under medical guidance, or for intravenous administration if administered by a physician. For emergency use with Penfill®/InnoLet®, the insulin must first be withdrawn into a syringe. Discard Penfill/InnoLet cartridge/syringe after emergency use. Suitable for treatment of diabetic ketoacidosis, hyperosmolar non-ketotic syndrome, initial stabilisation of diabetes, severe infection, major trauma and/or surgery in people with diabetes. Not suitable for CSII pumps. **Protaphane®, Mixtard® 30/70, Mixtard® 50/50:** Subcutaneous injection. Intramuscular injection in emergency under medical supervision. For such use with Penfill/NovoLet/InnoLet the insulin must first be withdrawn into a syringe. Discard Penfill/NovoLet/InnoLet cartridge/syringe after emergency use. **Presentation:** 100 IU/ml.

Penfill® 3 mL cartridge – Actrapid, Protaphane, Mixtard 30/70, Mixtard 50/50. For use with Novo Nordisk insulin delivery systems and NovoPen® needles. *NovoLet® 3 mL* – Protaphane. *InnoLet®* 3 mL – Protaphane, Mixtard 30/70. *10 mL vial* – Actrapid, Protaphane.

Refer to full Product Information before prescribing. Available on request.
Approved by TGA 9 October 2002.
Abridged 02 October 2007.
Novo Nordisk Pharmaceuticals Pty Ltd
A.B.N. 40 002 879 996
Level 3, 21 Solent Circuit
Baulkham Hills NSW 2153

MINIMUM PRODUCT INFORMATION*
Levemir® (insulin detemir) (rys)
Levemir® (100U/ml) is a clear, colourless solution for injection. **Indications:** Treatment of diabetes mellitus where used as basal insulin in combination with meal-related short- or rapid-acting insulin. Not recommended for diabetes mellitus type 2 patients who still respond to oral hypoglycaemic agents. (See 'Clinical Trials' in full PI/datasheet.) **Contraindications:** Hypersensitivity to insulin detemir or excipients. **Precautions:** Inadequate dosing may lead to hyperglycaemia and DKA. Hypoglycaemia may occur if dose too high in relation to requirements – see full PI/datasheet. Avoid i.m. administration. I.v. administration may result in a severe hypo. Mixed with other insulins the action profile of either or both may change. Do not use in infusion pumps. No studies in children under 6 years. No clinical experience during lactation. Studies do not suggest clinically relevant albumin binding interactions between insulin detemir and fatty acids or other protein-bound drugs. Do not add to infusion fluids. **Adverse Effects:** hypoglycaemia. **Dosage and Administration:** Adjust dose individually. Administer once or twice daily depending on needs.

* Note changes in Product Information

Nordisk Pharmaceuticals Pty Ltd, Level 3, 21 Solent Circuit, Baulkham Hills, NSW 2153, Australia.

novo nordisk®

Figure 5.4 (a) Range of NovoNordisk insulins with their time action characteristics and insulin profiles and (b) the delivery systems available with each insulin. Reproduced with permission from NovoNordisk (Australia). PBS information refers to Australian prescribing information.

Table 5.3 Some examples of commonly used insulin delivery devices and some of the issues to consider when helping the individual decide which device to use.

Device	Issues to be aware of
(a) *Insulin syringes* 30, 50, and 100 unit sizes	• There is still a place for syringes • Patients need to be able to recognise different dose increments on different sized syringes • Select size appropriate for dose • Needles are usually longer than other devices ○ Can be used with all available insulins but it is not advisable to withdraw insulin from penfills with a syringe ○ May lead to dose errors in hospital settings and in some hospitals only one routine stock size is available ○ A retractable syringe is available, which was designed to reduce needle stick injuries.
(b) *Insulin 'pens'*	• Insulin 'pens' are not suitable for people who need to mix insulins • They make injecting simpler because there is no need to draw up the dose • They can sometimes be difficult to manage for people with manual dexterity problems
SanofiAventis devices Apidra SolorStar Lantus SoloStar	Prefilled disposable devices
Novo Devices NovoPen 3 A new device, NovoPen, 4 is under development	• Dose range 2–70 units • Accurate dosing • Uses 3 mL insulin cartridges • Small, fine needles • Replacing the insulin cartridge can be difficult for some people • Has a function to check the accuracy of the device • Pen is reusable
NovoPen Demi	• Similar to NovoPen 3, but 1/2 unit dose increments are possible • Useful for children and insulin-sensitive patients who require very small doses
INNOLET	• Dose range 1–50 units • Accurate dosing • Small, fine needles • Device is preloaded and disposable • Limited range of insulins available • Contains 3 mL of insulin • Clear, easy to see numbers on the dose dial, which is an advantage for vision impaired people • Is easier for older people to manage • Larger than other devices – takes up less storage space in fridge
PenMate 3	• Automatic needle insertion device • Used with NovoPen 3 • Hides needle and injects insulin quickly and automatically • May benefit people with needle phobia and children

Table 5.3 Continued.

Device	Issues to be aware of
FlexPen	• Contains 3 mL of insulin • Disposable, preloaded device • Small, fine needles • A range of insulin is available
Eli Lilly devices Humapen Luxura	• Dose range 1–60 units • Accurate dosing • Easy to correct if an incorrect dose is dialed up without wasting insulin • Uses 3 mL insulin cartridges • Small, fine needles • Replacing the insulin cartridge can be difficult for some people • Has a function to check the accuracy of the device • Pen is reusable • Pen has audible clicks representing each unit dialled
Insulin pumps	• Provide continuous basal insulin with a facility for giving bolus doses with meals • Uses only short-acting insulin • Uses small, fine needles • Expensive • Requires considerable expertise and time to be used effectively

Note: Other devices may be available. The devices should only be used with the insulin specified by the manufacturer. Needles and syringes should only be used once and then discarded into an appropriate sharps container.

Injection sites and administration

Administer at the appropriate time before the meal. The abdomen is the preferred site; but upper arms, thighs, and buttocks can also be used. Injection sites must be rotated to avoid lipoatrophy and lipodystrophy and should be checked on a regular basis.

How to inject

The insulin injection technique can influence insulin absorption and, therefore, its action. Insulin should be administered subcutaneously. IM injections lead to unstable blood glucose levels (Vaag *et al.* 1990).

- Pinch up a fold of skin (dermis and subcutaneous tissue) between the thumb and index finger.
- Inject at 90-degree angle. If the needle is long, pinch up may not be needed and a 45-degree angle can be used to avoid giving an IM injection.
- Release the skin, remove the needle, and apply gentle pressure to the site.

- Document dose and time of the injection.
- Injection sites should be regularly checked for swelling, lumps, pain or leakage of insulin.

Practice points

(1) A range of needle sizes is available. Needle size is important to people with diabetes.
    They usually prefer small, fine gauge needles.
(2) Injection with fine gauge needles is relatively painless.
(3) Giving the first injection is often very difficult for people with diabetes. Support and encouragement and allowing them to take their time and inject at their own pace is important.
(4) If insulin tends to leak after the injection, release the skin fold before injecting. Pressure from holding the skin fold sometimes forces the insulin back out of the needle track. Withdraw the syringe quickly to allow the skin to seal. Do not cover so that any insulin leakage can be observed.
(5) The loss of even small amounts of insulin can result in unpredictable increases in the blood glucose and inappropriate dose adjustment especially in lean people and children. Careful observation and estimation of the amount of insulin lost is necessary to make appropriate adjustments to the individual's injection technique – this applies to both patients and nurses.
(6) The larger the volume of insulin to be injected the greater the likelihood of some insulin leaking back along the needle track. Likewise, leakage can occur if the injection is too shallow, or given intradermally.
(7) To minimise the risk of insulin loss during injection, inject slowly and leave the needle in place for 3–6 seconds after the insulin is delivered.
(8) Long-acting and pre-mixed insulins dispensed in insulin pens must be mixed gently before administration.

Instructions for teaching people how to draw up and administer insulin appear in Chapter 16. Refer also to the manufacturer's instructions and patient information material.

Practice points

(1) Insulin syringes and pen needles are approved for single use only.
(2) Pen needles should be removed after administering an insulin dose and a new needle used for the next dose especially with premixed insulins, which can block the needle.
(3) Most insulin administration devices, except syringes, were designed to enable patients to administer their own insulin. In hospital, patients should remove the needle and place it in the sharps container after injecting to avoid needle stick injury to staff.

(4) In hospital, aged care and community settings staff should NOT recap needles.
(5) If the patient cannot remove the needle from the pen, a removal device should
    be used, or the insulin administered using a syringe until the patient is well
    enough to self-inject again.

Mixing short- and intermediate-acting insulins

General points

There is less need to 'mix insulins' now, due to the range of modern premixed insulin
combinations and insulin analogues. However, it is still necessary in some settings and
in some countries. Mixing short- and intermediate-acting insulins before injecting may
diminish the effect of the short-acting peak, which is more marked when there is sub-
stantially more long-acting insulin in the mixture (as is usually the case), especially if
the insulin is left to stand for a long time before use.

The clinical significance of these changes is unknown. It is more likely to apply to
in home situations where home-care/domicillary nurses or relatives draw up doses for
several days for patients to self-administer, see Chapter 18. This practice may not be
ideal but it does enable people to retain a measure of independence where syringes are
still the device of choice.

The long-acting insulin analogues cannot be mixed with other insulin or injected into
the same site.

Commonly used insulin regimens

Daily injection

A combination of:

- Rapid or short- and long-acting insulin combinations, which are usually given before
  breakfast. Biphasic premixed insulins such as Mixtard 30/70 and Humulin 30/70 are
  often used.
- Long or intermediate acting insulin is often given at bedtime when it is combined
  with OHAs for Type 2 diabetes. Daily regimes are commonly used for:
  ○ older people.
  ○ those not willing to have more than one injection per day.
  ○ some situations where people require assistance to inject are living in aged care
    facilities or depending on home nursing care when staff are not available to inject
    more than once per day.
- Daily regimens are not recommended for people with Type 1 diabetes.

It can be difficult to attain good control using biphasic insulin because the amount of
individual insulin in the mix cannot be altered, which can increase the risk of hypoglycaemia if eating is erratic, the carbohydrate intake is low, or after vigorous exercise.

BD regimens

A combination of rapid or short- and intermediate or long-acting insulin is usually given before breakfast and before the evening meal. Biphasic insulins are commonly used but do not allow a great deal of flexibility in adjusting doses. The evening dose may effectively control overnight hyperglycaemia. There is a risk of nocturnal hypoglycaemia, see Chapter 6. Usually two-thirds of the total dose is given in the morning and one-third in the evening.

Figure 5.5 depicts the action profiles of the various insulins. Understanding the action profile enables hypoglycaemia risk times to be identified so that meals, activity, and medication administration times can be planned accordingly. They also help decide which insulin to adjust when considered in conjunction with the blood glucose profile. Consideration should always be given to other factors that affect blood glucose levels, see Chapter 3.

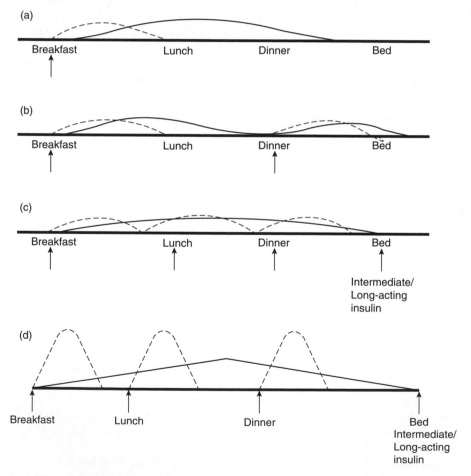

Figure 5.5 Diagrammatic representation of insulin action showing different regimens: (a) daily, (b) twice daily, (c) basal bolus using short-acting insulins and (d) basal bolus using rapid-acting insulins. *Note:* The broken line depicts short-acting insulin, the unbroken line intermediate/long-acting insulin. The arrows indicate the time of injection.

Practice point

Rapid-acting insulins act very quickly. They should be given immediately before a meal, or within 15 minutes after the meal to avoid hypoglycaemia.

Basal bolus regimen

Basal bolus regimens simulate the normal pattern of insulin secretion, that is a small amount of circulating insulin is present in the blood and restrains gluconeogenesis and glycogenolysis, this is the basal insulin. A bolus amount of insulin is stimulated by the blood glucose rise after a meal. Bolus injections of rapid or short-acting insulin are given before each meal. The longer-acting insulin, often an analogue, is often given before bed to supply the basal insulin requirement and restrain hepatic glucose output overnight and control the pre-breakfast blood glucose (fasting) level. This regimen offers more flexibility in insulin dose adjustment and meal times, and therefore lifestyle is less restricted. The amount of insulin given at each dose is usually small; therefore, the likelihood of hypoglycaemia is reduced. Basal bolus regimens are commonly used for young people with Type 1 diabetes and increasingly for Type 2. Despite the number of injections per day, basal bolus therapy using analogues may be safer for older people, with a lower risk of hypoglycaemia and falls. Nocturnal hypoglycaemia is less frequent when long-acting analogues are used.

Interpreting morning hyperglycaemia

There are three main reasons for fasting hyperglycaemia:

(1) Insufficient basal insulin to restrain overnight hepatic glucose output. It is a common finding with daily insulin regimens when the insulin is given in the morning. A larger dose of insulin may be needed or a second dose of insulin introduced at lunch or bedtime, or if the person is on OHA and insulin, the insulin could be given at night.
(2) The Somogyi effect, which is due to the counter-regulatory response to nocturnal hypoglycaemia. The cause needs to be sought (see Chapter 6) but the basal insulin dose may need to be reduced.
(3) 'Dawn phenomenon' reflects insufficient insulin and insulin resistance. There is a normal physiological increase in many hormones early in the morning. However, elevated fasting blood glucose may indicate general hyperglycaemia. A thorough assessment is needed and the medication regimen adjusted.

Continuous subcutaneous insulin infusion (CSII)

Insulin pumps continuously deliver subcutaneous insulin, usually a short-acting analogue, at a pre-programmed steady basal rate through a subcutaneous needle, which stays in place for 3 days. Bolus doses before meals or corrective doses for hyperglycaemia can be performed manually as needed. They enable a more physiological insulin profile to be attained and greater flexibility in meeting individual insulin requirements. They use rapid or short-acting insulin only, and therefore if they malfunction or are removed, for example, for surgery, the patient must be given insulin via another method to avoid hyperglycaemia. This can be subcutaneously or via an IV depending on the circumstances.

Modern insulin pumps are generally reliable and have an inbuilt alarm system that identifies a number of faults such as kinks/blockages in the tubing, tubing disconnections from the pump and low batteries, so that malfunctions can be identified early and appropriate steps taken to avoid hyperglycaemia. Some do not alarm if the tubing disconnects from the insertion site. If this occurs insulin is not delivered and can go unnoticed until the blood glucose is tested. In people with Type 1 diabetes hyperglycaemia can occur quickly and increase the risk of DKA. Reported rates vary between 2.7 and 9 episodes per 100 patient years.

Pumps are expensive and require a great deal of commitment on the part of the person with diabetes to use them safely and effectively. Health professional support and the ready availability of advice are vital. People need time to adjust to the pump regime and become accustomed to not having intermediate-acting insulin. Pumps offer a great deal of flexibility and can have significant psychological benefits. However, pumps do not suit everybody and some people dislike the thought of being constantly connected to a device.

People need to learn to carbohydrate count once they commence using an insulin pump. Structured education programmes such as Dose Adjustment for Normal Eating (DAFNE) (DAFNE Study Group 2002) are often used to help individuals learn how much insulin is required per meal (~0.5 units/10 g of carbohydrate). DAFNE is based on 10 g of carbohydrate.

Practice points

(1) Insulin pumps are not a cure for poor metabolic control but they can help some people achieve better control.

(2) They enable the insulin regimen and food intake to be matched to individual requirements and greater flexibility.

(3) Hypoglycaemia unawareness may be reversed and hypoglycaemia frequency and severity may be reduced.

(4) Insulin injections are not required.

(5) Blood glucose monitoring at least 4-hourly is necessary.

(6) Training and readily available support and advice from skilled pump experts are essential.

(7) People with existing psychological problems do worse on pumps than on other insulin regimes (DCCT 1993).

(8) Pumps are expensive to purchase and the ongoing cost of consumables is high. In Australia some health insurance funds subsidise the initial outlay for the pump according to specified guidelines. The cost of consumables is subsidised by the Commonwealth government under the National Diabetes Supply Scheme.

Currently there is no national Australian guideline for selecting which patients will benefit from using a pump but most diabetes centres offering pump therapy have guidelines for selecting patients and initiating pump therapy. The UK National Institute for Clinical Excellence (NICE) (2003) recommended that pumps be funded for people with Type 1 diabetes who suffer recurrent severe hypoglycaemia.

Continuous blood glucose sensors

Continuous glucose monitoring is step towards a closed-loop system that links continuous blood glucose measurements to a computer-driven insulin infusion system to approximate normal glucose homeostasis. Modern sensors consist of a disposable sensor probe, which is inserted into subcutaneous tissue using an insertion device and connected to a battery-powered transmitter. The transmitter sends a signal to a receiver, which displays the blood glucose reading. The sensors last for ~3–5 days.

After the sensor is attached to the transmitter warm-up periods between 2 and 10 hours are required and capillary blood glucose testing is required to calibrate the system. There are at least three sensors on the market and each manufacturer recommends ongoing calibration. In addition, abnormal sensor readings need to be confirmed with a capillary test before corrective action is taken. Thus, the current sensors are adjuncts to rather than replacements for capillary blood glucose testing but they enable people to have several days break from finger pricking. The cost is prohibitive for many people.

The choice of regimen and insulin delivery system depends on personal preference, management targets and the willingness and ability of the patient to monitor their blood glucose. Many factors can influence insulin absorption and consequently blood glucose; some of these factors are shown in Table 5.4.

Subcutaneous insulin sliding scales and top-up regimes

A sliding scale refers to subcutaneous insulin doses administered to reduce hyperglycaemia detected on routine blood glucose monitoring. Such sliding scales are reactive and retrospective rather than prospective and proactive (Hirsch *et al*. 1995). Sliding scales should not be confused with supplemental insulin administered at meal times based on blood glucose tests according to an algorithm (Hirsch *et al*. 1995).

Table 5.4 Some commonly encountered factors that affect insulin absorption.

Accelerated	*Delayed*
Type of insulin	Type of insulin
Exercise	Low body temperature
High body temperature	Condition of injection sites
Condition of injection sites	Poor circulation
Massage round injection site	Smoking
Depth of injection	Long-acting insulins

Sliding scales continue to be used in hospital despite there being no evidence of any benefit. In fact, diabetes experts have been advocating for a proactive prospective approach to managing hyperglycaemia in hospital rather than using sliding scales since 1981 (Walk *et al.* 1981; Gearhart *et al.* 1994; Hirsch 1997; Queale *et al.* 1997).

Sliding scales treat hyperglycaemia after it occurs. They may predispose the patient to hyperglycaemia-related adverse events, particularly given the fact that insulin doses are rarely adjusted and the underlying causes and predisposing factors that lead to hyperglycaemia are not addressed (Queale *et al.* 1997). Using subcutaneous sliding scales in day-to-day management can lead to disassociation between the insulin regimen and the other parameters that affect the blood glucose such as the timing of meals, effects of illness, and medications, for example, steroids. They may have a place in the very short term to re-establish acceptable blood glucose levels.

Using sliding scales to stabilise blood glucose for newly diagnosed, unstable or brittle diabetes is *not* generally recommended (Katz 1991). It is preferable to monitor the blood glucose over 24–48 hours and adjust the insulin regimen according to the emerging pattern considering the action profile of the various insulins.

Top-up or stat doses of insulin

Top-up or stat doses of insulin refer to temporary supplementary doses of insulin, usually rapid or short acting, given to correct existing hyperglycaemia found on routine blood glucose monitoring. Like traditional sliding, scales top-up dosing is reactionary and does not address the underlying causes of hyperglycaemia. When necessary, extra insulin is best added to the next due dose of insulin rather than being given in isolation.

Adopting a proactive problem-solving approach, considering the management regimen and nursing/medical actions occurring at the time will provide important insight into the cause/s of the hyperglycaemia, which can be appropriately treated. For example, hyperglycaemia might be a consequence of pain or fear in which case the most effective strategy would be to manage the pain/fear. In addition, non-medicine options might be effective. Often, top-up doses continue for days before the overall blood glucose profile and medicine requirements or the underlying causes are considered.

Practice points

(1) There are no documented benefits of insulin sliding scales in people in hospital (Walk *et al.* 1981; Gearhart *et al.* 1994; Hirsch 1997; Queale *et al.* 1997) or top-up doses.

(2) Insulin sliding scales are associated with a 3-fold higher risk of hyperglycaemia especially when basal insulin is not used (Queale *et al.* 1997).

(3) Sliding scales could help maintain acceptable blood glucose levels in hospital if they are used proactively according to a logical algorithm based on the action profiles of the relevant insulin regimen.

IV insulin infusions do require a sliding scale and are an example of proactive hyperglycaemia management.

Intravenous insulin infusions

The IV route is preferred for very ill patients because the absorption of insulin is rapid and more reliable than from poorly perfused muscle and fat tissue. Absorption may be erratic in these patients, especially if they are hypotensive. The aims of the insulin infusion are to:

• Prevent the liver converting glycogen and fatty acids into glucose and therefore avoid hyperglycaemia, that is restrain hepatic glucose output.
• Prevent utilisation of fatty acids and therefore limit ketone formation.
• Reduce protein catabolism and therefore limit production of glucose substrates.
• Enhance wound healing by limiting protein catabolism and normalising neutrophil function.
• Reduce peripheral resistance to insulin.
• If hyperglycaemia is present, gradually lower the blood glucose concentration to 10–12 mmol/L without subjecting the patient to hypoglycaemia.

Intravenous insulin infusions are associated with lower morbidity and mortality in surgical settings (see Chapter 9), during acute illness such as MI (see Chapter 8), in patients requiring parenteral nutrition (Cheung *et al*. 2005) and in intensive care settings (Quinn *et al*. 2006). In fact, Van den Berghe *et al*. (2001) demonstrated improved outcomes using insulin infusions in acutely ill non-diabetics as well as people with diabetes.

Two main insulin delivery methods are used:

(1) Insulin, given via an infusion pump and fluid administered separately.
(2) Insulin, glucose, potassium, and fluids are combined (GIK), which is efficient and safe. The glucose component is usually 5 or 10% dextrose depending on the calories required (Dagogo-Jack & Alberti 2002).

The medication order for the infusion must be clearly and legibly written on the treatment sheet. Insulin doses for IV insulin infusions are usually 0.1 unit/kg/hour. Sometimes an initial bolus of 5–10 units is given. In general, a low-dose infusion such as this has been shown to reduce the blood glucose and prevent ketosis and acidosis as effectively as high-dose regimens, without the added risk of hypoglycaemia. The rate at which the insulin is to be administered should be written in mL/hour and units to be delivered. Several protocols exist; the following is one example. Insulin-treated Type 2 may require 1–2 units/hour.

The infusion rate is adjusted according to the patient's blood glucose results (tested 1–2-hourly). This is a proactive sliding scale of insulin. For example:

Blood glucose (mmol/L)	Insulin (units/hour)
0–5.9	0
6–11.1	1
12–15.1	2
16–19	3
>19.1	4
>24	Notify doctor

The insulin order and blood glucose results should be reviewed regularly. The duration of the infusion depends on the clinical status of the patient.

Preparing the insulin solution to be infused

Two people should check and make up the solution according to the medication order and hospital protocols. In many cases it is prepared in pharmacy.

Practice points

(1) Only clear rapid or short-acting insulin is used for insulin infusions. Great care should be taken not to use long-acting insulin analogues in insulin infusions.
(2) Insulin is known to bind to plastic. Flushing the first 50 mL through the giving set prevents this non-specific absorption into the infusion equipment.

Uses of insulin infusions

General use (during surgical procedures)

Insulin is added to 4% dextrose in 1/5 normal saline or 5% dextrose. The infusion is often given via *burette* or more commonly an infusion pump at 120 mL/hour (i.e. 8-hourly rate; see previous example scale). Monitor blood glucose 1–2-hourly and review with medical staff *regularly*.

Special needs

- Myocardial infarction. In many areas an IV insulin infusion is commenced when the patient presents to the emergency department and continues for ~24 hours, after which time subcutaneous insulin is commenced (Malmberg 1997), see Chapter 8.
- Open heart surgery.
- Ketoacidosis.
- Hyperosmolar coma.
- Intensive care unit (ICU) situations.

These situations always require the use of a controlled-rate infusion pumps to ensure accurate insulin dosing. It is often necessary to limit the amount of fluid administered to avoid cerebral oedema in these situations especially in young children and the elderly. Standard regimes include:

(1) Haemaccel 100 mL + 100 units rapid or fast-acting insulin = 1 unit/1 mL, used in ICU and administered via an infusion pump.
(2) Haemaccel 500 mL + 100 units rapid or short-acting insulin = 1 unit/5 mL via an infusion pump.

People who are insulin-resistant, such as those who:

- have liver disease
- are on corticosteroid therapy
- are obese
- have a serious infection

may require more insulin, that is, a high-dose infusion (more units per hour).

Practice points

(1) Subcutaneous insulin must be given before removing the infusion and the patient must be eating and drinking normally to avoid hyperglycaemia because of the short half-life of insulin given IV.
(2) Ceasing the infusion before a meal enables a smooth transition to subcutaneous insulin.

Risks associated with insulin infusions

- Hypoglycaemia
- Cardiac arrhythmias
- Sepsis at the IV site
- Fluid overload and cerebral oedema especially in children, which is associated with high morbidity and mortality rates.

Factors affecting insulin delivery via IV infusions

- Accuracy of the system, including blood glucose testing.
- Stability of the solution.
- Circulatory insufficiency.

Mistakes associated with insulin infusions

(1) Where a burette is used and if insulin is added to the burette rather than the bag of IV fluid, refilling the burette from the bag results in no insulin being administered and hyperglycaemia results.
(2) An incorrect amount of insulin added to the bag/burette can be a result of inadequate checking, not using an insulin syringe to draw up the insulin or failing to check illegible medical orders, especially where insulin doses are written as U/s instead of 'units' and the dose is misinterpreted.
(3) Problems can arise if the insulin infusion is run at the same time through the same site as other intravenous fluids, for example, 4% dextrose in 1/5 normal saline. The most common method is to infuse the different fluids through the one IV cannula using a three-way adaptor (octopus), see Figure 5.6.

Usually, the dextrose or saline is running at a faster rate than the insulin infusion. Problems can arise if there is a complete or partial blockage of the cannula. The force

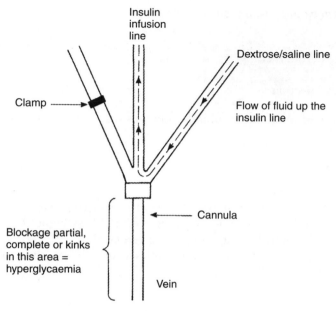

Figure 5.6   Possible results of a blockage in the IV cannula and three-way adaptor during the concurrent administration of insulin and dextrose/saline.

of gravity pushing the fluid towards the vein can actually cause the dextrose/saline to flow back up the slower-flowing insulin line resulting in high blood glucose levels. Figure 5.6 depicts the result of a blockage in the IV cannula and three-way adaptor during the concurrent administration of insulin and dextrose/saline.

If hyperglycaemia occurs during an insulin infusion check:

- That the tubing and adaptors are patent;
- That insulin has been added to the burette/bag;
- That the amount of insulin added is correct;
- Possible sources of infection, for example, UTI, the feet.

Clinical observation

Indicating insulin doses by writing U/s is common practice and can be very unclear when written by hand. Incorrect, usually excess, insulin has been administered where this is common practice and serious hypoglycaemia resulted. In one case, in Australia, in an aged care facility, a patient died and a court case ensued. Both the nurse who administered the insulin and the doctor who wrote the prescription were found to have contributed to the death. There were other issues involved with the particular patient but the case highlights the importance of accurate documentation and the nurse's responsibility to check.

Insulin doses should always be indicated by writing or typing 'units' after the amount to be given.

Insulin allergy

Insulin allergies are rare with modern, highly purified insulins but they do sometimes occur.

Two types of reaction have been reported:

(1) Localised weal and flare with itching due to antihistamine reactions;
(2) Generalised anaphylaxis, which is rare.

Allergic reactions are most likely to occur where people have been on insulin previously, for example, during GDM, surgery or acute illness in people with Type 2 diabetes where insulin is used intermittently, for example, during surgery and with steroid medications, and when injection sites are not rotated.

To diagnose insulin allergy a careful case history is required. The person should be given insulin and observed where resuscitation equipment is available. Any reaction should be carefully documented. Blood test for IgG and other immune response factors can be helpful.

If insulin allergy is present a desensitisation programme may be required. Local reactions can be managed by using a different insulin and antihistamine creams (Williams 1993; Dunning *et al.* 1998).

Transplants

Pancreas transplants of either the whole pancreas or islet cells or the pancreas and kidneys is available to some people with diabetes, for example, those with autonomic neuropathy causing life-threatening hypoglycaemic unawareness and end-stage renal failure. Immunosuppresive therapy is required, and if rejection does not occur, the response is good. The transplanted pancreas secretes insulin and HbA_{1c} normalises in ~ three months.

Obtaining pancreases for transplantation or to harvest islet cells is difficult, as is actually separating the islet cells from pancreatic tissue, and other options are under study. For example, beta cell engineering and stem cell cloning. Islet cell transplants have been undertaken successfully in Canada, Australia, USA, and in the UK and an international islet cell consortium has been established to try to reproduce positive results.

Stabilising diabetes

Rationale

Optimal blood glucose control can prevent or delay the onset of long-term complications. Insulin is frequently required by people with Type 2 diabetes to achieve optimal control.

Stabilisation of diabetes refers to the process of achieving an optimal blood glucose range, appropriate diabetes knowledge and managing diabetic complications, either acute or chronic, and usually specifically refers to commencing insulin

(NHMRC 1991). Stabilisation may occur at initial diagnosis of diabetes, when a change of treatment is indicated, for example, transfer from OHA to combination therapy or insulin, and for antenatal care.

In most cases, stabilisation of diabetes can be achieved without admitting the person to hospital. Managing diabetes in primary care settings as far as possible is a core component of both the Australian and UK diabetes management strategies (MacKinnon 1998; NDS 1998). This process is known as outpatient stabilisation. Outpatient stabilisation requires specialised staff, specific protocols and ample time if it is to be successful. It can result in considerable cost benefits, and reduces the stress and costs associated with a hospital admission.

There are considerable psychological and quality of life benefits for the person with diabetes. Home/outpatient stabilisation enables insulin to be adjusted according to the individual's usual lifestyle and reduces the risk of the person having to assume 'sick role' behaviours.

However, some patients will continue to be admitted to hospital for stabilisation of their diabetes, for example, complex issues that cannot be identified in outpatient settings, where clinical observation is necessary, for patient convenience or where the person is admitted with a concurrent illness or is diagnosed during an admission and commences insulin while in hospital.

Stabilisating diabetes in hospital

People admitted to improve their metabolic control (stabilisation) are not generally ill and should be encouraged to:

- Keep active;
- Wear clothes instead of pyjamas;
- Perform diabetes self-care tasks such as blood glucose monitoring and insulin administration.

They will require support, encouragement and consistent advice. The time spent in hospital should be kept to a minimum.

Nursing responsibilities

(1) Inform the appropriate staff about the person's admission especially the diabetes nurse specialist/diabetes educator, specialist team, and dietitian soon after they are admitted.
(2) Assess the patient carefully (refer to Chapter 2).
(3) Monitor blood and urine glucose according to usual protocols; for example, 7 AM, 11 AM, 4 PM, and 9 PM. In some cases postprandial levels are also performed (see Chapter 3 Appendices).
(4) Supervise and assess the patient's ability to test their own blood glucose and/or administer insulin, or teach these skills if the person is newly diagnosed.
(5) Ensure diabetes knowledge is assessed and updated, and select an appropriate diet: new learning may include insulin techniques, sharps disposal, hypoglycaemia and home management during illness.

(6) TPR daily, or every second day.
(7) BP, lying and standing, daily.
(8) Ensure all blood samples, urine collections and special tests are performed accurately. The opportunity is often taken to perform a comprehensive complication screen while the person is in hospital, especially if they often miss appointments with health professionals or it has not been performed for some time. Inspection of injection sites and assessment of the person's psychological status should be included. These tests include ECG, eye referral, spot urine collection for creatinine and microalbumin and blood tests such as lipids, HbA_{1c} and kidney function.
(9) Ensure the patient has supplies, for example, test strips, lancets, insulin device, before discharge and that the appropriate follow-up appointments are made.
(10) Ensure they have a contact telephone number in case they need advice.

Community and outpatient stabilisation

The types of outpatient service provided for people with diabetes include:

- Diabetes education;
- Commencement on diabetes medication (OHA, insulin);
- Complication screening and assessment;
- Blood glucose testing;
- Consultations with dietitian, diabetes nurse specialist/diabetes educator or diabetes specialist;
- Clinical assessment;
- Education is a key factor in a person's understanding and acceptance of diabetes. Diabetes educators often know the person well from the outpatient service and can assist ward nurses to plan appropriate nursing care and understand the person's needs.

Practice point

The specific protocol and policy of the relevant health care setting should be followed and all contacts including telephone advice documented. An example protocol for insulin stabilisation in the community or on an outpatient basis is shown on pages 158 and 159.

Objectives of outpatient stabilisation onto insulin

Short-term objectives:

(1) To reassure the individual and their family and allay the fear that everything about diabetes must be learned at once.
(2) Lifestyle should be modified as little as possible.
(3) To establish trust between the patient and the diabetes team.

(4) To gradually normalise blood glucose.
(5) To teach the 'survival skills' necessary for the person to be safe at home:
  • how to draw up and administer insulin;
  • blood glucose monitoring;
  • recognising and treating hypoglycaemia;
  • how to obtain advice – contact telephone number.

Long-term objectives
The aim in the long term is for the patient to:

(1) Accept diabetes as part of their life and recognise their part in the successful management of the diabetes.
(2) Be able to make appropriate changes in insulin doses, carbohydrate intake and activity to maintain acceptable blood glucose levels.
(3) Be able to maintain an acceptable range of blood glucose, HbA_{1c}, and lipids.
(4) Be able to maintain a healthy weight range.
(5) Modify risk factors to prevent or delay the onset of the long-term complications of diabetes and therefore the need for hospital admissions.
(6) Attend regular medical/education appointments.
(7) Receive ongoing support and encouragement from the diabetes team.
(8) Maintain psychological wellbeing and quality of life.

Clinical observations

People are often overwhelmed, unsure what to do and confused by conflicting or inaccurate advice given by health professionals, family and friends and the media or obtained on the Internet.

These issues frequently need to be addressed and clarified before commencing the insulin stabilisation process.

The therapeutic relationship and trust between health professional and the person with diabetes is a vital aspect of their adjustment to having diabetes and changes in their diabetic management or status. Therapeutic relationships should be cultivated and treasured.

Rationale for choosing community/outpatient stabilisation

Community/outpatient stabilisation onto insulin is preferred for the following reasons:

(1) To avoid the 'sick role', which is often associated with a hospital admission.
(2) It is cost effective, that is, does not require a hospital bed.
(3) It involves less time away from work and usual activity for the patient, who can therefore be stabilised according to their usual routine, rather than hospital routines and food.
(4) To encourage self-reliance and confidence.

Patient criteria

The patient must be:

- Able to attend the service for the required period, which depends on the individual service. In some cases twice daily visits may be necessary. Telephone contact should be maintained as long as necessary;
- Physically and mentally capable of performing blood glucose monitoring and insulin administration, or have assistance to do so.

In addition, some social/family support is helpful initially for older people and is required for children.

The process of stabilisation

(1) It should involve members of the diabetes team and relatives/carers as appropriate.
(2) Communication, especially between the doctor, practice nurses, diabetes nurse specialist/diabetes educator, dietitian and patient, is essential.
(3) Patients should be assessed on an individual basis, so that appropriate education goals and blood glucose range can be determined. The insulin regime and insulin delivery system will depend on individual requirements; follow-up advice and early assessment must be available.
(4) Formal teaching times should take account of the individual's commitments as far as is practicable.
(5) Adequate charting and documentation of progress should be recorded after each session: blood glucose results, ability to manage insulin technique, goals of management.
(6) Effective education strategies should be used. Stabilisation might be undertaken in groups (see Chapter 16).

A sample protocol for outpatient stabilisation is shown at the end of this chapter. It is included here to give nurses an overview of the kind of information required and the complex issues people with diabetes have to deal with, often when they feel vulnerable.

(2) People with Type 1 diabetes are at risk of ketoacidosis but often do not have ketone testing equipment at home or if they do it is out of date (Sumner *et al.* 2000; Tay *et al.* 2001). Constant, diplomatic reminders are important. An episode in hospital is one such opportunity.

Traditionally, initiation of insulin occurred on an individual basis. Recent reports suggest that group education programmes for commencing insulin can be effective and achieve reductions in HbA_{1c} and competent insulin self-care by individuals (Almond *et al.* 2001; Yki-Jarvinen *et al.* 2007). Such programmes could be a cost effective way to manage the increasing numbers of people being commenced on insulin as a result of the DCCT and UKPDS trials, provided competent facilitation is available.

Lipid lowering agents

Normalising the lipid profile is an essential component of diabetes management guidelines. People with diabetes, especially Type 2, are at significant risk of cardiovascular disease, which is often present at diagnosis, unless the blood glucose and lipids can be kept within normal limits. Generally, the aim is to reduce cholesterol, especially LDL-c and triglycerides, and increase HDL-c. HDL aids in the removal of LDL cholesterol but it might also have anti-inflammatory and antithrombotic properties. HDL-c is inversely related to triglycerides in that high triglyceride levels are associated with the removal of cholesterol from HDL-c to more atherogenic lipoproteins and lipoprotein precursors. HDL-c is often low in Type 2 diabetes, partly because of the increased production of triglyceride-rich lipoproteins. LDL-c may not be elevated because of the increased level of cholesterol LDL, which suggests relying on LDL-c levels may underestimate the cardiovascular risk in people with Type 2 diabetes (Sullivan 2008).

High LDL significantly increases the risk of myocardial infarction, but other risk factors such as obesity and inflammatory processes are important and are often exacerbated by low levels of HDL (Colquhoun 2002). The cholesterol content of HDL, HDL-c, could be protective in that it reflects removal of cholesterol from atherosclerotic plaque. Low HDL-c is an independent risk factor for cardiovascular disease (Anderson *et al.* 1991). Weight loss, reducing saturated fat in the diet, exercise, and stopping smoking all effectively raise HDL-c. Alcohol increases HDL-c but excess consumption is associated with significant health risks because it causes weight gain especially around the abdomen, liver damage, contributes to malnutrition, and reduces LDL-c and triglycerides, and increases the risk of breast cancer in women. Controlling blood glucose is integral to controlling lipids (Lipid Study Group 1998). Current lipid targets aim for total cholesterol <4 and triglyceride and LDL <3 in patients with existing heart disease (National Heart Foundation 2001).

The American Diabetes Association (2006) recommended using statins to prevent cardiovascular disease in all people with Type 2 diabetes, particularly reducing LDL-c 100 mg/dL, and initiating statins in people with diabetes >40 years without cardiovascular disease to reach the LDL-c target. Likewise, the CARDS study suggested statins are indicated in most people with Type 2 diabetes, whereas The ASPEN study (Knopp *et al.* 2006) suggested people at low risk of cardiovascular disease might receive less benefit for statin therapy. Not all people with diabetes have the same 10-year risk of cardiovascular disease, thus, lipid lowering therapy needs to be commenced according to individual level of risk (Grundy 2004).

Major cardiovascular prevention trials include:

- Antihypertensive and Lipid-Lowering Treatment to Prevent Heart Attack Trial (ALLHAT), which was one of the first trials to assess the efficacy of statins (Pravostatin) in people with and without diabetes. It failed to show a significant reduction in mortality but there was a trend towards a higher mortality risk in people with LDL-c >130 mg/dL. The findings were similar for those with and without diabetes.
- Heart Protection Study, which also included people with and without diabetes. The all-cause mortality and major cardiovascular event rate were significantly lower in the simvastatin group. The outcomes were similar for those with and without diabetes in the simvastatin group but people with diabetes in the placebo group had more vascular events than non-diabetics and the risk was additive. The researchers suggested people with diabetes have a risk equivalent to those with pre-existing cardiovascular disease and that statin therapy is beneficial for people with diabetes without cardiovascular disease and LDL-c close to the target.
- Anglo-Scandinavian Cardiac Outcomes Trial-Blood Pressure Lowering Arm (ASCOT-BPLA) compared two antihypertensive regimens in people with at least three cardiovascular risk factors. A substudy (LLA-ASCOT), compared atorvastatin to placebo. ASCOT was stopped after an average of 3.3 years because there was no significant difference in the primary endpoints. There was an overall benefit from using atorvastatin but it was not significant in people with diabetes. However, the researchers recommended statin therapy should be considered in people with Type 2 diabetes and hypertension.
- CARDS included people with Type 2 diabetes, LDL-c, no history of cardiovascular disease and one additional cardiovascular risk factor and used 10 mg of atorvastatin. There was a trend, which failed to reach significance, towards lower all-cause mortality and LDL-c was lower (<100 mg/dL) in the atorvastatin group than in the placebo group. CARDS researchers suggested that there was no specific LDL-c threshold at which statins should be initiated in people with Type 2 diabetes. CARDS was used as the basis of American Diabetes Association (2007) recommendation that people with diabetes >age 40 and no cardiovascular diseases should be commenced on a statin regardless of their LDL-c level. The Canadian Diabetes Association (CDA) (2006) recommended the LDL-c target for people with diabetes be lowered to 2 mmol/L from 2.5 mmol/L and placed less emphasis on the LDL/HDL ratio as a primary endpoint of treatment. The triglyceride level at which treatment should be commenced was also revised to >10 mmol/L from 4.5 mmol/L. The CDA suggested fenofibrate be commenced to reduce the risk of pancreatitis and a second lipid lowering agent be added if targets were not achieved after 4–6 months.
- ASPEN included people with Type 2 diabetes and a history of cardiovascular disease and compared 10 mg atorvastatin with placebo. The protocol was amended to include people with no history of cardiovascular disease following changes in the cardiovascular management guidelines. The results were not statistically significant but there was a trend towards clinical improvements. The researchers concluded that

the level of risk (presence of multiple risk factors) affects the degree to which statins reduce the cardiovascular risk in Type 2 diabetes without cardiovascular disease.

- Veterans Affairs High-Density Lipoprotein Cholesterol Intervention Trial (VA-HIT) indicated low HDL-c is a treatable risk factor in people with and without diabetes. VA-HIT results indicate fibrates reduce cardiovascular risk by lowering LDL-c but only had a small effect on increasing HDL-c.
- FIELD study, which used fenofibrate showed reductions in the rates of macular oedema and proliferative retinopathy but did not show a significant increase in HDL-c. It lowered LDL-c and there was a reduction in major cardiovascular events in the intervention group. Statins were added in the placebo group, which may have influenced the results.
- Framingham Study indicated low HDL-c is an independent risk factor for cardiovascular disease in people with diabetes and non-diabetics and developed a cardiovascular disease risk calculator (Anderson *et al.* 1991).
- PROSPER, which studied the effects of pravastatin on all-cause mortality in people aged 70–82 years with cardiovascular risk factors or cardiovascular disease, but failed to show a reduction in all-cause mortality. However, a later meta-analysis that included the 4S, CARE, LIPID, HPS trials and unpublished data from PROSPER showed a reduction in all-cause mortality by 22%, as well as cardiovascular mortality by 30%, non-fatal MI by 26% and the need for revascularisation by 30% and stroke by 25% (Afilalo *et al.* 2008). Afilalo *et al.* also suggested older people do not have higher rates of serious adverse events than younger people but they did experience higher rates of myalgia in the statin and placebo groups. Masoudi (2007) showed rosuvastatin reduced LDL-c and C-reactive protein but did not significantly reduce the combined risk of cardiovascular disease in older people, mean age 73 years and there were fewer admissions to hospital than in the placebo group.

Management strategies should be based on the absolute risk rather than the lipid level alone. Individual risk assessment should include cardiovascular status, age, gender, the presence of hypertension, smoking, and family history of hyperlipidaemia, hypertension, and cardiac disease. Management strategies consist of:

- Dietary modification including reducing salt, alcohol and saturated fat in the diet and increasing omega-3 fatty acids (see Chapter 4).
- Low-dose aspirin to reduce platelet aggregation.
- ACE inhibitors to control blood pressure and other antihypertensive agents as indicated.
- Stopping smoking, see Chapter 10.
- Lipid lowering agents. Most people will be commenced on a statin unless they are contraindicated. Diet and exercise therapy must continue, even when lipid lowering medicines are indicated. Metformin and TZDs might have some small effect on increasing HDL-c and rimonabant is associated with significant improvements in HDL-c, possibly because of the associated weight loss.
  - Statins reduce LDL-c and have some effect on HDL. However, long-term adherence to statins is poor and many older people are not commenced on these agents despite the improved cardiovascular outcomes (Diamond & Kaul 2008).
  - Nicotinic acid very effectively increases HDL-c, but is associated with side effects and non-adherence is significant. In addition, it increases blood glucose. Although

the increase is not significant it contributes to overall increased cardiovascular risk.

o Ezetimibe, can be administered with a statin but it only has a modest effect on HDL-c. Authority is required to prescribe Ezetimibe in Australia.

o A new class of lipid lowering agents, Cholesterol Ester Transfer Protein (CEPT), which block the transfer of cholesterol from HDL-c to more atherosclerotic lipo-proteins, is under trial. The first agent, Torcetrapib, significantly raised HDL-c but did not prevent the progression to atherosclerosis. The trial (ILLUMINATE) was stopped early due to the rate of cardiovascular events in the treatment group (Nissen *et al.* 2007). The adverse results triggered debate about the advisability of using medicines to treat HDL. Other lipid lowering agents under trial include Liver-X-receptor agonists, which promote cholesterol transport and reduce atherosclerosis in animal models, Endothelial Lipase Inhibitors, which raise HDL-c and Apolipoprotein A-1 mimetic peptides that improve HDL function in animal models (Rader 2007).

- Coaching.

Table 5.5 depicts the major classes of lipid lowering agents (Colquhoun 2001).

Side effects

The side effects of lipid lowering agents often contribute to non-adherence to these medicines:

- Statins: tendonitis and myositis occurs in ~2% of people (Marie *et al.* 2008). Regular assessment to detect these side effects should occur especially during the first year. Poor sleep quality has been associated with simvastatin but not pravastatin (Golomb 2007). Taking simvastatin earlier in the day may reduce these effects. Simons (2002) suggested measuring creatine kinase (CK) before commencing statins and then 6-monthly when lipids are checked could help interpret minor changes in muscle enzymes especially in people at risk of muscle effects such as in women, and those with a small body frame, multisystem disease, polypharmacy, perioperative, interactions with medicines such as cyclosporin, azole antifungals, macrolide antibiotics, some antidepressants, large amounts of grapefruit juice, and alcohol. The American College of Cardiology, American Heart Association, and National Heart Lung and Blood Institute (2002) recommended:
  o Advising people with no symptoms and raised CK to immediately report generalised muscle aches and pains.
  o Monitoring the individual if the CK is normal and the muscle effects are mild or change to another statin or another lipid lowering agent.
  o Referring people with very high CK to a lipid specialist but continue statin therapy until the individual is assessed.
  o Carefully monitoring muscle enzymes in people with raised CK and muscle aches. Discontinue statin therapy if clinically indicated, for example, severe symptoms such as fatigue, significant pain or an interaction with statin occurs.
  o Stop statins if CK is ≥10 (upper limit of normal).
- GIT disturbances (Clofibrate).

Many people discontinue taking their lipid lowering agents because they are unconvinced about the need, perceive that they have poor efficacy or dislike the

Table 5.5 Lipid lowering agents.

Lipid lowering agent and main action	Management considerations

HMG-CoA reductase inhibitors (statins): reduce LDL-c and have a modest effect on triglycerides and HDL, may increase bone mineral density, for example:
    Atorvastatin
    Simvastatin
    Fluvastatin
    Rouvastatin
	Test liver function on commencing and 6 months after commencing
	Use caution if liver disease is present
	Reduce the dose if the patient commences cyclosporine.
	Monitor creatinine kinase (CK) and effects on muscles and tendons.
	Generally not recommended during pregnancy[a]

Ezetimebe reduces LDL-c by ~18% and by up to 20% if combined with a statin Ezetimebe combined with simvastatin	Prescribing authority is required in Australia and specific criteria need to be met.

Fibrates: Reduce cholesterol and triglycerides and increase HDL-c, for example:
    Fenofibrate
    Gemfibrosil
	Can be combined with HMG-CoA after a trial on monotherapy but the risk of muscle toxicity is increased if used with statins or other fibrates
	Monitor CK and liver function 6 weeks after starting and again in 6 months

Bile acid sequestrants (Resins) Enhance LDL-c lowering effects of HMG-CoA agents – reduce triglyceride and HDL-c, for example:
    Cholestyramine
    Cholestyramine hydrochloride
	Allows lower doses of the resins to be used
	Slows absorption of oral hypoglycaemic agents
	Increases hypoglycaemia risk when used with these agents. Administer 1.5 hours apart.
	They can impair the absorption of other medicines such as statins, fat-soluble vitamins, and thyroxine.
	Can be used with a statin

Low-dose nicotinic acid	Can be given with HMG-CoA agents

Note: The main classes of lipid lowering medicines are depicted. Relevant prescribing information should be consulted. Combinations of statins and antihypertensive agents are also available, for example, Amlopipine bensylate with atorvastatin in eight dose combinations, which are indicated for people with hypertension and/or angina who meet the prescribing criteria for lipid lowering agents. Educating and supporting the person to maintain a healthy lifestyle and enhance their medication self-management and improve medication adherence is essential.

[a]Karamermer & Roos-Hesselink (2007).

associated side effects. Nurses can play a key role in encouraging people to adhere to their medications by explaining the reason they need them and suggesting ways to limit minor side effects. For example, Tai Chi might help reduce the muscle effects of statins.

Monitoring lipid medicines

Current lipid management guidelines recommend that blood lipids should be tested at diagnosis and then at least yearly. People using lipid lowering agents should have their lipid levels measured more frequently. Lipid targets were discussed in Chapter 3. Not achieving targets is not necessarily failure: any reduction in lipid levels has a beneficial effect.

Blood glucose should also be monitored and glucose lowering medicines adjusted as needed to reach blood glucose targets. Persistant hyperglycaemia can cause hypertriglyceridaemia, which usually falls along with cholesterol if blood glucose and weight improve. Mixed hyperlipidaemia is best treated with a statin or a fibrate initially depending on the underlying lipid abnormality. Doses are usually adjusted at four-week intervals. For example, more than 80% of the lipid lowering effect of statins is achieved at 50% of the maximal dose (Jackowski 2008).

Liver function tests and creatine kinase (CK) should be tested before commencing therapy, then in ~4–8 weeks and subsequently when doses are adjusted or if clinically indicated. For example, renal impairment, older people, severe muscle weakness. Statins may need to be temporarily ceased if the person requires macrolide antibiotics. Stopping statins is associated with an increased risk of a cardiac event, especially in the first weeks (Rossi *et al.* 2007).

If the triglycerides are <4.0 mmol/L or between 2 and 4 mmol/L and HDL is <1 mmol/L, gemfibrozil is the medicine of choice. Consider vitamins A, D, E, and K supplements if bile acid resins are used in high doses for long periods of time.

Omega-3 fish oils 2–5 mg/day effectively lower triglycerides (Rossi 2007) and may be a beneficial addition to other agents for hypertriglyceridaemia or mixed hyperlipidaemia. However, several products are available on the market and doses are not the same in all products. It is important that people read labels and seek professional advice when using these medicines.

Antihypertensive agents

Hypertension is a significant risk factor for cardiovascular disease. Thus, achieving and maintaining normotension is a major therapeutic goal. There are many medicines that reduce blood pressure. Therefore, the particular antihypertensive agent used depends on the underlying cardiovascular abnormality/ies and specific benefits and risks to the individual. Diabetes is associated with several cardiovascular abnormalities, thus several agents are often required. Generally, beta blockers are started at a low dose the dose gradually increased depending on the agent used to improve left ventricular function and reduce the risk of death in patients with heart failure (Jackowski 2008). Side effects of beta blockers include:

- Fluid retention, which might be exacerbated by concomitant use of TZDs, NSAIDs, and COX –2 selective agents.
- Hypotension, which might increase the risk of falls and may be the result of an interaction with another antihypertensive agent or tricyclic antidepressants.
- Bradycardia.
- Severe fatigue, other causes should be considered such as depression, hypothyroidism and hyperglycaemia.
- Bronchospasm can occur with beta blockers in patients with asthma and COPD.

ACE inhibitors (ACEI) are considered first-line therapy in diabetes because they have renoprotective, cardioprotective and probably retinoprotective properties as well as reducing blood pressure. In addition, they might improve insulin sensitivity. ACEI and metabolites are predominantly excreted via the kidney and doses may need to be adjusted or another antihypertensive agent used if renal function is impaired.

Post hoc data analysis suggests ACEI and angiotensin 11 receptor blockers reduce the risk of progression to Type 2 diabetes, however there may be different effects in different racial groups. For example, Wright *et al.* (2006) reported lower risk of progression to diabetes in African-Americans receiving ramipril compared to amlodipine and metoprolol. However, in the DREAM trial ramipril did not reduce the incidence of diabetes in non-African-Americans with impaired fasting glucose or glucose tolerance, although it did increase the regression to normoalbuminuira (Bosch *et al.* 2006).

The ACCOMPLISH trial (2008) to determine the effects of the ACE inhibitor benazepril and a calcium channel blocker, amlodipine on morbidity and mortality was stopped early because the combination treatment was more effective than an ACE inhibitor and a diuretic (Jamerson 2008). Cardiovascular morbidity and mortality was reduced by 20%.

The main side effects of ACEI are:

- The 'ACEI cough' is a well-known side effect that is benign but often irritating to the individual and family/friends. It is less common with some of the newer agents.
- Diabetes is often associated with hyporeninaemic hypoaldosteronism syndromes particularly if renal impairment is present. The syndrome presents with unexplained hyperkalaemia, which can be exacerbated by concomitant ACEI use.
- Using an ACEI in the presence of renal artery stenosis (RAS) may critically reduce glomerular filtration. Prevalence of RAS does not appear to be higher in people with diabetes but it may be associated with but not a cause of hypertension. Risk factors include male gender, smoking, and peripheral vascular and coronary artery disease. Ensuring absence of RAS is important in such patients before commencing ACEI. Plasma potassium and creatinine should be regularly monitored in all patients on ACEI prior to and within one week commencing therapy (Gilbert *et al.* 1998).

The main types of antihypertensive medicines are shown in Table 5.6.

Antiplatelet agents

Antiplatelet agents are indicated to reduce cardiovascular risk. Commonly used antiplatelet agents are:

- Aspirin (Salicylate). Salicylates were traditionally used to reduce inflammation, fever, and pain. They are also commonly used as antiplatelet agents to reduce the risk of cardiovascular disease particularly in people at high risk such as those who had a MI, smoke, have hypertension, and/or high cholesterol. Aspirin may be contraindicated if the individual has a bleeding disorder and sometimes asthma. Aspirin occasionally causes indigestion and a tendency to bleed freely, for example, from blood glucose testing, nosebleeds, and bruises.
- Clopidogrel hydrochloride sulphate is used if aspirin poses a significant risk of bleeding and is usually used to prevent recurrent stroke, TIA, or ischaemic event.
- Dipyridamole can be used alone or with low-dose aspirin or where aspirin represents a bleeding risk. A combination formulation is available – Dipyridamole with aspirin. These agents are used to prevent recurrent stroke, TIA, or ischaemic event.
- Warfarin and heparin. These agents are rarely combined with antiplatelet agents except when the individual is at high risk.

Table 5.6 Antihypertensive medications. Often more than one antihypertensive agent will be required in diabetes to manage the underlying cardiovascular abnormalities. Prescribing information should be followed.

Class of medicine	Generic name
Diuretics used for hypertension	
Thiazide diuretics	Hydrochlorothiazide
Sulphonamide diuretics	Chlorthalidone
	Indapamide hemihydrate
Diuretics used for heart failure	
High ceiling diuretics	Frusemide
Aryloxyacetic acid derivatives	Ethacrynic acid usually used if the person is sensitive to other oral diuretics
Potassium sparing agents:	Eplerernone
Aldosterone antagonists	Amiloride hydrochloride
Amiloride hydrochloride	
Combination potassium sparing agents and low ceiling diuretics	Hydrochlorothaizide with amiloride hydrochloride
	Hydrochlorothaizide with triamterene
Non-selective beta blockers used for hypertension	Oxyprenolol
	Hydrochloride
	Pindolol
	Propranolol hydrochloride
Selective beta blockers used for hypertension	Atenolol
	Metoprolol tartarate
Alpha beta blocking agents	Labetalol hydrochloride
Beta blocking agents used in heart failure	
Alpha and beta blocking agents	Carvedilol
Selective beta blocking agents	Bisoprolol fumarate
	Metropolol succinate
Beta blocking agents used as antiarhythmics	Sotalol hydrochloride
Calcium channel blockers[a]	
Selective calcium channel blockers with predominantly vascular effects – Dihydropyridine derivatives	Amlodipine bensylate
	Felodipine
	Lercanidipine hydrochloride
	Nifedipine
Selective calcium channel blockers with direct cardiac effects – phenylalkylamine derivatives	Verapamil hydrochloride
Calcium channel blockers with cardiac and vascular effects	Diltiazem hydrochloride
Agents acting on the Renin–Angiotensin System (ACE inhibitors (ACEI))[a]	
Plain ACEI	Captopril
	Enalapril maleate
	Fosinopril sodium
	Lisinopril
	Perindopril
	Quinapril hydrochloride
	Ramipril
	Tandolapril

(Continued)

Table 5.6 Continued.

Class of medicine	Generic name
ACEI and diuretic combinations	Enalapril maleate with Hydrocholorothiazide Fosinopril sodium with Hydrocholorothiazide Perindopril erbumine with Indapamide hemihydrate Quinapril hydrochloride with Hydrocholorothiazide
Angiotensin 11 antagonists	Candesartan cilexetil Eprosartan mersylate Irbesartan Telmisartan
Angiotensin 11 antagonist combinations	Candesartan cilexetil with Hydrocholorothiazide Eprosartam mesylate with Hydrocholorothiazide Irbesartan with Hydrocholorothiazide Telmisartan with Hydrocholorothiazide
Centrally acting antiadrenergic agents	Methyldopa
Imidazoline receptor antagonists	Clonidine Moxonidine
Peripherally acting antiadrenergic agents	Prazosin hydrochloride
Hydrazinophthalazine derivatives	Hydralazine hydrochloride
Pyramidine Derivatives	Minoxidil

[a] May be contraindicated in pregnancy.

It is important for people to understand how their medicines work and the potential interactions with complementary medicines such St John's wort and glucosamine, which might potentiate the action of warfarin and lead to bleeding. Regular INR monitoring is essential and frequent dose adjustment may be required. Home INR monitoring systems are available but regular medical review is essential.

Complementary cardiovascular medicines

Research over the past few years supports the cardiovascular benefits of CAM lifestyle measures such as the Ornish diet and fish oil supplements, which have similar triglyceride lowering capacity to fibrates, and vitamin D supplements. More recently, research has confirmed the positive inotrophic properties of hawthorn (extract WS® 1442 from *Crataegus monogyna*) independently of an increase in c-AMP. WS®1442 prolongs the action potential and refractory period, has antiarrhythmic properties, improves coronary blood flow, and induces vasorelaxation, which reduces pre and after load in heart failure (Pittler *et al.* 2008), see also Chapter 8.

Medication safety and medication self-management

Medication self-management is an essential aspect of diabetes self-care. It becomes increasingly complex as more medicines are added to the regimen, often, as the individual grows older. The preceding information indicates that polypharmacy is common and is probably best practice diabetes care. Polypharmacy is variously defined as using ≥2–10 medicines depending on the source sometimes including prescribed, over-the-counter and CAM medicines. Polypharmacy contributes to:

- Difficulty remembering the medicine regimen, which affects medication review and complicates prescribing.
- Increased risk of medicine interactions.
- Increased risk of non-adherence. Approximately half the medicines prescribed for people with chronic conditions are not taken. Krapek *et al.* (2004) reported people with high scores on the Moirsky Scale (denoting adherence) had lower HbA_{1c} levels. Non-adherence results in high HbA_{1c} and the related health risks (Grant *et al.* 2007). Non-adherence to cardiovascular medications is high: 10–25% discontinue medicines within six months of starting increasing to 21–47% by 24 months (Australian Institute of Health and Welfare (AIHW) 2007). Significantly people who do not have their prescriptions filled after discharge from hospital post-MI are more likely to die within a year than those who have their prescriptions filled (Jackevicius *et al.* 2008). Non-adherence to lipid lowering agents is also high, often because people are not sure they have any benefits, feel health professionals are not interested in the individual's input into their management plan, and the associated side effects (McGinnis *et al.* 2007). This finding suggests actually prescribing and monitoring medicines in the spirit of the newer term, 'concordance', which denotes shared decision-making and agreement might be more effective than current strategies.
- Increased likelihood of presenting to emergency or being admitted to hospital with a medication-related event. Budnitz & Knight (2007) reported one third of all presentations to emergency in the US involved older people with adverse medication events.
- Increased risk of a medication-related error in hospital. As already stated insulin, warfarin and digoxin are the top three high-risk medicines, all of which are frequently prescribed in diabetes. Adverse medicine-related events occurred in 28 500 hospital admissions in 2004–2005 predominantly in people >65 years and is probably under estimation (AIHW 2007).
- High medicine costs.
- Increased risk of falls.
- Increased risk of driving accidents.
- Relying on medicines rather than continuing mandatory healthy lifestyle.
- Reduced quality of life and well being.
- Health professionals not prescribing needed medicines on the basis of inadequate patient self-care (Grant *et al.* 2007) or because they do not want to complicate the regimen.

Enhancing medication self-care

Barriers to appropriate medication self-care include the complexity of the regimen, the number of medicines prescribed, the dose frequency, not understanding the regimen or when or how to take the medicines, poor communication, inadequate information or information in a format the individual does not understand, beliefs and attitudes to medicines. Adherence to beneficial medicines reduces morbidity and mortality, which suggests adherence is a surrogate marker of healthy behaviour (Johnson *et al.* 2007). Several meta-analysis have been undertaken but few show a benefit of any one strategy, which is not surprising given the complex and changing nature of managing diabetes medicines and more importantly, the fact that most strategies focus on changing patient's behaviour rather than also considering health professional's contribution to non-adherence. A truly concordant strategy would/should also address health professional- and systems-related factors.

Nevertheless, a number of strategies for measuring and promoting medication adherence have been proposed. Some show short-term benefits, but long-term benefits are unclear. Strategies include:

- AIDES method based on a meta-analysis of 53 studies, which suggested no single strategy is more effective than any other but strategies that combine cognitive, behavioural, and affective interventions are more likely to be effective (Roter *et al.* 1998). However, the AIDES method appears complicated and there is limited evidence to support its benefit.
- Federal Study of Adherence to Medications in the Elderly (FAME) (Taylor *et al.* 2006), which specifically addressed people >65 years and encompasses education, regular follow up, and customised blister packs. The strategy was based on a review of 12 interventions and was associated with improved adherence over six months from 61% at baseline to >96% and significant reductions in systolic blood pressure and LDL-c.
- Education materials such as those developed by the Australian National Prescribing Service, Consumer Medicines Information (CMI), which are available for all PBS listed medicines in Australia, Internet sites such as familydoctor.org, and the International Alliance of Patient Organisations, however, these are largely passive and their effect on medicines use is unclear. Part of medicines education is helping people understand risks and benefits and putting these into their individual context. Woloshin & Schwartz (2007) developed a booklet designed to help people understand risks using colon cancer and medical investigations as examples. It was said to be user-friendly and used 8th grade literacy level. The booklet was tested in a high socioeconomic group and the investigators reported 'significant improvements in participants' ability to interpret risk'. It is not clear whether the information would be applicable to lower socioeconomic groups or whether behaviour changed as a consequence of enhanced ability to interpret risk.

From these strategies, relevant meta-analysis and my clinical experience using a QUM approach, the following strategies are useful. They can be used alone or in combination depending on the individual's need and agreement. That is, patient-centred medication self-management.

- Understand the health professionals' impact on patient adherence.
- Understand the individual's beliefs and attitudes towards medicines and their life goals.
- Understand their usual lifestyle and daily activities.
- Assess their physical and mental capability to manage medicines, whether help is available, and whether they will accept it if it is.
- Identify triggers to non-adherence, for example, on >5 medicines, complex dosing regimen, sound alike medicine names, look alike medicines, low literacy, cognitive deficits.

- Develop strategies to address specific issues. These should be developed in consultation with the individual, for example, 'How do you think you could remember to take your insulin?' Some useful strategies include personal cues, reminders, and medicine boxes such as blister packs.
- Provide medicine information in a relevant format and language level suitable for the individual. Work through the information with the individual and ask them to repeat back what they learned. Explain the benefits and risks but apply them to the individual's context, that is, personalise the information. Information could include:
  - Why the medicines were prescribed. For diabetes this will include medicines prescribed for prevention, but maintaining healthy lifestyle is mandatory.
  - The name of the medicine, the difference between generic and other medicines, and what brand names mean.
  - What the medicine is expected to do (outcomes) and how they will know if it is effective
  - How soon an effect will show
  - The dose and dose frequency
  - Special instructions such as take before meals
  - What to do if they forget a dose
  - When to stop taking the medicine, if relevant
  - Where and when to seek medicine advice, for example, fasting for a procedure or investigation
  - Common side effects
  - Storing and disposing of unused medicines or medicines that have past their use by date.
- Help them use other self-care information to interpret the effects of medicines adherence, non-adherence on relevant outcomes, for example, blood glucose pattern.
- Help them keep their medication list up-to-date and ensure it includes over-the-counter and CAM medicines.
- Help them formulate questions to ask their doctor at the next appointment if necessary.
- Follow-up medicines self-management regularly.

Example protocol for outpatient stabilisation onto insulin

SUGGESTED PROTOCOL

These are guidelines only and should be modified to suit individual needs.

The information can be delivered individually or in groups and over various time frames and include other information relevant to the individual.

(1) Introduce the diabetes team and area facilities.
(2) Test blood glucose.
(3) Insulin dose/frequency is determined in consultation with the doctor.
(4) The educator demonstrates insulin technique and explains the procedure to the patient and encourages the patient to practice them
(5) It is important to encourage the patient to discuss their feelings about diabetes and to assess current diabetes knowledge, learning capacity, style, psychological status and social situation.

Education goals

(1) To give a basic explanation of what diabetes is and what an acceptable blood glucose range is.
(2) To explain the reason for instituting insulin therapy.
(3) To explain the effects of insulin on blood glucose levels, that is insulin action and the role of long- and short-acting insulin in control of blood glucose levels.
(4) To explain insulin technique:
 • preparing the dose depending on the insulin delivery system chosen
 • sites for injection
 • expiry dates of insulin bottles/cartridges
 • care and storage
 • appropriate sharps disposal.
(5) To explain why insulin must be given by injection and allow patient to handle insulin device or bottles and practise preparing the insulin dose.
(6) To explain hypoglycaemia:
 • recognising symptoms of low blood glucose levels
 • causes and prevention
 • effective management
 • patient should carry carbohydrate for 'emergencies'.
(7) Blood glucose monitoring should be encouraged, to provide feedback to the patient and enable them to telephone in the afternoon with a result if necessary. The role of monitoring should be explained as well as the timing of testing and how to record results.
(8) Basic introduction to a food plan: role of carbohydrate in blood glucose control and the need to reduce fat and the need for regular meals.
(9) Explain and enrol the patient in the National Diabetes Supply Scheme[a]
 Explain responsibilites with respect to self-care, medicine management, complication screening, and driving.
(10) Ensure patient has the equipment to administer insulin and monitor blood glucose and knows how and where to obtain future supplies and knows who to contact for advice.

(1) Discuss how to manage illness at home, in relation to:
   - who to contact
   - effects of illness on blood glucose
   - emergency diet
   - monitoring and recording of blood glucose and urine or blood ketones
   - adjusting/continuing insulin
   - need to rest.
(2) Discuss precautions to be taken relating to driving, work, etc.
(3) Discuss the role of exercise/activity in controlling blood glucose levels.

(6) Encourage patient to wear some form of identification.
(7) Ensure that patient has a contact telephone number and knows who to contact for advice.
(8) Provide appropriate follow-up appointments for doctor, nurse specialist/educator according to patient needs.
(9) Provide ongoing individual teaching as required.
(10) Ensure patient knows about other services available for people with diabetes, for example, Diabetes Associations and relevant support groups.
(11) Arrange for consultation with family if necessary.

[a]*Point (10) above:* the National Diabetes Supply Scheme only applies in Australia.

References

Abraham, E., Leech, C., Lin, J., Zulewski, H. & Habener, J. (2002) Insulinotrophic hormone glucagons-like peptide-I differentiation of human pancreatic islet-derived progenitor cell into insulin producing cells. *Endocrinology*, **143**, 3152–3161.

Afilalo, J., Duque, G. & Steele, R. (2008) Statins for secondary prevention in elderly patients. *Journal American College Physicians*, **51**, 37–45.

Almond, J., Cox, D., Nugent, M., Day, J., Rayman, G. & Graham, A. (2001) Experience of group sessions for converting to insulin. *Journal of Diabetes Nursing*, **5** (4), 102–105.

American Diabetes Association (2007) Standards of medical care in diabetes. *Diabetes Care*, **30**, S4–S41.

Australian Diabetes Society (ADS) (2007) ADS Position Statement on Rosiglitzone (AVANDIA®) May 28th, 2007. ADS, Canberra.

Australian Government Department of Health and Ageing (2001). *Smoking, Nutrition, Alcohol and Physical Activity (SNAP) Framework for General Practice. Integrated Approaches to Supporting the Management of Behavioural Risk Factors of Smoking, Nutrition, Alcohol and Physical Activity (SNAP) in General Practice.*

Australian Institute of Health and Welfare (AIHW) (2007) *Medicines for Cardiovascular Health: Are They Used Appropriately?* Report 23rd May. AIHW, Canberra.

Bergman-Evans, B. (2006) AIDES to improving medication adherence in older adults. *Geriatric Nurse*, **27**, 174–182.

Braddon, J. (2001) Oral hypoglycaemics: a guide to selection. *Current Therapeutics*, Suppl. 13, 42–47.

Budnitz, D. & Knight, S. (2007) Common drugs trigger most ER visits by seniors www.medicinenet.com/script/main/art.asp?articlekey=85633.

Buse, J. (2001) Insulin analogues. *Current Opinion in Endocrinology*, **8** (2), 95–100.

Calabrese, A., Coley, K., Da Pos, S., Swanson, D. & Rao, H. (2002) Evaluation of prescribing practice: risk of lactic acidosis with Metformin. *Archives of Internal Medicine*, **162**, 434–437.

Campbell, M., Anderson, D., Holcombe, J. & Massey, E. (1993) Storage of insulin: a manufacturer's view. *Practical Diabetes*, **10** (6), 218–220.

Cefalu, W., Skyler, J., Kourides, I., Landschulz, W., Balagatas, C. & Cheng, S. (2001) Inhaled insulin treatment in patients with Type 2 diabetes. *Annals of Internal Medicine*, **134**, 242–244.

Cheung, N., Napier, B., Zaccaria, C. & Fletcher, J. (2005) Hyperglycaemia is associated with adverse outcomes in patients receiving total parenteral nutrition. *Diabetes Care*, **28**, 2367–2371.

Colquhoun, D. (2000) Unstable angina – a definitive role for statins in secondary prevention. *International Journal of Clinical Practice*, **54**, 383–389.

Colquhoun, D. (2002) Lipid lowering agents. *Australian Family Physician*, **31** (1), 25–30.

Commonwealth Department of Health and Ageing (2000) *National Medicines Policy 2000.* http://www.health.gov.au

Dadona, P., Topiwala, S., Chaudhuri, A. & Ghanim, S. (2008) Insulin is an antiatherogenic hormone. *International Diabetes Monitor*, **20** (1), 9–16.

DAFNE Study Group (2002) Training in flexible, intensive insulin management to enable dietary freedom in people with type 1 diabetes: Dose Adjustment of Normal Eating (DAFNE) randomized controlled trial. *British Medical Journal*, **325**, 746.

Dagogo-Jack, S. & Alberti, G. (2002) Management of diabetes mellitus in surgical patients. *Diabetes Spectrum*, **15**, 44–48.

DCCT (Diabetes Control and Complications Trial Research Group) (1993) Effects of intensive insulin therapy on the development and progression of long-term complications in IDDM. *New England Journal of Medicine*, **329**, 977–986.

Delafenetre, M. & Massey, N. (2008) Tendinous disorders attributed to statins: a study on ninety six spontaneous reports in the period 1990–2005 and review of the literature. *Arthritis Care Research*, **59**, 367–372.

Dornhorst, A., Luddeke, H.-J., Sreenan, S., Koenen, C., Hanssen, J., Tour, A. & Landstedt
   Hallin, L. on behalf of the PROACTIVE Study Group (2007) Safety and efficacy of insulin
   detemined in clinical practice: 14-week follow-up data from type 1 and type 2 diabetes patients
   in the PREDICTIVE™ European Cohort. *Clinical Practice*, **61** (3), 52–58.

DREAM (Diabetes Reduction Assessment with ramipril and rosiglitazone Medication Investigators
   (2006) Effect of rosiglitazone on the frequency of diabetes in patients with impaired glucose
   tolerance or impaired fasting glucose: a randomized controlled trial. *Lancet*, **355**, 2427–2443.
   (correction *Lancet*, 2006, **368**: 1770).

Dornhorst, T. (2001) Insulinotropic meglitinide analogues. *Lancet*, **17** (358), 1709–1716.

Dormandy, J., Charbonnel, B. & Eckland, D. (2005) Secondary prevention of macrovascular events in patients with type 2 diabetes in the PRO active Study (PROspective pioglit-
   AzoneClinical Trial in Macrovascular Events): a randomised controlled trial. *Lancet*, **366**,
   1279–1289.

Dunning, T. & Martin, M. (1997) Using a focus group to explore perceptions of diabetes
   severity. *Practical Diabetes International*, **14** (7), 185–188.

Dunning, T. & Martin, M. (1999) Health professional's perceptions of the seriousness of
   diabetes. *Practical Diabetes International*, **16** (3), 73–77.

Dunning, T., Rosen, S. & Alford, F. (1998) Insulin allergy: a diagnostic dilemma. *Journal of
   Diabetes Nursing*, **2** (6), 188–190.

Gabbay, R., Hu, P., Bode, B. & Garber, A. (2005) The INITIATE Study group: initiating
   insulin therapy in type 2 diabetes: a comparison of biphasic insulin analogs. *Diabetes Care*,
   28, 254–259.

George, L. (1993) Sociological-perspectives on life transitions. *Annual Review of Sociology*, **19**,
   353–373.

Gilbert, R., Cooper, M. & Krum, H. (1998) Drug administration in patients with diabetes
   mellitus. *Drug Safety*, **1** (6), 441–456.

Golomb, B. (2007) Simvastatin but not pravastatin, may reduce sleep quality. American Heart
   Association Scientific Sessions. Abstract 3725, November, Orlando.

Grant, R., Adams, A., Trinacty, C., Zhang, F., Kleinman, K., Soumerai, S., Meigs, J. &
   Ross-Degnan, D. (2007) Relationship between patient medication adherence and subsequent
   clinical inertia in type 2 diabetes glycemic management. *Diabetes Care*, **30**, 807–812.

Greaves, C., Brown, P., Terry, R., Eiser, C., Lings, P. & Stead, P. (2003) Converting to insulin
   in primary care: an exploration of the needs of practice nurses. *Journal of Advanced Nursing*,
   42 (5), 487–496.

Grundy, S., Cleeman, J. & Merz, C. (2004) Implications of recent clinical trials for the National
   Cholesterol Education treatment Panel 111 Guidelines. *Circulation*, **110**, 227–239.

Hamilton, J., Cummings, E. & Zdravkovic, V. (2003) Metformin as an adjunct therapy in
   adolescents with type 1 diabetes and insulin resistance: a randomized controlled trial.
   Diabetes Care, **26**, 138–143.

Jackevicius, C., Li, P. & Tu, J. (2008) Prevalence, predictors, and outcomes of primary non-adherence after acute myocardial infarction. *Circulation*, DOI 10.1161/
   CIRCULATIONAHA.107.706820.

Jackowski, L. (2008) Lipid lowering therapy. *Australian Family Physician*, **37** (1/2), 39–41.

Jain, R., Allen, E. & Wahl, I. (2005) Premixed insulin analogues for the treatment of diabetets.
   Diabetes, **54** (Suppl. A69).

Jerrall, M. (2002) Warning over Metformin use. *Archives of Internal Medicine*, **162**, 434–437.

Hirsch, I., Paaun, D. & Brunzell, J. (1995) Inpatient management of adults with diabetes.
   Diabetes Care, **18** (6), 870–877.

Home, P., Pocock, S. & Beck-Nielsen, H. (2005) Rosaglitazone evaluated for cardiac outcomes
   and regulation of glycaemia in diabetes (RECORD): study design and protocol. *Diabetelogia*,
   48, 1726–1735.

Inzucchi, S. (2002) Oral antihyperglycemic therapy for type 2 diabetes: scientific review. *Journal
   American Medical Association*, **287**, 360–372.

Jamerson, K. for the ACCOMPLISH investigators (2008) Avoiding cardiovascular events in combination therapy in patients living with systolic hypertension. American College of Cardiology Scientific Sessions, March, Chicago.

Jackowski, L. (2008) Beta blockers in systolic heart failure. *Australian Family Physician*, **37** (3), 137–139.

Janka, H., Plewe, G., Riddle, M., Kliebe-Frisch, C., Schweitzer, M. & Yki-Jarvinen, H. (2005) Comparison of basal insulin added to oral agents versus twice daily premixed insulin as initial therapy for type 2 diabetes. *Diabetes Care*, **28**, 254–259.

Johnson, G. & Shalansky, S. (2007) Predictors of refill non-adherence in patients with heart failure. *British Journal of Clinical Pharmacology*, **63** (4), 488–493.

Katz, C. (1991) How efficient is sliding scale insulin therapy? Problem with a 'cookbook' approach in hospital patients. *Postgraduate Medicine*, **5** (5), 46–48.

Krapek, K., King, K., Warren, S., George, K., Caputo, D., Mihelich, K., Holst, E. & Nichol, B. (2004) Medication adherence and associated hemoglobin A_{1c} in type 2 diabetes. *The Annals of Pharmacotherapy*, **38** (9), 1357–1362.

Kuritzky, L. (2006) Addition of basal insulin to oral antidiabetic agents: a goal-directed approach to type 2 diabetes. *Medscape General Medicine*, **8** (4), 34–48.

Keech, A., Simes, R. & Barter, P. (2005) Effects of long term fenofibrate therapy on cardiovascular events in diabetes mellitus (the FIELD study): randomized controlled trial. *Lancet*, **366**, 1649–1861.

Knopp, R., D'Emden, M. & Smilde, J. (2006) Efficacy and safety of atorvastatin in the prevention of cardiovascular disease in people with type 2 diabetes: The Atorvastatin Study for the Prevention of Coronary heart Disease Endpoints in Non-Insulin dependent Diabetes mellitus (ASPEN). *Diabetes Care*, **29**, 1478–1485.

Kuritzky, L. (2006) Addition of basal insulin to oral antidiabetic agents: a goal directed approach to type 2 diabetes therapy. *Medscape General Medicine*, **8** (4), 34–47.

La Rosa, J., He, J. & Vupputuri, S. (1999) Effect of statins on risk of coronary disease: a meta-analysis of randomised controlled trials. *Journal of the American Medical Association*, **282**, 2340–2346.

Lee, J., Grace, K. & Taylor, A. (2006) Effect of a pharmacy care program on medication adherence and persistence, blood pressure, and low density lipoprotein cholesterol. *Journal American Medical Association*, DOI:10. 100/jama.296.21.joc60162.

Lipid Study Group (1998) The long term intervention with pravastatin in ischaemic disease. Prevention of cardiovascular events and death with pravastatin in patients with coronary heart disease and a broad range of initial cholesterol levels. *New England Journal of Medicine*, **339**, 1349–1357.

Malone, J., Campaigne, B., Reviriego, J. & Augendre-Ferrrante, B. (2005) Twice daily pre-mixed insulin rather than basal insulin therapy alone results in better overall glycaemic control in patients with type 2 diabetes. *Diabetic Medicine*, **22**, 374–381.

Malmberg, K. (1997) Prospective randomised study of intensive insulin treatment on long-term survival after acute myocardial infarction. *British Medical Journal*, **314**, 1512–1515.

Masoudi, F. (2007) Can statins benefit elderly patients with ischeamic heart disease? *Journal Watch Cardiology*, **6** (11), 10–16.

Mayfield, J. & White, R. (2004) Insulin therapy for type 2 diabetes: rescue, augmentation, and replacement of beta-call function. *American Family Physician*, **70** (3), 100–115.

Montori, V. & Isley, W. (2007) Waking up from the DREAM of preventing diabetes with drugs. *British Medical Journal*, **334**, 882–884.

MacKinnon, M. (1998) *Diabetes Care in General Practice*. Class Publishing, London.

McGinnis, B., Olson, K., Magid, D., Bayliss, E., Korner, E., Brand, D. & Steiner, J. (2007) Factors related to adherence in statin therapy. *Annals of Pharmacotherapy*, **41** (11), 1805–1811.

National Diabetes Strategy (NDS) (1998) *National Diabetes Strategy and Implementation Plan*. Diabetes Australia, Canberra.

NHMRC (National Health and Medical Research Council) (1991a) *Stabilisation of Diabetes.*
National Health and Medical Research Council, Canberra.

NHMRC (National Health and Medical Research Council) (1991b) *The Role of Ambulatory Services in the Management of Diabetes.* Document No. 1. Australia.

Nathan, D. & Buse, J. (2006) Management of hypertension in type 2 diabetes: a consensus algorithm for the initiation and adjustment of therapy. A consensus statement from the American Diabetes Association and the Diabetes Association for the Study of Diabetes. *Diabetologia,* **49,** 1711–1721.

National Heart Foundation (2001) *Lipid Management Guidelines.* National Heart Foundation, Melbourne.

National Prescribing Service (NPS) (2000) What is Polypharmacy? *NPS News.* NPS, Canberra.

National Prescribing Service (NPS) (2008) Managing hyperglycaemia in type 2 diabetes. *NPS News.* NPS, Canberra.

Nichols, G., Hillier, T. & Erbey, J. (2001) Congestive heart failure in type 2 diabetes: prevalence, incidence, and risk factors. *Diabetes Care,* **24,** 1614–1619.

Nicholson, G. (2002) Statins decrease fractures and increase bone mineral density. *Archives of Internal Medicine,* **163,** 537–540.

Nisbet, J., Sturtevant, J. & Prons, J. (2004) Metformin and serious adverse events. *Medical Journal of Australia,* **180** (2), 53–54.

Nissen, S. & Wolski, K. (2007) Effect of rosiglitazone on the risk of myocardial infarction and death from cardiovascular causes. *New England Journal of Medicine,* 10.1056/NEJMoa072761.

Nissen, S., Tardif, J. & Nicholls, S. (2007) Effect of torcetrapib on the progression of coronary atherosclerosis. *New England Journal of Medicine,* **356,** 1304–1316.

Phillips, P. (2000) Tablet tips for Type 2 diabetes. *Current Therapeutics,* **41** (9), 71–77.

Pittler, M., Guo, R. & Ernst, E. (2008) Hawthorn extract for treating chronic heart failure: a meta-analysis of randomised trials. *Cochrane Database of Systematic Reviews,* Issue 1, Art. No. CD005312.DOI:10.1002/14651858.CD005312.pub.2

Prochaska, J. & Velicer, W. (1997) The transtheoretical model of health behaviour change. *American Journal of Health Promotion,* **12,** 38–48.

Raskin, P., Rendell, M. & Riddle, M. (2001) A randomised trial of Rosiglitazone therapy in patients with inadequately controlled insulin treated Type 2 diabetes. *Diabetes Care,* **24** (7), 1226–1232.

Rossi, S. (ed.) (2007) *Australian Medicines Handbook.* Australian Medicines Handbook Pty Ltd, Adelaide.

Leiter, L. (2006) Can thiazolidinediones delay disease progression in type 2 diabetes? *Current Medical Research and Opinion,* **22** (6), 1193–1201.

Queale, W., Seidler, A. & Brancati, F. (1997) Glycaemic control and sliding scale insulin use in medical inpatients with diabetes mellitus. *Archives of Internal Medicine,* **157,** 545–552.

Quinn, J., Snyder, S., Berghoff, J., Colombo, C. & Jacobi, J. (2006) A practical approach to hyperglycaemia management in the intensive care unit: evaluation of an intensive insulin infusion protocol. *Pharmacotherapy,* **26** (10), 1410–1420.

Raskin, P., Allen, E., Hollander, P., Lewin, A., Gabbay, R., Hu, P., Bode, B. & Garber, A. (2005) The INITIATE study group: initiating insulin therapy in type 2 diabetes: a comparison of biphasic and basal insulin analogues. *Diabetes Care,* **28,** 260–265.

Riddle, M., Rosenstock, J. & Gerich, J. (2003) The insulin glargine 2004 study investigators; the treat-to-target trial: randomized addition of glargine to human NPH insulin to oral therapy in type diabetes patients. *Diabetes Care,* **26,** 3080–3086.

Rosenstock, J., Schwartz, S., Clark, C., Park, G., Donley, D. & Edwards, M. (2001) Basal insulin therapy in type 2 diabetes: 28-week comparison of insulin gargine (HOE 901) versus NPH insulin. *Diabetes Care,* **24,** 631–636.

Roter, D., Hall, J., Mersica, R., Nordstrom, B., Cretin, D. & Svarstad, B. (1998) Effectiveness of interventions to improve patient compliance: a meta-analysis. *Medical Care,* **36,** 1138–1161.

Rutherford, E., Wright, E., Hussain, Z., Colagiuri, R. on behalf of the DAWN Committee (2004) *DAWN: Diabetes Attitudes, Wishes and Needs. The Australian Experience.* NovoNordisk, Australasia, Sydney.

Shenfield, G. (2001) Drug interactions with oral hypoglycaemic agents. *Australian Prescriber*, **24** (4), 83–84.

Simons, L. (2002) Test CK before starting on statins. *Medical Observer*, 30th Augsust, 5.

Skyler, J., Cefalu, W., Kourides, I., Landschulz, W., Balagatas, C. & Cheng, S. (2001) Efficacy of inhaled human insulin in Type 1 diabetes mellitus. *Lancet*, **357**, 331–335.

Sullivan, D. (2008) Raising HDL cholesterol in diabetes. *Diabetes Management Journal*, **22**,16.

Sumner, J., Baber, C. & Williams, V. (2000) What do people with Type 1 diabetes know about hypoglycaemia? *Practical Diabetes International*, **17** (6), 187–190.

Strowig, S., Aviles-Santa, L. & Raskin, P. (2004) Improved glycaemic control without weight gain using triple therapy in type 2 diabetes. *Diabetes Care*, **27**, 1577–1583.

Tan, Y. (2006) Initiating insulin in patients with type 2 diabetes. *Diabetes Management Journal*, **14**, 28–29.

Tay, M., Messersmith, R. & Lange, D. (2001) What do people on insulin therapy remember about safety advice? *Journal of Diabetes Nursing*, 5 (6), 188–191.

Ting, R. (2006) Metformin use increases vitamin B 12 deficiency in patients with diabetes. *Archives of Internal Medicine*, **166**, 1975–1079.

Turner, R., Cull, C., Frighi, V. & Holman, R. (1999) Control with diet, sulphonylurea, metformin, or insulin in patients with type 2 diabetes mellitus: progressive requirement for multiple therapies (UKPDS 49). *Journal American Medical Association*, **281**, 2005–2012.

United Kingdom Prospective Diabetes Study (UKPDS 33) (1998) Intensive blood glucose control with sulphonylureas or insulin compared with conventional treatment and risk of complications in patients with type 2 diabetes. *Lancet*, **352**, 837–853 (correction *Lancet* 1999; **354**: 602).

Vaag, A., Handberg, A., Lauritzen, M., Henriksen, J., Pedersen, K. & Beck-Neilsen, H. (1990) Variation in insulin absorption of NPH insulin due to intramuscular injection. *Diabetes Care*, **13** (1), 74–76.

Wah, C. (2008) Improved glycaemic control after surgical procedures. *Diabetes Management Journal*, **22**, 28–29.

Williams, G. & Pickup, J. (1992) *Handbook of Diabetes*. Blackwell Science, Oxford.

Williams, P. (1993) Adverse effects of exogenous insulin: clinical features, management and prevention. *Drug Safety*, **8**, 427–444.

Willi, C., Bodenmann, P., Ghali, W., Faris, P. & Cornuz, J. (2007) Active smoking and the risk of Type 2 diabetes: a systematic review and meta-analysis. *Journal of the American Medical Association*, **298**, 2654–2664.

Wright, J., Randall, O., Miller, E., Lash, J., Grassman, J., Contreras, G., Appel, L., Agodoa, L. & Cheek, D. for the African-American Study of Kidney Disease and Hypertension (2006) Differing effects of antihypertensive drugs on the incidence of diabetes mellitus among patients with hypertensive kidney disease. *Archives of Internal Medicine*, **166**, 797–805.

Woloshin, S. & Schwartz, L. (2007) The effectiveness of a primer to help people understand risk. *Annals of Internal Medicine*, **146**, 256–265.

Worthington, B. (2003) The nurses' role in patient-centred medicines management. *Professional Nurse*, **19** (3), 142–144.

Zeolla, M. (2007) Are novoLog and Humalog interchangeable? *Medscape Pharmacist*, 4.2.2007.

Yki-Jarvinen, H., Ryysky, L., Nikkila, K., Tulokas, T., Vanamo, R. & Heikkila, M. (1999) Comparison of bedtime regimens in patients with type 2 diabetes mellitus: a randomized controlled trial. *Archives of Internal Medicine*, **130**, 389–296.

Yki-Jarvinen, H., Juurinen, L., Alvarsson, M., Bystedt, T., Caldwell, I., Davies, M., Lahdenpera, S., Nijpels, G. & Vahatalo, M. (2007) Initiate insulin by aggressive titration and educate (INITIATE). *Diabetes Care*, **30**, 1364–1369.

Chapter 6

Hypoglycaemia

Key points

- Hypoglycaemia is one of the most common short-term complications of diabetes treatment with insulin and some oral glucose lowering medicines.
- The brain depends on a constant supply of glucose because it is unable to synthesise or store glucose. Severe hypoglycaemia is associated with cognitive impairment that affects the person's ability to manage the hypoglycaemia and function normally.
- Hypoglycaemia is the most feared side effect of insulin especially in the presence of hypoglycaemic unawareness.

Rationale

Hypoglycaemia can be prevented by proactive self-care including regular blood glucose monitoring, appropriate nursing care, and recognising impending hypoglycaemia and managing it appropriately. The prevalence of hypoglycaemia is increasing due to the focus on achieving blood glucose levels as close to normal as possible.

Introduction

Hypoglycaemia is the most common and the most serious side effect of insulin. The prevalence of hypoglycaemia has increased since the results of the Diabetes Control and Complications Trial DCCT (DCCT 1997 and 2003) and the United Kingdom Prospective Diabetes Study (UKPDS) (UKPDS 1998) demonstrated that keeping blood glucose in the normal range reduced the risk of long-term complications and glucose targets were revised.

Severe hypoglycaemia was three times more frequent in the intensive insulin treatment group compared to conventional treatment in the DCCT (61 events per 100 people). Hypoglycaemia was more common in men than women and in adolescents than adults. The risk of severe hypoglycaemia was 1 in 3 and the risk of coma 1 in 10 (DCCT 1991). Concern about hypoglycaemia was thought to contribute to the difficulty achieving glycaemic targets. Likewise, Pramming *et al.* (1991) reported mild hypoglycaemia was 1.8 episodes per patient per week and 1.4 episodes of severe hypoglycaemia per patient per year.

The increased rate of hypoglycaemia is largely due to the focus on achieving normoglycaemia by intensifying management in both Type 1 and Type 2 and transferring people with Type 2 diabetes onto insulin sooner since the results of these studies were released. In early reports from the UKPDS, major hypoglycaemia occurred between 0.4 and 2.3% of insulin-treated patients per year compared with 0.4% of those treated with diet or sulphonurylureas (UKPDS). Later studies also show the frequency and severity of hypoglycaemia in people with Type 2 diabetes is lower than Type 1 (Yki-Jarvinen *et al.* 1999).

Wright *et al.* (2006) recorded self-reported hypoglycaemia rates and severity grade (transient (1), temporarily incapacitated (2), requiring assistance (3), requiring medical attention (4) in various treatment groups who remained on their allotted therapy for six years from diagnosis as part of the UKPDS). Grades 1 and 2 occurred in 0.8% in the diet and 1.7% in the metformin groups per year and 0.1% and 0.3% respectively for grades 2–4 per year. Rates for those on sulphonylureas were 7.9% and 1.2%; 21.2% and 3.65 on basal insulin and 32% and 5.5% on basal and pre-meal insulin.

Younger people (<45 years), women, those with HbA_{1c} <7%, and islet autoantibody-positive people were twice as likely to report hypoglycaemia. Wright *et al.* claimed the low rates of hypoglycaemia in Type 2 diabetes was unlikely to have a major negative impact on people's ability to achieve glycaemic targets. Despite ~30% of people initially recruited were lost from the study, possibly due to intensifying treatment to achieve optimal glycaemic control so the numbers of people in each treatment group was small, the overall hypoglycaemia rate was low. Not surprisingly, hypoglycaemia risk was greater in people on insulin with poorer control but lower doses of insulin were associated with a 35% lower rate of hypoglycaemia. Older people (>65) were not included in the study, thus their risk and ability to recognise hypoglycaemia is unclear from the study.

A number of researchers suggest the rate of mild and severe hypoglycaemia is lower in insulin-treated Type 2 diabetes than in Type 1. However, hypoglycaemia risk increases once insulin is commenced and with increasing duration of diabetes (Henderson *et al.* 2003). Hypoglycaemic unawareness is uncommon in Type 2 diabetes, but when present, it is associated with a higher incidence of severe hypoglycaemia. Ziemer *et al.* (2007) suggested intensifying insulin treatment is not associated with increased hypoglycaemia, even when the HbA_{1c} is close to the target.

The rate of severe hypoglycaemia is higher in young children: 0.49 in children <6 years compared to 0.16 in children >6 (Davis *et al.* 1997). Daneman *et al.* (1989) reported 31% of children (*n* = 311); mean age 11.6 and mean duration of diabetes 4.6 years, had at least one coma or convulsion since diagnosis. Other researchers report rates ranging from 6.8 to 12%.

In contrast, Nordfeldt & Ludvigsson (1997) stated the incidence of hypoglycaemic coma did not increase when HbA_{1c} improved from 8.1% to 6.9%, but episodes of severe hypoglycaemia increased from 1.01 to 1.26 per patient per year. Early recognition and treatment of hypoglycaemia in young children is essential because their brains are vulnerable to hypoglycaemia, which may cause permanent cognitive deficits (Tattersall 1999).

Normal glucose homeostasis was discussed in Chapter 1. Counter-regulatory hormones, especially glucagon, the catecholamines, growth hormone, and cortisol are released when the blood glucose falls below the normal range to maintain the blood glucose level and ensure a constant supply of energy to the brain. Glucagon and the catecholamines stimulate gluconeogenesis and reduce glucose utilisation. The severity and duration of hypoglycaemia determines the magnitude of the counter-regulatory response and begins as the blood glucose falls to ~3.5–3.7 mmol/L before cognitive function is impaired around 3.0 mmol/L (Heller & Macdonald 1996).

The counter-regulatory hormones are largely responsible for the signs and symptoms of hypoglycaemia through activating the autonomic nervous system. Several researchers have compiled lists of hypoglycaemic symptoms (Hepburn 1993; Cox *et al.* 1993). Recognising the signs enables early treatment to be initiated. Significantly, symptoms are specific to the individual and are interpreted differently from health professionals. For example, people report symptoms differently if they are asked to indicate the relevance of each symptom to themselves (Tattersall 1999, p. 57). In the author's experience, some people think 'a hypo means you go into a coma' and do not associate mild symptoms with hypoglycaemia, other people and their relatives associate trembling, vagueness and aggressive behaviour as 'having a fit', which suggests some information included in hypoglycaemia education programmes may not be appropriate to everybody. The most commonly reported symptoms are: sweating, trembling, difficulty concentrating, nervousness, feeling tense, light-headedness and dizziness (Cox *et al.* 1993).

When the blood glucose is <3.0 mmol/L, fine motor coordination, mental speed and concentration, and some memory functions become impaired. Reaction times are slower especially when the individual needs to make decisions: mental arithmetic and short-term verbal memory and working memory are impaired (Sommerfield *et al.* 2003). McAulay *et al.* (2001) also demonstrated significant impairment of attentional abilities during hypoglycaemia but found fluid intelligence (problem-solving ability) was not impaired. Thus, many everyday tasks appear to be impaired during hypoglycaemia including the individual's ability to manage the episode.

Factors associated with increased cognitive deficits include male gender, hypoglycaemic unawareness, Type 1 diabetes, and high IQ. These findings have implications for effective hypoglycaemia self-management and safety. For example, people drive slowly, swerve more, steer inappropriately, spend more time driving off the road and position the car badly on the road when the blood glucose is <2.6 mmol/L (Cox *et al.* 1993). The counter-regulatory response to recurrent hypoglycaemia may be blunted in subsequent hypoglycaemia and the individual may not recognise the signs and symptoms. Often, people do not recall severe hypoglycaemic episodes.

Results from continuous glucose monitoring systems (CSII) suggest people taking four insulin injections per day have at least one blood glucose level <2.8 mmol/L of varying duration per day, which may not cause symptoms (Thorsteinsson *et al.* 1986). This is affected by a number of factors including the number of injections per day, the type of insulin, variations in absorption within individuals and among injection sites.

Emotions are also affected and mood changes in the three basic mood types: energetic arousal (feel active), tense arousal (feel anxious), and hedonic state (feel happy) occur during or in anticipation of hypoglycaemia. People with diabetes fear hypoglycaemia, which can lead them to inappropriately lower their insulin doses to reduce the risk of hypoglycaemia, see Chapter 15.

Thus, the effects of hypoglycaemia are complex and multifactorial. Education and strategies to prevent/manage hypoglycaemia should be individualised and accompany changes in medication management and include family and significant others.

Definition of hypoglycaemia

Hypoglycaemia is defined in several ways:

- Biochemical: blood glucose below a specific level, which is common especially overnight and is often unrecognised.
- Mild symptomatic where the individual is able to self-treat. The symptoms are often vague and may not be related to the actual blood glucose level. The most commonly reported initial symptoms that closely reflect the actual blood glucose level are trembling, sweating, tiredness, difficulty concentrating and hunger.
- Severe symptomatic associated with neuroglycopenia where help is required to treat. People do not always remember a severe hypoglycaemic episode because of retrograde amnesia or denial. Severe hypoglycaemia can occur without coma.
- Profound associated with coma and sometimes convulsions (Tattersall 1999, pp. 55–87). Some experts associate severe hypoglycaemia with coma and convulsions.

In addition, a grading system is often used, especially in research, as follows:

- Grade 1 – mild: the person recognises and self-treats.
- Grade 2 – moderate: the person requires assistance but oral treatment normalises the blood glucose.
- Grade 3 – severe: the person is semiconscious and requires assistance, and glucagon or IV glucose may be needed.

Clinically, hypoglycaemia is often defined as blood glucose low enough to cause hypoglycaemia signs and symptoms and/or a blood glucose level of <3.0 mmol/L in people with diabetes treated with insulin or oral hypoglycaemic agents.

Practice points

(1) People with diabetes managed by diet alone do not usually require treatment of low blood glucose levels.
(2) People treated with insulin are at the greatest risk of hypoglycaemia.
(3) Hypoglycaemia is the most significant side effect of insulin.

In addition to insulin and/or OHA treatment, age, gender, and associated medical conditions such as liver disease, cerebrovascular disease, autonomic neuropathy, and the rate at which the blood glucose falls influences the development and recognition of symptoms. In general, a rapid fall in blood glucose results in the development of the classic symptoms of hypoglycaemia described in Table 6.1. The classic presentation is more likely to occur in insulin-treated patients.

The onset of hypoglycaemia is usually slower with sulphonylureas especially in older people and can be prolonged and recur for >24 hours despite treatment. Mortality rates between 4 and 10% are reported and permanent neurological damage is present in 5% of those who survive (Salas *et al.* 2002). Long-acting sulphonylureas increase the risk because of their long duration of action, active metabolites, and the reduced

Table 6.1 Signs and symptoms of hypoglycaemia. These symptoms are so common that they are used in the Edinburgh Hypoglycaemia Scale (Deary *et al.* 1993). Symptoms are different in young children and may vary between episodes in the same individual.

Sympathetic or adrenergic[a]	Neuroglycopaenic[b]
Weakness	Headache
Pale skin	Tiredness
Sweating	Hypothermia
Tachycardia	Visual disturbances
Palpitations	Difficulty concentrating
Shaking	Difficulty speaking
Tremor	Confusion
Nervousness or feeling anxious	Amnesia
Irritability	Seizures
Tingling of the mouth and fingers	Coma
Hunger	Inappropriate behaviour

[a] Caused by increased activity of the autonomic nervous system triggered by a rapid fall in blood glucose. Also referred to as sympathetic and sympathomedullary.
[b] Caused by decreased activity of the central nervous system because of very low blood glucose. Psychomotor function deteriorates. Some people appear withdrawn others become restless and irritable. They may refuse treatment. Recovery can be slow or rarely the person may die if they do not have help.

Nausea and vomiting may occur but are unusual.

ability to mount a counter-regulatory response that occurs with increasing age. Presenting symptoms may be neuroglycopenic, often confusion, dizziness, and altered behaviour, rather than sympathetic and the hypoglycaemia can be mistaken for stroke, transient ischaemia, or early dementia and lead to unnecessary investigations and delayed treatment (Sinclair *et al.* 2006).

Risk factors for hypoglycaemia in older people include:

- Treatment with sulphonylureas or insulin, especially long-acting agents, although long-acting insulin analogues have significantly lower risk, see Chapter 5.
- Recent discharge from hospital especially if the glucose lowering medicine regimen was changed in hospital and discharge planning is inadequate and the person lives alone.
- Renal or liver disease.
- Excess alcohol consumption.
- Inadequate knowledge of the signs and symptoms of hypoglycaemia.
- Inability to self-treat the hypoglycaemia, for example, due to confusion.
- On multiple medicines.
- Using glucose lowering conventional and complementary medicines together.

Recognising hypoglycaemia

Some, or all, of the signs and symptoms listed in Table 6.1 can be present. A number of factors affect the individual's ability to recognise hypoglycaemia as indicated.

In addition, some commonly consumed substances such as caffeine, which can increase the intensity of the symptoms, and alcohol, which clouds judgement, can make it difficult for people to recognise hypoglycaemia.

Symptoms are more varied in children than adults and between hypoglycaemic episodes in the same child, and they have more difficulty recognising the symptoms. Young children may become naughty, aggressive, complain of abdominal pain, feeling 'awful', yawning, daydreaming, and warm to the touch (Ross *et al.* 1998). As indicated, older people with Type 2 diabetes commonly present with neurological symptoms. Many emergency departments now have a policy of testing the blood glucose in unconscious patients.

Gonder-Frederick *et al.* (1997) described a number of factors that affect the individual's ability to detect and treat hypoglycaemia including:

- The blood glucose level.
- Usual metabolic control.
- Recent hypoglycaemia.
- Chronic hypoglycaemia, which can occur 'acutely' in older people as a result of repeated unrecognised hypoglycaemia or as a result of hypoglycaemic unawareness, see Chapter 8.
- Counter-regulatory response and amount of adrenaline secreted. The counter-regulatory response, especially glucagon release, diminishes over time in Type 1 diabetes.
- Medications such as beta blockers can mask the sympathetic warning signs, and caffeine can cause trembling and sweating that can be mistaken for hypoglycaemia. Smoking confers a 2.6 times greater risk of severe hypoglycaemia in Type 1 diabetes (Klein *et al.* 2007) as well as contributing to the long-term complications of diabetes and other diseases.
- Distractions such as concentrating on work, when anxious and stressed, which also activates the autonomic nervous system ('fight or flight' response).
- Knowledge such as not recognising the symptoms.
- Hypoglycaemic unawareness or impaired mental function, which inhibits appropriate management.
- Cognitive impairment.

Other research shows older people, especially those living alone, young children who depend on their parents (McCrimmon *et al.* 1995), adolescents (DCCT 1997), those determined to achieve strict glycaemic control, lower social class (Muhlhauser *et al.* 1998), and pregnant women with Type 1 diabetes, experience more hypoglycaemia. For example, 45% of pregnant women with Type 1 diabetes experience severe hypoglycaemia during pregnancy particularly in the first trimester and 3–5 mild hypoglycaemic events per patient-week especially in the presence of previous severe hypoglycaemia and impaired or hypoglycaemia unawareness (Ringholm Nielsen *et al.* 2008).

Counter-regulatory hormonal response to hypoglycaemia

The brain requires 120–140 g glucose per day to function normally and has a very limited capacity to manufacture its own glucose. Therefore it is dependent on adequate

Table 6.2   The counter-regulatory hormonal response to hypoglycaemia.

Hormone	Action
Glucagon	Increases glucose output from liver and muscle (glycogenolysis)
Adrenaline and noradrenaline	Enhances glycogenolysis in liver and muscle Enhances gluconeogenesis Reduces insulin secretion Causes many of the signs and symptoms of hypoglycaemia (autonomic response; see Table 6.1)
Cortisol	Mobilises the substrates for gluconeogenesis
Growth hormone	Acts with cortisol and adrenaline to inhibit peripheral glucose utilisation

levels of circulating blood glucose. When the blood glucose falls below normal the body releases hormones to counteract the effects of hypoglycaemia. This is known as the counter-regulatory response. Glycogen stores are liberated and new glucose is formed in the liver from precursors, for example, fatty acids and protein. The hormones released are shown in Table 6.2, along with their resultant action, the net result being an increase in blood glucose.

Causes of hypoglycaemia

Although hypoglycaemia is associated with insulin and OHA use, the relationship among these agents and food intake, exercise, and a range of other contributory factors is not straightforward. Some episodes can be explained by altered awareness or mismatch between food intake and/or food absorption and insulin. It should be noted that serum insulin levels and glucose clearance following insulin injections varies in the same individual even when the same dose is injected at the same time, dose and approximate site each day (Galloway & Chance 1994), even with modern purified insulins.

Exercise is also a contributing factor in many cases but the effect of exercise is also difficult to predict and depends on exercise intensity and duration, planned or spontaneous, time of the day, previous food intake, when it occurred in relation to insulin/OHA dose, and the insulin injection site. For example, absorption is enhanced if exercise commences immediately after injecting insulin but not if exercise commences >35 minutes after injecting.

As indicated, sulphonylureas cause hypoglycaemia but less commonly than insulin. However, when it does occur it causes significant morbidity and mortality, may be prolonged and may accompany or precipitate a stroke or myocardial infarction. Interactions with other medicines including complementary medicines should be considered especially in the setting of compromised renal function, see Chapters 8 and 19. Alcohol may be a contributing factor.

Frequent hypoglycaemia might indicate changing renal function and insulin doses may need to be reduced. OHAs may be contraindicated. Lowered appetite and nausea accompanying renal disease may contribute to hypoglycaemia risk.

If no reasonable common contributing factor can be identified less common causes such as endocrine disorders, gastroparesis, and coeliac disease should be considered. Psychological factors need to be considered, see Chapter 15.

A specific reason for the episode cannot always be found, which makes prevention difficult; unknown rates ranging between 19 and 38% have been reported.

Various authors attribute hypoglycaemia to 'patient non-compliance' such as manipulating insulin doses, reducing intake, or omitting meals. While these behaviours do occur, health professionals need to understand the reason for the behaviour rather than attaching a label to the individual. They need to appreciate the complexity of achieving diabetes balance and the frustration it causes many people with diabetes. The view that achieving blood glucose balance is an equation where:

insulin/OHAs + appropriate diet + appropriate exercise = target glucose

is simplistic, and ignores significant individual factors.

Hypoglycaemic unawareness

Hypoglycaemic unawareness means people no longer recognise the early autonomic hypoglycaemic signs and do not recognise hypoglycaemia thus do not treat it and are at risk of severe hypoglycaemia and coma. Recurrent episodes of hypoglycaemia reduce the counter-regulatory response, associated symptoms and cognitive responses, which affects the individual's ability to recognise and treat the episode. People with Type 1 diabetes have compromised counter-regulatory response and a cycle of hypo-glycaemia where each episode becomes increasingly severe may develop. If counter-regulation is compromised endogenous insulin secretion is not inhibited. Significantly, glucagon release in response to hypoglycaemia is impaired soon after diagnosis of diabetes and becomes progressively defective in Type 1 diabetes. Adrenaline release is also reduced, which ultimately results in hypoglycaemic unawareness (DCCT Research Group 1991).

Hypoglycaemic unawareness may develop when the usual blood glucose is in the low/normal range and people may begin to recognise the symptoms again if the blood glucose targets are raised. Chronic hypoglycaemic unawareness develops with long duration of diabetes usually as a result of autonomic neuropathy and diminished coun-ter-regulatory response. Both acute and chronic hypoglycaemic unawareness can be aggravated by medicines such as non-selective beta blockers, alcohol, and stimulants such as caffeine. Hypoglycaemic unawareness increases the risk of severe and profound hypoglycaemia and is one criterion for islet cell transplants.

Indicators that chronic hypoglycaemia might be present in elderly people, especially those on OHAs, include failing mental function, personality changes, and disordered behaviour and must be distinguished from other less easily reversible causes of these signs. Accurately monitoring the blood glucose levels is important to detect chronic hypoglycaemia and CGMS can be useful. Management consists of revising the care plan and checking:

- That carbohydrate intake is adequate and evenly distributed;
- The individual is able to accurately prepare and administer their insulin;

- Whether any new medications or complementary therapies were commenced and reviewing the individual's medication self-management practices;
- Teeth/dentures to ensure there is no infection or mouth ulcers and that false teeth fit and are worn;
- Presence of diabetic complications or comorbidities that can affect self-care ability.
- Knowledge, which might mean relatives and friends need information about managing hypoglycaemia including how and when to use. People may benefit from education programmes such as BGATT and some regain the ability to recognise hypoglycaemia or new body cues after a period free from hypoglycaemia.

Nocturnal hypoglycaemia

Nocturnal hypoglycaemia is particularly worrying in children because they have a blunted counter-regulatory response (Jones *et al.* 1998). It is defined as blood glucose, 3.3 mmol/L occurring during the night and mainly occurs in Type 1 diabetes, usually as a consequence of relative insulin excess and impaired glucose production overnight. Increased insulin sensitivity overnight plays a role. More than 80% of people treated with insulin experience nocturnal hypoglycaemia; 40% of these episodes are severe and are associated with significant morbidity and rarely, death. Continuous blood glucose monitoring (CGSM) suggests the prevalence of nocturnal hypoglycaemia is 10–56%, lasts for ~6 hours, the time of the lowest level (nadir) depends on the insulin type and regimen (Raju *et al.* 2006). Raju *et al.* (2006) did not find differences in mean nocturnal blood glucose or mean nadir using CGSM to compare four insulin regimens in people with Type 1 diabetes with HbA$_{1c}$ <7.1%, but detected high rates of under- and overestimation of the glucose level.

Pramming *et al.* (1985) tried to identify predictors of early morning hypoglycaemia. They suggested if the blood glucose was <6 mmol/L at 11 PM there was an 80% chance of nocturnal hypoglycaemia compared to 12% risk if the blood glucose was >5 mmol/L. Other researchers report similar predictive blood glucose levels but the likelihood increases if multiple injections are used compared to CSII (Whincup & Milner 1987; Bendtson *et al.* 1988). Vervoort *et al.* (1996) found the bedtime blood glucose level predicted hypoglycaemia in the early part of the night but not hypoglycaemia occurring in the early morning. They also found a fasting blood glucose (before breakfast) <5.5 mmol/L indicated early morning hypoglycaemia.

However, the only risk factor Young *et al.* (2007) identified in a study to determine the amount of glucose needed to prevent exercise-induced hypoglycaemia was frequent exercise. In Young *et al.*'s study, nocturnal hypoglycaemia occurred on both exercise and sedentary nights. Blood glucose 7.2 mmol/L at 9 PM predicted overnight hypoglycaemia on sedentary days. Exercise has multifactorial effects on fuel utilisation and mobilisation. Initially, in the first 5–10 minutes muscle glycogen is the primary fuel source, followed by circulating glucose and then fuel derived from gluconeogenesis and oxidation of fatty acids (Silverstein 2008). Due to the counter-regulatory deficits, children with Type 1 diabetes are unable to mobilise glucose stores for gluconeogenesis.

In many cases the individual does not recognise the signs of nocturnal hypoglycaemia and does not wake up especially in Type 1 (Veneman *et al.* 1993; Raju *et al.* 2006). Repeated episodes of nocturnal hypoglycaemia reduce the counter-regulatory response to hypoglycaemia. Undetected autonomic dysfunction and nocturnal hypoglycaemia can increase the risk of fatal cardiac ventricular dysrrhythmias ('dead in bed' syndrome).

Indicators of nocturnal hypoglycaemia

- Night sweats.
- Nightmares or vivid dreams.
- Unaccustomed snoring.
- Morning lethargy or chronic fatigue.
- Headaches or 'hung over' feeling.
- Mood change, particularly depression.
- High blood glucose before breakfast (Somogyi effect).
- Morning ketouria.

Factors that contribute to nocturnal hypoglycaemia include preceding physical activity that may have occurred many hours previously, insufficient carbohydrate in meals, excess insulin as a result of these factors, enhanced sensitivity to insulin and/or inappropriate insulin dose, alcohol consumption.

The Somogyi effect refers to pre-breakfast hyperglycaemia following an overnight hypoglycaemic episode. If any of the above symptoms occur, the blood glucose should be measured at 2 to 3 am over several nights to establish whether nocturnal hypoglycaemia is occurring. The insulin is then adjusted accordingly by decreasing the morning long-acting dose for those on a daily insulin, the afternoon long-acting dose for those on BD insulin or the pre-evening meal or bedtime dose for basal bolus regimes.

Clinical observations

(1) Sometimes the evening short-acting insulin, rather than the intermediate-acting insulin, causes the hypoglycaemia episode.
(2) Stress and illness are usually associated with hyperglycaemia; however, they can induce hypoglycaemia in Type 1 diabetes.

Practice point

The Somogyi effect should be distinguished from another condition that results in morning hyperglycaemia, the 'dawn phenomenon'. The dawn phenomenon refers to a situation where insulin requirements and blood glucose concentration increase between 5 AM and 8 AM, which occurs in up to 75% of diabetic patients. Treatment consists of *increasing* the insulin dose.

Many other hormones have a normal physiological rise in the early morning, for example, testosterone, which causes early morning erections.

Managing nocturnal hypoglycaemia

Not surprisingly, people with diabetes and their relatives are very fearful of hypoglycaemia at any time, but particularly at night, and careful explanations about the possible causes and suggestions of ways to prevent nocturnal hypoglycaemia are essential. Families/significant others need to know how to manage the hypoglycaemia by maintaining the person's airway and calling an ambulance. If they have glucagon at home, they should give the injection.

Various methods have been used to prevent nocturnal hypoglycaemia, these include providing carbohydrate snacks at bedtime, although there is no real evidence to support the practice (Allen & Frier 2003) or demonstrate efficacy (Raju *et al.* 2006), and adjusting the insulin regimen. The long-acting insulin analogues, with their more predictable action profile, are associated with significantly lower rates of nocturnal hypoglycaemia. Helping the individual and their family/carers to recognise cues to hypoglycaemia through hypoglycaemia training programmes such as HYATT and BGATT may be effective (Cox *et al.* 2004). Despite Raju *et al.*'s (2006) findings, CGSM may provide important clues to assist in such training.

More recently, antihypoglycaemic agents such as ß$_2$-adrenergic agonists (terbutaline) were trialled and a significant reduction in the frequency and severity of nocturnal hypoglycaemia was demonstrated (Raju *et al.* 2006). The morning blood glucose was significantly higher after terbutaline and the pulse rate was elevated. Acarbose with a carbohydrate bedtime snack also reduced the mean blood glucose nadir but did not prevent nocturnal hypoglycaemia.

Relative hypoglycaemia

People who are accustomed to high blood glucose levels for long periods of time may experience the symptoms of hypoglycaemia when blood glucose control improves and blood glucose levels normalise. In general, it is not necessary to treat the symptoms once the blood glucose is recorded, but reassurance, support, and education are necessary until the patient adapts to the new blood glucose range.

Medicine interactions

Some commonly prescribed medicines can interact with sulphonylureas and increase the possibility of hypoglycaemia (see Table 6.3).

Practice point

Consider complementary medicines such as herbs, supplements and other complementary therapies such as massage and relaxation therapies. These therapies can exert hypoglycaemic effects themselves, interact with conventional medicines or cause liver or renal damage that alters the pharmacokinetics and pharmacodynamics of medicines and predisposes the person to hypoglycaemia, or indirectly affect the blood glucose by reducing stress (see Chapter 19).

Table 6.3   Commonly prescribed medicines that can increase the hypoglycaemic effect of sulphonylurea medicines.

Medicines	Means of potentiation
Sulphonamides Salicylates Warfarin Clofibrate Phenylbutazone	Displaces sulphonylureas from protein binding sites
Coumarin derivatives Chloramphenicol Phenylbutazone	Inhibits/decreases hepatic metabolism of the sulphonylurea
Probenecid Salicylates Tuberculostatics Tetracyclines	Delays urinary excretion of the sulphonylurea
MAO inhibitors	Increases action by an unknown mechanism

Objectives of care

In hospital settings staff need to be alert to the possibility of hypoglycaemia in all patients on insulin or OHAs, and should it occur to:

(1) Supply quick-acting carbohydrate to immediately raise blood glucose levels.
(2) Maintain blood glucose levels within the acceptable range of 4–10 mmol/L.
(3) Ascertain the cause of the hypoglycaemic episode.
(4) Limit further episodes of hypoglycaemia.
(5) Allay fear and anxiety including that of relatives.
(6) Prevent trauma occurring as a result of hypoglycaemia, for example, falls.
(7) Assess knowledge and educate if necessary. In particular people should be assisted to recognise their personal risk of hypoglycaemia and learn to recognise their individual 'hypo symptoms' rather then being provided with a list of textbook signs and symptoms.

Treatment

Rapid treatment is important to prevent mild hypoglycaemia progressing to severe hypoglycaemia and limit the potential adverse risks associated with severe episodes. The following management refers to patients in hospital but can be applied in other settings.

Mild hypoglycaemia

Test and record the blood glucose level.

First: 10–15 g of carbohydrate as quick acting glucose or other high glycaemic index carbohydrate to raise the blood glucose immediately, for example:

3 level teaspoons sugar in 1/2 cup water
or   1/2 regular sugary/soft drink (*not low calorie* (joule))
or   proprietary glucose preparation such as glucose gels/tablets or person's usual remedy, for example, jelly beans.

Second: follow with long-acting carbohydrate to maintain blood glucose until the next meal time, for example:

1/2 sandwich
or   2 to 4 dry biscuits (unsweetened)
or   1 piece of fruit.

Check blood glucose in one hour and then as necessary. The next dose of insulin or OHA is not usually withheld following a mild hypoglycaemic episode. However, if hypoglycaemia occurs frequently, the management regimen might need to be adjusted, for example, extra carbohydrate in the diet, reduced medication dose.

Severe hypoglycaemia with impaired conscious state

Note: Do not give anything by mouth if the person is unconscious. Confused patients often spit fluids out or refuse to swallow. Gels are preferable and can be smeared onto the buccal mucosa but the dose may not be sufficient to reverse the hypoglycaemia.

(1) Place patient on side.
(2) Clear airway.
(3) Notify the doctor in hospital settings or call an ambulance.
(4) Test the blood glucose level and confirm with chemical pathology (i.e. urgent glucose).
(5) Assemble glucagon and IV tray containing 50% dextrose. Instructions for glucagon administration appear in section Guidelines for administering glucagon. Fifty per cent glucose should be given into an antecubital vein because injection into hand veins often results in extravasation and thrombophlebitis. Ten per cent glucose is recommended for children to reduce the risk of hyperosmolality. Dose: adult 20–30 mL 50% glucose; child 2–5 mL/kg bolus 10% glucose then 0.1 mL/kg/minute until the child regains consciousness. Consciousness usually returns within five minutes (Therapeutic Guidelines (TG) 2004).
(6) Monitor blood glucose 1–2 hourly until blood glucose level is stable above 5 mmol/L and then revert to the usual testing regimen.
(7) Give complex carbohydrate low glycaemic index food to maintain the blood glucose level when consciousness returns. The patient may still be confused and may need to be reminded to chew and swallow.

The patient should be monitored for at least 36 hours. Ascertain the time and dose for the next insulin injection/OHA dose. Provide education, counselling and support to the individual and their family/carers.

Prolonged hypoglycaemia

Recovery from hypoglycaemia can be prolonged if the episode is severe, prolonged, and/ or associated with coma and/or seizures. Other causes of impaired consciousness should be considered such as stroke and insulin overdose. Insulin overdose should be excluded when high doses of IV glucose are needed to maintain the blood glucose >5 mmol/L.

Hypoglycaemia related to long-acting sulphonylureas is a medical emergency and the person should be managed in hospital. Prolonged infusion of 10% IV and 1–2 hourly blood glucose monitoring is often necessary. Some experts recommend using 50 µg of subcutaneous octreotide 8 hourly for three doses (TG Guidelines 2004). In some cases a brain scan will be indicated, and if cerebral oedema is present, IV mannitol is administered. Shorr *et al.* (1996) suggested the crude rate for long-acting sulphonylurea-related hypoglycaemia is 16.6% per 1000 person years compared to 1.9% in second-generation agents.

Significantly, recent hospital discharge is a significant predictor of serious medicine-associated hypoglycaemia in older people (days 1–30), especially the very old, frail, those of ≥5 medicines (Schorr *et al.* 1997).

In both cases recovery should be rapid. If recovery does not occur in 10–15 minutes, exclude other causes of unconsciousness.

(1) Record episode and blood glucose level on the appropriate chart/s and in patient's medical record. Consider whether an 'alert sticker' should be attached to their record.
(2) Monitor progress/recovery from the episode.
(3) Look for cause of hypoglycaemia, for example, meal delayed or missed, inadequate intake of carbohydrate, unaccustomed activity, excessive medication, medication/ medication, medication/herb or herb/herb interactions.
(4) Reassure the patient and relatives.
(5) Ensure patient has an understanding of causes and management of hypoglycaemia (refer to diabetes nurse specialist/diabetes educator).
(6) See Chapter 12 for information about managing hypoglycaemia in older people.

Patients most at risk of hypoglycaemia

A number of factors significantly increase the risk of hypoglycaemia. These include:

- Those taking insulin or OHAs, especially long-acting formulations and intensive insulin therapy, see Chapter 12. However, the long-acting insulin analogues have lower hypoglycaemia risk than the other long-acting and biphasic insulins.
- Medicine doses not adjusted for changes such as weight loss, increased activity, following acute illness, and reducing oral corticosteroid doses.
- Beginning an exercise/diet regimen or prolonged aerobic exercise. Hypoglycaemia can occur many hours after exercise, often during the night. Unaccustomed activity such as rehabilitation programmes should be considered 'exercise'.
- People on insulin achieving blood glucose within the normal range.
- History of hypoglycaemia.
- People with an irregular lifestyle and irregular meal and exercise patterns and when carbohydrate content of the meal is low.
- Eating disorders.

- Young children. It is difficult to predict their activity levels and food intake and the presenting signs may be difficult to distinguish from other causes such as tiredness and misbehaving. It is important to support and educate the family.
- Adolescents, possibly because of their erratic eating patterns and experimentation with alcohol and striving for 'good control'.
- The elderly especially those who live alone.
- Insulin-treated pregnant women and newborn babies of women with GDM or on insulin.
- Those with renal or hepatic disease.
- Those with long-standing diabetes who may have autonomic neuropathy are at risk of hypoglycaemic unawareness, and effects on the gastrointestinal tract that may delay gastric emptying and thus food absorption.
- People fasting for a procedure/surgery or religious reasons, for example, Ramadan.
- People with diarrhoea and vomiting where food absorption is impaired. Hypoglycaemia may impair gastric emptying (Russo *et al.* 2005).
- Those with an impaired conscious state.
- Those sedated or on narcotic infusions.
- Endocrine diseases such as hypothyroidism and hypoadrenalism.
- Alcohol may also cause hypoglycaemia particularly if food is not eaten at the same time. The hypoglycaemia can occur hours after consuming alcohol.
- People taking a lot of medications and/or complementary medicines, especially those that lower blood glucose.
- Social class.

Practice points

(1) The signs of alcohol intoxication can make hypoglycaemia difficult to recognise. Alcohol impairs cognitive function and reduces the ability to recognise and effectively treat hypoglycaemia. Self-care and diet are often inadequate. In addition, chronic alcohol abuse leads to malnutrition and limited glucose stores to mount an effective counter-regulatory response.
(2) People with chronic alcohol addiction are very difficult to manage because OHAs are often contraindicated and insulin puts them at high risk of hypoglycaemia.

Psychological effects of hypoglycaemia

Hypoglycaemia is feared and hated by many people with diabetes and the effects are often under-rated by health professionals. The importance of recognising and accepting these concerns cannot be overemphasised. Hypoglycaemia has profound effects on people's quality of life, social activities, for example, driving and work, and they fear brain damage and death from hypoglycaemia. It is not unusual for people to deliberately run their blood glucose levels high to avoid hypoglycaemia (Dunning 1994) (see Chapter 15). They can then be termed 'non-compliant' and placed in a conflict situation. Commonly expressed concerns about hypoglycaemia are:

- Loss of control of the situation;
- Reminder that they have diabetes;
- Losing face and making a fool of themselves;

- Blood glucose rising too high after treatment;
- Sustaining brain damage however, the DCCT and EDIC studies did not show a relationship between hypoglycaemia and declining cognitive function (DCCT 1993). The DCCT is not relevant to older people. Hershey *et al.* (2005) found impaired spatial long-term memory performance and repeated episodes of severe hypoglycaemia, particularly when the hypoglycaemia commenced before age 5. Severe, repeated hypoglycaemia has also been associated with a lower volume of grey matter in the left superior temporal region of the brain, which is associated with episodic memory, in young people with Type 1 diabetes (Perantie *et al.* 2007).
- Recovery can take days following serious hypoglycaemia and leave residual headache and tiredness;
- Dying: 2–45 of deaths occurring in people on insulin, mostly Type 1, are attributed to hypoglycaemia (Laing *et al.* 1999).

Hypoglycaemia can affect the individual's confidence in their ability to cope. Support and understanding, and exploring all of the issues, physical, mental, and social that affect coping is an important part of management.

Clinical observation

Pet dogs sometimes recognise their owner's hypoglycaemia and alert them in time to be able to treat it early or rouse another family member.

Guidelines for administering glucagon

Glucagon is a hormone produced by the alpha cells of the pancreas. Glucagon stimulates glycogenolysis and hepatic glucose output. It is available as a medicine. Glucagon is available in a single dose pack containing one vial of glucagon hydrochloride powder (1 mg) and a glass syringe prefilled with sterile water (water for injection).

Indication

Glucagon is used to treat severe hypoglycaemia in people with diabetes treated with insulin or OHAs, primarily those unable to take glucose orally who are unconscious or uncooperative. It can be administered by relatives.

Instructions for use

(1) Individual patients must be assessed to determine the appropriate dose and route of administration. Glucagon is given according to body weight and muscle bulk (intramuscularly or subcutaneously). The buttock is the ideal injection site.
(2) The intravenous route may be the preferred route in hospital settings in profound hypoglycaemia to ensure rapid absorption and reversal of the hypoglycaemia. Tattersall (1999) suggested glucagon takes ~10 minutes longer than IV glucose to restore consciousness. However, DCCT data suggest unconscious patients recover within ~6 minutes. In addition, it may be ineffective in people with low glycogen stores such as thin frail older people and alcoholics.

(3) Check the expiry date. Glucagon should be used soon after reconstitution. Do not use if reconstituted solution is not clear and colourless.
(4) Follow the instructions in the package to prepare the injection and the medical order for the dose.
(5) Record the time and route of administration, the dose, and the patient's response.

Dosage

- Adults and children of weight >25 kg full dose (1 mg).
- Children of weight <25 kg half dose (0.5 mg).

Practice points

(1) Glucagon can be repeated; however, repeated injections can cause nausea, making subsequent food intake difficult and repeat dosing is not recommended.
(2) If recovery does not occur within 10–15 minutes, IV glucose might be required. It could indicate limited glucose stores but other causes of unconsciousness should be considered.
(3) Glucagon may be contraindicated where glycogen stores are low, for example, in fasting states, chronic hypoglycaemia, chronic adrenal insufficiency and malnutrition where the individual is unable to mount an effective counter-regulatory response.

Adverse reactions

These are rare. Occasionally transient nausea occurs that can make it difficult to consume sufficient oral carbohydrate, which is necessary to avoid the blood glucose dropping again. Vomiting occurs occasionally, usually only after a second dose.

Glucagon is a peptide so theoretically hypersensitivity is possible and is more likely in atopic patients. In reality hypersensitivity is rare.

Clinical observation

Hypothermia can prolong recovery from hypoglycaemia especially in the elderly in winter. Management of the hypothermia as well as the hypoglycaemia is usually required.

References

Allen, K. & Frier, B. (2003) Nocturnal hypoglycaemia: clinical manifestations and therapeutic strategies towards prevention. *Endocrine Practice*, 9, 530–543.
Bendtson, I., Kverneland, A., Pramming, S. & Binder, C. (1998) Incidence of nocturnal hypoglycaemia in insulin-dependent diabetic patients on intensive therapy. *Acta Medica Scandinavica*, 223, 543–548.
Cox, D., Clarke, W., Gonder-Frederick, L., Pohl, S., Hoover, C., Snyder, A., Zimbelman, I., Catrer, W., Bobbitt, S. & Pennebaker, J. (1985) Accuracy of perceiving blood glucose in IDDM. *Diabetes Care*, 8, 529–536.

Cox, D., Kovatchev, B. & Koev, D. (2004) Hypoglycaemia anticipation, awareness training (HYATT) reduces occurrences of severe hypoglycaemia among adults with Type 1 diabetes. *International Journal Behavioural Medicine*, **11**, 212–218.

Davis, E., Keating, B., Byrne, G., Russell, M. & Jones, T. (1997) Hypoglycaemic incidence and clinical predictors in a large population based sample of children and adolescents with IDDM *Diabetes Care*, **20**, 22–25.

Daneman, T., Frank, M., Perlman, K., Tamm, J. & Ehrlich, R. (1989) Severe hypoglycaemia in children with insulin dependent diabetes: frequency and predisposing factors. *Journal of Paediatrics*, **115**, 681–685.

Deary, I. (1993) Effects of hypoglycaemia on cognitive function. In: *Hypoglycaemia and Diabetes: Clinical and Pyysiological Aspects* (eds B. Frier and B. Fisher), pp. 80–92. Edward Arnold, London.

Dunning, P. (1994) Having diabetes: young adult perspectives. *The Diabetes Educator*, **21** (1), 58–65.

Galloway, J. & Chance, R. (1994) Improving insulin therapy: achievements and challenges. *Hormone and Metabolic Research*, **26**, 591–598.

Gonder-Frederick, L., Cox, D., Driesen, N., Ryan, C. & Clarke, W. (1994) Individual differences in neurobehavioural disruption during mild to moderate hypoglycaemia in adults with IDDM. *Diabetes*, **43**, 1407–1312.

Henderson, J., Allen, K., Deary, I. & Frie, H. (2003) Hypoglycaemia in insulin-treated type 2 diabetes: frequency, symptoms and impaired awareness. *Diabetic Medicine*, **20** (12), 1016–1021.

Hepburn, D. (1993) Symptoms of hypoglycaemia. In: *Hypoglycaemia and Diabetes: Clinical and Pyysiological Aspects* (eds B. Frier and B. Fisher), pp. 93–103. Edward Arnold, London.

Hershey, T., Perantie, D. & Warren, S. (2005) Frequency and timing of severe hypoglycaemia affects spatial memory in children with type 1 diabetes. *Diabetes Care*, **28**, 2372–2377.

Jones, T., Porter, P. & Sherwin, R. (1998) Decreased epinephrine responses to hypoglycaemia during sleep. *New England Journal of Medicine*, **338**, 1657–1662.

Klein, R. (2007) Smoking is linked to hypoglycaemia in type 1 diabetes. *Diabetes Care*, **30**, 1437–1441.

Laing, S., Swerdlow, A. & Slater, S. (1999) The British Diabetic Cohort Study 1. All-cause mortality in patients with insulin-treated diabetes mellitus. *Diabetic Medicine*, **16**, 459–465.

McAuley, V., Deary, I., Ferguson, S. & Frier, B. (2001) Acute hypoglycaemia in humans causes attentional dysfunction while nonverbal intelligence is preserved. *Diabetes Care*, **24**, 1745–1750.

McCrimmon, R., Gold, A., Deary, I., Kelnar, C. & Frier, B. (1995) Symptoms of hypoglycaemia in children with IDDM. *Diabetes Care*, **18**, 851–861.

Muhlhauser, I., Overmann, H., Bender, R., Bott, U. & Berger, M. (1998) Risk factors of severe hypoglycaemia in adult patients with type 1 diabetes – a prospective population based study. *Diabetologia*, **14**, 1274–1282.

Morris, A. DARTS/MEMO Collaboration (2003) Frequency of severe hypoglycaemia requiring emergency treatment in type 1 and type 2 diabetes: a population-based study of health service resource use. *Diabetes Care*, **26**, 1176–1180.

National Health and Medical Research Council (1991) *Hypoglycaemia and Diabetes*. Australian Government Printers, Canberra.

Nordfeldt, S. & Ludvigsson, J. (1997) Severe hypoglycaemia in children with IDDM. A prospective study, 1992–1994. *Diabetes Care*, **20**, 497–503.

Perantie, D., Wu, J. & Koller, J. (2007) Regional brain volume differences associated with hyperglycaemia and severe hypoglycaemia in youth with type 1 diabetes. *Diabetes Care*, **30**, 2331–2337.

Pramming, S., Thorsteinsson, B., Ronn, B. & Binder, C. (1985) Nocturnal hypoglycaemia in patients receiving conventional treatment with insulin. *British Medical Journal*, **291**, 376–379.

Pramming, S., Thorsteinsson, B., Bendtson, I. & Binder, C. (1991) Symptomatic hypoglycaemia in 411 type 1 diabetic patients. *Diabetic Medicine*, **8**, 217–222.

Raju, B., Arbelaez, A., Breckenridge, S. & Cryer, P. (2006) Nocturnal hypoglycaemia in type 1 diabetes: an assessment of preventative bedtime treatments. *Journal Clinical Endocrinology and Metabolism*, **91**, 2087–2092.

Ringholmn Nielsen, L. (2008) Hypoglycaemia most common in early pregnancy in women with type 1 diabetes. *Diabetes Care*, **31**, 9–14.

Ross, L., McCrimmon, R., Frier, B., Kelnar, C. & Deary, I. (1998) Hypoglycaemic symptoms reported by children with type 1 diabetes mellitus and by their parents. *Diabetic Medicine*, **15**, 836–843.

Russo, A., Stevens, J., Chen, R., Gentilcore, D., Burnet, R., Horowitz, M. & Jones, K. (2005) Insulin-induced hypoglycaemia accelerates gastric emptying of solids and liquids in long standing type 1 diabetes. *Journal Clinical Endocrinology and Metabolism*, **90**, 4489–4495.

Salas, M. & Caro, J. (2002) Are hypoglycaemia and other adverse effects similar among sulphonylureas? *Adverse Drug Reactions Toxicology Review*, **21**, 205–217.

Silverstein, J. (2008) The lows of exercise: another piece of the puzzle. *International Diabetes Monitor*, **20** (1), 44–46.

Shorr, R., Daugherty, W. & Griffin, M. (1996) Individual sulfonylureas and serious hypoglycaemia in older people. *Journal American Geriatric Society*, **44** (7), 751–755.

Shorr, R., Ray, W., Daugherty, J. & Griffin, M. (1997) Incidence and risk factors for serious hypoglycaemia in older persons using insulin or sulphonylureas. *Archives of Internal Medicine*, **157** (15), 1681–1686.

Sinclair, A. (2006) Special considerations in older adults with diabetes: meeting the challenge. *Diabetes Spectrum*, **19**, 229–233.

Sommerfield, A., Deary, I., McAuley, V. & Frier, B. (2003) Short-term delayed, and working memory are impaired during hypoglycaemia in individuals with type 1 diabetes. *Diabetes Care*, **26**, 390–396.

The Diabetes Control and Complication trial Research Group (1991) Epidemiology of severe hypoglycaemia in the Diabetes Control and Complications Trial. *American Journal of Medicine*, **90**, 450–459.

The Diabetes Control and Complication Trial Research Group (1997) Hypoglycaemia in the Diabetes Control and Complications Trial. *Diabetes*, **46**, 271–286.

Therapeutic Guidelines (2004) Hypoglycaemia. http://www.tg.com.au/etg_demo/tcg/edg/1473.htm (accessed December 2007).

Thorsteinsson, B., Pramming, S., Lauritzen, T. & Binder, C. (1986) Frequency of daytime biochemical hypoglycaemia in insulin-treated diabetic patients: relation to daily median blood glucose concentrations. *Diabetic Medicine*, **3**, 147–151.

UKPDS (1998) Intensive blood glucose control with sulphonylureas or insulin compared with conventional treatment and risk of complications in patients with type 2 diabetes (UKPDS 33). *Lancet*, **352**, 837–853 (correction *Lancet* 1999; **354**: 602).

Vervoort, G., Goldschmodt, H. & van Doorn, L. (1996) Nocturnal blood glucose profiles in patients with type 1 diabetes on multiple (>4) daily insulin injection regimens. *Diabetic Medicine*, **13**, 794–799.

Veneman, T., Mitrakou, A., Mokan, M., Cryer, P. & Gerich, J. (1993) Induction of hypoglycaemia unawareness in asymptomatic nocturnal hypoglycaemia. *Diabetes*, **42**, 1233–1237.

Wright, A., Cull, C., Macleod, K. & Holman, R. (2006) Hypoglycaemia in type 2 diabetic patients randomized to and maintained on monotherapy with diet, sulphonylurea, metformin, or insulin for six years form diagnosis UKPDS 73. *Journal of Diabetes Complications*, **20**, 395–401.

Yki-Jarvinen, H., Ryysy, L., Nikkila, K., Tulokas, T., Vanamo, R. & Heikkila, M. (1999) Comparison of bedtime insulin regimens in patients with type 2 diabetes mellitus. A randomised, controlled trial. *Archives of Internal Medicine*, **130**, 399–396.

Yogev, Y., Chen, R. & Ben-Haroush, A. (2003) Continuous glucose monitoring for the evaluation of gravid women with Type 1 diabetes mellitus. *Obstetrics and Gynaecology*, **101**, 633–638.

Ziemer, D., Barnes, C. & Tsui, C. (2007) Hypoglycaemia is not associated with intensification of diabetes therapy. *American Diabetes Association Scientific Sessions*, June 24, Chicago, Illinois.

Chapter 7
Hyperglycaemia, Acute Illness, Diabetic Ketoacidosis (DKA), Hyperosmolar Coma (HONK), and Lactic Acidosis

Key points

- Acute illness most commonly causes hyperglycaemia and less commonly, hypoglycaemia.
- Untreated hyperglycaemia can precipitate ketoacidosis and hyperosmolar coma, which are serious short-term complications of diabetes, even if they are managed competently.
- Meticulous attention to detail and proactive insulin use reduces morbidity and mortality.
- Monitor hydration status closely especially in children.
- *Gradually* lower the blood glucose level to avoid hypoglycaemia.
- Monitor ketone clearance in blood.
- Educate the person with diabetes and their family about how to manage illness.
- Consider psychological and social issues especially if there are repeated admissions for DKA.

Rationale

Hyperglycaemia, DKA, and HONK are preventable short-term complications of diabetes. When hyperglycaemia does occur, effective proactive management can reduce the progression to DKA and HONK and limit the attendant metabolic derangements should these conditions occur. People with well controlled diabetes do not usually experience higher rates of intercurrent illness than non-diabetics. However, those with persistent hyperglycaemia may have lower immunity and are at increased risk of infections including infections caused by organisms that are not normally pathogenic, tuberculosis, and have a poorer response to antibiotics (Australasian Paediatric Endocrine Group 2005). Infection is the most common cause of DKA and HONK.

Prevention: proactively managing intercurrent illness

Prevention strategies consist of educating the person with diabetes and their family about how to prevent intercurrent illness or proactively managing intercurrent illnesses to limit the metabolic consequences. Illness prevention/management strategies should be individualised and based on a thorough physical, psychological, and social assessment using a risk management approach. Illness prevention education should encompass:

- Proactive health care such as identifying key illness risk times, for example, colds and flu during winter, having a documented plan for managing illness, and a kit containing essential equipment and information such as ketone test strips and relative's and health professional's telephone numbers.
- Recognising and managing the signs and symptoms of DKA and HONK, which includes the importance of monitoring blood glucose and ketones and using the information to adjust glucose lowering medicine doses or seek medical advice and how to maintain fluid intake.
- How to adjust insulin/OHAs and dietary intake to control blood glucose levels.
- When to seek assistance.

In addition, health professionals should regularly reassess the individual's illness self-care capability including:

- Knowledge, according to the factors outlined in the preceding list.
- Physical ability to manage such as mobility, sight, manual dexterity, and other activities of daily living, bearing in mind these may all be compromised by hyperglycaemia. This is an important aspect of long-term complication screening programmes. Groups likely to need assistance are children, pregnant women, frail older people who live alone, those who are acutely ill and those who are depressed. The most effective management strategy for these people may be to seek health professional advice quickly.
- Psychosocial factors such as mental health and coping skills, cognitive function, and available support from family of other carers considering their state of health and coping ability especially in older people.
- Preventative health care strategies such as vaccinations, mammograms, prostate checks, usual metabolic control, and their sick day management plan and kit. Annual influenza and pneumococcal vaccinations are recommended for people with diabetes, COPD, cardiovascular disease including children with these conditions (National Asthma Council 2005). Mortality increases by 5–15% in people with diabetes during influenza epidemics especially those with cardiovascular and renal complications (Smith *et al.* 2004). The increased risk may be due to older age cardiovascular disease or to the diabetes itself due to the impaired immune response due to DKA/HONK (Diepersloot *et al.* 1990). Kornum (2007) suggested Type 2 diabetes predicted mortality associated with pneumonia and further, hyperglycaemia on admission, >11 mmol/L in diabetics and >6 mmol/L in non-diabetics, predicts pneumonia-related mortality.
- Observational data suggest influenza vaccination prior to and during an influenza epidemic reduces the associated hospital admissions and mortality in people with diabetes (Wang *et al.* 2004). Thus, all people with diabetes aged 6 months and older

should receive annual influenza vaccination unless contraindicated. Contraindications include allergy/anaphylactic reaction to eggs and/or the vaccine, intercurrent illness with fever >38°C.

- Regular medicine reviews including complementary and over-the-counter medicines. In particular, assessing the continued need for diabetogenic medicines such as atypical antipsychotic medications, glucocorticoids and thiazide diuretics. If these medicines are necessary and there are no alternatives, the lowest effective dose should be used.
- Early recognition of new presentations of diabetes.
- Good access to competent medical and nursing care and ongoing education.
- Good knowledge on the part of people with diabetes and health professionals.
- Good communication/therapeutic relationship between the person with diabetes and their health professionals (see Munro *et al.* 1973: this is an old reference but it is still pertinent in the light of the frequent presentations to hospital with hyperglycaemia-associated conditions).
- Psychological screening should be incorporated into routine complication assessment programmes (Ciechanowski *et al.* 2000; Dunning 2001).

Self-care during illness

People with Type 1 diabetes are at greatest risk of DKA but DKA can occur in seriously ill Type 2 and HONK is associated with significant morbidity and mortality. A suggested plan for monitoring blood glucose and ketones is shown in Table 7.1 (International Society for Paediatric and Adolescent Diabetes 2000; Kitabchi *et al.* 2001; American Diabetes Association 2004; Laffel *et al.* 2005; Australian Diabetes Educators Association (ADEA) 2006; Dunning 2007). In the early stages of the illness people may be able to be managed at home if they are capable of self-care, have support and can telephone their doctor at least every 1–2 hours. Admission to hospital is advised in the following situations:

- Children especially younger than 2 years.
- Persistent vomiting and/or bile-stained vomitus.
- Persistent diarrhoea.
- Blood glucose persistently, 4 mmol/L or >15 mmol/L and ketones present
- Severe localised abdominal pain.
- Hyperventilation (Kussmaul's respirations)
- Dehydration.
- Coexisting serious illness.
- Impaired conscious state.
- The individual, parent or care providers are unable to cope

Hyperglycaemia

Hyperglycaemia refers to an elevated blood glucose level (>10 mmol/L) due to a relative or absolute insulin deficiency. The symptoms of hyperglycaemia usually occur when the blood glucose is persistently above 15 mmol/L. In people with an established diagnosis of diabetes. The cause of the hyperglycaemia should be sought and corrected to avoid

Table 7.1 Self managing blood glucose, ketones and fluid during illness. These recommendations should be tailored to the individual's self-care capabilities, available assistance, and their physical condition. Ketosis can develop rapidly in people using insulin pumps. The underlying cause needs to be ascertained and treated.

	Type 1	Type 2
Blood glucose (BG)	Monitor 2 hourly Monitor ketones 2 hourly if >15 mmol on two consecutive occasions in a 2–6 hour period	Monitor 2 hourly If >15 mmol on two consecutive occasions in an 8–12 hour period increase monitoring frequency to 2–4 hourly QID testing may be adequate in people managed with diet and exercise.
# Blood ketones <1 mmol/L	BG 4–15 mmol/L recheck in 2 hours	Follow the same test procedure as described for Type 1 diabetes.
1–1.4 mmol/L:	BG, <8 mmol/L extra sweet fluids: >8 mmol/L extra 5% insulin	Ketones are less common in Type 2 diabetes but do occur.
>1.5 mmol/L:	BG, <8 mmol/L extra sweet fluids: >8 mmol/L extra	
<1 mmol/L	5–10% insulin BG 15–22 mmol/L 5% extra insulin	
1–1.4 mmol/L	10% extra insulin	
>1.5 mmol/L	15–20% extra insulin and hospitalise if ketones persist	
<1 mmol/L	BG >22 mmol/L 10% extra insulin	
1 –1.4 mmol/L	15% extra insulin	
>5 mol/L	20% extra insulin and hospitalise if ketones persist	
Medicines	Give supplemental doses of quick/rapid acting insulin 2–4 hourly	*OHAs* Consider ceasing metformin Increase sulphonylurea dose unless on maximal doses or on slow release preparation when insulin is preferred[a] *OHA and insulin* Supplemental doses of quick/rapid acting insulin *Insulin treated* Supplemental doses of quick/rapid acting insulin
Refer to hospital	Unable to maintain fluid intake Blood glucose and ketones not falling despite supplemental insulin Unable to self-care and no support available Condition deteriorating	Unable to maintain fluid intake Blood glucose and ketones not falling despite supplemental insulin Unable to self-care and no support available Condition deteriorating

(Continued)

Table 7.1   Continued.

	Type 1	Type 2
Fluids	BG <4 mmol/L usual meals and extra sweet fluids if tolerated ~10–12 mmol/L and able to tolerate food 150 mL easily digested fluid every 1–2 hours, for example, soup, fruit juice, ice cream. BG >12 mmol and unable to tolerate food 100–300 mL low calorie fluids every hour, for example, gastrolyte, low calorie soft drink, mineral water, water. Unable to tolerate fluids at any BG level refer to hospital	BG <4 mmol/L usual meals and extra sweet fluids if tolerated ~10–12 mmol/L and able to tolerate food 150 mL easily digested fluid every 1–2 hours, for example, soup, fruit juice, ice cream. BG > 12 mmol and unable to tolerate food 100–300 mL low calorie fluids every hour, for example, gastrolyte, low calorie soft drink, mineral water, water. Unable to tolerate fluids at any BG level refer to hospital

[a]If the person has no experience of insulin they will need reassurance and a careful explanation about why insulin is needed. If they are not able to manage or do not have assistance and home nursing is not available they may need to be managed in hospital.

the development of diabetic ketoacidosis (DKA) or HONK. Hyperglycaemia, DKA and HONK are often referred to as short-term complications of diabetes. DKA develops relatively quickly. HONK usually evolves over several days to weeks.

Hyperglycaemia disrupts multiple organ systems and needs to be treated to reduce the morbidity and mortality associated with acute illness. Fluid resuscitation corrects dehydration, improves microcirculation, and reduces tissue damage during acute sepsis, which helps correct hyperglycaemia, but increased insulin doses and/or dose frequency or rescue insulin therapy in Type 2 diabetes is usually required.

Many researchers have demonstrated that hyperglycaemia is associated with adverse outcomes in hospitalised people both diabetics and non-diabetics and that controlling the blood glucose improves outcomes (Abourizk *et al.* 2004; Clement *et al.* 2004; ACE Taskforce 2004; ACE/ADA Taskforce 2006). There is still debate about whether continuous IV insulin infusion is the safest and most effective therapy despite the well described benefits in both diabetic and non-diabetics (Van den Berghe *et al.* 2001). Intensive insulin therapy protects renal function in critically ill patients and reduces the incidence of oliguria and the need for renal replacement therapy in surgical patients. Intensive insulin infusion is also associated with improved lipid and endothelial profile (Schetz 2008).

The greatest concern appears to be causing hypoglycaemia (Schulman *et al.* 2007; Brunkhorst 2008). Likewise, it is not clear whether less stringent blood glucose targets achieve similar morbidity and mortality reductions (Schulman *et al.* 2007). Laboratory or capillary blood glucose tests are the best method of monitoring blood glucose during illness. Capillary tests are undertaken more frequently except in intensive care situations and may give better insight into the blood glucose pattern (Cook *et al.* 2007).

Quality management organisations in the US are currently developing hospital outcome measures for managing hyperglycaemia in hospitalised patients (Joint Commission on Accreditation of Healthcare Organisations 2006). Despite the evidence that insulin requirements increase during illness, insulin doses are often reduced, even in the presence of significant hyperglycaemia, because health professionals are concerned about causing hypoglycaemia, whereas the factors contributing to hypoglycaemia are only rarely investigated and addressed (Cook *et al.* 2007).

Diabetic ketoacidosis (DKA)

Diabetic ketoacidosis is a life-threatening complication of diabetes. The basic pathophysiology consists of a reduction in the effective action of circulating insulin and an increase in counter-regulatory hormones. Glucose is unable to enter the cells and accumulates in the blood. Insulin deficiency leads to catecholamine release, lipolysis and the mobilisation of free fatty acids and subsequently ketone bodies, B-hydroxybutyrate, acetoacetate, and acetone, resulting in metabolic acidosis (ADA Position Statement 2002). Protein catabolism also occurs and forms the substrate for gluconeogenesis, further increasing the blood glucose. At the same time, glucose utilisation in tissues is impaired. DKA usually only occurs in Type 1 patients, but may occur in Type 2 people with severe infections or metabolic stress. The mortality rate in expert centres is <5% but is higher at the extremes of age and if coma and/or hypotension are present (Malone *et al.* 1992; Chiasson *et al.* 2003).

Diabetic ketoacidosis is characterised by hyperglycaemia, osmotic diuresis, metabolic acidosis, glycosuria, ketonuria and dehydration. The definition by laboratory results is blood glucose >17 mmol/L; ketonaemia (ketone bodies) >3 mmol/L; acidosis, pH <7.30 and bicarbonate <15 mEq/L.

The signs, symptoms, and precipitating factors for DKA are shown in Table 7.2, while Figure 7.1 outlines the physiology and the signs and symptoms that occur as a result of impaired glucose utilisation, and the biochemical manifestations found on blood testing.

Late signs, that is severe DKA

The initial signs and symptoms of DKA (polyuria, polydipsia, lethargy, and Kussmaul's respirations) are an attempt by the body to compensate for the acidosis. If treatment is delayed the body eventually decompensates. Signs of decompensation (late signs) include:

- Peripheral vasodilation with warm, dry skin.
- Hypothermia.
- Hypoxia and reduced conscious state.
- Reduced urine output (oliguria).
- Reduced respiratory rate – absence of Kussmaul's respirations.
- Bradycardia.

The signs and symptoms can be masked by intercurrent illness. For example, pneumonia can cause tachyapnoea, dry mouth and dehydration, abdominal pain and

Table 7.2 Early signs, symptoms, and precipitating factors of diabetic ketoacidosis (DKA).

Symptoms and signs	Precipitating factors

Thirst
Polyuria
Fatigue
Weight loss
Nausea and vomiting
Abdominal pain
Muscle cramps
Tachycardia
Kussmaul's respirations (early sign)
	(1) Newly diagnosed Type 1 (5–30%)
	(2) Omission of insulin therapy/OHAs (33%)
	(3) Inappropriate insulin/OHA dose reduction. DKA has also been associated with inaccurate use of insulin delivery devices after changing devices in both older people and adolescents (Bhardwaj *et al.* 2006).
	(4) Eating disorders
	(5) Severe emotional distress, either directly or by insulin manipulation
	(6) Relative insulin deficiency due to:
	(7) Insulin pump failure
	(8) Severe morning sickness during pregnancy
	  (a) Acute illness:
	    Infection (10–20% of cases)
	    Myocardial infarction
	    Trauma, burns
	    Cerebrovascular accident
	    Surgical procedures
	  (b) Endocrine disorders (rare):
	    Hyperthyroidism
	    Pheochromocytoma
	    Acromegaly
	    Cushing's disease
	  (c) Medications:
	    Glucocorticoids
	    Thiazide diuretics
	    Sympathomimetic agents
	    Alcohol
	    Illicit drugs
	Brittle diabetes: life disrupting blood glucose lability associated with frequent admission to hospital (Benbow *et al.* 2001)

vomiting are symptoms of gastrointestinal disease, likewise, abdominal pain is usual in appendicitis and labour. Polyuria and polydipsia can be difficult to detect in toddles not yet toilet trained, bed wetters, and incontinent older people. Unexplained bed wetting in these groups needs to be investigated and DKA considered when the onset is sudden. Hypothermia as a result of peripheral vasodilation can mask fever due to underlying infection.

Differential diagnosis

- Starvation ketosis, which can be determined by taking a careful clinical history of the presentation.
- Alcoholic ketosis where the blood glucose is usually only mildly elevated or low.

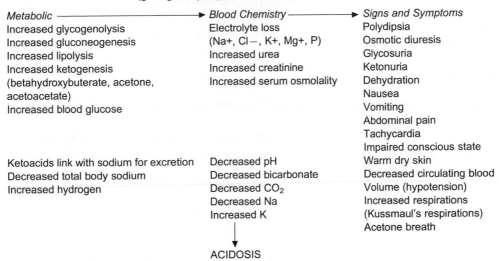

Figure 7.1 An outline of the physiology, signs, and symptoms and biochemical changes occurring in the development of diabetic ketoacidosis (DKA).

The implications of the metabolic and physiological changes associated with DKA are shown in Table 7.3.

Assessment

The following factors should be established:

- Whether the person has known diabetes;
- Usual insulin/OHA dose, dose interval and type/s of insulin/OHA;
- The time the last dose was taken and dose administered;
- Presence of fever, which can be a sign of myocardial infarction as well as infection;
- Duration of the deteriorating control/illness;
- Remedial action taken by the patient;
- Whether the person has taken any other medications, complementary medicines, alcohol or illegal drugs;
- Conscious state.

A thorough physical assessment should be undertaken and blood taken to:

- Establish the severity of the DKA: glucose, urea and electrolytes, pH and blood gases, degree of ketonaemia. If severe acidosis is present, pH <7.1, and the blood glucose is not significantly elevated alcohol, aspirin overdose or lactic acidosis need to be

Table 7.3 The metabolic consequences of diabetic ketoacidosis and associated risks. Many of these changes increase the risk of falls in older people.

Metabolic consequences of ketoacidosis	Associated risk
Metabolic acidosis	Nausea and vomiting Cardiac arrest
Hyperlipidaemia	Thrombosis/embolism
Haemoconcentration and coagulation changes	Myocardial infarction, stroke, thrombosis
Dehydration	Volume depletion Renal hypoperfusion Can cause acute tubular necrosis
Gastric stasis	Inhalation of vomitus, aspiration pneumonia
Hyperkalaemia but overall deficit in total potassium due to loss in osmotic diuresis.	Cardiac arrhythmias
Hyperglycaemia, which is exacerbated by glycogenolysis and gluconeogenesis	Plasma hyperosmolality Cellular dehydration Osmotic diuresis Compromised immune function leading to infection and delayed wound healing, also thrombosis, low mood, visual changes
Glycosuria	Hyponatraemia and ketonaemia, which contributes to sodium, potassium, and chlorine loss Hyponatraemia is common but if sodium is <120 mmol/L may indicate hypertriglyceridaemia
Abdominal pain	Unnecessary surgery, inappropriate pain relief causing further respiratory distress, missed labour Death

excluded especially in older people. Ketones in the presence of low blood glucose can indicate starvation.

- Assess the cause: full blood count, cardiac enzymes, blood cultures, ECG, chest X-ray, urine culture.

Aims of treatment of DKA

Treatment aims to:

(1) Correct:
- dehydration
- electrolyte imbalance
- ketoacidosis
- hyperglycaemia by slowly reducing the blood glucose to 7–10 mmol/L). Hyperglycaemia, relative insulin deficiency, or both, predispose people with and without diabetes to complications such as severe infection, polyneuropathy, multiorgan failure and death (Van den Bergh *et al.* 2001).

(2) Reverse shock.
(3) Ascertain the cause of DKA and treat appropriately.
(4) Prevent complications of treatment.
(5) Educate/re-educate the patient and their family/carers.

Objectives of nursing care

To support the medical team to:

(1) Restore normal hydration, euglycaemia and metabolism.
(2) Prevent complications of DKA including complications occurring as a result of management.
(3) Pay meticulous attention to detail.
(4) Document progress of recovery.
(5) Re-educate/educate the patient and their family/carers about the management of illness at home or general diabetes education if in a new diagnosis. Patient education about managing diabetes during illness can be found in this chapter.
(6) Ensure follow-up care after discharge, in particular: review of diabetes knowledge, nutritional assessment and physical and psychological assessment.

Preparing the unit to receive the patient

Assemble:

(1) Oxygen and suction (tested to ensure they are in working order).
(2) Intravenous trolley (IV) containing:
   • dressing tray and antiseptic solution
   • local anaesthetic
   • selection of intravenous cannulae
   • IV fluids – normal saline, SPPS
   • giving sets, burette
   • IMED pump or syringe pump
   • clear short or rapid acting insulin, preferably administered as an IV infusion
   • blood gas syringe
   • blood culture bottles.
(3) Cot sides and IV pole.
(4) Blood glucose testing equipment (cleaned, calibrated).
(5) Blood ketone testing equipment.
(6) Appropriate charts:
   • fluid balance
   • diabetic
   • conscious state.
(7) Urinary catheterisation equipment.
(8) Nasogastric tubes may or may not be used. Some experts recommend passing a nasogastric tube to prevent gastric dilatation and aspiration.
(9) Initial care in the intensive care unit is preferable for moderate to severe ketoacidosis.

If the patient is admitted to the intensive care unit, central venous pressures, continuous blood gas, and electrocardiogram monitoring is usually performed.

Practice point

Rapid and short-acting insulin has a rapid onset of action and quickly promotes transport of glucose into the cells. Intravenous administration is preferred because absorption is more predictable than by the subcutaneous route.

Nursing care/observations

The nursing management of DKA involves traditional nursing actions as well as monitoring the response to medical therapy.

Initial patient care

Initial patient care is often given in the intensive care unit. The procedure is:

- Maintain the airway.
- Nurse the patient on their side, even if the patient is conscious, because gastric stasis and inhalation of vomitus is a possible and preventable complication of DKA.
- Ensure strict aseptic technique.

Nursing observations (1–2 hourly)

(1) Observe 'nil orally'. Provide pressure care especially in the elderly patient.

(2) Provide mouth care to protect oral mucous membranes and relieve the discomfort of a dry mouth.

(3) Administer IV fluid according to the treatment sheet usually initially isotonic saline until the blood glucose is <12 mmol/L then 10% dextrose. However, the first litre of saline may be 0.45% in the presence of hypernatraemia (sodium >150 mmol/L).

(4) Administer insulin according to the treatment sheet; it is usually given via an insulin infusion and the dose adjusted according to blood glucose tests, see Chapter 7. Intensive insulin therapy maintains the blood glucose within a narrow range and thereby reduces the morbidity and mortality asociated with critical illness (Van den Burghe *et al.* 2001). In some cases rapid or short-acting insulin is given intramuscularly, usually in remote areas where ICU units are not available.

(5) Replace serum potassium. If the initial biochemical result is >5.0 mmol/L potassium is not required initially. It should be added to the second or third litres of IV fluid or when levels fall to <4.5 mmol/L depending on expected potassium loss, for example, from vomiting. Initially potassium levels should be monitored on an hourly basis.

(6) There is general agreement that bicarbonate replacement is not required if the pH is >7.0. There is no consensus about pH <7.0. Some experts state that bicarbonate should be given to minimise respiratory decompensation. Others believe bicarbonate automatically corrects as the acidosis resolves with fluid and insulin (Hamblin 1995). Some experts use bicarbonate if the pH is <7.1, if the patient presents with a cardiac arrest, or cardiac arrest is imminent.

(7) Estimate blood glucose levels 1–2 hourly and confirm biochemically in the early stages.

(8) Observe strict fluid balance. Record second hourly subtotals of input/output *from admission*. Urine output should be >30 mL per hour measured hourly in a calibrated collecting device. Report a urine output of <30 mL per hour. Measure specific gravity (SG). Be aware that some creatinine assays cross react with ketones and creatinine may not reflect renal function in DKA.
   - *Heavy* glycosuria invalidates SG readings.
   - Record fluid loss, for example, vomitus.

(9) Monitor central venous pressure.

(10) Monitor conscious state. In children with DKA the level of consciousness initially, is significantly associated with pH as well as age but not blood glucose or sodium levels (Edge *et al.* 2006). Therefore, cerebral function in DKA is related to the severity of the acidosis in children even when cerebral oedema is not present. Cerebral oedema is a serious complication of DKA and has a high morbidity rate in children and older people. If coma is prolonged heparin might be indicated to prevent thrombosis and pulmonary embolism.

(11) Record pulse, respiration, and blood pressure. Fever associated with DKA indicates sepsis. But it should be noted that an elevated white cell count can be due to metabolic abnormalities and does not necessarily indicate the presence of infection.

(12) Administer oxygen via face mask or nasal catheter.

(13) Monitor and report all laboratory results (electrolytes and blood gases).

(14) Report any deterioration of condition immediately.

(15) Physiotherapy may be helpful to prevent pneumonia and emboli due to venous stasis, and to provide passive mobilisation.

(16) Administer other medications as ordered (potassium, calciparine, broad-spectrum antibiotics to treat underlying infections, mannitol to reduce cerebral oedema).

(17) Reposition and provide skin care to avoid pressure areas and/or venous stasis.

Subsequent care

As the patient's condition improves:

- Review the frequency of blood glucose testing, decreasing to 4-hourly including the night time.
- Allow a light diet and ensure the patient is eating and drinking before the IV is removed.
- Administer subcutaneous insulin before the IV is removed. Often the infusion is turned off before a meal but the IV line left *in situ* until the person can eat and drink normally and the blood glucose level is stable within the normal range.
- Continue to monitor temperature, pulse and respiration every 4 hours.
- Provide support and comfort for the patient.
- Establish the duration of deteriorating control and identify any precipitating factor such as infection.

Plan for:

- Medical follow-up appointment after discharge.
- Nutrition review.

- Education/re-education about appropriate management (for days when the patient is unwell); see Chapter 16.
- Review medication dosage, especially insulin. DKA can occur as a result of incorrect use of insulin delivery devices, which highlights the importance of checking insulin administration technique particularly given hospital staff do not consider incorrect technique as a potential cause (Bhardwaj *et al.* 2006).
- Consider sexual assault. Sexual assault is an uncommon but important cause of DKA and should be considered when repeated admissions occur. This is a difficult area to assess and should be undertaken by people with the appropriate skills and with consideration of the legal implications and the effect on the individual and their family.

Practice point

Psychiatric consultation should be considered if a patient repeatedly presents in DKA. Eating disorders complicate 20% of recurrent cases of DKA (Polonsky *et al.* 1994). People, especially young women, reduce their insulin doses to avoid weight gain and hypoglycaemia. Reducing or stopping insulin is also a form of risk taking and rebellion at having diabetes (Dunning *et al.* 1994).

Brittle diabetes and hyperglycaemia

Brittle diabetes is difficult for people with diabetes and their carers and health professionals to manage. Brittle diabetes most commonly occurs between 15 and 30 years of age and leads to frequent hospital admissions for DKA. However, brittle diabetes also occurs in older people. Criteria for 'elderly brittle diabetes' are >60 years, treated with insulin, experiencing unstable blood glucose associated with frequent, often prolonged admissions to hospital (Gill & Lucas 1996; Benbow *et al.* 2001). In the older group, women are more likely to present with brittle diabetes than men but the preponderance of women may reflect the proportion of men and women in older people. There does not appear to be consistent underlying causative factors but cognitive behavioural factors appear to play a role (Benbow *et al.* 2001). See also Chapter 10.

Complications that can occur as a result of DKA

Most complications of DKA are due to complications of treatment and most are avoidable:

(1) Hypoglycaemia due to overzealous treatment.
(2) Inhalation of vomitus causing aspiration pneumonia.
(3) Hypokalaemia, which may lead to cardiac arrhythmias.
(4) Cerebral oedema is rare and often fatal. It occurs in 0.7–10% of children especially on the first presentation of diabetes and any morbidity that occurs is permanent (Rosenbloom 1990).

(5) Myocardial infarction.
(6) Deep venous thrombosis.
(7) Adult respiratory distress syndrome.

Be extra vigilant with:

(1) Elderly patients, especially those with established vascular and coronary disease. Risks include myocardial infarction and deep venous thrombosis.
(2) Children are at increased risk of cerebral oedema, which has a high mortality rate in this group of patients.

Euglycaemic DKA

Munro *et al.* originally documented euglycaemic DKA in 1993. Euglycaemic DKA refers to ketoacidosis in the setting of near normal blood glucose levels. This condition indicates that the blood glucose level and development of DKA do not necessarily correlate. De & Child (2001) postulated that heavy glycosuria triggered by counter-regulatory hormone activity or reduced hepatic glucose production could result in lower than expected blood glucose levels. Although euglycaemic DKA is a rare condition it highlights the importance of monitoring serum ketones and blood gases and using low-dose IV insulin infusions in all people with diabetes during illness.

Ketosis without hyperglycaemia occasionally occurs postoperatively in the presence of repeated vomiting. Rehydration with dextrose/saline and controlling the vomiting are required to restore depleted hepatic glycogen stores.

Hyperosmolar non-ketotic coma (HONK)

HONK is a metabolic disturbance characterised by a marked increase in serum osmolality, the absence of ketones, hyperglycaemia (usually >40 mmol/L) and extreme dehydration caused by a concomitant illness (often infection) that leads to inadequate fluid intake. It most commonly occurs in Type 2 diabetes, usually in older people >65, however, HONK has been reported in a 9-month-old baby and an 18-month old toddler (Goldman 1979; Sagarin *et al.* 2005). People with Type 2 diabetes usually secrete enough endogenous insulin to prevent lipolysis and ketoacidosis (Kitabchi *et al.* 1994) but not sufficient to prevent hyperglycaemia and hepatic glucose output.

In addition, the hyperosmolality may limit ketogenesis and the level of free fatty acids available for ketogenesis (Sagarin *et al.* 2005). Type 2 diabetes is associated with progressive beta cell loss so the risk of DKA and HONK may be higher with long duration of Type 2 diabetes or people with LADA; see Chapter 1. Approximately one third of cases occur in people with no previous diagnosis of diabetes. Dehydration is usually severe. The patient is often confused, and focal and general neurological signs are usually present, however, despite the name, coma is rare, occurring in < 10% of cases (Sagarin *et al.* 2005).

Practice point

People with Type 2 diabetes usually still have sufficient endogenous insulin production to prevent the formation of ketones.

HONK occurs in ~17.5 cases per 1000 000 in the US and has a mortality rate of 10–20% with a slightly higher prevalence in women (Sagarin *et al.* 2005). The onset is associated with severe stress such as infection, for example, pneumonia and UTI, extensive burns, myocardial infarction, stroke and/or reduced fluid intake. People in aged care facilities are at the highest risk of HONK because they are often unaware of thirst and are not always offered fluids in hot weather. Other precipitating factors include:

- Some medications such as diuretics, for example, IV diazoxide and furosemide in the surgical setting, corticosteroids, beta blockers, Histamine$_2$ blockers immunosuppressant agents.
- Dialysis.
- Parenteral nutrition.
- IV fluids that contain dextrose.
- Non-adherence with OHA.

There is a high mortality rate associated with HONK. The mortality rate has decreased since the 1960s but is still 10–20% (ADA 2002; Sagarin *et al.* 2005).

Presenting signs and symptoms

A thorough physical examination should be carried out to detect sources of infection and include eyes, ears, nose, throat and teeth and gums, pneumonia, UTI, skin, meningitis, pelvic infection, and triggers such as CCF, and acute respiratory distress syndrome.

- Neurological signs such as drowsiness and lethargy, delirium, seizures, visual disturbances, hemiparesis, diminished reflexes, unsteady gait, and sensory deficits.
- Dehydration indicated by: reduced skin turgor, sunken eyes, and dry mouth.
- Tachycardia is an early sign; hypotension is a late sign and indicates profound dehydration. Tachycardia could also indicate thyrotoxicosis.
- Tachypnoea as a consequence of respiratory compensation for the metabolic acidosis.
- Hypoxaemia, which may compound the effects of dehydration on mental function.
- Signs of infection such as enlarged lymph nodes. Warm moist skin is an early indication of infection whereas cool dry skin indicates late sepsis.

Specific investigations depend on the results of the physical assessment. Laboratory investigations include blood glucose, ketones, electrolytes, renal function (BUN and creatinine, which can be elevated due to the dehydration), osmolality, creatine phosphokinase (CPK), blood cultures, coagulation studies, arterial blood gases (pH is usually ⩾7.25), and urine cultures. Other investigations such as ECG, cardiac enzymes and troponins, lumbar puncture and CSF studies, chest X-ray, head and abdominal CT, and HbA$_{1c}$ as an indication of preceding metabolic control may be useful to plan future management.

The nursing care and objectives are similar to those for DKA, but extra vigilance is needed because of the age of these patients.

Monitor closely:

- Record strict fluid balance.
- IV fluid rate. Central venous access may be used. In some cases Swan-Ganz catheter is inserted to monitor intravascular volume. There is usually a large fluid deficit (~10 L). Replacement: In the first 2 hours 1–2 L isotonic saline but the rate depends on the degree of dehydration, if severe a higher volume may be indicated; lower volumes may be used if there is no urine output. Half normal saline is used once the blood pressure and urine output are normalised and stable.
- An arterial line may be inserted in ICU settings to monitor blood gases.
- Blood glucose may fall with rehydration alone over the first 1–3 hours but usually insulin is indicated to correct the hyperglycaemia and is usually given as an IV insulin infusion adjusted according to the blood glucose level (tested 1–2 hourly).
- ECG.
- Urine output. A urinary catheter may be indicated to accurately measure output and obtain a clean urine specimen to detect infection but can introduce infection.
- Neurological observations.
- Manage the airway.
- Maintain skin integrity including the feet. Compromised peripheral circulation and peripheral neuropathy increases the risk of foot ulcers, which are slow to heal and increase length of stay and the risk of amputation. Nursing on air mattresses may be indicated.
- Observe for deep venous thrombosis or embolism.
- Administer medications as indicated, which might include antibiotics, which might be administered IV. Subsequent care as for DKA.

Education may be more difficult initially because of the mental confusion associated with HONK and the age of these patients. Ensuring that the family/caregivers understand how to care for the patient and ensuring follow-up education occurs in 2–3 weeks is important.

Figure 7.2 outlines the factors involved in the development of hyperosmolar coma. There are similarities with DKA, and some important differences. Ketone production is absent or minimal because the patient is usually producing enough endogenous insulin to allow the ketone bodies to be metabolised and utilised. The degree of dehydration is often greater in HONK and the serum and urine osmolality is increased.

Lactic acidosis

Lactic acidosis is another uncommon condition that sometimes occurs in people with diabetes. Lactic acidosis occurs in 0.06 cases per 1000 patient years, usually those with predisposing factors (Pillans 1998). Lactate is a product of anaerobic glucose

Figure 7.2   An outline of the development of hyperosmolar coma.

metabolism. Disordered lactate metabolism frequently occurs in critically ill people who are at risk of multiorgan failure and the mortality rate is ~70% if the serum lactate remains >2 mmol/L for >24 hours (Nicks 2006). It is primarily cleared from the blood by the liver, kidney, and skeletal muscles.

Lactic acidosis is defined as metabolic acidosis associated with serum lactate >5mmol/L. It occurs due to either an increase in hydrogen ions or reduction in bicarbonate with increased acid production, loss of alkali and reduced renal clearance of acids. Lactic acidosis should be considered during acute illness in patients with vasoconstriction, hypotension and with underlying diseases associated with poor tissue perfusion and hypoxia such as:

- Recent myocardial infarction.
- Cardiac failure and cardiogenic shock.
- Pulmonary disease.
- Cirrhosis
- Sepsis.
- Renal impairment.

- Medicines and toxins such as isoniazid, salicylates, beta-adrenergic agents, alcohol and biguanides especially in older people with hypoxic diseases and/or dehydration.
- Surgery.
- Inborn errors of metabolism such as fructose 1, 6-diphosphatase deficiency.

Excess lactate is produced in ischaemic skeletal muscle and to a lesser extent in the intestine and erythrocytes and accumulates due to a fall in lactate consumption in the liver, which overwhelms the buffering system (Nicks 2006). Lactate levels correlate with tissue hypoperfusion and mortality and the duration and degree of lactic acidosis predicts morbidity and mortality. Lactate >4 mmol/L for >24 hours carries an 11% mortality rate in critically ill patients. After 48 hours, only 14% survive.

Signs and symptoms

- Signs that the cardiovascular system is compromised, for example, cyanosis, cold extremities, tachycardia, hypotension, dyspnoea.
- Lethargy, confusion, stupor.
- Dry mucous membranes.

Biochemistry shows an anion gap, lactate 4–5 mmol/L (normal ~1 mmol/L) low pH, usually <7.1 but only moderate, if any ketones, and mildly elevated blood glucose, usually <20 mmol/L.

Lactic acidosis should be managed in ICU settings.

Lactic acidosis associated with metformin

Ninety per cent of metformin is excreted unchanged via the kidneys and the half-life is prolonged and renal clearance reduced in patients with renal impairment where creatinine clearance is reduced. Renal impairment may develop slowly as a complication of diabetes or acutely. Metformin is contraindicated when the creatinine >0.16 mmol/L, hepatic disease, and conditions associated with hypoxia (Pillans 1998). Some experts suggest 0.15 mmol/L (Nesbit *et al.* 2004) and that age, muscle mass, and protein turnover influence the creatinine clearance rate. Although, metformin-associated lactic acidosis is rare, it remains the most frequently reported cause of medicine-associated mortality (Pillans 1995). It may present as respiratory failure and shock, cardiac arrhythmias, hypothermia and hypoglycaemia (Cohen 2008).

In Australia, 48 cases of metformin-induced lactic acidosis were reported to the Australian Adverse Drug Reactions Advisory Committee (ADRAC) between 1985 and 2001 (ADRAC 2001). Thirty-five had known risk factors for lactic acidosis. An average of six metformin-related adverse events are reported to ADRAC per year. Nisbet *et al.* (2004) calculated the prevalence of lactic acidosis in Australia to be 1 in 30 000 based on ~200 000 metformin prescriptions per year and the reported adverse event rate. They caution that the actual rate may be higher due to under-reporting.

In the US 204 of 263 patients admitted to hospital were taking metformin; 27% had at least one contraindication and metformin was continued in 41% of these despite the contraindication (Calabrese *et al.* 2002). Emslie-Smith *et al.* (2001) identified contraindications to metformin in 24.5% of 1847 of people taking the medicine.

Regular physical assessment to identify patients at risk of lactic acidosis including monitoring renal function, structured medication reviews, adhering to metformin prescribing guidelines, and reporting medicine adverse events are important aspects of care.

Management

Management consist of:

- IV fluid replacement with normal saline to maintain the circulating volume and tissue perfusion.
- Oxygen therapy.
- Bicarbonate given early to correct the acidosis and should be administered slowly to avoid causing metabolic alkalosis and ventillatory failure.

Thiamine 50–100 mg IV followed by 50 mg orally for 1–2 weeks in some cases where thiamine deficiency is likely such as malnourished older people and alcoholics.

- IV insulin at a rate of 10–12 units/hour in dextrose solution.
- Monitoring renal and cardiac status.
- The mental status should be monitored as well as monitoring the physical status.
- Withdrawing precipitating medicines or toxins, which might include haemodialysis in some cases.
- Antibiotics if sepsis is present.
- Medication review and discontinuing medication or reducing the dose if contraindications exist. Metformin is the medicine of choice in overweight Type 2 patients but doses >500 mg per day should be used with caution in older people with renal, liver, and cardiac disease or other hypoxic diseases (Nisbet *et al.* 2004).

References

American Diabetes Association (ADA) (2002) *Hyperglycaemic Crisis in Patients with Diabetes Mellitus*. American Diabetes Association, USA.

Australian Diabetes Educators Association (ADEA) (2006) *Guidelines for Sick Day Management for People with Diabetes*. ADEA, Canberra.

Australian Drug Reactions Bulletin (ADRAC) (2001) Incidence of lactic acidosis between 1985–2001. ADRA 20 (1) http://.www.tga.gov.au/aarb/aadr9505/htm (accessed December 2007).

Benbow, S., Walsh, A. & Gill, G. (2001) Brittle diabetes in the elderly. *Journal of the Royal Society of Medicine*, **94**, 578–580.

Bhardwaj, V. & Metcalfe, N. (2006) Diabetic ketoacidosis after changing insulin pens: check technique to avoid complications. *British Medical Journal*, **332**, 1259–1260.

Brunkhurst, F. (2008) Intensive insulin therapy, Pentastarch may be harmful for patients with severe sepsis. *New England Journal Medicine*, **358**, 125–139.

Calabrese, A. & Turner, R. (2002) Evaluation of prescribing practices: risk of lactic acidosis with metformin therapy. *Archives of Internal Medicine*, **162**, 434–437.

Ciechanowski, P., Katon, W. & Russo, J. (2000) Depression and diabetes. Impact of depressive symptoms on adherence, function and costs. *Archives of Internal Medicine*, **160**, 3278–3285.

Cohen, Z. (2008) Lactic acidosis. American Thoracic Society. http://www.thoracic.org/sections/
clinical-information/critical-care/critical-care-cases/ (accessed 9 February 2008).

Cook, C., Castro, J., Schmidt, R., Gauthier, S., Whitaker, M., Roust, L., Agueta, R., Hull, B. &
Zimmerman, R. (2007) *Journal Hospital Medicine*, 2 (4), 203–211.

De, P. & Child, D. (2001) Euglycaemic ketoacidosis – is it on the rise? *Practical Diabetes
International*, 18 (7), 239–240.

Diepersloot, R., Bouter, K. & Hoekstra, J. (1990) Influenza infection and diabetes mellitus.
Case for annual vaccination. *Diabetes Care*, 13, 876–882.

Dunning, P., Ward, G. & Rantzau, C. (1994) Effect of alcohol swabbing on capillary blood
glucose measurements. *Practical Diabetes*, 11 (4), 251–254.

Dunning, T. (2001) Depression and diabetes, summary and comment. *International Diabetes
Monitor*, 13 (5), 9–11.

Dunning, T. (2007) Diabetes: managing sick days, a patient-centred approach. *General Practice
Continuing Education Conference Proceedings*. Exhibition Centre, Melbourne.

Edge, J., Roy, Y., Bergomi, A., Murphy, N., Ford-Adams, M., Ong, K. & Dunger, D. (2006)
Conscious level in children with diabetic ketoacidosis is related to severity of acidosis and not
to blood glucose concentration. *Pediatric Diabetes*, 7, 11.

Emslie-Smith, A., Boyle, D. & Evans, J. (2001) Contraindications to metformin therapy in
patients with type 2 diabetes – a population based study of adherence to prescribing guidelines.
Diabetic Medicine, 18, 483–488.

Gill, G., Lucas, S. & Kent, L. (1996) Prevalence and characteristics of brittle diabetes in Britain.
Quarterly Journal of Medicine, 89, 839–843.

Goldman, S. (1979) Hyperglycaemic hyperosmolar coma in a 9-month-old child. *Archives of
Paediatrics and Adolescent Medicine*, 133 (2), 30.

Hamblin, S. (1995) Diabetic ketoacidosis. *Australian Diabetes Educator's Association Journal*,
Spring, 17.

Kitabchi, A., Fisher, J., Murphy, M. & Rumbak, M. (1994) Diabetic ketoacidosis and the
hyperglycaemic hyperosmolar nonketotic state. In: *Joslin's Diabetes Mellitus* (eds C. Kahn &
G. Weir), pp. 738–770. Lea & Febiger, Philadelphia.

Kornum, J. (2007) Type 2 diabetes linked to higher pneumonia-related mortality. *Diabetes Care*,
30, 2251–2257.

Malone, M., Gennis, V. & Goodwin, J. (1992) Characteristics of diabetic ketoacidosis in older
versus younger adults. *Journal of the American Geriatric Society*, 40, 1100–1104.

Munro, J., Campbell, I., McCuish, A. & Duncan, L. (1973) Euglycaemic ketoacidosis. *British
Medical Journal*, 2, 578–580.

National Asthma Council Australia (2005) *Roles of Influenza and Pneumococcal Vaccinations
in Subgroups with Asthma, COPD, Diabetes or Heart Disease*. CSL Pharmaceuticals,
Canberra.

Nicks, B. (2006) Lactic acidosis. E medicine http://www.emedicine.com/emerg/topic 291.htm
(accessed January 2008).

Nisbet, J., Sturtevant, M. & Prins, J. (2004) Metformin serious adverse effects. *Medical Journal
of Australia*, 180 (2), 53–54.

Pillans, P. (1998) Metformin and fatal lactic acidosis. Center for Adverse Reactions Monitoring
(CARM) http://www.medsafe.govt.nz/profs/Puarticles/5.htm (accessed January 2008).

Polonsky, W., Anderson, B., Lohrer, P., Aponte, J., Jacobson, A. & Cole, C. (1994) Insulin
omission in women with IDDM. *Diabetes Care*, 17, 1178–1185.

Rosenbloom, A. (1990) Intracerebral crises during treatment of diabetic ketoacidosis. *Diabetes
Care*, 13, 22–33.

Sagarin, M., McAfee, A., Sachter, J., Talavera, F. Bessen, H., Feied, C. (2005) *Hyperosmolar
Hyperglycaemic Coma*. Emedicine http://www. Emedicine.com/emerg/topic24.htm (accessed
January 2008).

Schetz, M. (2008) Intensive insulin therapy may protect renal function in critically ill patients. *Journal of the American Society of Nephrologists Online* January 30 (accessed January 2008).

Shulman, R., Finney, J., O'Sullivan, C., Glynne, P. & Greene, R. (2007) Tight glycaemic control: A prospective observational study of computerized decision-supported intensive insulin therapy. *Critical Care*, **11** (4), R75(doi:10.1186/cc5964).

Smith, S. & Poland, G. (2004) American Diabetes Association: influenza and pneumococcal immunisation in diabetes. *Diabetes Care* 27 (Suppl. 1) S111–S113.

Van den Berghe, M., Wouters, P., Weekers, F. *et al.* (2001) Intensive insulin in critically ill patients. *New England Journal of Medicine*, 345, 1359–1367.

Wang, C., Wang, S. & Lai, C. (2004) Reducing major cause-specific hospitalization rates and shortening hospital stays after influenza vaccination. *Clinical Infectious Diseases*, **39**, 1322–1332.

Chapter 8

Long-Term Complications of Diabetes

Introduction

The long-term complications of diabetes are generally classified as:

- Macrovascular disease: cardiovascular disease, cerebrovascular disease, and peripheral vascular disease. These are common in Type 2 diabetes and are often present at diagnosis. Type 2 diabetes is often preceded by the metabolic syndrome, which confers a high level of cardiovascular risk. Significantly, myocardial infarction is often 'silent' and sudden.
- Microvascular disease: nephropathy and retinopathy. These are a major concern in Type 1 diabetes but the rate macrovascular disease risk is also increased.
- Neuropathy: peripheral, which predominantly affects the feet and legs and autonomic, which can lead to gastroparesis, erectile dysfunction (ED), and hypoglycaemic unawareness.

These conditions are inter-related and often occur concomitantly. For example, ED has vascular and nerve components. In the long term in the presence of persistent hyperglycaemia, diabetes can affect almost all body systems and is associated with a number of other disease processes, especially Type 2 diabetes where there is an association between obesity, some cancers, and sleep apnoea. Diabetes is also associated with a range of musculoskeletal diseases, osteoporosis, depression, and dementia although the causal links are not clear in all cases. The presence of other concomitant and age-related diseases such as arthritis contribute to reduced quality of life and depression and inhibit self-care.

Thus, a multifactorial approach to managing diabetes complication risk is needed and encompasses regular systematic, individualised risk assessment processes, effective self-care, optimising physical and mental health and diabetes education to prevent the morbidity and mortality and reduce the health costs associated with diabetes.

Pathophysiology of diabetes complications

It is becoming evident that the pathophysiology of diabetes complications is complex and that glycaemic control is the most important determinant of optimal mitochondrial function and therefore, long-term diabetic complications (Brownlee 2000). Changes in mitochondrial function result in oxidative stress and play a key role in the development and progression of both micro and macrovascular complications associated with diabetes. Thus, maintaining normoglycaemia to preserve normal oxidative mitochondrial function is needed to delay or prevent the progression of complications (Forbes & Cooper 2007).

Increases in HbA_{1c} from normal to 9.5% confer a 10-fold increased risk of microvascular disease. The relationship between macrovascular disease and hyperglycaemia is not as clear; for example, only a twofold increase in macrovascular disease risk at the same HbA_{1c} was noted in the UKPDS (UKPDS 1998). This finding might be partly explained by the fact that free fatty acids can also be utilised as fuel for oxidative processes in the mitochrondria.

Hyperglycaemia initiates a cascade of pathological changes that underlie diabetes complications. Glucose is the major source of fuel for energy production by oxidative phosphorylation. Hyperglycaemia has significant effects on metabolic pathways concerned with generating cellular energy especially in the mitochondria. Most cells have the capacity to reduce glucose transport across the plasma membrane into the cytosol to maintain glucose homeostasis in the presence of hyperglycaemia. However, some cells are not able to adapt and reduce glucose transport sufficiently to prevent intercellular changes in glucose concentration. The cells are at particular risk include capillary endothelial cells in the retina, mesangial cells in renal glomeruli, neuronal and Schwann cells in peripheral nerves (Forbes & Cooper 2007).

An increasing body of research suggests reactive oxygen species (ROS) initiate the development of diabetic complications (Nishikawa *et al.* 2000). ROS are generated by damaged or dysfunctional mitochondria. The antioxidant chain is a complex pathway involving the metabolism of oxygen and the transfer of electrons from glucose and other fuels through the respiratory chain via a complex series of reactions. When excess fuel enters the respiratory chain, the mitochondrial membrane potential is overwhelmed and leaks electrons to oxygen to form superoxide (Nishikawa *et al.* 2000). However, despite the increasing evidence that ROS plays a role in the pathogenesis of diabetes complications the exact mechanisms are still being determined. Maintaining optimal mitochondrial function appears to be important to reduce the progression of diabetes complications.

Hyperglycaemia contributes to cell death, thickened basement membranes in blood vessels, stiffened vessels and reduces the functionality and structure of resistance vessels (proximal vessels before the blood flows into the capillaries). Calcium-regulated potassium channels are disrupted, which affects smooth muscle cell contraction, which contributes to hypertension. As a result, both under perfusion and over perfusion occur. The myogenic response is lost, so the resistance vessels no longer have the capacity to cope with the increased blood flow. Increased basement membrane dysfunction and reduced nerve fibre density is apparent in impaired glucose tolerance. Micro and macrovascular and endothelial cell damage and reduced lumenal size also occur.

Brownlee (2000) suggested that no 'unifying hypothesis' links the four main hypotheses proposed to explain the pathogenesis of diabetic complications shown below, but suggested either redox changes in the polyol pathway, or hyperglycaemia-induced formation of ROS, may account for all the underlying biochemical changes.

(1) Formation of advanced glycation endproducts (AGE). Products of glucose metabolism from glycolysis and the tricarboxylic acid cycle initiate protein

glycosylation more rapidly than glucose. The protein–glucose complex is broken down by proteosomes or form AGE that become cross-linked and resistant to proteosome activity. Tissues become stiffened and function is compromised. AGE formation may be due to the effects of glucose metabolites rather then glucose itself (Wells-Knecht *et al.* 1995).

(2) Activation of protein kinase C (PKC) isoforms. Hyperglycaemia stimulates diacylglycerol, the lipid second messenger, which activates isoforms of PKC and alters gene and protein expression in organs prone to complications. Inhibiting PKC prevents renal and retinal damage in animal models and a number of clinical trials are in progress involving ruboxisataurin (Forbes & Cooper 2008).

(3) Increased flux through the polyol pathway. In the polyol pathway glucose is converted into sorbitol via aldose reductase and subsequently oxidised to fructose, which eventually contributes to the mitochondrial respiratory chain. Intracellular hyperglycaemia results in increased production of sorbitol and reduces the level of other important enzymes involved in detoxifying toxic aldehydes such as glutathione and adenine dinucleotide phosphate, and compounds oxidative stress. Sorbitol does not cross cell membranes and causes osmotic stress. Inhibiting aldose reductase delays or prevents diabetes complications especially neuropathy (Kaiser *et al.* 1993). To date, aldose reductase inhibitor medications have been disappointing despite improvements in nerve physiology and nerve fibre density, largely due to poor tissue penetration and side effects (Hotta *et al.* 2001).

(4) Increased flux through the hexosamine pathway. When intracellular glucose is high, the normal glucose-6-phosphate metabolic cascade is disrupted and a series of moieties are produced that bind to transcription factors and increase the synthesis of some proteins such as transforming growth factor-β_1 and plasminogen activator inhibitor type 1, both of which have adverse effects on blood vessels (Du *et al.* 2000). The role of the hexosamine pathway in the pathogenesis of diabetic complications is still evolving.

CARDIOVASCULAR DISEASE AND DIABETES

Key points

- Cardiovascular disease is a leading cause of death in people with diabetes.
- People with diabetes need to be treated as if they have heart disease, especially Type 2 diabetes.
- Chest pain may be atypical in people with diabetes.
- Watch for weakness, fatigue, increased blood glucose, congestive cardiac failure (CCF).
- Counsel about how to reduce cardiac risk factors.
- Smoking increases micro- and macrovascular damage. Smoking cessation is imperative.
- Depression is common.
- Transient ischaemic attacks (TIA) may indicate impending stroke.

Rationale

Diabetes is a significant risk factor for cardiovascular disease, for example, coronary heart disease, cardiomyopathy, peripheral vascular disease and stroke (Australian Institute of Health and Welfare (AIHW) 2007). Cardiovascular disease is a major cause of hospital admissions and mortality in people with diabetes. It is often associated with other vascular disease and depression. Complex metabolic abnormalities are present and the need for surgical intervention is high. Autonomic neuropathy can give rise to atypical presentations of cardiovascular disease and heart attack and lead to delayed treatment.

The major clinical manifestations of cardiovascular disease involve:

- The heart and coronary circulation
- The brain and cerebral circulation
- The lower limbs – peripheral vascular disease.

Cardiac disease is a common complication of diabetes, and carries a higher mortality rate than for people without diabetes. The World Health Organisation (WHO) (2003) estimated ~16.7 million people die from cardiovascular disease each year. Myocardial infarction may be a diabetes risk equivalent in non-diabetics. Diabetes often occurs within 3.5 years of an infarct particularly in older people, those with a high BMI, hypertension and smokers. Risk is lower in people consuming a Mediterranean diet and those on lipid-lowering medicines (Mozaffarian *et al.* 2007).

There is an association among increasing age, duration of diabetes, the presence of other complications and mortality. Cardiac disease is associated with diffuse atherosclerosis, coexisting cardiomyopathy, autonomic neuropathy, hyperglycaemia and hyperlipidaemia, the metabolic consequences being hypercoaguability, elevated catecholamines and insulin resistance. Atherosclerosis is more frequent and more severe in people with diabetes. It occurs at a younger age than in people without diabetes and is more prevalent in women.

Cardiac disease accounts for >50% of deaths in Type 2 diabetes (Standl & Schnell 2000; Huang *et al.* 2001) and half of these people die before they reach hospital. The mortality rate has not been reduced despite new therapeutic measures and preventative health programmes.

A number of clinical trials demonstrate the importance of reducing lipids, blood pressure, and blood glucose to reduce the risk of cardiovascular disease (Hansson *et al.* 1998; UKPDS 1998). Hypertension leads to thicker, less elastic blood vessel walls and increases the strain on the heart. There is a linear relationship between the diastolic blood pressure and the eventual outcome of Type 2 diabetes. Reducing the blood pressure below 90 mmHg significantly improves the outcome (UKPDS 1998).

Subtle changes occur in the heart as a result of ischaemia-induced remodelling and the effects of hyperglycaemia on the endothelium of large blood vessels that predispose the individual to heart failure (Standl & Schnell 2000). Heart muscle metabolism is critically dependent on glucose during ischaemia, and heart muscle performance is improved in the presence of insulin, which stimulates glucose uptake, which support the use of IV insulin in acute myocardial infarction (Malmberg *et al.* 1995). However, impaired heart performance is multifactorial and blood pressure, lipids, and

Table 8.1 Diabetes specific cardiovascular abnormalities that predispose an individual to heart disease.

Abnormality	Relevance to cardiovascular disease
Microvascular disease	Often occurs concomitantly with macrovascular disease Affects nutrient and oxygen exchange Nephropathy, frequently in association with retinopathy
Autonomic neuropathy	Postural hypotension Abnormal cardiovascular reflexes Loss of sinus rhythm Resting sinus tachycardia Painless myocardial ischaemia and infarction 'silent MI' Delayed recognition and treatment Increased anaesthetic risk Increased risk in critical care situations Sudden death
Endothelial damage in basement membrane or outer lining of large blood vessels	Weak vessel walls, stiffened vessels contributing to hypertension Impaired blood flow Reduced tissue oxygenation and nourishment
Hypertension	Thickening of blood vessel walls Increased strain on the heart Risk of stroke and MI

prothrombin imbalance all play a part. Table 8.1 outlines some of the diabetic-specific abnormalities linked to the development of cardiovascular disease.

Myocardial infarction is 'silent' in 32% of people with diabetes, which leads to delay in seeking medical attention and may be a factor in the increased mortality rate. 'Silent' infarct means that the classic pain across the chest, down the arm and into the jaw is absent. Only mild discomfort, often mistaken for heartburn, may be present. The atypical nature of the chest pain may make it difficult for people to accept that they have had a heart attack. Risk factor modification may not be seen as essential. The person may present with hypertension, heart failure, cardiogenic shock or, in the elderly, diabetic ketoacidosis or hyperosmolar coma.

Diabetes may be diagnosed at the time of an infarct or during cardiac surgery. Emotional stress, and the associated catecholamine response, leads to increased blood glucose levels in 5% of patients admitted to coronary care units (CCUs). The blood glucose may normalise during convalescence; however, counselling about diabetes and its management is important especially if other diabetes risk factors are present. Tact and sympathy are necessary when informing the patient about the diagnosis of diabetes in these situations.

Medicines and cardiovascular disease

Many types of medicines are needed to prevent and manage cardiovascular disease (see also Chapter 5). The choice of medicines depends on the clinical indication, patient factors such as contraindications and risk of medicine interactions, availability, and cost. Commonly used medicine types include:

- Antithrombotic medicines to prevent thromboembolism generally and during coronary procedures and surgery, prevent stroke in patients with atrial fibrillation, prevent thromboembolism in patients with prosthetic heart valves, and treat acute MI. Types of medicines include Vitamin K antagonists (warfarin), heparin (enoxaparin), platelet aggregation inhibitors (aspirin), and thrombolytic enzymes (alteplase). These medicines require frequent monitoring and interact with many other medicines including complementary medicines (CAM).
- Cardiac medicines to treat arrhythmias (cardiac glycosides such as digoxin), heart failure antiarrythmics such as amiodarone), relieve cardiac symptoms such as angina (vasodilators such as isorbide), treat high and low blood pressure, cardiogenic shock and MI (cardiac stimulants such as adrenaline).
- Antihypertensive agents often used as primary prevention to reduce the risk of microvascular disease. These include low dose diuretics as first-line treatment (frusemide), peripheral vasodilators (oxpentifylline), calcium channel blockers (amlodipine). Antihypertensive therapy is usually selected according to the comorbidities present to achieve blood pressure 130/80 in people with cardiovascular disease. The first-line medicine for people with diabetes and hypertension is an ACE or an ARB; the most appropriate choice in an older person following a MI is a calcium channel blocker to reduce the risk of stroke, however, most people require several antihypertensive medicines (European Society of Hypertension 2007).
- Beta blocking agents (atenolol, metorpolol, propanolol), which can be used with a diuretic and an ACE inhibitor.
- Medicines acting on the renin–angiotensin system such as ACE inhibitors, which are first-line treatment in heart failure, left ventricular dysfunction following MI, and diabetes in the presence of microalbuminuria (ramipril); angiotensin 11 antagonists (irbesartin), which are used if the person cannot tolerate ACE. For example, ACE inhibitors are associated with a three times higher rate of cough.
- Lipid lowering agents such as HMG-CoA reductase inhibitors (statins, e.g., atorvastatin), which reduces LDL cholesterol, fibrates, which are first choice if triglycerides are elevated, nicotinic acid, which lowers both cholesterol and triglycerides but is not tolerated very well (*Australian Medicines Handbook* 2006). Ongoing trials using statins include CORONA, GISSI-HF, and UNIVERSE (Leite-Moreira & Castro-Chaves 2008) that will further clarify the place of these medicines in managing heart failure.

However, these medicines are not always prescribed optimally. For example, anithrombotic medicines, ACE inhibitors, ACE, and beta blocker combinations, and antihypertensive agents are under utilised (National Institute of Clinical Studies 2005). Patient non-adherence with many medicines is high and is a significant limiting factor in achieving optimal outcomes.

Complementary medicines (CAM)

Recently, WS 1442, a formula of *Crataegus monogyna* (hawthorn) was shown to increase intracellular calcium concentration, contractile force, action potential and the refractory period, improve coronary blood flow and reduce preload and after load (Pittler *et al.* 2008). Animal studies have also demonstrated a smaller area of infarction after induced MI. These findings suggest WS 1442 may have a place in managing cardiovascular disease, but that place is not yet defined.

Coenzyme Q_{10} (CQ_{-10}) lowers systolic and diastolic blood pressure and reduces inflammation, suggests individuals with mild-to-moderate hypertension and cardiac disease may benefit from CQ_{-10} supplements (Rosenfeldt *et al.* 2007), but like W1442, its place is under researched. CQ_{-10} is an antioxidant and is present in LDL-c where it reduces the potential for LDL-c to be oxidised and become atherogenic. Some experts suggested CQ_{-10} might be a useful addition to statins to reduce myotoxicity. However, while it may have a place in some people, at present there is no recommendation to use it in all patients taking statins (Barenholtz & Kohlhaas 2006).

Other complementary therapies such as massage, meditation, and Tai Chi can help reduce stress, improve quality of life and manage pain, see Chapter 19. But should be used within a quality of medicine framework.

Patients with an acute cardiovascular event are usually cared for in CCUs or stroke units, but patients in other wards may develop cardiovascular problems. A longer stay in CCU may be indicated for people with diabetes, because 35% of patients die, often in the second week after the infarct (Karlson *et al.* 1993). People with diabetes and unstable angina, MI without ST elevation or STEMI have a higher mortality risk within one year of the onset of acute coronary syndrome than non-diabetics (Donahoe 2007).

Silent MI may be relatively common in common critical care settings and the diagnosis can be difficult and is often missed due to analgesia controlling chest pain, intubation, sedation, and coma (Lim *et al.* 2008). Cook (2008) suggested screening for elevated troponin levels in critically ill patients together with and ECG could reduce mortality and that elevated troponins might be predicative of mortality. Although more research is needed, these findings might be particularly relevant to people with diabetes where the risk of cardiovascular disease is likely to be high.

Short- and long-term morbidity and mortality can be improved by IV insulin/glucose infusion followed by multidose subcutaneous insulin injections (Malmberg *et al.* 1995). Acute myocardial infarction causes a rapid increase in catecholamines, cortisol, and glucagon. Insulin levels fall in the ischaemic myocardium and tissue sensitivity to insulin falls and impairs glucose utilisation by cardiac muscle. Free fatty acids are mobilised as fuel substrates and potentiate ischaemic injury by direct toxicity or by increasing the demand for oxygen and inhibiting glucose oxidation. IV insulin during acute episodes and subcutaneous insulin for three months after the infarct may restore platelet function, correct lipoprotein imbalance, reduce plasminogen activator inhibitor-1 activity and improve metabolism in non-infarcted areas of the heart.

The need for invasive procedures depends on the severity at presentation and the results of relevant investigations. Pfisterer (2004) showed invasive treatment provided short-term symptomatic relief, reduced the rate of revascularisation and hospitalisation and less frequent use of antianginal medicines, compared to medicine treatment. In the longer term, both strategies were effective in older patients with angina. Mortality risk factors included age >80 years, prior heart failure, left ventricular ejection <45%, and the presence of two or more comorbidities.

Mental health and cardiovascular disease

Anxiety is common among people with cardiac disease and can have serious consequences for self-care and long-term outcomes if it is not recognised and managed to prevent depression. However, anxiety can be life saving if it prompts the person to seek help early (Moser 2007). Significantly depression is an independent risk factor for cardiovascular disease and its prognosis. Both depression and heart disease are associated with social isolation and lack of social support (Bunker *et al.* 2003). These factors need to be considered when estimating cardiovascular risk.

Several trials have investigated the cardiovascular benefit of treating depression. These include ENRICH (cognitive behaviour therapy and SSRI medicines), which is difficult to interpret but which showed no significant difference between treatment and usual care. SADHART (SSRI), which showed improvements in mild-to-moderate depression but no significant differences in cardiac events. The results of CREATE (SSRI (citalopram) and interpersonal psychotherapy) are not yet available but suggest depression improves but HbA_{1c} does not significantly improve (Reddy 2008).

The effects on mental health may change; for example, Gudjhar & Dunning (2003) found people with diabetes were most concerned about the implications of the MI immediately after the event and less concerned about the impact of diabetes on their long-term physical health, mental health, and quality of life. Patient generated quality-of-life tools were used. As people recovered and realised they would survive, about four months after the MI, concern about the MI began to diminish and pre MI worry about diabetes re-emerged.

Depression may increase cardiovascular risk and vice versa via several mechanisms:

- Risk behaviours such as inadequate diet and inactivity, smoking and non-compliance with medicines.
- Effects on autonomic function by enhancing sympathetic nervous system activity and heart rate variability.
- Consequence Model – Inflammatory processes with sub-chronic elevation of cytokines activate the stress response and inhibit serotonin. MI might also induce physical changes in the brain that are mediated by the inflammatory response and cause depression.
- Coincidence model – autonomic dysregulation decreased heart rate variability and increased risk of ventricular arrhythmias, changes in platelets, inflammation and changes in endothelial function some of which might be linked to dietary factors. For example, increasing omega-3 fatty acids improves cardiac function (Lesperance & Frasure-Smith 2007).

Objectives of care in hospital

Nursing care should be planned to avoid constantly disturbing the patient and allow adequate rest and sleep. The objectives of care are to:

- Treat the acute attack according to medical orders and standard protocols.
- Stabilise cardiac status and relieve symptoms.

- Prevent extension of the cardiac abnormality and limit further episodes.
- Retain independence as far as possible.
- Achieve and maintain euglycaemia.
- Provide psychological support.
- Prevent complications while in hospital.
- Counsel about risk factor modification.
- Educate/re-educate about diabetes.

Nursing responsibilities

(1) To be aware that myocardial infarction can present atypically in people with diabetes and may present as CCF, syncope, vomiting, abdominal pain, and fatigue that improves with rest. An ECG should be performed urgently if any of these symptoms are present. A high resting heart rate is associated with mortality in people with diabetes. Sanchis (2007) developed a risk assessment process for patients without an increase in troponins or ST deviation that was able to identify patients with a similar prognosis to patients with elevated troponins and ST depression that might be useful in people with diabetes.

(2) To provide psychological, educational, and physical care.

(3) To monitor blood glucose, 2–4 hourly depending on stability and route of insulin administration.

(4) To provide adequate pain relief, and to control vomiting, which can exacerbate high blood glucose levels.

(5) To perform treatment according to the medical orders for the specific cardiac abnormality.

(6) To administer insulin:
  - Many patients on OHAs are changed to insulin during the acute phase to improve blood glucose control.
  - Insulin is usually administered via an infusion at least for the first 48 hours. Only clear insulin is used. Insulin infusions are discussed in Chapter 7. The patient should be eating and drinking normally before the infusion is removed, and a dose of subcutaneous insulin given to prevent hyperglycaemia developing.

  Some endocrinologist/cardiologist teams have adopted Malmberg *et al.*'s recommendations, the so-called DIGAMI protocol, or some variation of it. This usually involves commencing an IV insulin infusion for people with diabetes presenting with MI from the time of presentation in the emergency room. IV insulin is usually continued for 24 hours after which time subcutaneous insulin is commenced and maintained for three months.

  The aim of the DIGAMI regime is to normalise glucose utilisation in the myocardium, achieve normoglycaemia and reduce morbidity and mortality.

(7) Medications: OHAs should be stopped while the patient is having insulin to reduce the risk of hypoglycaemia and lactic acidosis. Thiazide diuretics can:
  - increase blood glucose levels.
  - cause hypokalaemia.
  - Beta blockers reduce mortality by >30%. Ace inhibitors improve blood pressure and cardiac remodelling and stabilise the rate of progression of renal disease. There is a close association between cardiac and renal disease in diabetes.

Non-cardiac-specific beta-blocking agents may mask the signs of hypoglycaemia. Patients who are normally tablet controlled will require support and education about the use of insulin. It should be explained that insulin is being given to increase the glucose available to the myocardium and decrease free fatty acids in the blood. Units where the DIGAMI regime is used usually discharge the patient on subcutaneous insulin that is continued for three months then reassessed.

(8) Physical status:
- Monitor fluid balance and maintain accurate charts, to help assess kidney function.
- Monitor blood pressure, lying, and standing. Some antihypertensive medications can cause orthostatic hypotension. Counsel the patient to change position gradually, especially on getting out of bed or out of a chair.
- Monitor ECG.
- Observe for weakness, fatigue, CCF or unexplained hyperglycaemia, which may indicate a further infarct.
- Provide appropriate skin care to prevent dryness and pressure areas.

(9) Blood tests:
- Monitor serum electrolytes, cardiac enzymes, blood gases and potassium levels. Report abnormalities to the doctor promptly. Fluctuating potassium levels can cause or exacerbate cardiac arrhythmias.
- Prevent hypoglycaemia by careful monitoring of blood glucose and carbohydrate intake.

(10) Thrombolytics are beneficial to reduce plaque. Low-dose aspirin reduces emboli and reduces the risk of cardiac disease and stroke.

(11) If relevant, consider end-of-life care and support the family to cope with the crisis.

Clinical observation

Introducing the DIGAMI protocol requires collaboration between the cardiology, emergency room, and endocrinology teams. It does increase the workload of nurses especially diabetes nurse specialists/diabetes educators, but the benefits to the person with diabetes are significant.

In many cases previous metabolic control was suboptimal and insulin therapy indicated for some time before the infarct occurred.

Some OHAs are contraindicated if cardiac, renal, and/or liver disease is present (see Chapter 5).

Practice points

(1) The patient may not recognise the signs of hypoglycaemia if:
- Autonomic neuropathy is present.
- Non-selective beta-blocking agents are used.

(2) Neuroglycopenic signs of hypoglycaemia (confusion, slurred speech or behaviour change) may predominate. Alternatively, these signs may indicate a cardiovascular event.

Medical tests/procedures (see Chapter 9)

(1) The eyes should be assessed *before* thrombolytic medications are commenced. If proliferative retinopathy is present, bleeding into the back of the eye may occur, requiring urgent treatment.
(2) Diagnostic procedures that require the use of contrast dyes, for example, angiograms, have been associated with renal complications.
Ensure adequate hydration before and after procedures and monitor urine output, especially in elderly people or those with renal disease.
(3) There is a high prevalence of cardiovascular disease in people with renal disease (Levin 2001).

Rehabilitation

Structured rehabilitation after an acute cardiovascular event and heart failure improves long-term outcomes, reduces social isolation, and improves function and quality of life.

(1) Encourage activity within tolerance limits. Refer for physiotherapy/occupational therapy.
(2) Encourage independence.
(3) Counsel about resumption of normal activity, including sexual intercourse, after discharge home.
(4) Explain restrictions on driving after cardiac surgery.
(5) Ensure diabetes education/re-education is available. Refer to diabetes nurse specialist/diabetes educator, dietitian, and physiotherapist. Education should include the need to protect kidney function and also address the risk factors involved in the development of cardiac disease. Particular areas of concern are:
   • Recognition of hypoglycaemia.
   • Correct insulin technique.
   • Correct blood glucose monitoring technique.
   • Possible indicators of further cardiac problems.
   • Dietary assessment and advice.
   • Risk factor modification.
(6) Explain the need for multi-medicine therapy and the importance of adhering to the medicine regimen.
(7) Monitor to detect anxiety and depression and treat early.

Modifying risk factors associated with the development of cardiac disease

Current cardiovascular management guidelines focus on reducing global cardiovascular risk, which requires a proactive approach and attention to multiple risk factors taking age into account. Cardiovascular risk can be stratified and individualised to enable personalised teaching using tools such as the QRISK and ASSIGN in the UK and the Framingham algorithm, which is sex-specific and is based on the presence of hypertension, dyslipidaemia, and smoking. The Systematic Coronary Risk Evaluation (SCORE) based on cholesterol, blood pressure, and age was developed for European countries (Zannad 2008). Significantly, research suggests that doctors do not adequately assess cardiovascular risk and this contributes to patients not achieving management targets (Bohm 2008). Other researchers found general practitioners overestimate the risk of diabetes complications but the impact on patient care and service utilisation or outcomes was not reported (Haussler *et al.* 2007).

Patients require both information and support to manage diabetes and reduce the risk of adverse health outcomes. Personalised information is more effective than generalised information. Management targets are described in Chapter 2. As indicated in Chapter 16, helping people determine their cardiovascular age could be a useful way to help people understand their cardiovascular risk and enhance their adherence to risk reduction strategies.

Key messages are to:

- Stop smoking.
- Avoid high calorie foods and high fat intake especially trans fats to achieve sensible weight reduction. Include omega-3 fatty acids in the diet. Reduce salt intake. Suitable diets are described in Chapter 4 and include the DASH and Mediterranean diets
- Limit alcohol intake.
- Maintain a healthy weight range suitable to age and developmental stage. In particular reduce abdominal obesity.
- Increase regular exercise/activities.
- Achieve acceptable blood glucose levels. However, the ACCORD trial in Type 2 diabetes was halted after 18 months when an interim analysis showed an increased number of deaths in the intensive control versus (HbA_{1c} target <6%) control groups.
- Reduce blood lipids. If this is not achieved by diet and exercise lipid lowering agents are needed, see Chapter 5. High LDL-c, low HDL-c, and mixed hyperlipidaemia significantly increase the risk of developing cardiovascular disease (Hansel 2007).
- Reduce blood pressure by an appropriate diet and exercise and stopping smoking. Tight blood pressure control is important and people are often prescribed three or more antihypertensive agents. The choice of medication is individualised and includes reducing blood glucose as part of a comprehensive cardiovascular risk management plan (Lowe 2002). Hypertension is also a risk factor for poorer performance on verbal and concept formation tests in Type 2 diabetes (Elias *et al.* 1997), which has implications for self-care and activities of daily living.
- Secondary prevention programmes such as cardiac rehabilitation are important to help individuals regain the best possible functioning.
- Manage stress. Long-term stress is associated with increased risk of cardiovascular disease in both men and women and high level of trait anger in middle aged men with hypertension is associated with increased risk of hypertension progression to a cardiovascular event (Player *et al.* 2007).
- Seek treatment for depression.
- Patients with known cardiac disease should have a written action to plan to follow if they experience chest pain. They should know early management is important and not to delay presenting to hospital. The plan might include using short-acting nitrate medicines, resting, taking aspirin if they are not already prescribed this medicine, calling an ambulance, notifying their doctor, and wearing medic alert information.

Telephone coaching

Telephone coaching patients with coronary heart disease and suboptimal lipids improves adherence to medication therapy and dietary advice. It contributes to an improved lipid profile and could be an important aspect of cardiac rehabilitation programmes (Vale *et al.* 2002). The COACH protocol is currently under investigation in a general practice setting with practice nurses providing coaching with support for the COACH investigators (Young *et al.* 2007).

Cerebrovascular disease

The brain is supplied with blood by four main arteries: two carotids and two vertebral arteries. The clinical consequences of cerebrovascular disease depend on the vessels or combination of vessels involved.

Transient ischaemic attacks (TIAs) arise when the blood supply to a part of the brain is temporarily interrupted without permanent damage. Recovery from a TIA usually occurs within 24 hours. If TIAs occur frequently they can indicate impending stroke. Small repeated strokes that cause progressive brain damage can lead to multi-infarct dementia, which is common in diabetes. Signs that this is occurring are:

- Gradual memory loss.
- Diminished intellectual capacity.
- Loss of motor function.
- Incontinence.

Strokes are classified as thrombotic or haemorrhagic and occur when a major vessel is blocked. They frequently cause permanent damage requiring prolonged rehabilitation and often significantly reduced self-care potential and quality of life. In these cases diabetes management should be discussed with the family or carers who will be responsible for assisting the person with diabetes.

The risk factors for cerebrovascular disease are similar to those for cardiovascular disease. High BMI >25 kg/m^2 and systolic hypertension increase risk of death after a stroke among men (Chen 2008). However, there appears to be some significant differences between man and women. Women may have worse outcomes after acute stroke than men if they do not receive thrombolytic therapy and women are more likely to benefit from thrombolytic therapy than men (Lutsep 2008). Likewise, healthy women over age 65 benefit from alternate day aspirin (100 mg) to prevent stroke but aspirin has not been shown to prevent strokes in healthy men (Ridker *et al.* 2005).

There are also gender differences in response to treatment and outcome following acute stroke. Women with carotid artery stenosis have a lower risk of recurrent stroke than men and receive less benefit from surgical treatment of moderate carotid artery stenosis than men (Alamowitch *et al.* 2005). Women with intracranial stenosis are at higher risk of recurrent stroke than men (Williams *et al.* 2007).

Poor sleep quality is also linked to increased risk of vascular events including stroke and daytime sleepiness may be an independent risk factor for stroke conferring a 4.5-fold increased risk (Boden-Albala 2008).

Signs and symptoms

- A careful history will elicit failing mental function.
- Carotid bruits are usually present and can be evaluated using Doppler studies.
- Angiography is required in symptomatic cases.

Management

The preventative measures outlined for cardiovascular disease apply to cerebrovascular disease. Carotid endarterectomy is indicated if the carotid arteries are significantly narrowed. Low-dose aspirin may be beneficial.

Nursing responsibilities include care during investigative procedures (see Chapter 9). Rehabilitation focuses on returning the person to optimal functioning and independence within their capabilities.

Driving assessment needs to be undertaken and assessed regularly, see Chapter 10.

DIABETES AND EYE DISEASE

Key points

- Encourage independence. People with visual loss are capable of caring for themselves if they are provided with appropriate tools and information. However, visual impairment has a profound impact on an individual's ability to learn diabetes self-care tasks and on their psychological wellbeing.
- Maintain a safe environment.
- Orient patient to the environment and staff.
- Explain procedures carefully and fully recognising the person is not a visual learner
- Return belongings to the same place.
- Use appropriate teaching style to the individual's learning style.

Rationale

Retinopathy is a significant complication of diabetes. Prevention and early identification of people at risk are essential. Nurses need to be aware of the impact of visual loss on the self-care and psychological wellbeing of people with diabetes and their role in preventative care. Other vision changes occur in people with diabetes in addition to diabetic retinopathy, for example, macular degeneration is common in older people. Age-related macular degeneration might be related to elevated levels of high-sensitivity CRP. Cataracts and glaucoma have a higher incidence in diabetes but also occur in non-diabetics.

Introduction

Visual impairment and blindness are significant complications of diabetes. The specific cellular mechanisms that lead to reduced visual acuity have not been defined. (Antonetti *et al.* 2006) proposed a combined nerve and vascular mechanism that causes loss of neurons, which compromises neurotransmission and altered structure and function of retinal cells types. Macular cysts could scatter light and reduce the quality of the image and/or visual function could decline as a result of fluid accumulation in the retina. The neurons are susceptible to circulating amino acids, antibodies and/or inflammatory cells that reach the retina through leaking capillaries. The vascular leakage can affect vision even when macular oedema is not present (Antonetti *et al.* 2006). There is also evidence that cognitive ability declines over time in people with diabetes and may be linked to complications such as proliferative retinopathy (Ryan *et al.* 2003).

Key changes in the eye include:

- Maculopathy: macular oedema and macular ischaemia. The macular may be distorted or elevated or vitreous haemorrhages may occur and distort the ocular media (Antonetti *et al.* 2006).
- Retinopathy – stages of retinopathy have been described based on a system of photographic grading that requires comparison with a standard set of photographs showing different features and stages of retinopathy (DRS 1981; EDTRS 1991)
- Generalised ocular oedema
- Lens opacity – cataract
- Papillopathy – optic disc swelling that occurs in Type 1 diabetes.

Retinopathy occurs in almost all people with Type 1 diabetes after 20 years duration of diabetes and 70% of people with Type 2 diabetes (DRS 1981; DCCT 1993). Retinopathy occurs as a result of microvascular disease that manifests as increased capillary permeability and closure of the retinal capillaries, which causes vascular leakage, retinal oedema, and accumulation of lipids that is seen as hard exudates in the retina and retinal ischaemia.

Risk factors for retinopathy

The factors that lead to an increased risk of retinopathy include:

- Long duration of diabetes.
- Poor metabolic control.
- Renal disease.
- Pregnancy in people with diagnosed diabetes. Pregnancy may exacerbate existing retinopathy, see Chapter 14 (but it does not usually develop in women with gestational diabetes).
- Smoking.
- Hypertension.

People with diabetic eye disease are at greater risk of developing other diabetes-related complications unless they are screened regularly, take appropriate preventative action and treatment is commenced early.

Visual impairment from non-diabetic causes can coexist with diabetes. People with diabetes also have an increased incidence of glaucoma and cataracts and there is an increasing correlation with age-related macular degeneration. Many of the underlying causes that lead to macular degeneration are also associated with diabetes, see Table 8.2. Poor vision can be a significant disadvantage during diabetes education and

Table 8.2   Risk factors for age-related macular degeneration (Lim 2006). Many of these are similar to the risk factors for diabetic retinopathy and the same risk reduction strategies apply to both conditions. The table shows modifiable and non-modifiable factors. Sun exposure, and iris and hair colour do not appear to be associated with AMD (Khan *et al.* 2006).

Modifiable factors	Non-modifiable factors
Cigarette smoking, the risk increases with long duration of smoking.	Increasing age: for both exudative and non-exudative AMD[a]
Diet high in fats especially monounsaturated and polyunsaturated fats. Linoleic acid increases the risk for advanced AMD. Omega-3 fatty acids are associated with lower risk. High GI[b] foods is related to the development of retinal pigmentation abnormalities (Chui *et al.* 2006). Emerging research suggests a diet rich in fruit and vegetables especially carotenoids may help prevent AMD. Vitamins C and E and zinc (van Leeuwen *et al.* 2005).	Ethnicity. AMD is more prevalent in whites. Especially for the components of late AMD, increased retinal pigmentation and retinal pigment epithelial depigmentation. Cataracts and glaucoma are more common in Blacks.
High BMI[c]. The risk of developing AMD increases with increasing BMI and geographic atrophy could be associated with high BMI, low education and antacid use (Clemons *et al.* 2005).	Genetic inheritance
Hypertension is associated with exudative AMD but not non-exudative AMD Hypercholesteraemia is also associated with exudative AMD.	
Inflammation. Recent studies suggest C-reactive protein is associated with intermediate and advanced AMD (Seddon *et al.* 2004).	

[a] AMD: age-related macular degeneration.
[b] GI: glycaemic index.
[c] BMI: body mass index.

general living because most diabetic and general health information contains essential visual components (IDF-DECS 2000).

Practice points

(1) The shape of the lens changes with changes in blood glucose concentrations, leading to refractive changes and blurred vision. This usually corrects as the blood glucose is normalised, but may take some time if the blood glucose has been high for a long time.

(2) Vision can worsen in the short term when blood glucose control begins to improve, for example, when commencing insulin and during pregnancy.

(3) The temporary vision disturbance creates significant stress for the person with diabetes and a careful explanation is needed.

Eye problems associated with diabetes

(1) One-third of people with diabetes have retinopathy as a result of microvascular disease. The incidence is related to the duration of diabetes. Sixty per cent of people with diabetes and a duration of more than 15 years have some degree of retinopathy, this especially applies to women. There is increasing evidence that ACE inhibitors can reduce the risk of microvascular disease (see Chapter 5).

(2) People can have severe eye damage without being aware of it. Vision is not always affected and there is usually no pain or discomfort.

(3) Cataracts are more common in people with diabetes.

(4) Maculopathy is the most common cause of visual loss in people with diabetes.

(5) Sudden loss of vision is normally an emergency. It may be due to:
   - vitreous haemorrhage
   - retinal detachment
   - retinal artery occlusion.

   Reassurance, avoidance of stress and sudden movement, and urgent ophthalmological assessment are required.

(6) Prevention and early detection are important aspects in the management of visual impairment. It involves:
   - good blood glucose control can slow the rate of progression in Type 1 diabetes (DCCT 1993)
   - regular eye examinations (commencing at diagnosis in Type 2 and within 5 years in Type 1)
   - non-mydriatic fundus photography, as the name suggests, does not require mydriatic eye drops to be used. This means people do not have to wait long periods to have their eyes examined and can drive themselves home after the procedure. The procedure is not painful but the patient should be warned that the flash of light is very bright. Retinopathy screening committees in both Australia and the UK recommend indirect fundoscopy and digital photography to screen for retinopathy
   - retinal photography
   - confocal microscopy is increasingly being applied to diabetes complication screening, especially to detect eye changes and neuropathy. Confocal microscopy enables greater contrast to be achieved and three-dimensional images to be created that show great detail. The technique uses a spatial pinhole to eliminate out of focus light and flare. It enables faster diagnosis, is non-invasive and painless.
   - fluorescein angiography.

(7) Laser treatment is very effective in preventing further visual loss.

Clinical observation

Eye drops occasionally cause pain and increased pressure in the eye some hours after they were instilled. If this occurs the patient should be advised to call the doctor.

Resources for people with visual impairment

People with significant visual loss often require assistance to perform blood glucose monitoring and to administer their own insulin. It is important to encourage independence as far as possible. Careful assessment is important and should include assessment of the home situation.

Vision Australia and the Royal National Institute for the Blind in the UK offer a variety of services for people who have degrees of visual loss. These services include:

- Assessment of the home situation to determine if modifications are necessary to ensure safety at home.
- Low vision clinics.
- Talking library and books in Braille.
- Training on how to cope in the community with deteriorating vision.

Other help includes:

- Services such as pensions, which may be available from the government.
- Seeing eye dogs (guide dogs for the blind).
- A range of diabetes products are available that can help visually impaired people remain independent (see next section).

The community nurses and home-based services play a major role in maintaining visually impaired people in their own homes.

Aids for people with low vision

Various magnifying devices are available to help people continue to care for themselves. They can be obtained from diabetes associations and some pharmacies specialising in diabetic products. Other aids include:

(1) Insulin administration:
   - clicking syringes, Instaject devices, clicking insulin pens
   - chest magnifying glass (available from some opticians); Magniguide – fits both 50 and 100 unit syringes and enlarges the markings
   - location tray for drawing up insulin if syringes are used.
(2) Blood glucose monitoring:
   - strip guides for accurate placement of the blood onto the strips
   - talking blood glucose meters, blood pressure monitors, and talking weight scales
   - meters with large result display areas.
(3) Medications:
   - dosette boxes, which can be prefilled with the correct medication.

Practice point

People with visual problems and/or red/green colour blindness may have difficulty interpreting the colours on visual test strips where they are still used.

Nursing care of visually impaired patients

Aims of care
- To encourage independence as far as possible.
- To ensure the environment is safe when the patient is mobile.

Patients confined to bed
 (1) Introduce yourself and address the patient by name, so the patient is aware that you are talking to them.
 (2) Ascertain how much the patient is able to see. (Few patients are totally blind.) Assess if the blood glucose fluctuates at certain times. High and low levels can interfere with clear vision. Plan education to avoid these times and determine measures that can avoid such fluctuations, for example, appropriate timing of meals and medications. Dexterity and cognitive function may also be impaired especially in the elderly and hamper diabetes education. Visual impairment increases the risk of falls in elderly patients (see Chapter 12).
 (3) Some patients prefer a corner bed because it makes location easier, avoids confusion with equipment belonging to other patients and enables greater ease in setting up personal belongings.
 (4) Introduce the patient to other people in their ward or close by.
 (5) If you move the patient's belongings they must be returned to the same place.
 (6) Explain all procedures carefully and fully before commencing. (An injection when you can't see it and don't expect it can be very unnerving.)
 (7) If eye bandages are required, make sure the ears and other sensory organs are not covered as well.
 (8) Consider extra adjustable lighting for those patients with useful residual vision.
 (9) Mark the patient's medication with large print labels or use a dosette.
 (10) A radio, talking clock, talking watch, Braille watch, or a large figured watch, helps the patient keep orientated to time and place.
 (11) Indicate when you are leaving the room and concluding a conversation.

Patients who are mobile
 (1) A central point like the patient's bed assists with orientating a patient to a room.
 (2) When orientating a patient to a new area, walk with them until they become familiar with the route.
 (3) Keep obstacles (trolleys, etc.) clear of pathways where possible.

Meal times
 (1) Describe the menu and let the patient make a choice.
 (2) Ensure the patient knows their meal has been delivered.
 (3) Ask 'Do you need assistance with your meal?' rather than say, 'I will cut your meat for you.'
 (4) Colour contrast is important for some patients. A white plate on a red tray-cloth may assist with location of place setting.

DIABETES AND RENAL DISEASE

Key points

- Diabetes may be the underlying cause of renal disease.
- Measurement of microalbuminuria and overt proteinuria is the most useful method of detecting abnormal renal function.
- Elevated blood pressure is an early indicator of renal disease.
- There is a strong association between retinopathy and renal disease.
- Microalbuminuria indicates early renal disease and predicts cardiovascular disease in people with diabetes.

Introduction

Diabetic nephropathy is a significant microvascular complication of diabetes and diabetes is the second most common cause of end-stage renal disease in Australia and the UK (ANZDATA 2000; Department of Health 2001). There is a similar initial disease progression in both Type 1 and Type 2 diabetes. Eventually, microalbuminuria occurs in up to 20% of people with Type 1 diabetes and in a similar percentage of people with Type 2. Some cultural groups are at significant risk, for example, Aboriginal and Torres Strait Islander peoples and Afro-Caribbeans.

Risk factors for renal disease

There is a strong link between hypertension and the progression of renal disease. The risk of end-stage renal failure increases as the diastolic blood pressure increases to >90–120 mmHg (Klag *et al.* 1996). Other risk factors include:

- Smoking, which represents a significant and dose-dependent risk.
- Hyperglycaemia, predialysis control is an independent predictor of the outcome in people with Type 2 diabetes on haemodialysis (Wu *et al.* 1997). The Diabetes Control and Complications Trial (DCCT) demonstrated that good control of blood glucose delayed the rate and progression of microvascular disease including renal disease (DCCT 1993).
- The presence of microalbuminuria and proteinuria are independent risk factors for the development and progression of renal disease in people with diabetes (Keane 2001). People with diabetes are at risk of microalbuminuria if they have any of the following. The more of these factors present the greater the risk:
  - A urine albumin excretion rate in the upper range of normal (20–30 mg/day)
  - Systolic blood pressure >130 mmHg
  - HbA_{1c} >9%
  - Total cholesterol >5.2 mmol/L (Sheldon *et al.* 2002)

Incipient renal disease is present when the albumin excretion rate reaches 20–200 μg/ minute and becomes overt when it exceeds 200 μg/minute. Once macroproteinuria is present the decline in renal function is regarded as irreversible. In addition, proteinuria is an important marker for cardiovascular disease in Type 2 diabetes. Tests for microalbuminuria include timed urine collections (12- or 24-hour collections) usually on an outpatient basis, but compliance is poor. Initial screening can be achieved by testing the first early morning specimen voided (50 mL). Another method is the use of dipsticks such as Micral test (Gilbert *et al.* 1998). Recently the eGFR was introduced and is widely used in Australia (Chadban & Lerino 2005).

- Hypertension, which is a risk factor for cardiovascular disease and kidney disease and the risk is continuous independent of other cardiovascular risk factors (Committee on the Prevention, Detection, Evaluation, and Treatment of High Blood Pressure: Chobanian *et al.* 2003). Most people with advanced renal disease develop hypertension. If not controlled, hypertension can accelerate the rate of decline in renal function. If the cycle from hypertension to renal impairment can be halted, fewer people would require dialysis (Nurko 2004).
- Presence of retinopathy (Gilbert *et al.* 1998).
- Long duration of diabetes.
- Male gender.
- Increasing age.

People with Type 2 diabetes often have microalbuminuria at diagnosis, which is consistent with the fact that impaired glucose tolerance or diabetes is often present for many years before it is diagnosed. Thus screen should begin at diagnosis in Type 2 diabetes. Microalbuminuria is rarely present in Type 1 diabetes at diagnosis so screening usually begins at ~5 years duration of diabetes. However, patients with LADA may present differently and screening might need to be commenced earlier in these patients.

Practice points

(1) False-positive results can occur after heavy exercise or if the person has an UTI.
(2) Women with diabetes may develop proteinuria during pregnancy and the cause should be investigated to ensure the protein is not an early sign or preeclampsia especially if they also present with hypertension.
(3) If a person develops heavy proteinuria in a short period of time other cause should be investigated.
(4) Serum creatinine alone is a poor indicator of renal status in older people. Underweight and overweight are risk factors for misclassifying the degree of renal dysfunction (Gianelli *et al.* 2007)

Renal failure

Early referral to a nephrologist is imperative to improve the long-term outcomes especially when dialysis or transplantation may be needed. However, collaboration with diabetes and other relevant experts must still occur. Late referral is associated with higher morbidity and mortality rates in people on dialysis even when they survive the first year on dialysis (Cass *et al.* 2002).

Renal failure, often requiring dialysis, occurs in 25% of people diagnosed with diabetes before the age of 30. The presence of mild renal disease increases the risk of cardiovascular disease even with only small elevations of urinary protein, but the relationship is not clear. The presence of other cardiovascular risk factors increases the risk, and endothelial cell dysfunction may play a part. Angiotensin converting enzyme (ACE) inhibitors have been shown to delay or stabilise the rate of progression of renal disease and to decrease cardiac events (Keane 2001).

The development of renal problems is insidious and frank proteinuria may not be present for 7–10 years after the onset of renal disease. Microalbuminuria, on the other hand, is detectable up to 5–10 years before protein is found in the urine. Regular urine collections to screen for microalbuminuria controlling blood glucose and blood pressure, the use of ACE inhibitors (Type 1) and angiotensin receptor blockers (Type 2) and avoiding nephrotoxic agents can attenuate renal and cardiac disease (Gilbert & Kelly 2001).

ACE inhibitors have been shown to be more effective than other antihypertensive agents in reducing the time-related increase in urinary albumin excretion and plasma creatinine in Type 2 diabetes and in people with other cardiovascular risk factors, heart failure and myocardial infarction (Ravid *et al.* 1993). Likewise, the HOPE and MICRO-HOPE studies demonstrated that ACE inhibitors reduced cardiovascular events and overt nephropathy whether or not microalbuminuria was present (HOPE 2000).

Great care should be taken if IV contrast media are required for diagnostic purposes, see Chapter 9. Contrast-induced nephropathy (CIN) is defined as renal dysfunction following any investigative procedure where radi-opaque contrast media were used (Rudnick *et al.* 2006). Most episodes of CIN do not cause oliguria but result in a rise in serum creatinine ~2 days after the procedure, which usually returns to pre-procedure levels within a week. CIN occurs in 7–15% of patients and up to 50% in high risk groups such as people with diabetes, with a mortality rate of 14% (Rudnick *et al.* 2006).

Risk factors for CIN are:

- Pre-existing renal disease.
- Increasing age.
- Congestive heart failure.
- Hypotension.
- Using large volumes of contrast media.
- The type of contrast media used.
- Presence of anaemia.
- Diabetes.

In addition to diabetes *per se*, people with diabetes are likely to have greater than two other risk factors for CIN, which puts them in a very high-risk group. A rise in serum creatinine by 25% is an indicator of CIN but the inaccuracy of creatinine in various states has been outlined. Therefore, eGFR may be a better marker.

The Australian Adverse Drug Reactions Bulletin (2008) issued a warning about using gadolinium-containing contrast agents in people with renal impairment because of the risk of nephrogenic systemic fibrosis (NSF). The incidence of NSF may vary between the different gadolinium agents available. Renal function should be assessed in all patients before using gadolinium, especially if they are in a high-risk category and the risks and benefits of using gadolinium carefully considered.

Using as low a volume of contrast media as possible and ensuring the person is well hydrated are important preventative measures (Meschi *et al.* 2006). However, recent research suggests IV sodium bicarbonate administered seven hours before procedures involving radio contrast media reduces the incidence of CIN from 15% to 2% (Briguori 2007). Research is currently underway to determine whether oral sodium bicarbonate will be effective.

Renal function can decline in critically ill patients especially people with diabetes and is associated with high morbidity and mortality (Schetz *et al.* 2008). For example, hyperglycaemia and insulin resistance are common in critically ill patients with and without diabetes. Associations between interoperative hyperglycaemia during cardiac surgery, cardiac catherisation, total parenatal nutrition, and acute kidney injury have been noted. Intensive insulin therapy in these settings is renoprotective. The incidence of oligouria, and the need for renal replacement therapies (dialysis) is reduced (Schetz *et al.* 2008). The authors suggested as well as controlling hyperglycaemia insulin improves the lipid profile and reduces nitric oxide levels, which reduces oxidative damage.

Over 50% of patients on OHAs with significant renal disease require insulin therapy. Insulin requirements often decrease in people already on insulin because insulin, like many other drugs, is degraded and excreted by the kidney. Kidney damage can delay degradation and excretion of many drugs and prolong their half-life, increasing the risk of unwanted side effects and drug interactions. The dose, or dose interval, of drugs may need to be altered.

Renal disease and anaemia

Anaemia occurs as a consequence of chronic renal insufficiency. Renal anaemia occurs earlier in people with diabetes than in people without diabetes. It is more severe and is associated with other factors such as erythrocyte abnormalities and increased osmotic stress that are associated with decreased erythropoietin production (Bosman *et al.* 2001; Ritz 2001). As renal function declines the anaemia becomes more marked.

Anaemia is associated with fatigue, decreased quality of life, depression, left ventricular hypertrophy, decreased exercise capacity, malaise, and malnutrition. It is treated with recombinant human erythropoietin (rhEPO) in conjunction with intravenous iron.

Clinical observation

To date there has been little, if any, focus on monitoring haemoglobin as part of routine biochemical monitoring or diabetes complication screening in patients with renal impairment.

Diet and renal disease

Improving nutritional status can delay end-stage renal failure (Chan 2001). Nutritional needs are individual and depend on the stage and type of renal disease. The aim is to maintain homeostasis and electrolyte balance, decrease uraemic symptoms and regularly reassess dietary requirements to ensure changing needs are addressed (National Kidney Foundation 2002).

Protein and energy malnutrition are common and need to be corrected to prevent catabolism, lipid metabolism, and anaemia. Sodium restriction is often recommended, but salt substitutes should not be used because they are usually high in potassium and can increase the serum potassium, usually already elevated in renal disease. Water-soluble vitamin supplementation may be required when dialysis commences, for example, B group and vitamin C.

Anorexia is often a feature of renal disease and food smells can further reduce appetite and predispose the patient to malnutrition. Small frequent meals may be more appealing. Malnutrition has implications for the individual's immune status and phagocyte function and increases the risk of infection (Churchill 1996). Referral to a dietitian is essential.

Malnutrition is prevalent in haemodialysis patients and has a high mortality rate (Lopes *et al.* 2007). Lack of appetite is a significant predictor of malnutrition and is related to inflammation and may link protein-energy malnutrition in these patients. However, appetite varies and is often lower on haemodialysis days. This predisposes the person to hypoglycaemia in the short term and malnutrition in the long term. Lopes *et al.* (2007) suggested asking people with diabetes on haemodialysis about their appetite in the past four weeks or asking them to keep a food and appetite diary for 3–4 days is helpful. The Kidney Disease Quality of Life-Short Form (KDQOL-SF) (Hays *et al.* 1994) includes questions about appetite.

Depression, the presence of several coexisting comorbidites, cachexia, using oral medicines, being older and women on haemodialysis are particularly at risk of malnutrition. As anorexia increases markers of malnutrition decreases (serum albumin, creatinine, nPCR, and BMI) (Lopes *et al.* 2007).

Renal disease and older people

Older people with renal disease are at increased risk of adverse medicine events. A wide range of medicines are used in older people and some may need dose adjustments especially digoxin, ACE inhibitors, narcotics, antimicrobials, and OHAs (Howes 2001). Long-acting agents are contraindicated because of the risk of hypoglycaemia (see Chapter 6).

Medicine therapy needs to be closely monitored along with monitoring renal function and nutritional status and non-medicine alternatives used where possible.

Practice points

(1) Lower rates of creatinine are produced by older people and creatinine clearance rates can be misleading especially in people with low muscle mass.
(2) Renal disease is an important cause of medicine toxicity necessitating a hospital admission.

Kidney biopsy

See Chapter 9. Extra care is required for people with renal disease undergoing renal biopsy. A pressure dressing should be applied to the site and the patient should lie supine after the procedure for six hours. The blood pressures should be monitored and fluids encouraged to maintain urine output unless fluid is restricted. Activity should be reduced for two weeks.

Renal dialysis

Dialysis can be used in the management of diabetic kidney disease. Dialysis is a filtering process, which removes excess fluid and accumulated waste products from the blood. It may be required on a temporary basis or for extended periods of time. Some patients may eventually receive a kidney transplant.

Several forms of dialysis are in use as shown below.

Haemodialysis (artificial kidney)

Blood is pumped through an artificial membrane then returned to the circulation. Good venous access is required and special training in management. Haemodialysis is usually administered three times per week. A recent Canadian study suggests frequent nocturnal haemodialysis (six times per week) is associated with improved left ventricular mass, fewer antihypertensive agents, improved mineral metabolism and improvements in some aspects of quality of life (Culleton 2007).

Hypotension is common when haemodialysis therapy is first commenced. Management consists of:

- An appropriate haemodialysis prescription.
- Minimising interdialytic fluid gains by setting limits on fluid intake.
- Elevating the foot of the bed.
- Differentiating between disequilibrium syndrome and hypoglycaemia.
- Advising the patient to sit on the edge of the bed or chair to allow the blood pressure to stabilise before standing (Terrill 2002).
- Maintaining good glycaemic control. Significantly, >50% of people with diabetes on haemodialysis have HbA_{1c} >7%, especially those with long duration of diabetes, microvascular disease and on insulin (Lliescu 2007). These findings probably reflect advanced diabetes and may not be due to haemodialysis. However, given the amount of glucose in dialysate it is imperative that HbA_{1c} be as close to normal as possible without causing excess hypoglycaemia to reduce the risk of infection and other complications. Lliescu (2007) suggested it may not be possible to achieve good control with medicines and suggested insulin pumps might be a useful strategy. Significantly poor glycaemic control is linked to lower survival rates in patients on haemodialysis (Oomichi *et al.* 2006).

Strict aseptic technique and careful patient education are essential when managing dialysis therapies. Patients with CKD are susceptible to infections due to abnormal immune function, which is likely to be worse in people with diabetes and hyperglycaemia where neurophil function is abnormal and malignancies (Chaudhury & Luna-Salazar 2008).

Mucocutaneous barriers are often disrupted secondary to skin excoriation from pruritis, xerosi and sweat gland atrophy. Common bacterial infections include *Staphylococcus species, Escherichia coli, Klebsiella* and *Mycobacterium tuberculosis*. Viral infections are also common. Strict aseptic technique and careful patient education are essential when managing dialysis therapies.

Peritoneal dialysis

The filtering occurs across the peritoneum. This form of dialysis is an excellent method of treating kidney failure, in people with and without diabetes. The uraemia, hypertension, and blood glucose can be well controlled without increasing the risk of infection, if aseptic techniques are adhered to.

Continuous ambulatory peritoneal dialysis (CAPD)

CAPD is a form of peritoneal dialysis in which dialysate is continually present in the abdominal cavity. The fluid is drained and replaced 4–5 times each day or overnight if the patient is on automated peritoneal dialysis (APD). The patient can be managed at home, which has psychological advantages, once the care of equipment is understood and the patient is metabolically stable.

CAPD can also be used postoperatively to control uraemia related to acute tubular necrosis or early transplant rejection.

Insulin added to the dialysate bags achieves smoother blood glucose control because the insulin is delivered directly into the portal circulation and is absorbed in the dwell phase, which is closer to the way insulin is normally secreted after a glucose load.

The usual insulin dose may need to be increased because of glucose absorption from the dialysate fluid and to account for insulin binding to the plastic of the dialysate bags and tubing. The continuous supply of glucose and lactate in the dialysate fluid are calorie-rich energy sources and can lead to weight gain and hyperglycaemia. The art is to calculate insulin requirements to avoid hyperinsulinaemia, which carries its own complication risks. Glucose-free solutions such as Nutrimeal and glucose polymers may help reduce complications associated with high insulin and glucose levels (Rutecki & Whittier 1993). Insulin is usually administered subcutaneously if the person is on APD. Many renal dialysis units do not advocte adding insulin to dialysate bags due to the increased risk of infection.

Priorities of dialysis treatment

(1) Remove waste products and excess fluids from the blood (urea and creatinine).
(2) To provide adequate nutrition and safe serum electrolytes, and to prevent acidosis.
(3) Patient comfort.
(4) To prevent complications of treatment.
(5) To provide information and support to the patient.
(6) To ensure privacy.

Objectives of care

The individual's ability to carry out self-care tasks needs to be assessed early when considering renal replacement therapies. Changed joint structure due to oedema and tissue glycosylation (e.g. carpel tunnel syndrome) can limit the fine motor skills required to manage CAPD. Visual impairment due to retinopathy frequently accompanies renal disease and if present, can limit self-care abilities.

(1) To assess the patient carefully in relation to:
- knowledge of diabetes
- preventative healthcare practices
- ability to use aseptic technique
- usual diabetic control
- presence of other diabetic complications
- support available (family, relatives)
- motivation for self-care
- uraemic state.

(2) To ensure thorough instruction about administration of dialysate and intraperitoneal medication (insulin).

(3) To ensure a regular meal pattern with appropriate carbohydrate in relation to dialysate fluid.

(4) To maintain skin integrity by ensuring technique is aseptic especially in relation to catheter exit site and skin care.

(5) To monitor urea, creatinine, and electrolytes carefully.

(6) To provide psychological support.

(7) To encourage simple appropriate exercise.

(8) To ensure adequate dental care and regular dental assessments. Poor oral health causes chronic inflammation and is a site of infection. Untreated uraemia is associated with stomatitis and patients on dialysis are prone to gingivitis and peridontitis. Prophylactic antibiotics for dental procedure may be advisable (Choudhury & Luna-Salazar 2008).

(9) To prevent pain and discomfort, especially associated with the weight of the dialysate.

(10) To ensure the patient reports illness or high temperatures immediately.

(11) Monitor for infections and advise people to have preventative vaccines such as influenza and pneumococcal vaccination and an annual screen for Tuberculosis. Regular screening for nasal *staphylococcal* infections, certain types of malignancy may also be indicated, for example, renal cell carcinoma, prostate cancer, breast, and cervical cancer.

Nursing responsibilities

(1) Meticulous skin care.

(2) Inspect catheter exit site daily, report any redness, swelling, pain or discharge.

(3) Monitor fluid balance carefully:
- measure all drainage
- maintain progressive total of input and output
- report a positive balance of more than 1 litre – the aim generally is to achieve a negative balance to maintain the dry weight.

(4) Monitor blood glucose.

(5) Monitor temperature, pulse, and respiration, and report abnormalities.

(6) Monitor nutritional status – intake and biochemistry results.

(7) Weigh daily to monitor fluid intake and nutritional status.
(8) Ensure patency of tubes and monitor colour of outflow. Report if:
   • cloudy
   • faecal contamination
   • very little outflow (tube blocked).
(9) Report lethargy and malaise that can be due to uraemia or high blood glucose levels.
(10) Warm dialysate before the addition of prescribed drugs and before administration to decrease the possibility of abdominal cramps.
(11) Oral fluid intake may be restricted – provide mouth care and ice to suck.
(12) Assess self-care potential:
   • blood glucose testing
   • adding medication to bags
   • aseptic technique
   • psychological ability to cope.
(13) Protect the kidney during routine tests and procedures by avoiding dehydration and infection (Chapter 9).

Practice point

Overestimation of blood glucose levels can occur using some blood glucose meters and hypoglycaemia can be missed in patients using Icodextrin for dialysis. It is recommended that meters, which use glucose oxidase reagent strips be used in these patients (Oyibo *et al.* 2002).

Commencing CAPD in patients on insulin

Prior to commencing intraperitoneal insulin, most patients require a 24-hour blood glucose profile to assess the degree of glycaemia in order to calculate insulin requirements accurately. The glucose profile should be carried out following catheter implantation, with the patient stabilised on a CAPD regime.

Suggested method

(1) Obtain venous access for drawing blood samples.
(2) Obtain hourly blood glucose levels for 24 hours.
(3) At each bag exchange send:
   • 10 mL new dianeal fluid for glucose analysis
   • 10 mL drained dianeal fluid for glucose and insulin analysis to the appropriate laboratory.

Protocol for insulin administration in people with diabetes on CAPD based on four bag changes each day

(1) Calculate usual daily requirement of insulin and double it.
(2) Divide this amount between the four bags.

Note: The overnight bag should contain half of the daytime dose. Some centres add only 10% to the overnight bags.

Example

usual total insulin units	= 60 units
multiply this amount by 2	= 120 units
divide 120 units by 4 exchanges	= 30 units
3 daily exchanges	= 30 units/bag
overnight exchange	= 15 units/bag

Adjustments for the dextrose concentration of the dialysate may be necessary. Intraperitoneal insulin requirements are usually one-third higher than the amount needed before CAPD.

Note: Many renal units do not recommend adding insulin to dialysis bags.

Educating patient about CAPD

The patient should be instructed to:

(1) Not have a shower or bath for the first 5 days after the catheter is inserted.
(2) Always carefully wash hands prior to changing the bags.
(3) Wear loose fitting clothes over exit site.
(4) Examine feet daily for signs of bruising, blisters, cuts or swelling.
(5) Wear gloves when gardening or using caustic cleaners.
(6) Avoid hot water bottles and electric blankets because sensory neuropathy can diminish pain perception and result in burns.
(7) Avoid constrictive stockings or wearing new shoes for a long period of time.
(8) Wash cuts or scratches immediately with soap and water and apply a mild antiseptic (e.g., betadine ointment). Any wound that does not improve within 24–36 hours or shows signs of infection (redness, pain, tenderness) must be reported promptly.
(9) Bag exchanges should be carried out 4–6 hours apart. The person may be on APD having overnight exchanges.
(10) Only short-acting clear insulin must be used in bags.
(11) Adjust insulin doses according to diet, activity, and blood glucose levels and at the physician's discretion.
(12) Accurately monitor blood glucose 4-hourly. A blood glucose meter may be required.
(13) Provide written information.

Immediate help should be sought if any of the following occur:

- Decreased appetite.
- Bad breath/taste in mouth.
- Muscle cramps.
- Generalised itch.
- Nausea and vomiting, especially in the morning.
- Decreased urine output.
- Signs of urinary infection such as burning or scalding.

Renal disease and herbal medicine (see also Chapter 19)

People with end-stage renal failure often try complementary therapies to alleviate the unpleasant symptoms of their disease. Some therapies, for example, aromatherapy to reduce stress and maintain skin condition, or counselling for depression, are beneficial and usually safe. Herbal medicines are popular with the general public but they may not be appropriate for people with renal disease (Myhre 2000).

The kidneys play a key role in eliminating medicines and herbal products from the system. Some of these medicines and herbs can cause kidney damage that may be irreversible and put already compromised renal function at great risk. In addition, some herbal products, particularly those used in traditional Chinese medicine (TCM) are often contaminated with drugs, heavy metals and other potentially nephrotoxic products (Ko 1998). Frequently these contaminants are not recorded in the list of ingredients in the product. As well as the direct effect of the herbs on the kidney, the intended action of particular herbs can complicate conventional treatment.

An herb, *Taxus celebica*, used in TCM to treat diabetes, contains a potentially harmful flavonoid and has been associated with acute renal failure and other vascular and hepatic effects (Ernst 1998). Kidney damage can be present with few specific overt renal symptoms; therefore, it is vital that kidney and liver function is closely monitored in people taking herbs, especially if kidney function is already compromised by diabetes.

Practice points

(1) Nurses must know when their renal patients are taking herbal medicines so that their kidney function can be closely monitored. Patients should be asked about the use of complementary therapies periodically.

(2) Conventional medicines can also cause significant renal damage and dose adjustments may be needed or alternative medicines used, for example, NSAID, statins, OHA.

The potentially adverse renal effects are:

- electrolyte imbalances, for example, *Aloe barbedensis*
- fluid imbalances, for example, *Liquorice root*
- hypokalaemia, for example, *Aloe, Senna*
- kidney damage, for example, *Aristolochia*

In addition, herbal and conventional medicine interactions may occur, see Chapter 19.

PERIPHERAL AND AUTONOMIC NEUROPATHY

Many subgroups of neuropathy occur and these include mononeuropathy, peripheral, and autonomic neuropathy. The two most common forms are discussed here: peripheral and autonomic.

Peripheral

Key points

- Lower limb problems represent a significant physical, psychological, social, and economic burden for people with diabetes and the health system.
- Forty to seventy per cent of lower limb amputations occur in people with diabetes.
- Peripheral neuropathy, vascular disease, infection, foot deformity, and inappropriate footwear predispose people to foot disease.
- Screening for foot disease and preventative self-care practices is essential.
- Foot complications are common in the older people.
- A multidisciplinary team approach and good communication are essential to optimal management.

Introduction

Peripheral neuropathy is present in >20% of people with Type 1 diabetes after 20 years duration of diabetes and is already present at diagnosis in 10% of people with Type 2 at diagnosis and 50% by 20 years duration of diabetes. Peripheral neuropathy leads to inability to sense pressure and pain in the feet, dry skin, reduced joint mobility, bony deformity, and problems with balance, which increases the risk of falling. Common foot deformities associated with diabetes are claw toes, hammer toes, *hallus valgus, haalus rigidus* callus, flattened or high foot arches, Charcot's feet and amputation sites. These changes mean the normal cushioning that protects the feet during usual activities are deficient and the foot is at high risk of injury.

Foot ulcers occur in ~25% of people with diabetes: ~25% develop an infection, 20–60% of ulcers involve bone (osteomyelitis) and 34% present with a recurrent ulcer/year. Careful assessment, consideration of the causative factors, and managing the existing problems can limit further exacerbation of diabetic foot disease. Appropriate nursing care can prevent foot problems occurring as a result of hospitalisation or placement in an aged care facility.

Diabetic foot disease is a common cause of hospital admissions and is associated with long length of stay: 59% longer than for non-foot admissions, and significant morbidity and mortality. Significantly, foot ulcers also occur during hospital admissions. Diabetic foot disease is a heterogeneous disease entity, defined as a group of syndromes that lead to tissue breakdown. Infection, neuropathy, and ischaemia are usually present and increase the risk of infection (Apelqvist & Larsson 2000).

Foot disease and its management, have an adverse impact on the wellbeing and quality of life of people with diabetes (Brod 1998). The disease itself and some management practices, for example, non-weight-bearing regimes restrict physical activity and social interaction and often result in non-adherence.

Foot care is an extremely important aspect of the nursing care of people with diabetes in any setting. Significantly, preventative foot care is often neglected in acute care settings. The combination of mechanical factors and vascular and nerve damage as a complication of diabetes leads to an increased risk of ulceration, infection, and amputation. In older people, these factors increase the risk of falling. An estimated 40% of people with diabetes have peripheral neuropathy but it occurs in up to 50% of older people (Boulton 2005) and 20% of hospital admissions are for foot-related problems. Not surprisingly, peripheral neuropathy is associated with significantly impaired quality of life and effects on energy, pain, mobility, and sleep (Benbow *et al.* 1998).

Forty to seventy per cent of lower limb amputations occur in people with diabetes and most begin with an ulcer. The amputation rate can be reduced by preventative foot care. The spectrum of diabetic foot disease varies globally depending on socioeconomic circumstances, but the basic underlying pathophysiology is the same (Bakker 2000). Charcot's deformity is a severe form of diabetic foot disease that is often missed through misdiagnosis in the early stages and delay in appropriate management. The possibility of Charcot's deformity should be considered in any person with long-standing diabetes, neuropathy, and foot disease.

Foot disease and its management, have an adverse impact on the wellbeing and quality of life of people with diabetes (Brod 1998). The disease itself and some management practices, for example, non-weight-bearing regimes, restrict physical activity and social interaction and often result in non-compliance.

Foot care is an extremely important aspect of the nursing care of people with diabetes in any setting and is often neglected in acute care settings. The combination of mechanical factors and vascular and nerve damage as a complication of diabetes leads to an increased risk of ulceration, infection, and amputation.

It is estimated that 40% of people with diabetes have peripheral neuropathy but it occurs in up to 50% in older people (Boulton 2005) and 20% of hospital admissions are for foot-related problems.

Vascular changes

People with diabetes and peripheral vascular disease are predisposed to atherosclerosis, which is exacerbated by chronic hyperglycaemia, endothelial damage, nonenzymatic tissue glycosylation, and polyneuropathy. These conditions impair vascular remodelling.

(1) *Macrovascular* (major vessel) disease may lead to:
   • intermittent claudication and rest pain
   • poor circulation to the lower limbs which leads to malnutrition, tissue hypoxia, and delayed healing if any trauma occurs in this area. The injured tissue is prone to infection and gangrene can result.
(2) *Microvascular* (small vessel) disease leads to thickening of capillary basement membranes, poor blood supply to the skin and tissue hypoxia, predisposing the feet to infection and slow healing.

Infection

Foot infections are a common and serious problem in people with diabetes. They are prone to infections and non-healing wounds. Foot infection occurs as a result of skin ulceration or deep penetrating injuries, for example, standing on a drawing pin. These injuries can go unnoticed for days because the person does not feel pain if they have peripheral neuropathy. They act as a portal for infection that can involve tissues at all levels and foot structures including bone. The diagnosis of an infected wound is based on clinical signs. These include purulent discharge or two or more of erythemia, swelling, local heat, and pain. These signs may also indicate the presence of Charcot's foot rather than infection and alkaline phosphatase, ESR, X-ray, and/or MRI may be indicated (Wraight 2008), samples should also be collected to detemine what organisms are present in the wound. The samples need to be collected from deep within the wound after the wound has been debrided or biopsy samples from the base of the wound rather than superficial swabs.

Acute infections are usually due to aerobic Gram-positive cocci such as *Staphylococcus aureus* or β-*haemolytic streptococci* especially if the individual has limited exposure to antibiotics previously. Chronic ulcers and deep infections are often due to Gram-negative bacilli and anaerobic organisms such as *Escherichia coli, Klebsiella, Proteus, Bacteroides,* and *Peptostreptococcus* with *Staphylococcus aureus* is also likely to be present, sometimes as the only pathogen but usually in combination with other pathogens (Lipsky & Berendt 2000; Wraight 2008).

Charcot's foot is a relatively common, under diagnosed condition that complicates management of the neuropathic foot and can lead to significant pain, mobility deficits, and amputation (Piaggesi *et al.* 2005). Charcot's foot is due to the progressive destruction of the bones and joints in neuropathic diabetic feet secondary to inflammation following trauma, which is usually not recognised by the person with diabetes. Inflammation is followed by sclerosis, which leads to changes in the bony architecture of the foot and reduces the capacity to reduce subsequent everyday stress such as walking. Reactivation of the inflammatory process increases bone reabsorption and increases the risk of further trauma. Higher rates of foot fractures and Charcot's feet have been observed in patients following successful pancreas transplants and those on long-term corticosteroid therapy possibly because these medicines reduce bone resistance to minor trauma (Jeffcoate *et al.* 2000). Regular assessment of bone densitometry may be indicated in people on long-term corticosteroids.

Managing the diabetic foot requires a collaborative team approach and includes:

- Admission to hospital for a thorough foot and clinical assessment including self-care ability, bed rest, administration of broad-spectrum antibiotics, which needs to be continued after the acute phase resolves and surgical procedures if indicated.
- Broad-spectrum antibiotics are usually commenced initially until the results of the wound swabs are known and may be given IV for severe infections. Antibiotic therapy may be required for 1–2 weeks and up to 6 weeks if osteomyelitis is present. The risk of the person developing antibiotic resistance must be considered and every effort made help them to prevent recurrent foot infections. The parson should be asked whether they are allergic to penicillin before commencing antibiotic therapy. Flucloxacillin can be used for superficial infections and cellulitis if the person is not allergic to penicillin. Cephalexin can be used for minor infections and Clindamycin for severe infections. If the infection is deep, Augmentin or a combination of ciprofloxacin and Clindamycin may be indicated.
- X-ray (although the classical finding of osteomyelitis are not usually seen on plain X-ray until 10–21 days after the onset of bone infection), MRI bone scans to

determine whether osteomyelitis is present and determine the extent of the soft-tissue injury. If it is a long course of antibiotics and/or amputation is indicated. Alkaline phosphatase 135U/L, ESR >70 mm/hour and/or being able to feel bone when probing the base of the wound are suggestive of osteomyelitis.

- Bone densitometry or ultrasound may be indicated
- Surgical débridement to clean the wound and appropriate dressings. Referral to the wound care nurse and/or infectious disease team may be warranted.
- Revascularisation, for example, femoral/popliteal bypass, or amputation if indicated.
- Selection and application of appropriate wound dressings (Edmonds *et al.* 2000; Harding *et al.* 2000).
- Pressure off-loading to improve blood supply to the foot. Biomechanical measures such as total contact casts to relieve pressure in high-pressure ulcers and Charcot's foot deformity. Casts enable the person to remain mobile thus improving their social and psychological wellbeing. Infection and subsequent oedema must be managed because they aggravate the pressure on muscles and can lead to muscle necrosis. In hospital settings high specification foam mattresses make a significant difference in preventing neuropathic foot ulcers.
- Improving blood glucose control and diet to ensure optimal neutrophil functioning and nutrition to promote wound healing.
- Dietetic assessment.
- Counselling to stop smoking if relevant.
- Rehabilitation including regular podiatric assessment. Modification of foot wear and orthotics may be required.

Practice points

(1) Swabs need to be taken from deep in the ulcer cavity. This can be painful and analgesia may be required. Superficial swabs often do not identify all the organisms present, particularly anaerobes.
(2) Hyperglycaemia inhibits wound healing. Thus people undergoing amputations and other surgical procedures are at high risk of post-operative infections. Good metabolic control, optimal nutrition and aseptic technique reduce the risk.

Diabetic peripheral neuropathy

Diabetic neuropathy is defined as the presence of clinical or subclinical evidence of peripheral nerve damage, which cannot be attributed to any other disease process (Boulton *et al.* 1998). Neuropathy can affect the sensory nerves resulting in pain, tingling, pins and needles, or numbness. These symptoms are often worse at night. The sensory loss results in insensitivity to pain, cold, heat, touch, and vibration. The patient may not detect trauma, pressure areas, sores, blisters, cuts, and burns. Callous formation, ulceration and bone involvement can occur.

The motor nerves can also be affected, resulting in weakness, loss of muscle fibres and diminished reflexes. Both types of nerves can be affected at the same time. Medications may not be effective in the treatment of neuropathic pain, but some commonly used medicines prescribed to manage the discomfort are shown in Table 8.3.

Differentiating between the different types of nerve fibres involved allows a more targeted approach to pain management. Where unmyelinated c fibres are affected, characterised by burning, dysthetic pain, capsaicin or Clonidine may be effective. Where the alpha fibres are involved the pain is often deep and boring and insulin infusion, lignocaine or gabapentin may be effective (Vinik *et al.* 2000). Often both types of fibres are affected.

Medicines under study include α-Lipoic acid, an antioxidant that scavenges free radicals and has been shown to reduce pain when administered parenterally (Ziegler *et al.* 2004). Preliminary studies suggest the protein kinase C inhibitor (LY33531) improves allodynia, and prickling pain (Litchy *et al.* 2002). C-peptide has recently been shown to improve early neurological abnormalities in people with Type 1 diabetes with established clinical neuropathy (Brismar *et al.* 2007). It is given subcutaneously QID and appears to be most effective when baseline neuropathy is mild. Aldose reductase inhibitors have been under study for many years with various degrees of success. Recent research suggests Epalrestat improves objective and subjective measures of peripheral neuropathy and might slow the progression of retinopathy (Hotta 2006).

Other pain management strategies

Other non-medicine options with varying degrees of evidence to support their benefits include:

- Physiotherapy and exercise such as Tai Chi to maintain muscle tone and strength.
- Percutaneous nerve stimulation, static magnetic field therapy, low intensive laser therapy, bodyflow technology, and monochromatic infrared light. These techniques might improve peripheal circulation, and reduce local oedema, which reduces some of the local pressure and relieves local pain.
- Acupuncture, which has benefits up to six months (Abusaisha *et al.* 1998).

Other non-medicine measures include improving blood glucose control, stopping smoking, reducing alcohol intake, and eating a healthy diet.

The autonomic nervous system may also be affected by diabetes. Autonomic nervous system involvement may lead to an absence of sweating, which causes dry, cracked skin, and increases the risk of infection. Other effects of autonomic neuropathy include gastric stasis, erectile dysfunction, hypoglycaemic unawareness, and incontinence.

The small muscle wasting secondary to longstanding neuropathy can lead to abnormal foot shapes, for example, clawing of the toes, making the purchase of well fitting shoes difficult.

Vascular disease, neuropathy, and infection are more likely to develop if there is longstanding hyperglycaemia, which contributes to the accumulation of sorbitol through the polyol pathway, leading to damage to the nerves and small blood vessels. Figure 8.1 illustrates the interaction of factors leading to foot problems in people with diabetes.

Table 8.4 lists changes in feet due to the normal ageing process. These factors should all be incorporated in the nursing assessment to ensure that appropriate foot care is part of the overall management of the patient.

Table 8.3 Medicines used to manage diabetic peripheral neuropathy. Usually medicines are started at a low dose and titrated up to maximal doses over a few weeks depending on symptoms (Semla *et al.* 2002; Boulton 2005).

Medicine	Dose range and frequency	Side effects	Cautions and contraindications
Antidepressants **Tricyclic** Amitriptylline[a] Desipramine[b] Doxepin[a] Imipramine[a] Nortriptyline[b]	10–25 mg QID maximum dose 300 mg/day When ceasing these medicines the dose should be reduced slowly over 2–4 weeks to prevent withdrawal syndrome	Constipation, dry mouth, blurred vision, cognitive changes, tachycardia, urinary hesitation, sedation. Secondary amines have fewer effects. Older people are more likely to experience side effects and lower doses and slower titration is recommended.	**Caution:** angle-closure glaucoma, benign prostatic hyperplasia, urinary retention, constipation, cardiovascular disease, impaired liver function **Contraindications:** second- or third-degree heart block, arrhythmias, prolonged QT interval, severe liver disease, recent acute MI
Venlafaxine	75 mg	Nausea	
Anticonvulsants Carbamazepine	100 mg BD or QID maximum 1200 mg/day		**Caution:** liver function tests and full blood count before commencing and repeat 2-monthly for 2 months then annually **Contraindication:** bone marrow depression **Caution:** renal dysfunction
Gabapentin Approved for people over 18 years Lamotrigine	300 mg QID maximum 3600mg/day pain relief may only occur at higher doses 50 mg QID maximum 700 mg/day	Somnolence, dizziness, ataxia, fatigue, occasionally tremor, diplopia, nystagmus Ataxia, blurred vision, incoordination, diplopia Rarely Stevens–Johnson syndrome, angioedema	

Miscellaneous medicines Clonidine Oral or Weekly transdermal patch	0.1 mg maximum 2.4 mg/day Usually a last resort	Hypotension, dry mouth, dizziness, sedation, constipation, sexual dysfunction	**Cautions:** cardiac abnormalities, cardiac symptoms should be evaluated before commencing **Contraindicated:** second- or third-degree heart block
Mexiletine	200 mg 8 hourly maximum 1200 mg/day An IV 'lidocaine test' may be performed to predict the response to mexiletine (an oral congener of lidocaine). It targets superficial pain: allodynia, burning and tingling	Local skin irritation with patches Gastrointestinal symptoms, dizziness, tremor, irritability, nervousness and headache, seizures at high doses	
Topical agents Lidocaine patch Topical nitrate to the feet may relieve burning	5% maximum 4 patches/day		
Capsaicin	Depletes substance P and may be most effective for localised pain Wear gloves to apply Sustained relief for up to 6 months		
Opoid analgesics Recent trials support some efficacy and they may have a role as add on therapy Tramadol Controlled release oxycodone		Somnolence, nausea, constipation, dependence	

PN: peripheral neuropathy; QID: four times per day; BD: twice per day.
a Secondary amines.
b Tertiary amines.

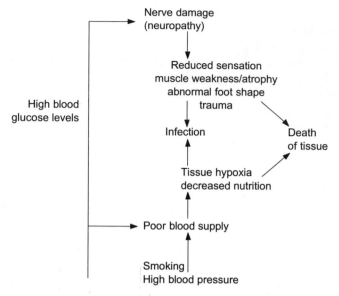

Figure 8.1 Diagrammatic representation of the factors leading to foot problems in people with diabetes.

Table 8.4 Changes in feet due to normal ageing.

(1)	Skin becomes thin, fragile
(2)	Nails thick and often deformed
(3)	Blood supply is reduced
(4)	Nerve function often impaired
(5)	Muscle weakness and wasting
(6)	Arthritis, may lead to pain and deformity

Stages of peripheral neuropathy

- Chronic and painful – improve metabolic control.
- Acute and painful – analgesia.
- Painless – education, orthoses, regular assessment.
- Late complications (Vinik *et al.* 2000).

Risk factors for the development of foot problems in people with diabetes

(1) Diabetes, especially if blood glucose is continually high.
(2) Smoking people with chronic neuropathic pain are twice as likely to smoke as those with chronic nociceptive pain but this might not represent a causative effect (Todd *et al.* 2008). Some studies suggest nicotine has a mild analgesic effect.

(3) Obesity.
(4) High blood pressure.
(5) Cardiovascular disease.
(6) Lack of or inadequate foot care, which is likely to be multifactorial including inability to reach the feet and lack of knowledge.
(7) Visual impairment.
(8) Inappropriate footwear.
(9) Delay in seeking help.
(10) Previous foot problems and amputation.
(11) Depression.

These factors should be part of the nursing assessment. The more risk factors present the greater the likelihood of amputation (Pecorara 1990). Routine assessment to detect neuropathy and associated foot changes should be part of regular health assessment in primary care.

Objectives of care

(1) To identify feet most at risk of trauma, ulceration and infection in aged care, rehabilitation, and hospital settings by assessing vascular, nerve, and diabetic status:
  - *Sensation* using 10 g Semmes–Weinstein monofilaments, 128 Hz tuning forks and disposable pin prickers (Apelqvist *et al.* 2000); recently, a new non-invasive test that can be undertaken by the person with diabetes was developed and is said to have 87% sensitivity and 66% specificity (Tentolouris 2008). The test, the indicator plaster neuropad (IPN) can be performed in 10 minutes and might be a useful screening tool to incorporate into the individual's foot self-care regimen.
  - *Presence of vascular insufficiency* by checking capillary return and the presence of foot and peripheral pulses; Doppler ultrasound, toe pressures, and transcutaneous oxygen measurement are used in some centres.
  - *Foot deformity.*
(2) To assess patient knowledge of foot care.
(3) To reinforce appropriate preventative foot care.
(4) To prevent trauma, infection, and pressure ulcers.
(5) To treat any problem detected.
(6) To refer to podiatry, orthotics, physiotherapy, rehabilitation, diabetes nurse specialist/diabetes educator or specialist foot clinic as necessary.
(7) To control or eliminate any factors which predispose the patient to the risk of foot problems in hospital.
(8) Risk of falls in the elderly (see Chapter 12).
(9) Pain management.

Nursing responsibilities

(1) Prevent neuropathic ulcers occurring in people with diabetes and peripheral neuropathy during a hospital admission.

(2) To assess the feet carefully on admission. Assess self-care potential (can the patient reach the feet, see clearly?). When assessing the feet, obtain information about:
   (a) Past medical history:
   - glycaemic control
   - previous foot-related problems/deformities
   - smoking habits
   - nerve and vascular related risk factors
   - claudication, rest pain
   - previous foot ulcer/amputation
   - alcohol intake.
   (b) Type of footwear (socks, shoes):
   - hygiene
   - activity level.
   (c) Social factors:
   - living alone
   - elderly.
(3) When examining the feet:
   Check both feet
   - check pulses, dorsalis pedis, posterior tibial
   - assess toenails: thick, layered, curved, ingrowing toenails will need attention
   - note foot structure; overlapping toes, prominent metatarsal heads on the sole of the foot
   - check for callus, cracks and fungal infections that can indicate inadequate foot care and poor hygiene.
(4) Note also:
   - pallor on elevation of leg
   - capillary return (normally 1–2 seconds)
   - any discoloration of legs
   - hair loss on the feet.
(5) To ensure appropriate foot hygiene:
   - wash in lukewarm water – use pH neutral soap products that do not dry the skin especially in elderly people or people on steroid medications and those with atopic skin
   - check water temperature with wrist before putting the patient into a bath
   - dry thoroughly, including between toes
   - apply cream to prevent dryness and cracks (urea cream, sorbelene).
(6) Ensure Elastoplast/Band Aids, bandages do *not* encircle toes as they can act like tourniquets and reduce the circulation, which could result in gangrene. Apply elastic support stockings correctly.
(7) Maintain a safe environment:
   - use a bed cradle
   - ensure shoes are worn if walking around the ward
   - strict bed rest may be necessary while the ulcer is healing
   - maintain aseptic technique.
(8) Check feet daily and report any changes or the development of any callus, abrasion or trauma.
(9) Monitor blood glucose control.
(10) Attend to dressings and administer antibiotics according to treatment order. Antibiotics are often given intravenously if foot infection is present.

(11) Take the opportunity to ensure self-care knowledge is current and that complication screening has been attended to. Ensure preventative foot care education is provided, to give the patient with diabetes:
- an understanding of effects of diabetes on the feet
- a knowledge of appropriate footwear
- the ability to identify foot risk factors
- an understanding of the principal effects of poor control (continual hyperglycaemia) on foot health
- knowledge about the services available for assistance with their diabetes care and how to obtain advice about foot care
- knowledge about appropriate foot care practices, in particular that they must inspect their feet daily and seek help early if any problems are found
- odour control can be an issue when infection and gangrene are present. Some wound dressings have an absorbent layer that eliminates odour by absorbing bacteria. Good foot hygiene helps reduce the odour.

Classification of foot ulcers

A number of ulcer classification systems are in existence and nurses are advised to follow the system in their place of employment. In 2002 an international working party was established to develop an international consensus foot ulcer classification system. Foot ulcers can be loosely classified as:

(1) Clean, superficial ulcer.
(2) Deeper ulcer, possibly infected, but no bone involvement.
(3) Deep ulcer, tracking infection and bone involvement.
(4) Localised gangrene and necrosis (usually forefoot, heel).
(5) Extensive gangrene of foot.

The depth and width of the ulcer should be recorded regularly; a plastic template, dated and filed in the patient's history, aids in the assessment of changes in ulcer size. The presence, amount, and type of exudate must be recorded.

Clinical observation

Aromatherapy essential oils on the *surface of the secondary dressing* can help reduce wound odour. They should not be applied directly to the wound. They can be used in a vapouriser for environmental fragrancing. Some essential oils can help improve mood.

Practice point

Painting the area with a betadine or other skin antiseptic is of little value. Coloured antiseptics can obscure some of the signs of infection.

Wound management

Dressings may be needed to absorb the exudate and protect the foot. No dressing is appropriate for all wound types. Surgical débridement, amputation or an occlusive dressing may be required. It is important to keep the temperature at 37°C, the dressing moist and the pH acidic to promote healing. Choose a dressing that does not cause tissue damage when it is removed, that is does not stick to the wound and protects the wound from infection. The moisture aids in pain relief, decreases the healing time and gives a better cosmetic result. An acidic environment promotes granulation tissue. The management of ulcers in hospital and other specific foot problems are listed in Table 8.5.

Diabetic foot ulcers heal slowly and bed rest is important. The patient may be otherwise well. Encourage independence with blood glucose testing and insulin administration. Refer for occupational therapy. The person may benefit from counselling if they are depressed.

Careful discharge planning is imperative:

- To ensure mobilisation and rehabilitation and that there is a safe environment at home.
- Interim placement in an extended care facility may be necessary.
- Assess the physical and social support available after discharge.

Practice point

Orthopaedic patients with diabetes and foot or leg plasters should be encouraged *not* to scratch under the plaster, especially if they have 'at risk' feet. Damage can occur and remain undetected until the plaster is removed.

Wound management techniques under study

Several new wound management products for hard-to-heal ulcers are under study:

- Platelet-derived growth factor applied topically to increase granulation;
- Hyaff;
- Dermagraft;
- Apilgraf;
- Granulocyte-colony stimulating factor (Edmonds *et al.* 2000).

Hyperbaric oxygen may be beneficial in some serious ulcers. Oxygen is necessary for wound healing and hyperbaric oxygen can increase tissue oxygen levels and improves the killing power of phagocytes (Bakker 2000).

Rehabilitation

Despite the best care, amputations are required in 5–15% of people with diabetes presenting with a foot problem particularly in the presence of gangrene, non-healing

Table 8.5 Management of specific foot problems while the person is in hospital or community settings.

Problem	Treatment
Burning, paraesthesia, aching	Assess neuropathic status Encourage person to walk Maintain euglycaemia Appropriate analgesia Manage depression if present.
Pain	Foot cradle, sheepskin analgesia
Dry skin, cracks	Clean, dry carefully, apply moisturiser, for example, urea cream, sorbelene A duromet can be used to evaluate skin hardness and identify areas of where plantar hyperkeratosis is likely to develop Plantar pressures, which can indicate force and workload
Claudication	Medications as ordered Rest Elevate feet cardiovascular assessment; peripheral pulses, ankle/brachial pressure index (APBI), transcutaneous oxygen tension (Tcp O_2) Angiography
Foot deformity	Clinically evaluate and describe Estimate joint mobility refer to podiatrist Physiotherapy Orthotist
Charcot's deformity	
Ulcers, infection	The presence of a lesion transform an at-risk foot into an acute clinical emergency. Grade the ulcer, for example, University of Texas Staging System for Diabetic foot ulcers. X-ray and MRI may be indicated to assess the depth. Record the width and depth, for example, using a polyurethane sheet. Refer to specific medical order Assess daily Make template to note change in size of ulcer Antibiotics Débridement, amputation

ABPI >0.9 normal; 0.9–0.5 indicates peripheral vascular disease is present; <0.5 indicates critical limb ischaemia. ABPI >1.3 usually indicates medial artery calcification (Monckerberg sclerosis), an indirect sign of autonomic neuropathy (Piaggesi *et al.* 2005).

TcpO$_2$ pressure <60 mmHg indicates local ischaemia; <40 mmHg indicates critical ischaemia (Piaggesi *et al.* 2005).

ulcers, which may be associated with osteomyelitis and severe foot infection. A rehabilitation process is necessary once the acute stage has settled. Below-knee amputations give a favourable result even if the popliteal pulses are diminished (Steinberg 1991). The goals of rehabilitation are:

- Appropriate stump care. In the early stages this may involve bandaging to reduce oedema. Circular bandages should be avoided because they tend to act like tourniquets and reduce the blood supply to the stump. Analgesia should be available. Later, correctly fitting the stump into the socket of the prothesis and regular inspection for the presence of infection or pressure areas.
- Prevent muscle contracture with regular physiotherapy.
- Help the person be as independent and active as possible.
- Ambulation with a prothesis or wheelchair depending on the individual assessment. However, not all people with diabetes benefit from having a prothesis, people who have advanced neurological disease such as stroke, Parkinson's disease, CCF, obstructive pulmonary disease, unstable angina, knee and hip contractures may not be suitable for a prothesis. These people often have limited ability to mobilise even before an amputation. High risk of gangrene or infection in the other limb may warrant delaying an amputation.
- Early mobilisation in whatever capacity is usually desirable after amputation to reduce postoperative complications. The person will need to learn how to manage whatever mobilisation method is appropriate.
- Care of the stump is important to prevent wound contractures.

Practice points

(1) Amputation should not always be seen as treatment failure. It can relieve pain, enable the person to return home and enjoy an improved quality of life. Amputation is distressing for the person with diabetes and their family and careful explanation, support, and counselling are essential. The patient should be included in the decision-making process and make the final decision. Their social and psychological situation should be considered as well as their physical needs.

(2) Amputation does increase the risk of a second amputation.

Autonomic neuropathy

Key points

- Often several organs are involved.
- Signs and symptoms are often non-specific.
- Autonomic neuropathy is often undiagnosed.
- Postural hypotension is the most significant sign of autonomic neuropathy.

- People with postural hypotension and nocturnal diarrhoea should be investigated for autonomic neuropathy.
- The progression to autonomic neuropathy is related to poor metabolic control.
- It is more common in people over 65 but it can occur in the first year after diagnosis.

Rationale

Autonomic neuropathy is a distressing condition for people with diabetes. It can cause erratic blood glucose readings. People are often accused of manipulating their food and/or diabetic medications, which causes stress and anxiety. The symptoms associated with the various manifestations of autonomic neuropathy can be uncomfortable, painful and have an adverse impact on the individual's quality of life.

Introduction

The autonomic nervous system plays an important role in the regulation of carbohydrate metabolism. Many processes are affected by it, for example, it both facilitates and inhibits insulin secretion.

(1) Stimulation of the right vagus nerve, which innervates the pancreatic islet cells, or the beta-adrenergic receptors in the islet cells, stimulates insulin secretion.
(2) Stimulation of the alpha-adrenergic receptors in the islet cells decreases insulin secretion.

This is an aspect of blood glucose regulation essential to maintaining glucose homeostasis.

The autonomic nervous system also has a role in the conversion of glycogen into glucose in the liver where free fatty acids undergo further metabolism to ketones. Neurogenic stimulation of the hypo-pituitary axis results in cortisol secretion, one of the counter-regulatory hormones that have a role in correcting hypoglycaemia. In stress situations, especially prolonged stress, hyperglycaemia results (Feinglos & Surwit 1988).

Diabetes is the commonest cause of autonomic neuropathy but it also occurs in association with other diseases such as advanced Parkinson's disease and Guillain–Barre syndrome.

Autonomic neuropathy is a common, under-diagnosed condition associated with a range of signs and symptoms, depending on the specific nerves and organs affected (Vinik *et al.* 2000; Aly & Weston 2002). It has a slow onset and affects up to 30–40% of people with diabetes, and although many people only have mild, often subclinical features, significant functional abnormalities can be present.

Rarely, in <5% of cases, overt clinical features develop. Autonomic neuropathy can involve any system, but commonly affects the heart, GIT, and genitourinary systems (Spallone & Menzinger 1997). The GIT is one of the most frequently affected systems but GIT problems, not associated with autonomic neuropathy, occur in 50% of the general population and are more common in people with diabetes (Lock *et al.* 2000). Older people are at risk of having many neuropathic GIT changes but some GIT changes are age-related or associated with the use of vasoconstrictive drugs (Aly & Weston 2002). Therefore many factors can be involved in an individual.

> ### *Practice points*
>
> (1) Autonomic neuropathy is physically uncomfortable and treatment options are limited. Where the GIT is involved, frequent adjustment to the food and medication regimen is often needed. Blood glucose monitoring is important to allow such changes to be made appropriately.
> (2) Psychological distress is common. Support and understanding are important aspects of management.

The commonly affected systems and associated clinical manifestations are shown in Table 8.6.

Diagnosis and management

Special tests are required to make a definitive diagnosis. The particular test depends on which organs are being tested, for example, gastric emptying times for the GIT, Valsalva manoeuvre for the cardiovascular system and voiding cystourethrogram to determine the effects on the bladder. In many cases specific treatment is commenced on the basis of the clinical history and assessment.

Management consists of:

(1) Adopting preventative strategies early by:
  • improving blood glucose control and lipid levels.
  • treating hypertension.
  • regular complication screening.
  • adequate self-care.
  • being aware that antioxidants may have a role in preventing oxidative tissue damage.
(2) Direction when present.

Treatment is often by trial and error and is aimed at alleviating the unpleasant symptoms. Preventative measures should be continued. Treatment for specific autonomic neuropathic conditions consists of:

(1) Gastrointestinal tract
  Small, light, frequent meals that are low in fat. Fat delays gastric emptying and exacerbates the already slow gastric emptying time.
  • Using gluten-free foods could help some people.
  • Medications such as Metoclopramide and Cisapride may give some relief but should not be used continuously.

Table 8.6 Organs commonly affected by diabetic autonomic neuropathy and the resultant clinical features.

Affected organ	Main clinical features	Consequences
Gastrointestinal tract (gastroparesis)	Decreased peristalsis Abdominal distension and feeling of fullness Early satiety Postprandial nausea Vomiting undigested food Diarrhoea, especially at night Depression	Weight loss Erratic blood glucose control Stomach may not be empty even after fasting, for example, for procedures
Urinary tract	Distended bladder Urine overflow Feeling of incomplete bladder emptying Stress incontinence Nocturia Vaginal mucous membrane excoriation in women	Silent urinary tract infection Falls in elderly people Sleep disturbance Uncomfortable sexual intercourse
Genitals	Erectile dysfunction in men. Indeterminate, if any effect in women Possibly vaginal dryness in older women	Psychological sequelae including depression Negative impact on sexual health
Cardiovascular system	Blood pressure: Postural hypotension Loss of diurnal variation Dizziness when standing Resting tachycardia Reduced sympathetic tone Decreased beta-adrenergic responsiveness	Silent myocardial infarction Stroke Falls
Lower limbs	Reduced sweating Reduced blood flow Reduced pain Redness Defective thermoregulation	Foot ulcers and infection Sleep disturbance
Brain	Cognitive impairment	Reduced self-care ability
General	Excessive sweating, especially of the upper body, resembling a hot flush and sometimes mistaken for hypoglycaemia Slow pupillary reaction Heat intolerance	Trauma Depression

Note: Many of these conditions predispose elderly people to falls (see Chapter 12).

- Antibiotics such as Tetracycline or Trimethoprim, may be required to treat bacterial overgrowth that occurs as a consequence of gastric stasis.
- Cholestyramine can be used to chelate bile salts, which immobilise the gut.
- Treating constipation, nausea, and vomiting as they occur.
- Elevating the head of the bed to use gravity to assist gastric emptying.
- Jejunostomy is a last resort.

(2) Cardiovascular system
- Support garments such as stockings or a body stocking to support venous return and relieve stress on the heart. They should be put on while the person is lying down.
- Managing postural hypotension – finding a balance between increasing the pressure on standing and preventing hypertension when lying. Fludrocortisone or Midodrine can be used. Medications should be reviewed to exclude drugs that precipitate postural hypotension.

(3) Genitourinary
- Urinary catheterisation and self-catheterisation. Sometimes parasympathomimetic drugs are also used.
- Managing erectile dysfunction with drugs such as Sildenafil, intracavernosal injections or mechanical and implanted devices and counselling (see Chapter 17).

(4) General measures
- Adjusting insulin or OHAs and diet to cater for the erratic blood glucose profile.
- Topical glycopyrrolate to alleviate gustatory sweating.
- Stopping smoking.
- Careful explanations about autonomic neuropathy and counselling to address the psychological consequences and treatment options.
- Encouraging activity.

Nursing care

Nursing care is palliative and supportive in nature. Providing a safe environment and reducing the risk of falls is essential, especially in older people, to prevent trauma, for example, fractures. This could involve ensuring the home environment is safe before discharging patients.

Nurses can have a role in the early identification of autonomic neuropathy by having a level of suspicion and taking a careful history.

Important nursing responsibilities are:

(1) The prevention, early recognition, and management of hypoglycaemia.
(2) Taking care when moving the patient from a lying to a sitting position, and from sitting to standing. Give them time for the blood pressure to adjust. Ensure their footwear will not contribute to the risk of falling.
(3) Providing adequate foot care and appropriate advice to minimise the risk of ulcers, including advice about footwear.
(4) Arranging counselling if indicated.
(5) Using aseptic technique.

(6) Being alert to the possibility of silent pathology – myocardial infarction, urinary tract infection.

(7) Encouraging people to remain physically active within their individual limits. Physical activity aids many body systems and improves mental outlook.

Clinical observation

Gentle abdominal massage and warm compresses can help alleviate the discomfort of gastroparesis. Aromatherapy essential oils can be added to the compress. The abdomen is a vulnerable part of the body and this needs to be taken into consideration when offering an abdominal massage (see Chapter 19).

References

Cardiovascular disease and diabetes

ACCORD Trial Study Group (2008) Intensive glucose control group of ACCORD Trial halted for excess deaths. National Heart, Lung and Blood Institute. February 2008 reported in *US Today*.

Alamowitch, S., Eliasziw, M. & Barnett, H. (2005) The risk and benefit of endarterectomy in women with symptomatic internal carotid artery disease. *Stroke*, **36**, 27–31.

Australian Institute Health and Welfare (AIHW) (2007) *Medicines for Cardiovascular Health*. AIHW Cardiovascular Series No. 27. AIHW, Canberra.

Australian Medicines Handbook (2006). Australian Medicines Handbook PTY Ltd, Adelaide.

Barenholtz, H. & Kohlhaas, H. (2006) Considerations for supplementing with coenzyme Q_{10} during satin therapy. *Annals of Pharmacotherapy*, **40**, 290–294.

Boden-Albala, B. (2008) Ddaytime sleepiness is an independent risk factor for stroke. *Proceedings American Stroke Association International Stroke Conference*. Abstract '94. New Orleans.

Bohm, M. (2008) Treating to protect: current cardiovascular treatment approaches and remaining needs. *Medscape Journal Medicine*, **10** (Suppl. 3), 1–13.

Brownlee, M. (2000) Mechanisms of Hyperglycaemic damage in diabetes. Chapter 10. In: Kahn R (ed) *Atlas of Diabetes* (R. Kahn, ed.). Science Press, London.

Bruckert, E. & Hansel, B. (2007) HDL-c is a powerful lipid predictor of cardiovascular disease. *International Journal of Clinical Practice*, **61** (11), 1905–1913.

Bunker, S., Colquhoun, D., Esler, M., Hichie, I., Hunt, D., Jeleniek, M. & Oldenburg, B. (2003) 'Stress' and coronary heart disease: psychosocial risk factors. *Medical Journal of Australia*, **178**, 271–276.

Chen, Z. (2008) High BMI linked with streoke mortality in obese, overweight men. *Stroke Online* January 31. http://www.medscape.com/viewarticle/569864?src=mp (accessed February 2008).

Donahoe, S., Stewart G., McCabe C., Mohanavelu S., Murphy S., Cannon C., Antman E (2007) Diabetes mortality following acute coronary syndromes. *Journal American Medical Association*, **298** (7), 765–775.

Du, X., Edelstein, D. & Rossetti, L. (2000) Hyperglycaemia induced mitochondrial superoxide overproduction activates the hexosamine pathway and induces plasminogen activator inhibitor-1 expression by increasing Sp1 glycosylation. *Proceedings National Academy of Science USA*, **97**, 1222–1226.

Elias, P., Elias, M., D'Agostino, R., Cupples, L., Wilson, P., Silbershatz, H. & Wolf, P. (1997) NIDDM and blood pressure as risk factors for poor cognitive performance. The Framingham Study. *Diabetes Care*, **20** (9), 138–139.

European Society of Hypertension (2007) Guidelines on treatment of hypertension. *Journal of Hypertension*, **25**, 1105–1187.

Forbes, J. & Cooper, M. (2007) The role of mitochondrial dysfunction in diabetic complications. *International Diabetes Monitor*, **19** (6), 9–15.

Gujadhur, A., Dunning, T. & Alford, F. (2003) Metabolic and cardiac outcomes after acute myocardial infarction. *Journal of Diabetes Nursing*, 7 (6), 208–212.

Haussler, B., Fischer, G., Meyer, S. & Sturm, D. (2007) Risk assessment in diabetes management: how do general proaactitioners estimate risks due to diabetes? *Quality and Safety in Health Care*, **16**, 208–212.

Hotta, N., Toyota, T. & Matsouka, K. (2001) Clinical efficacy of fidarestat, a novel aldose reductase inhibitor, for diabetic peripheral neuropathy: a 52-week multicenter placebo-controlled double blind parallel group study. *Diabetes Care*, **24**, 1176–1182.

Kaiser, N., Sasson, S. & Feener, E. (1993) Differential regulation of glucose transports by glucose in vascular endothelial and smooth muscle cells. *Diabetes*, **42**, 80–89.

Leite-Moreira, A. & Castro-Chaves, P. (2008) Heart failure: statins for all? *British Medical Journal*, www.heartjnl.com (accessed February 2008).

Lesperance, F. & Frasure-Smith, N. (2007) Depression and heart disease. *Cleveland Clinic Journal of Medicine*, **74** (Suppl. 1), S63–S66.

Lim, W., Holinski, H., Devereaux, P., Tkaczyk, A., McDonald, E., Clarke, F., Qushmaq, I., Terrenato, I., Schunemann, H., Crowther, M. & Cook, D. (2008) Detecting myocardial infarction in critical illness using screening troponin measurements and ECG recordings. *Critical Care*, **12**, R36doi:10.1186/cc6815.

Lutesp, H. (2008) Stroke treatment and prevention are not the same in men and women. *Medscape Medical Journal*, **10** (2), 26–27.

Mose, D. (2007) 'The rust of life:' impact of anxiety on cardiac patients. *American Journal of Critical Care*, **16** (4), 361–369.

Mozaffarian, D. (2007) Acute myocardial infarction: a prediabetes risk equivalent? *The Lancet*, **25**, 667–675.

National Institute of Clinical Studies (NICS) (2005) *Evidence-Practice Gaps Report*, Vol. 2. NICS, Melbourne.

Nishikawa, T., Edelstein, D. & Du, X. (2000) Normalising superoxide production blocks three pathways of hyperglycaemic damage. *Nature*, **404**, 787–790.

Pfisterer, M. (2004) In elderly patients with chronic angina, drugs offer outcomes equal to invasive treatment. *Circulation on line* http://www.medscape.com/viewarticle/488214 (accessed August 2007).

Pittler, M., Guo, R. & Ernst, E. (2008) Hawthorn extract for treating chronic heart failure. *Cochrane Database of Systematic Reviews*, Issue 1, Art No. CD005312 DOI: 10. 1002/14651858.CD005312.pub2.

Player, M., King, D., Mainous, A. & Geesey, M. (2007) Psychosocial factors and progression from prehypertension to hypertension or coronary heart disease. *Annals of Family Medicine*, 5 (5), 403–411.

Reddy, P. (2008) Diabetes and depression. Practical tools for the diabetes educator. Sanofi-Aventis diabetes partnership seminar 12 April 2008. Novotel, Melbourne.

Ridker, P., Cook, N. & Lee, I. (2005) A randomized trial of low dose aspirin in the primary prevention of cardiovascular disease in women. *New England Journal of Medicine*, **352**, 1293–1304.

Rosenfeldt, F., Haas, S. & Krum, H. (2007) Coenzyme Q_{10} in the treatment of hypertension: a meta-analysis of the clinical trials. *Journal of Human Hypertension*, **21**, 297–306.

Sanchis, J. (2007) Risk score useful in assessing chest pain with normal troponin levels. *American Journal of Cardiology*, **99**, 797–801.

United Kingdom Prospective Study (UKPDS) Group (1998) Effect of intensive blood glucose control with metformin on complications in overweight patients with type 2 diabetes. *Lancet*, **352**, 854–865.

Vale, M., Jelinek, M., Best, J. *et al.* (2003) Coaching patients on achieving cardiovascular health (COACH): a multicenter randomized trial in patients with coronary heart disease. *Archives Internal Medicine*, **163**, 2775–2783.

Wells-Knecht, K., Zyzak, D. & Litchfield, J. (1995) Mechanism of autoxidative glycosylation: identification of glyoxal and arabinose as intermediates in the autooxidative modification of proteins by glucose. *Biochemistry*, **34**, 3702–3709.

Williams, J., Chimowitz, M., Cotsonis, G., Lunn, M. & Waddy, S. (2007) WASID Investigators. Gender differences in outcomes among patients with symptomatic intracranial arterial stenosis. *Stroke*, **38**, 2055–2062.

Young, D., Furler, J., Vale, M., Walker, W., Segal, L., Best, J., Dunning, T., Blackberry, I., Audehm, R., Dunbar, J. & Chondros, P. (2007) Patient engagement and coaching for health: the PEACH study – a cluster randomised controlled trial using the telephone to coach people with type 2 diabetes to engage with their GPs to improve diabetes care. *BMC Family Practice*, **8** (20), 8–13.

Zannad, F. (2008) cardiovascular high risk patients – treat to protect, but whom? *Medscape Journal of Medicine*, **10** (Suppl. 2), 1–11.

Diabetes and eye disease

Antonetti, D., Barber, A., Bronson, S., Freeman, W., Gardner, T., Kester, L., Kimball, S., Krady, K. *et al.* (2006) Diabetic retinopathy: seeing beyond glucose-induced microvascular disease. *Diabetes*, **55** (9), 401–411.

Chiu, C., Hubbard, L. & Armstrong, J. (2006) Dietary glycaemic index and carbohydrate in relation to early age-related macular degeneration. *American Journal of Nutrition*, **63**, 880–886.

Clemons, T., Milton, R., Klein, R., Seddon, J. & Ferris, F. (2005) Age-Related Eye Disease Study Research group. Risk factors for the incidence of advance age-related macular degeneration in the Age-Related Eye Disease Study (AREDS). AREDS report no. 19. *Ophthalmology*, **112**, 533–539.

Khan, J., Shahid, H. & Thurlby, D. (2006) Age-related macular degeneration and sun exposure, iris colour, and skin sensitivity to sunlight. *British Journal Ophthalmology*, **90**, 29–32.

Lim, J. (2006) Risk factors for age-related macular degeneration. *eMedicine*. http://www.medscape.com/viewarticle/532642 1–5 (accessed November 2007)

Ryan, C., Geckle, M. & Orchard, T. (2003) Cognitive efficiency declines over time in adults with Type 1 diabetes: effect of micro- and macrovascular complications. *Diabetologia*, DOI: 10.1007/soo125–003-1128–2, 940–948.

Seddon, J., Gensler, G., Milton, R., Klein, M. & Rifai, N. (2004) Association between C-reactive protein and age-related macular degeneration. *Journal American Medical Association*, **292**, 704–710.

Van Leeuwen, R., Boekhoorn, S. & Vingerling, J. (2005) Dietary intake of antioxidants and risk of age-related macular degeneration. *Journal American Medical Association*, **294**, 3101–3107.

Diabetes and renal disease

ANZDATA Registry (2000) *Australian and New Zealand Dialysis Transplant Registry*. Adelaide, South Australia.

Bosman, D., Winkler, A., Marsden, J., MacDougall, I. & Watkins, P. (2001) Anemia with erythropoietin deficiency occurs early in diabetic nephropathy. *Diabetes Care*, **24** (3), 495–499.

Briguori, C. (2007) Renal insufficiency following contrast media administration trial (REMEDIAL); a randomized comparison of 3 preventative strategies. *Circulation*, **115**, 1211–1217.

Cass, A., Cunningham, J., Arnold, P., Snelling, P., Wang, Z. & Hoy, W. (2002) Delayed referral to a nephrologist: outcomes among patients who survive at least one year. *Medical Journal of Australia*, **177** (3), 135–138.

Chadban, S. & Lerino, F. (2005) Welcome to the era of CKD and the eGFR. *Medical Journal of Australia*, **183** (3), 117–118.

Chan, M. (2001) Nutritional management in progressive renal failure. *Current Therapeutics*, **42** (7), 23–27.

Choudhury, D. & Luna-Salazar, C. (2008) Preventive health care in chronic kidney disease and end stage renal failure. *Clinical Practice Nephrology*, **4** (4), 3–16.

Churchill, D. (1996) Results and limitations of peritoneal dialysis. In: *Replacement of Renal Function by Dialysis* (eds C. Jacobs, C. Kjellstrand, K. Koch & F. Winchester). Kluwer Academic Publishers, Boston.

Culleton, B. (2007) Frequent nocturnal hemodialysis may have better outcomes than conventional hemodialysis. *Journal American Medical Association*, **298**, 1291–1299.

DCCT (Diabetes Control and Complications Trial Research Group) (1993) Effects of intensive insulin therapy on the development and progression of long-term complications in IDDM. *New England Journal of Medicine*, **329**, 977–986.

Department of Health (2001) *Diabetes National Service Framework: Standards for Diabetes Services*. Department of Health, London.

Duncan, H., Pittman, S., Govil, A., Sorn, L., Bissler, G., Schultz, T., Kant, S. & Roy-Chaudhury, P. (2007) Alternative medicine use in dialysis patients: potential for good and bad. *Nephrology and Clinical Practice*, **105** (3), 108–113.

Ernst, E. (1998) Harmless herbs? A review of the recent literature. *American Journal of Medicine*, **104** (2), 170–178.

Giannelli, S., Patel, K., Windham, G., Ferrucci, F., Guralnik, J. (2007) Magnitude of under-ascertainment of impaired kidney function in old: normal serum creatine. *Journal American Geriatric Society*, **55** (6), 816–823.

Gilbert, R. & Kelly, D. (2001) Nephropathy in Type 2 diabetes: current therapeutic strategies. *Current Therapeutics*, **6**, 266–269.

Gilbert, R., Akdeniz, A. & Jerums, G. (1992) Semi-quantitative determination of microalbuminuria by urinary dipstick. *Australian New Zealand Journal Medicine*, **22**, 334–337.

Gilbert, R., Akdeniz, A. & Jerums, G. (1997) Detection of microalbuminuria in diabetic patients by urinary dipstick. *Diabetes Research in Clinical Practice*, **35**, 57–60.

Gilbert, R., Tsalamandris, C., Allen, T., Colville, D. & Jerums, G. (1998) Early nephropathy predicts vision-threatening retinal disease in patients with Type I diabetes mellitus. *Journal of the American Society of Nephrology*, **9**, 85–89.

Hays, R., Kallich, J., Mapes, D., Coons, S. & Carter, W. (1994) Development of the kidney disease quality of life instrument (KDQOL-SF). *Quality of Life Research*, **3**, 329–338.

HOPE (Heart Outcomes Prevention Evaluation Study Investigators) (2000) Effects of ramipril on cardiovascular and microvascular outcomes in people with diabetes mellitus: results of the HOPE study and MICRO-HOPE substudy. *Lancet*, **355**, 253–259.

Howes, L. (2001) Dosage alterations in the elderly: importance of mild renal impairment. *Current Therapeutics*, **42** (7), 33–35.

Iliescu (2006) Glycaemic control often poor among hemodialysis patients. *Diabetes Care*, **29**, 2247–2251.

Keane, W. (2001) Metabolic pathogenesis of cardiorenal disease. *American Journal of Kidney Disease*, **38** (6), 1372–1375.

Ko, R. (1998) Adulterants in Asian patent medicines. *New England Journal of Medicine*, **339**, 847.

Lopes, A., Elder, S., Ginsberg, N., Andreucci, V., Cruz, J., Fukuhara, S., Mapes, D., Saito, A., Pisoni, R., Saran, R. & Port, F. (2007) Lack of appetite in haemodialysis patients_associations with patient characteristics, indicators of nutritional status and outcomes in the international DOPPS. *Nephrology Dialysis Transplant*, **22** (12), 3538–3546.

Meschi, M., Detrenis, S., Musini, S., Strada, E. & Savazzi, G. (2006) Facts and fallacies concerning the prevention of contrast medium-induced nephropathy. *Critical Care Medicine*, **34** (8), 2060–2068.

Myhre, M. (2000) Herbal remedies, nephropathies and renal disease. *Nephrology Nursing Journal*, **27** (5), 473–480.

National Kidney Foundation (2002) Clinical Practice Guidelines for Nutrition in Chronic Renal Failure. Kidney Outcome Quality Initiative, *American Journal of Kidney Disease*, **35** (6), Supp. 2.

Oomichi, T., Emoto, M., Tabata, E., Morioka, T., Tsujimoto, Y., Tahara, H., Shoji, T. & Nishizawa, Y. (2007) Impact of glycemic control on survival of diabetic patients on chronic regular hemodialysis: a 7-year observational study. *Diabetes Care*, **29**, 1496–1500.

Oyibo, S., Prichard, G., Mclay, L. *et al.* (2002) Blood glucose overestimation in diabetic patients on continuous ambulatory peritoneal dialysis for end-stage renal disease. *Diabetic Medicine*, **19**, 693–696.

Quellhorst, E. (2002) Insulin therapy during peritoneal dialysis: pros and cons of various forms of administration. *Journal American Society Nephrology*, **13**, S92–S96.

Ravid, M., Savin, H. & Jutrin, I. (1993) Long-term stabilising effect of angiotensin-converting enzyme on plasma creatinine and on proteinuria in normotensive Type II diabetic patients. *Annals of Internal Medicine*, **118**, 577–581.

Ritz, E. (2001) Advances in nephrology: success and lessons learnt from diabetes. *Nephrology Dialysis Transplant*, **16** (Suppl. 7), 46–50.

Rudnick, M., Kesselheim, A. & Goldfarb, S. (2006) Contrast-induced nephropathy: how it develops, how to prevent it. *Cleveland Clinic Journal of Medicine*, **73** (1), 75–87.

Rutecki, G. & Whittier, F. (1993) Intraperitoneal insulin in diabetic patients on peritoneal dialysis. In: *Dialysis Therapy* (eds A. Nissenson & R. Fine). Hanley & Belfus, Philadelphia.

Schetz, M., Vanhorebeck, I., Wouters, P., Wilmer, A. & Van der berghe, G. (2008) Tight blood glucose control is renoprotective in critically ill patients. *Journal American Society of Nephrology*, DOI:10.1681/asn2006101091.

Terrill, B. (2002) *Renal Nursing: A Practical Approach*. Ausmed Publications, Melbourne.

Wu, M., Yu, C. & Yang, C. (1997) Poor pre-dialysis glycaemic control is a predictor of mortality in Type II diabetic patients on maintenance haemodialysis. *Nephrology Dialysis Transplant*, **12**, 2105–2110.

Peripheral and autonomic neuropathy

Abusaisha, B., Constanzi, J. & Boulton, A. (1998) Acupuncture for treatment of chronic painful diabetic neuropathy: a long-term study. *Diabetes Research Clinical Practice*, **39**, 115–121.

Aly, N. & Weston, P. (2002) Autonomic neuropathy in older people with diabetes. *Journal of Diabetes Nursing*, **6** (1), 10–14.

Apelqvist, J. & Larsson, J. (2000) What is the most effective way to reduce incidence of amputation in the diabetic foot? *Diabetes/Metabolism Research and Reviews*, **16** (Suppl. 1), s75–s83.

Apelqvist, J., Bakker, K., Van Houtum, W., Nabuurs-Franssen, M. & Schaper, N. (2000) The international consensus and practical guidelines on the management and prevention of the diabetic foot. *Diabetes/Metabolism Research and Reviews*, **16** (Suppl. 1), s84–s92.

Bakker, D. (2000) Hyperbaric oxygen therapy and the diabetic foot. *Diabetes/Metabolism Research and Reviews*, **16** (Suppl. 1), s55–s58.

Boulton, A., Gries, F. & Jervell, J. (1998) Guidelines for the diagnosis and outpatient management of diabetic peripheral neuropathy. *Diabetes Medicine*, **15**, 508–514.

Boulton, A. & Jervell, J. (1998) International guidelines for the management of diabetic peripheral neuropathy. *Diabetic Medicine*, **15** (6), 508–514.

Boulton, A. (2000) The diabetic foot: a global view. *Diabetes/Metabolism Research and Reviews*, **16** (Suppl. 1), s2–s5.

Brod, M. (1998) Quality of life issues in patients with diabetes and lower limb extremity ulcers: patients and caregivers. *Quality Life Research*, 7, 365–372.

DCCT (1993) The effect of intensive treatment of diabetes on the development and progression of long-term complications in insulin-dependent diabetes mellitus. *New England Journal of Medicine*, **329**, 977–986.

DRS (1981) Photocoagulation treatment of proliferative diabetic retinopathy: clinical implications of DRS findings. DRS Report No. 8. *Ophthalmology*, **88**, 583–600.

Edmonds, M., Bates, M., Doxford, M., Gough, A. & Foster, A. (2000) New treatments in ulcer healing and wound infection. *Diabetes/Metabolism Research and Reviews*, **16** (Suppl. 1), s51–s54.

EDTRS (1991) Early photocoagulation for diabetic retinopathy: EDTRS Report No. 9. *Ophthalmology*, **98** (Suppl.), 767–785.

Foster, A., Eaton, C., McConville, D. & Edmonds, M. (1994) Application of Op-cite film: a new effective treatment for painful diabetic neuropathy. *Diabetic Medicine*, **11**, 768–772.

Harding, K., Jones, V. & Price, P. (2000) Topical treatment: which dressing to choose. *Diabetes/Metabolism Research and Reviews*, **16** (Suppl. 1), s47–s50.

Hemstreet, B. & Lapointe, M. (2001) Evidence for the use of gabapentin in the treatment of diabetic peripheral neuropathy. *Clinical Therapeutics*, **23** (4), 520–531.

Hotta, N. (2006) Epalrestat may delay progression and reduce symptoms of diabetic neuropathy. *Diabetes Care*, **29**, 1538–1544.

Huang, E., Meigs, J. & Singer, D. (2001) The effect of interventions to prevent cardiovascular disease in patients with Type 2 diabetes. *American Medical Journal*, **11** (8), 663–642.

International Diabetes Federation Consultative Section on Diabetes (2000) Position Statement *Diabetes Education for People who are Blind or Visually Impaired*. International Diabetes Federation, Brussels, pp. 62–72.

Karlson, B., Herlitz, J. & Hjalmarson, A. (1993) Prognosis of acute myocardial infarction in diabetic and non-diabetic patients. *Diabetic Medicine*, **10**, 449–454.

Larkins, R. (1995) Aspirin: the effects are complex. *Diabetic Communication*, **10** (3), 5–6.

Lipsky, B. & Berendt, A. (2000) Principles and practice of antibiotic therapy of diabetic foot infections. *Diabetes/Metabolism Research and Reviews*, **16** (Suppl. 1), s42–s46.

Litchy, W., Dyck, P., Tesfaye, S. for the MBBQ Study Group (2002) Diabetic peripheral neuropathy (DPN) assesses by neurological examination and composite scores is improved with LY333531 treatment. *Diabetes*, **45**, A197.

Locke, D., Ill, G. & Camileri, M. (2000) Gastrointestinal symptoms among persons with diabetes in the community. *Archives of Internal Medicine*, **160**, 2808–2816.

Lowe, J. (2002) Hypertension in diabetes. *Australian Prescriber*, **25** (1), 8–10.

Malmberg, K., Ryden, L., Efendic, S., Herlitz, J., Nicol, P. & Waldenstrom, A. (1995) Randomised trial of insulin–glucose infusion followed by subcutaneous insulin treatment in diabetic patients with acute myocardial infarction (DIGAMI study) effects on mortality at 1 year. *Journal of the American College of Cardiology*, **26**, 57–65.

Pecorara, R. (1990) Pathways to diabetic limb amputation. *Diabetes Care*, **13** (5), 513–530.

Ponchilla, S., Richardson, K. & Turner-Barry, M. (1990) The effectiveness of six insulin measurement devices for blind persons. *Journal of Visual Impairment and Blindness*, **84**, 364–370.

Semia, T., Beizer, J. & Higbee, M. (2002) (eds.) *Geriatric Dosage Handbook*. Hudson, Ohio.

Spallone, V. & Menzinger, G. (1997) Autonomic neuropathy: clinical and instrumental findings. *Clinical Neuroscience*, **4** (96), 346–358.

Standl, E. & Schnell, O. (2000) A new look at the heart in diabetes: from ailing to failing. *Diabetalogia*, **43**, 1455–1469.

Steinberg, F. (1991) Rehabilitation after amputation. *Diabetes Spectrum*, **4** (1), 5–9.

Surwit, R. & Feinglos, M. (1988) Stress and autonomic nervous system in Type 2 diabetes. A hypothesis. *Diabetes Care*, **11**, 83–85.

Sutton, M., McGrath, C., Brady, L. & Wood, J. (2000) Diabetic foot care: assessing the impact of foot care on the whole patient. *Practical Diabetes International*, **17** (5), 365–372.

UKPDS Group (1998) Intensive blood glucose control with sulphonylureas or insulin compared with conventional treatment and risk of complications in patients with Type 2 diabetes (UKPDS 33). *Lancet*, **352**, 837–853.

Vale, M., Jelinek, M., Best, J. & Santamaria, J. (2002) Coaching patients with coronary heart disease to achieve cholesterol targets: a method to bridge the gap between evidence-based medicine and the 'real world' – randomized controlled trial. *Journal of Clinical Epidemiology*, **55**, 245–252.

Vinik, A., Park, T., Stansberry, K. & Henger, P. (2000) Diabetic neuropathy. *Diabetologia*, **43**, 957–973.

Zhang, W., Kamiya, H. & Ekberg, K. (2007) C-peptide improves neuropathy in Type 1 diabetic BB/Wor-rats. *Diabetes Metabolism Reviews*, **12**, 1471–1488.

Ziegler, D., Nowak, H., Kempler, P., Vargha, P. & Low, P. (2004) Treatment of symptomatic diabetic neuropathy with antioxidant alpha-lipoicacid: a meta-analysis. *Diabetic Medicine*, **21**, 114–121.

Chapter 9
Management During Surgical and Investigative Procedures

Key points

- Surgery induces the counter-regulatory response that can increase the blood glucose to 6–8 times normal. Optimal control before, during, and after surgery reduces morbidity and mortality.
- Morning procedures are desirable.
- Insulin should never be omitted in people with Type 1 diabetes.
- Complications should be stabilised before, during, and after surgery.
- Cease oral agents 24–36 hours before the procedure depending on their duration of action (some experts recommend continuing oral agents until surgery).
- Ascertain whether the person is taking any complementary therapies especially herbal medicines.

Rationale

Diabetes is associated with an increased need for surgical procedures and invasive investigations and higher morbidity than non-diabetics. Anaesthesia and surgery are associated with a complex metabolic and neuroendocrine response that involves the release of counter-regulatory hormones and glucagon leading to insulin resistance, gluconeogenesis, hyperglycaemia and neutrophil dysfunction, which impairs wound healing. This response also occurs in people without diabetes but is more pronounced and difficult to manage in people with diabetes. Advances in diabetes management, surgical techniques, anaesthetic medicines and intensive care medicine have significantly improved surgical outcomes for people with diabetes.

Introduction

People with diabetes undergo surgery for similar reasons to those without diabetes; however, because of the long-term complications of diabetes they are more likely to require:

- Cardiac procedures:
- Angioplasty or stents

- Bypass surgery
- Ulcer debridement, amputations (toes, feet)
- Eye surgery such as cataract removal, repair retinal detachment, vitrectory
- Carpal tunnel decompression.

Surgery induces a stress response that results in endocrine, metabolic and long-term effects that have implications for the management of people with diabetes undergoing surgery, see Table 9.1. Stress induces hyperglycaemia, which causes osmotic diuresis, increased hepatic glucose output, lipolysis and insulin resistance. Unless controlled, surgical stress increases the risk of DKA, HONK, and lactic acidosis (see Chapter 7), infection, impaired wound healing, and cerebral ischaemia. The risk of HONK is high in procedures such as cardiac bypass surgery and has a high mortality rate (Dagogo-Jack & Alberti 2002).

Table 9.1 Hormonal, metabolic, and long-term effects of surgery.

Hormonal	Metabolic	Long-term effects if optimal blood glucose control is not achieved
↑ Secretion of[a] epinephrine, norepinephrine, ACTH, cortisol and growth hormone	Catabolic state and ↑ metabolic rate Hyperglycaemia Insulin resistance	Loss of lean body mass – impaired wound healing, ↓ resistance to infection Loss of adipose tissue
↓ secretion of insulin due to impaired beta cell responsiveness	↓ Glucose utilisation and glycogen storage ↑ Gluconeogenesis	Deficiency of essential amino acids, vitamins, minerals, and essential fatty acids
Insulin resistance	↑ Protein catabolism and reduced amino acid and protein synthesis in skeletal muscle	Surgical complications
	↑ Lipolysis and formation of ketone bodies	
	↓ Storage of fatty acids in the liver	
	Osmotic diuresis with electrolyte loss and compromised circulating volume	
	↑ Risk of cerebrovascular accident, myocardial arrhythmias infarction electrolyte disorders	
	↑ Blood pressure and heart rate	
	↓ Peristalsis	

[a] Norepinephrine is mostly augmented during surgery and epinephrine postoperatively. Stress stimulates glucagon secretion from the pancreatic alpha cells and together with growth hormone and cortisol, potentiates the effects of norepinephrine and epinephrine. Cortisol increases gluconeogenesis.

In addition, anaesthesia and surgical stress, as well as medicines, induce gastrointestinal instability that can compound gastric autonomic neuropathy and lead to nausea, vomiting and predispose the individual to dehydration and exacerbates fluid loss via osmotic diuresis and blood loss during surgery. As a result, electrolyte changes particularly in potassium and magnesium, increase the risk of cardiac arrhythmias, ischaemic events, and acute renal failure (Dagogo-Jack & Alberti 2002). The risk is particularly high in those with chronic hyperglycaemia, existing diabetes complications, older people, and those who are obese. All of which are associated with increased risk of postoperative complications (Dickersen 2004).

Obesity is associated with functional risks in addition to the metabolic consequences of surgery that need to be considered when positioning the patient. The respiratory system is affected and functional residual capacity and expiratory reserve volume may be reduced possibly due to excess weight on the chest wall and/or displacement of the diaphragm. Severe obesity can lead to hypoventilation and obstructive sleep apnoea. These factors predispose the individual to aspiration pneumonia. Various cardiac changes increase the risk of heart failure and inadequate tissue oxygenation. In addition, the risk of pressure ulcers is increased due to the weight, and activity level is often compromised increasing the risk of venous stasis and emboli.

The need for nutritional support may be overlooked in obese individuals and protein deprivation can develop because protein and carbohydrate are used as the main energy sources during surgery rather than fat. In addition, energy expenditure is higher due to the increase in lean body mass, which impacts on wound healing (Mirtallo 2008).

Different types of surgery present specific risks as do the age of the person, with the very young and older people being particularly at risk. These effects are summarised in Table 9.1. These factors must be controlled in order to prevent DKA and HONK, promote healing and reduce the risk of infection postoperatively. Hyperglycaemia inhibits white cell function and increases coagulability (Kirschner 1993).

Surgery is often performed as a day procedure often without appropriate consideration of the effects of surgical and the related psychological stress on metabolic control. A multidisciplinary approach to planning is important.

The magnitude of the metabolic/hormonal response depends on the severity and duration of the surgical procedure, metabolic control before, during, and after surgery, and the presence of complications such as sepsis, acidosis, hypotension, and hypovolaemia (Marks *et al.* 1998). Metabolic disturbances can be present in euglycaemic states (De & Child 2001).

Aims of management

(1) To identify underlying problems that could compromise surgery and recovery.
(2) To achieve normal metabolism by supplying sufficient insulin to counterbalance the increase in stress hormones during fasting, surgery, and postoperatively (blood glucose between 5 and 7 mmol/L) and avoid the need for prolonged fasting.
(3) To achieve this with regimens that minimise the possibility of errors.
(4) To supply adequate carbohydrate to prevent catabolism, hypoglycaemia, and ketosis.
(5) To ensure that the patient undergoes surgery in the best possible physical condition.

(6) To prevent:
- hypoglycaemia, children <5 years are prone to hypoglycaemia during anaesthesia and surgery (Kirschner 1993)
- hyperglycaemia predisposing the patient to dehydration, electrolyte imbalance, ketoacidosis, and hyperosmolar states
- complications of surgery
- electrolyte imbalance
- worsening of pre-existing diabetic complications
- infection.

(7) To avoid undue psychological stress.

Preoperative nursing care

Good preoperative nursing care is important for both major and minor procedures. Preadmission clinics have an important role in identifying and managing preventable surgical risks. Sometimes people need to be admitted 2–3 days before major surgery to stabilise blood glucose levels and manage complications, see Table 9.2. Because many procedures only require a day admission, careful explanation about what is required and *written* instructions about medication adjustment/withdrawal are vital.

The individual's blood glucose profile needs to be reviewed and their diabetes regimen may need to be adjusted prior to surgery to achieve good control. Erratic control could indicate the presence of infection that should be treated prior to surgery. If possible, schedule for a morning procedure to avoid the need for prolonged fasting and counter-regulatory hormone release that leads to hyperglycaemia.

Nursing actions

(1) Confirm time of operation.
(2) Explain procedure and postoperative care to the patient and/or family members if appropriate for example a child. Those patients controlled OHAs may require insulin *during surgery and immediately post-operatively*. They should be aware of this possibility. Insulin during the operative period does not mean that diet- or tablet-controlled patients will remain on insulin when they recover from the procedure. People controlled by diet and exercise with good metabolic control may not require an IV insulin infusion for minor procedures but 1–2 hourly blood glucose monitoring is necessary. If control is suboptimal, and for procedures longer than 1 hour, an IV insulin/dextrose infusion is advisable (Dagogo-Jack & Alberti 2002). It should be noted that suboptimal control is common in diet-treated individuals.
(3) Ensure all documentation is completed:
- consent form
- medication chart
- monitoring guidelines
- chest X-ray and other X-rays, scans, MRI (magnetic resonance imaging)
- ECG.
(4) Sulphonylureas are usually ceased 24 hours preoperatively and metformin and chlorpropamide 36 hours preoperatively. Check medical orders. Metformin should be withdrawn 3 days before surgery because any deterioration in renal function

Table 9.2 Common diabetic complications that can affect surgery and postoperative recovery. Many of these conditions may be documented in the person's medical record and they may undergo regular complication assessment but health status can change rapidly especially older people. Therefore, the current complication status should be assessed prior to surgery. Hyperglycaemia must be controlled.

Complication	Possible consequences	Preoperative evaluation
Cardiovascular	Hypertension Ischaemic heart disease Cardiomyopathy Myocardial infarction, which can be 'silent' and in the presence of autonomic neuropathy cause sudden tachycardia, bradycardia, and/or postural hypotension Cerebrovascular disease. Increased resting heart rate is associated with increased risk of death in older people. Daytime sleepiness is associated with 4.5-fold increased risk of stroke and other vascular events.	Careful history and examination ECG Manage existing conditions such as heart failure Assess for silent cardiac disease autonomic neuropathy, indicators include; Shortness of breath, palpitations, ankle oedema, tiredness, and atypical chest pain. Assess resting heart rate. Ask about daytime sleepiness or assess formally, for example, using the Epworth Sleepiness Scale (ESS).
Neuropathy Autonomic	Cardiac as above Inability to maintain body temperature during anaesthesia	Lying and standing blood pressure (abnormal if decrease >30 mmHg) Heart rate response on deep breathing (abnormal if increase >10 beats/min).
Peripheral	Pressure areas on feet and ulceration Foot infection Falls post operatively	Foot assessment, assess for active and occult infection and signs of neuropathy.
Renal	Nephropathy, which may affect medication excretion. Urinary tract infection (UTI), which may be silent and predispose to sepsis Acute renal failure and the need for dialysis. UTI if catheterisation is needed.	Urine culture to detect UTI, which should be treated with the relevant antibiotics Microalbuminuria and creatinine clearance, eGFR Blood electrolytes, correct potassium >5 mmol/L before surgery.
Respiratory Airway	Obese people and smokers are prone to chest infections Obesity may be associated with reduced respiratory reserve and displacement of the diaphragm Reduced tissue oxygenation. Soft tissue, ligament, and joint thickening that might involve the neck making it difficult to extend the neck and intubate and predispose the individual to neck injury and post operative pain	Counsel to stop smoking Chest physiotherapy Chest X-ray Blood gases Nebulised oxygen pre and postoperatively if indicated See test for musculoskeletal disease (see page 265) Take extra care of the neck

Gastrointestinal	Autonomic neuropathy leading to gastric stasis delayed gastric emptying, gastric reflux, regurgitation and aspiration on anaesthesia induction Ileus May need to modify nutritional support if required postoperatively and given enterally.	Assess history of heartburn or reflux and whether the person sleeps in an upright position A H_2 antagonist and metoclopramide might be indicated preoperatively Erratic food absorption can affect blood glucose levels
Eyes	Cataracts, glaucoma, and retinopathy can be exacerbated by sudden rise in blood pressure	Assess retinopathy stage.
Neutrophil dysfunction	Increased risk of infection Inability to mount an appropriate response to infection	Check for possible foci of infection: including feet, teeth, and gums, UTI, Ensure optimal blood glucose control Optimise vascular function.
Polypharmacy	Risk of medicine interactions with anaesthetic agents and postoperative medicines Risk of lactic acidosis with metformin Some medicines increase the risk of hyperglycaemia some hypoglycaemia	Medicine review Ask about complementary medicines Give the person clear, concise written instructions about how to manage their medicines preoperatively and postoperatively on discharge
Musculoskeletal	Difficulties with intubation and tube placement. Falls risk	Assess, for example, prayer sign, Dupuytren's contracture, trigger finger Foot abnormality including Charcot's foot
Obesity	Increased systemic vascular resistance leading to reduced tissue oxygenation and increased risk of lactic acidosis in people on metformin especially if renal function is compromised and those with surgical wound infections. Sleep apnoea and associated daytime sleepiness with associated risk of cardiovascular events. Difficulty intubating the person Assumption that the person is well nourished when in fact nutritional deficiencies especially protein are common. High prevalence of hypertriglyceridaemia Cardiovascular and respiratory effects, which affect postoperative nutrition support if it is required. Non-alcoholic fatty liver Risk of pressure ulcers	Assess nutritional status Assess cardiovascular and respiratory status. Ask about daytime sleepiness or assesss formally, for example, using the ESS. Skin condition

predisposes the patient to lactic acidosis (Gill 1997), see Chapter 7. However, some experts recommend continuing OHA up until surgery to counteract surgical stress (French 2000) depending on the extent of the surgery, diabetes type, and usual blood glucose control. Insulin therapy must be initiated before the procedure in people with Type 1 diabetes.

(5) Encourage patients who smoke to stop.
(6) Assess:
  - metabolic status: blood glucose control, ketones in blood and urine, hydration status, nutritional status, presence of anaemia, diabetic symptoms
  - educational level and understanding of diabetes
  - family support available postoperatively
  - any known allergies or medicine reactions, which should include asking about complementary therapies, particularly herbal medicines, because some herbs predispose the person to haemorrhage and/or interact with anaesthetic agents and should be stopped at least 7 days prior to surgery (see Chapter 19)
  - presence of diabetic complications and other comorbidities, for example, renal, hepatic, cardiac disease (ECG for people >50 years to detect the risk of silent infarction is performed in some units), presence of neuropathy. Patients with autonomic neuropathy pose special problems during anesthesia: gastroparesis delays gastric emptying and the stomach can be full despite fasting and increases the possibility of regurgitation and inhalation of vomitus; or the vasoconstrictive response to reduced cardiac output may be absent and they may not recognise hypoglycaemia
  - current medication regimen
  - presence of infection, check feet and be aware of silent infection such as UTI.
  - self-care potential and available home support.

Note: Complications should be managed before the operation where possible, see Table 9.2.

Major procedures

Major surgery refers to procedures requiring anaesthesia and lasting longer than 1 hour (Dagogo-Jack & Alberti 2002).

Day of the operation

Premedication and routine preparation for the scheduled operative procedure should be performed according to the treatment sheet and standard protocols.

Where insulin is required, for example, Type 1 diabetes, major surgery, and poor control, an IV insulin infusion is the preferred method of delivering the insulin. The insulin dose should be balanced with adequate calories to prevent starvation ketosis, for example, saline/dextrose delivered at a rate that matches the insulin dose (Alberti & Gill 1997), see Chapter 5. Fluid replacement should be adequate to maintain intravascular volume; normal saline/dextrose in water is the preferred solution for this purpose. Preoperative hyperglycaemia especially if polyuria is present can cause significant fluid deficits and intracellular dehydration. Clinical signs of dehydration are:

- Thirst and a dry mouth: water loss <5% of body weight.
- Capillary refill >2 seconds (normal <2 seconds), reduced skin turgor, sunken eyes, reduced urine output, orthostatic hypotension, fainting on standing, low CVP/JVP: water loss 5–10% of body weight.
- Unconscious or shock: water loss >10% of body weight (French 2000).

Morning procedure

(1) Ensure oral medications were ceased.
(2) Fast from 12 midnight.
(3) Ascertain insulin regimen: commence insulin infusion.
(4) Monitor blood glucose 1–2-hourly.

Afternoon procedure

(1) Fast after an early light breakfast.
(2) Ensure oral medications have been ceased.
(3) Ascertain insulin dose, usually 1/2 to 1/3 of usual dose (best given after IV dextrose has been commenced).
(4) It is preferable for IV therapy to be commenced in the ward to:
    - prevent hyperglycaemia and dehydration
    - reduce the risk of hypoglycaemia.
    This will depend on the surgical and anaesthetist and usual hospital procedure. Some anaesthetists prefer to commence the infusion in theatre. It is preferable to insert the IV line in theatre in children unless blood glucose is <4 mmol/L (Werther 1994).
(5) Monitor blood glucose.

The anaesthetist is usually responsible for the intraoperative blood glucose monitoring. The patient is dependent on this monitoring to detect hypo- or hyperglycaemia. The anaesthetic will mask the usual signs of hypoglycaemia. Precautions are needed to avoid regurgitation and aspiration, cardiac arrhythmias, and postural hypotension in young children and patients with autonomic neuropathy. Hypoglycaemia increases the risk of seizures. In all cases careful explanation to the patient and their family/carers is essential.

Postoperative nursing responsibilities

Immediate care

(1) Monitor and record vital signs.
(2) Monitor blood and urinary glucose/ketones initially 2-hourly.
(3) Observe dressings for signs of haemorrhage or excess discharge.
(4) Ensure drain tubes are patent and draining.

(5) Maintain an accurate fluid balance. Document all information relating to input and output, especially:

Input	Output
IV fluid	Drainage from wound
Oral	Vomitus
EN and TPN	Diarrhoea
	Urine

(6) Maintain care of IV insulin infusion.
(7) Ensure vomiting and pain are controlled.
(8) Ensure psychological needs are addressed, for example, body image change.
(9) Ensure referral to appropriate allied health professional, for example, physiotherapist.
(10) Insulin therapy is continued for tablet-controlled patients until they are eating a normal diet and blood glucose levels are stabilised.
(11) Provide pressure care including high-risk neuropathic feet.

Ongoing care

(1) Document all data accurately on the appropriate charts.
(2) Prevent complications:
  • infection – aseptic dressing technique including IV sites
  • venous thrombosis – anti-embolic stockings, physiotherapy, early ambulation, anticoagulants
  • hypo/hyperglycaemia
  • pressure ulcers.
(3) Diabetes education, instruct patient and their family/carers in wound care and medication management.
(4) Rehabilitation.

Antibiotics, heparin and other medicines should be administered according to individual patient requirements and medical orders.

Clinical observation

People sometimes complain of a sore throat for 24 hours after a general anaesthetic. They need to be reassured that this is normal and resolves spontaneously but advised to seek medical advice if it persists.

Minor procedures

Minor surgery may be performed on an outpatient basis. The metabolic risks are still a consideration if the patient is expected to fast for the procedure. Ensure that the procedure is fully explained to the patient at the time of making the appointment. Give *written* instructions about how to manage insulin, oral agents and other medications. Preoperative care is the same as for major surgery on the day of operation as regards:

- Diabetes medications.
- Complications screening and management when present.
- Morning procedure is preferred.

Guidelines for patient instructions

Examples of patient instructions for people undergoing outpatient procedures can be found in Example Instruction Sheets 2 (a) and (b) (see pages 279 and 280).

Note: These are examples only and protocols in the nurse's place of employment should be followed. Adjusting medications for investigations and day procedures is becoming more complex as the range of available insulin, oral agents, and other medicines increase, and multiple insulin injections and combining insulin and oral agents is common practice.

It is important to consider the individual's blood glucose pattern, the medication regimen they are on and the type of procedure they are having when advising them about preoperative medication self-care.

Where people are on basal bolus regimes and scheduled for a morning procedure, the bedtime insulin dose may need to be reduced and the morning dose omitted. If the procedure is scheduled for the afternoon the morning dose may be given and the lunchtime dose omitted.

When people are on a combination of insulin and oral hypoglycaemic agents, the oral agents are usually withheld on the night before the procedure and the morning dose of insulin will be withheld for morning procedures. A reduced dose of insulin will usually be given if the procedure is scheduled for the afternoon.

Practice point

Advice about medications should also include information about medications and complementary therapies the person may be taking besides insulin and oral hypoglycaemic agents.

Morning procedure

(1) Withhold insulin in the morning on the day of the procedure.
(2) Test blood glucose and ketones if Type 1 before coming to hospital.
(3) Fast from 12 midnight.
(4) Bring insulin to hospital.
(5) Advise patient to have someone available to drive them home after the procedure.

Afternoon procedure

(1) Light breakfast (e.g. tea and toast).
(2) Fast after this breakfast.
(3) Test blood glucose and ketones in Type 1 before coming to hospital.
(4) Give insulin dose according to blood glucose test as ordered by the doctor.

(5) Explain before discharge:
- the risk of hypoglycaemia if not eating
- what to take for pain relief
- when to recommence OHAs/insulin
- what and when to eat
- any specific care, for example, wound dressings or care of a biopsy site.

In both cases

(1) Test blood glucose at the end of the procedure and before discharge and administer OHA or insulin dose.
(2) Ensure the patient has appropriate follow-up appointments with doctors and other relevant health professionals, for example, diabetes educator, dietitian.
(3) Ensure the patient has someone to accompany him or her home.
(4) Allay concerns about the procedure.
(5) Provide appropriate care according to the medical orders.
(6) Inspect all wounds before discharge.
(7) It is not advisable to drive, operate machinery or drink alcohol until the following day.

Clinical observations

It is important to ensure the patient and their family/carers understand what is meant by 'fasting' and 'light breakfast'. People have stated that they will 'come as fast as I can but I can only move slowly because of my hips'.

Emergency procedures

Approximately 5% of people with diabetes will need emergency surgery at some stage of their lives. These may be for general surgical emergencies such as appendicitis or diabetes-specific such as acute foot ulcer. Abdominal pain in the presence of DKA may not be an abdominal emergency. However if the abdominal pain persist after the DKA is corrected an abdominal emergency should be considered. Likewise, functional problems associated with gastroparesis, gastroenteropathy and cyclical vomiting may be mistaken for a surgical emergency. Thus, even in an emergency situation it is important to undertake a thorough assessment and medical history.

The specific management will depend on the nature of the emergency. If possible, the metabolic status should be stabilised before surgery is commenced. Many patients requiring emergency surgery have suboptimal control. The minimum requirements are:

(1) Adequate hydration. IV access should be obtained and blood drawn for glucose, ketones, electrolytes, pH, and other tests as indicated by the presenting problem.
(2) If possible surgery should be delayed until the underlying acid–base derangement is corrected if ketoacidosis (DKA), hyperosmolar or lactic acidosis is present.

Dehydration is often severe in hyperosmolar states and the fluid volume needs to be replaced quickly taking care not to cause fluid overload or cerebral oedema. If the patient presents with an abdominal emergency ensure that it is not due to DKA before operating.

Specific treatment depends on:

- The nature of the emergency
- The time of the last food intake and the presence of autonomic neuropathy/gastric stasis.
- The time and type of the last insulin dose
- The blood glucose level, which should be monitored hourly.

Presence of complications such as cardiac arrhythmias and renal disease. Postoperative care will depend on the reason for the emergency and will encompass the care outlined earlier in the chapter.

Bariatric surgery

Bariatric surgery as a solution to obesity when other methods fail is becoming safer and more acceptable. A recent study demonstrated that laproscopic adjustable gastric banding (LAGB) and conventional diabetes management had five times the diabetes remission rate than other methods in 60 obese people with Type 2 diabetes (Dixon *et al.* 2008). Seventy three per cent achieved diabetes remission, there was an average weight loss of 20%, and average BMI fell from 36.6 to 29.5, and 80% achieved normoglycaemia.

People who successfully lose weight after gastric banding are more likely to have improved insulin sensitivity, reduced fasting blood glucose and HbA_{1c}, especially those with Type 2 diabetes, and the lipid profile improves in people with Type 2 diabetes and those with impaired glucose tolerance (Geloneze *et al.* 2001). However, the risks and benefits need to be carefully considered.

Investigative procedures

Key points

- Careful preparation and explanation to the patient and their family/carers.
- Never omit insulin in Type 1 diabetes.
- Radio-opaque contrast media may cause tubular necrosis in older people with diabetes so fluid balance must be monitored carefully.
- Complementary therapies especially herbs and topical essential oils may need to be stopped temporarily.

Rationale

Metabolic stress occurs to a lesser degree during investigative procedures than during surgical procedures but still occurs and needs to be managed appropriately to limit adverse outcomes.

Clear written instructions about managing medications and any specific preparation required can improve the individual's understanding and compliance with instructions.

Management protocols for patients undergoing medical tests/procedures such as X-rays, gastroscopy or laser therapy is not as intricate as those for ketoacidosis or major surgery. However, vigilant nursing care is equally important to prevent excursions in blood glucose levels and consequent metabolic effects, and psychological stress.

Note: Morning procedures are preferred.

The objectives of care

(1) As for surgical procedures.
(2) To ensure correct preparation for the test.
(3) To ensure the procedure has been explained to the patient.
(4) To provide written instructions for the patient especially if the test is to be performed on an outpatient basis. These instructions should include what to do about their diabetes medications (insulin and oral agents) and any other medications they are taking and how to recognise and manage hypoglycaemia should it occur while they are fasting. They should also warn the person that it may not be safe for them to drive home depending on the procedure.

Usually, the doctor referring the person for a procedure should explain the procedure to the individual as part of the process for obtaining informed consent to undertake the procedure. Nurses have a duty of care to ensure instructions have been given and were followed.

General nursing management

(1) Insulin/oral hypoglycaemic agents:
  • insulin is *never omitted* in Type 1 diabetics
  • if the patient needs to fast, insulin doses should be adjusted accordingly
  • OHAs are usually withheld on the morning of the test
  • ensure written medical instructions are available, including for after the procedure.
(2) Aim for a morning procedure if fasting is required and avoid prolonged fasting that results in a catabolic state and counter-regulatory hormone release (see Chapters 1 and 7).
(3) Monitor blood glucose before and after the test and during the night (3 AM) if fasting and in hospital.
(4) Observe for signs of dehydration. Maintain fluid balance chart if:
  • fasting is prolonged
  • bowel preparations are required – some may lead to a fluid deficit especially in the setting of hyperglycaemia.

- an IV infusion is commenced
- dehydration in older people may predispose them to kidney damage if a radio-opaque contrast medium is used.

An IV infusion may dilute some radio-opaque contrast media. The advice of the radiographer should be sought if IV therapy is necessary. Continue IV infusions and oral fluids after the procedure to wash out contrast medium.

(5) Control nausea and vomiting and pain, which can increase the blood glucose level.
(6) Ensure the patient can eat and drink normally after the procedure to avoid hypoglycaemia.
(7) Assess puncture sites (e.g. angiography) before discharge.
(8) Recommence medications as per the medical order.
(9) Counsel not to drive home if relevant.

Bowel procedures, for example, colonoscopy

(1) Iron, aspirin, and arthritis medications may need to be stopped one week before the procedure. Diabetes medications should be adjusted according to the procedures outlined for day procedures.
(2) The day before the colonoscopy only clear fluids are permitted and some form of bowel preparation is usually required to clean out the bowel and allow a better view of the lining. Bowel preparations should be diluted in water because cordial can contribute to diarrhoea. Older people are at risk of dehydration and should be carefully monitored. Modern preparations are not absorbed and do not usually lead to significant electrolyte disturbances.
(3) Fasting for at least 6 hours is usually necessary.

Eye procedures

People with diabetes are more prone to visual impairment and blindness than the general population. The eye manifestations of diabetes can affect all ocular structures. The time of appearance, rate of progression and severity of eye disease vary among individuals. However, most patients have some evidence of damage after 25 years of diabetes and vision is threatened in 10% of people with diabetes.

Retinopathy is symptomless and may remain undetected if an ophthalmologist or optician does not examine the eyes regularly. Retinal cameras are commonly used to assess the degree of retinopathy and do not require papillary dilation. Fluorescein angiography and retinal photography may aid in determining the severity of the disease. Management aims to conserve vision, and laser therapy is often effective in this respect.

Risk factors for eye disease include hypertension, pregnancy, nephropathy, hyperlipidaemia, and smoking (see Chapter 8).

Care of patient having fluorescein angiography

Fluorescein angiography is usually an outpatient procedure. The reasons for the test and the procedure should be carefully explained to the patient. They should be aware that:

- Transient nausea may occur.
- The skin and urine may become yellow for 12–24 hours.
- Drinking adequate amounts of fluid will help flush the dye out of the system.
- The dye is injected into a vein.

Care of the patient having laser therapy (photocoagulation)

'Laser' is an acronym for light amplification stimulated emission of radiation. There are many types of laser. The ones that are used to treat diabetic patients are the argon, krypton, and diode lasers. The lasers absorb light, which is converted into heat, which coagulates the tissue. Laser therapy is frequently used to treat diabetic retinopathy and glaucoma.

Goals of photocoagulation

To maintain vision:

- By allowing fluid exchange to occur and reducing fluid accumulation in the retina.
- By photocoagulating the retina, which is ischaemic, and thereby causing new vessels that are prone to haemorrhage, to regress.

Laser therapy is usually performed on an outpatient basis. Fasting is not required and medication adjustment is unnecessary.

Practice point

Laser therapy may not increase vision, but can prevent further loss of vision.

Nursing responsibilities

Ensure the purpose of laser therapy has been explained to the patient. Advise them to ask their doctor whether it is still safe to drive after the treatment – not just immediately after but generally. The majority can still drive safely but a driving assessment might be required.

(1) Before the procedure the patient should know that:
   - the procedure is uncomfortable
   - the pupil of the eye will be dilated
   - anaesthetic drops may be used
   - the laser beam causes bright flashes of light
   - vision will be blurred for some time after the laser treatment
   - they should test their blood glucose before and after laser treatment
   - they should not drive home and that they may have tunnel vision after the procedure, which can limit their visual field. The possible effects on driving should be explained (see Chapter 10).

(2) After the procedure the patient should know that:
   - sunglasses will protect the eye and help reduce discomfort
   - spots may be seen for 24–48 hours
   - there can be some discomfort for 2–3 weeks
   - headache may develop after the procedure
   - paracetamol may be taken to relieve pain

Practice point

Aspirin is best avoided because of its anticoagulant effect. If new vessels are present due to retinopathy they can bleed and threaten sight.

- activities that increase intraocular pressure, for example, lifting heavy objects, straining at stool, should be avoided for 24–36 hours
- night vision may be temporarily decreased
- lateral vision may be permanently diminished; this is known as 'tunnel vision'.

Other eye procedures include cataract operations.

Practice point

Blurred vision does not necessarily indicate serious eye disease. It can occur during both hypo- and hyperglycaemia. Vision often also becomes worse when diabetic control is improved, for example, after commencement of insulin therapy. Although this is distressing for the patient, vision usually improves in 6–8 weeks. Prescriptions for glasses obtained in these circumstances may be inappropriate. Glasses are best obtained when the eyes settle down.

The nursing care of people who are vision impaired is discussed in Chapter 14.

Care of the patient having radio-contrast media injected

Radio-contrast media are eliminated through the kidneys. Fasting is often required before the procedure and the patient can become dehydrated, especially if they are kept waiting for long periods, and kidney complications can occur. Patients most at risk:

- Are over 50 years old
- Have established kidney disease
- Have had diabetes for more than 10 years
- Are hypertensive
- Have proteinuria
- Have an elevated serum creatinine but note the limitations of serum creatinine discussed in Chapter 3.

Kidney problems caused by radiocontrast media may not produce symptoms. Reduced urine output following procedures requiring radiocontrast media may indicate kidney damage and should be investigated.

Management
(1) Ensure appropriate preparation has been carried out.
(2) Ensure the patient is well hydrated before the procedure (intravenous therapy may be needed).
(3) Maintain an accurate fluid balance chart.
(4) Avoid delays in performing the procedure.

(5) Monitor urine output after the procedure.
(6) Assess serum creatinine and/or other kidney function tests after the procedure.
(7) Maintain good metabolic control.
(8) Encourage the patient to drink water to help flush out the contrast media.

Complementary therapies and surgery and investigative procedures

A version of the following information was published in the *Australian Diabetes Educator* 2008, see also Chapter 19. Fifty per cent of patients undergoing surgical and investigative procedures use complementary medicines (CAM) and other CAM. Women aged 40–60 years are high users and often use CAM on the advice of friends (Tsen *et al.* 2000; Norred *et al.* 2000). Thus CAM use is an important consideration for people with diabetes having surgical and/or investigative procedures.

Significantly, despite the high rates of CAM usage, most conventional practitioners do not ask about CAM use (Braun *et al.* 2006). CAM use can improve health outcomes of patients undergoing surgery: for example, essential oil foot massage reduces stress and anxiety post CAGS (Stevenson 1994), essential oils lower MRI-associated claustrophobia and stress, acupuncture and peppermint or ginger tea reduce nausea, a range of strategies relieve pain and improve sleep and CQ10 prior to cardiac surgery improves post-operative cardiac outcomes (Rosenfeldt *et al.* 2005).

However, there are also risks, which need to be considered in the context of the particular surgery or investigation required and overall management plan. Bleeding is the most significant risk. Other risks include hypotension, hypertension, sedation, and cardiac effects such as arrhythmias, renal damage, and electrolyte disturbances (Norred *et al.* 2000, 2002). It is well documented that many conventional medicines need to be adjusted or ceased prior to surgery. Less information about managing CAM in surgical settings is available but a growing body of evidence suggests many CAM medicines may also need to be stopped or adjusted prior to surgery and some investigative procedures.

The following general information applies to people already using CAM medicines and those considering using them before or after surgery. Conventional practitioners may be able to provide general advice regarding CAM use but people with diabetes should be advised to consult a qualified CAM medicine practitioner because many therapies should be used under qualified supervision and for specific advice. Self-prescribing is not recommended in the surgical period because of the complex metabolic and neuroendocrine response to surgery.

Preoperative phase

People need written information about how to manage CAM medicines and conventional medicines in the operative period as well as any special preparation needed for the surgery or investigation. Conventional health professionals can provide such information if they are qualified to do so or refer the person to a qualified CAM practitioner. Such information should be provided in an appropriate format relevant to the individual's health literacy level, see Chapter 16.

Great care is needed for major and high risk such as heart, orthopaedic, or neurosurgery, if the person has renal or liver disease, or is very young or elderly.

The conventional medication list is unlikely to include CAM medicines or supplements, although it should, thus health professionals should discuss CAM use with people during all structured medicine reviews and preoperative health assessments.

Some CAM medicines such as evening primrose oil, bilberry, cranberry, fish oils, ginger, Gingko, liquorice, guarana, willow bark, meadowsweet, and ginseng need to be stopped at least one week before surgery. St John's Wort and supplements such as vitamin E should be stopped two weeks before surgery, primarily because of the risk of bleeding. In addition, medicines such as St John's Wort, need to be stopped gradually (like conventional antidepressants). However, when CAM medicines are the main form of treatment, alternative management may be required to prevent the condition deteriorating and affecting the surgical outcome, for example, glucose lowering herbal medicines.

In addition to the bleeding risk, some commonly used CAM medicines might/do interact with some anaesthetic agents and prolong their sedative effects, some affect blood pressure and heart rate, others cause changes in the major electrolytes, potassium, calcium, and sodium levels in the blood. Grapefruit juice interferes with the action of some antibiotics such as cyclosporine, which may be needed pre or postoperatively. These problems do not occur in everybody who uses CAM in the same way that not everybody experiences adverse events associated with conventional treatments. It is sometimes difficult to predict who will or will not have problems. Some hospitals have policies and guidelines about using CAM and people who wish to continue using CAM in hospital should clarify such policies with the relevant hospital and surgeon before they are admitted. Most do not prescribe or supply CAM.

In addition to managing CAM and conventional medicines, achieving the best possible health status before surgery improves postoperative recovery. The preoperative assessment is an ideal time to revise the importance of eating a healthy balanced diet and exercise within the individual's capability, controlling blood glucose and lipids, which will support immune system functioning and enhance wound healing. Most people should continue their usual physical activity unless it is contraindicated to maintain strength and flexibility. Stress management strategies such as meditation, guided imagery, essential oils administered in a massage or via an inhalation, and music help reduce anxiety and fear about the surgery. Ginger capsules or tablets taken one hour before surgery reduces postoperative nausea (Gupta & Sharma 2001).

The preoperative assessment is also an ideal time to discuss postoperative recovery including managing pain and promoting sleep. CAM may be a useful alternative to some conventional medicines provided a quality use of medicines framework is adopted, see Chapter 5. For example, valerian, hops, and lavender in a vapourised essential oil blend, administered via massage or as herbal teas or medicines promote restful sleep and have a lower side effect profile than most conventional sedatives.

Postoperative phase

CAM users need information about whether and when it is safe to start using CAM again postoperatively considering any new conventional medicines that were prescribed, for example anticoagulants, which could influence the choice and/or dose of CAM medicines. Likewise, some non-medicine CAM therapies might need to be used with care such as needle acupuncture and deep tissue massage because they can cause bruising and/or bleeding.

A range of CAM strategies can be used to manage pain in the immediate postoperative phase as well as in the longer term is needed. Most are less likely to cause constipation and drowsiness than pethidine and morphine-based medicines. Alternatively, if these medicines are the best method of managing pain, high fibre CAM food/ medicines such as *Aloe vera* juice, probiotics, and psyllium can reduce constipation once oral feeding is permitted. Probiotics also increase bowel health and support natural bowel flora. Peppermint or ginger tea reduces mild-to-moderate nausea. Lymphatic drainage massage is very effective after some surgery to reduce swelling and relieve pain.

Some CAM products promote wound healing, for example, *Aloe vera*, Medihoney, and calendula and could be used depending on the wound. Arnica ointment reduces bruising but should not be used on open wounds. Comfrey poultices are very effective at reducing local oedema and local pain but should not be used on open wounds or taken internally.

Implications for nursing care

- CAM has both risks and benefits for people with diabetes undergoing surgery and investigative procedures.
- Not all the CAM therapies people use are medicines and not all CAM carry the same level of risk or confer equal benefits.
- Adopting an holistic quality use of medicines (QUM) approach can optimise the benefits and reduce the risks. A key aspect of QUM is asking about and documenting CAM use.
- People with diabetes who use CAM need written advice about how to manage their CAM during surgery and investigations.
- People with diabetes and cardiac or renal disease and those on anticoagulants, older people, and children are at particular risk if they use some CAM medicines.

References

Alberti, G. & Gill, G. (1997) The care of the diabetic patient during surgery. In: *International Textbook of Diabetes Mellitus* (2nd edn.) (eds G. Alberti, R. DeFronzo & H. Keen). Wiley, Chichester, pp. 1243–1253.

Braun, L. *et al.* (2006) Use of complementary medicines by surgical patients. Undetected and unsupervised. In: *Proceedings of the Fourth Australasian Conference on Safety and Quality in Health Care*, Melbourne.

De, P. & Child, D. (2001) Euglycaemic ketoacidosis – is it on the rise? *Practical Diabetes International*, **18** (7), 239–240.

Dagogo-Jack, S. & Alberti, G. (2002) Management of diabetes mellitus in surgical patients. *Diabetes Spectrum*, **15**, 44–48.

Dickerson, R. (2004) Specialised nutrition support in the hospitalized obese patient. *Nutrition in Clinical Practice*, **19**, 245–254.

Dixon J., O'Brien P., Playfair J., Chapman L., Schachter L., Skinner S., Prietto J., Bailey J., Anderson M. (2008) Adjustable gastric banding and conventional therapy for type 2 diabetes: a randomized contolled trial. *Journal American Medical Association*, **299** (3), 316–323.

French, G. (2000) Clinical management of diabetes mellitus during anaesthesia and surgery. *Update in Anaesthesia*, **11** (13), 1–6.

Geloneze, B., Tambascia, M., Pareja, J., Repetto, E. & Magna, L. (2001) The insulin tolerance test in morbidly obese patients undergoing bariatric surgery. *Obesity Research*, **9**, 763–769.

Gill, G. (1997) Surgery and diabetes. In: *Textbook of Diabetes* (eds. G. Williams & J. Pickup). Blackwell Science, Oxford, pp. 820–825.

Gupta, Y., & Sharma, M. (2001) Reversal of pyrogallol-induced gastric emptying in rats by ginger (*Zingber officinalis*). *Experimental Clinical Pharmacology*, **23** (9), 501–503.

Kirschner, R. (1993) Diabetes in paediatric ambulatory surgical patients. *Journal of Post Anaesthesia Nursing*, **8** (5), 322–326.

Marks, J., Hirsch, J. & de Fronzo, R. (eds) (1998) *Current Management of Diabetes Mellitus*, C.V. Mosby, St Louis, pp. 247–254.

Mirtallo, J. (2008) Nutrition support for the obese surgical patient. *Medscape Pharmacist* http://www.medscap.com/viewarticle/566036(accessed February 2008).

Norred, C. *et al.* (2000) Use of complementary and alternative medicines by surgical patients. *Journal American Association of Nurse Anaesthetists*, **68** (1), 13–18.

Norred, C. (2002) Complementary and alternative medicine use by surgical patients. *AORN*, **76** (6), 1013–1021.

Rosenfeldt, F. *et al.* (2005) Coenzyme CQ-10 therapy before cardiac surgery improves mitochondrial function and *in vitro* contractility of myocardial tissue. *Journal of Thoracic and Cardiovascular Surgery*, **129**, 25–32.

Stevenson, C. (1994) The psychophysiological effects of aromatherapy massage following cardiac surgery. *Complementary Therapies in Medicine*, **2** (1), 27–35.

Tsen, I. *et al.* (2000) Alternative medicine use in presurgical patients. *Anaesthesiology*, **93** (1), 148–151.

Werther, G. (1994) Diabetes mellitus & surgery. Royal Children's Hospital Melbourne. http://www.rch.org.au/clinicalguide/cpg.cfm?doc_id=5190 (accessed February 2008).

Example Instruction Sheet 2(a): Instructions for diabetic patients on oral hypoglycaemic agents having procedures as outpatients under sedation of general anaesthesia

Patient's Name: ....   UR...
Time & Date of Appointment: ....

IT IS IMPORTANT THAT YOU INFORM NURSING AND MEDICAL STAFF THAT YOU HAVE DIABETES

Morning

If your diabetes is controlled by diet and/or diabetic tablets and you are going to the operating theatre in the morning:
- take nothing by mouth from midnight
- test your blood glucose
- omit your morning diabetic tablets.

Afternoon

If your diabetes is controlled by diet and/or diabetic tablets and you are going to the operating theatre in the afternoon:
- have a light breakfast only (coffee/tea, 2 slices of toast with spread), and nothing by mouth after that
- test your blood glucose
- omit your morning diabetic tablets.

If you have any questions:
Contact: ....   Telephone: ....

Note: The inappropriate paragraph can be deleted or, better still, separate forms can be produced for morning and afternoon procedures.

Example Instruction Sheet 2(b): Instructions for diabetic patients on insulin having procedures as outpatients under sedation or general anaesthesia

---

Patient's Name: .... UR: ....
Time & Date of Appointment:...

IT IS IMPORTANT THAT YOU INFORM NURSING AND MEDICAL STAFF THAT YOU HAVE DIABETES

Morning

If your diabetes is controlled by insulin and you are going to the operating theatre in the morning:
- take nothing by mouth from midnight
- test your blood glucose
- omit your morning insulin.

Afternoon

If your diabetes is controlled by insulin and you are going to the operating theatre in the afternoon:
- have a light breakfast only (coffee/tea, 2 slices of toast with spread), and nothing by mouth after that
- test your blood glucose
- take .... units of insulin.

If you have any questions:
Contact:....................................   Telephone: ....

Note: The inappropriate paragraph can be deleted or, better still, separate forms can be produced for morning and afternoon procedures.

Chapter 10

Managing Common Conditions Associated with Diabetes

Key points

- Some of the conditions described in this chapter are rare; others occur more often.
- Many are overlooked in the focus on achieving metabolic targets.
- Most could be identified as part of routine diabetes assessment programmes and preventative screening.
- The presence of these conditions may influence management choices and health outcomes.

Introduction

This chapter outlines some specific conditions that are associated with diabetes. They are often managed in specialised services and some are very rare. A basic knowledge about these conditions can alert nurses to the possibility that they could be present, allow appropriate nursing care plans to be formulated and facilitate early referral for expert advice, which ultimately improve the health and well being of the individual.

The conditions covered in this chapter are:

- Enteral and parenteral nutrition
- Diabetes and cancer
- Smoking and alcohol addiction
- Brittle diabetes
- Oral conditions
- Liver diseases
- Breast mastopathy
- Coeliac disease
- Musculoskeletal disorders
- Corticosteroid medications and diabetes
- Diabetes and driving

ENTERAL AND PARENTERAL NUTRITION

Practice point

The policies and procedures of the health service facility should be followed when caring for people with central lines, PEG tubes, and nasogastric tubes.

Enteral and parenteral nutrition is used to supply nutritional requirements in special circumstances such as malnourished patients admitted with a debilitating disease and where there is a risk of increasing the malnourishment, for example, fasting states. Malnourishment leads to increased mortality and morbidity thus increasing length of stay in hospital (Middleton *et al.* 2001). Often the patient is extremely ill or has undergone major gastrointestinal, head or neck surgery, or has gastroparesis diabeticorum, a diabetes complication that leads to delayed gastric emptying and can result in hypoglycaemia due to delayed food absorption, bloating, and abdominal pain. Alternatively, hyperglycaemia can occur. Gastroparesis is very distressing for the patient (see Chapter 8).

Aims of therapy

(1) Reduce anxiety associated with the procedure by thoroughly explaining the process and why it is necessary. In some cases family members/carers will need to be included in the education. Ample time should be allowed to enable people's concerns to be addressed.
(2) Prevent sepsis.
(3) Maintain an acceptable blood glucose range (4–8 mmol/L).
(4) Maintain normal urea, electrolytes, LFTs, and blood gas levels.
(5) Supply adequate nutrition in terms of protein, fat, and carbohydrate to support normal body functions and promote growth and repair.
(6) Achieve positive nitrogen balance.
(7) Prevent complications of therapy.
(8) The long-term aim of enteral/parenteral feeding is the return of the patient to oral feeding. However, life expectancy is reduced or in older people it may be permanent. In such cases decisions about discontinuing the feeding will eventually need to be made.

Complications of enteral nutrition

(1) Mechanical problems such as aspiration, poor gastric emptying and reflux can occur especially if the person has altered mental status and/or a suppressed gag reflex.
(2) Metabolic consequences include hyperglycaemia and hypernatraemia depending on the feed used, the supplements added to the feed, and when a high feeding rate is used. Feeding into the small bowel rather than the stomach minimises these disturbances. People who cannot indicate that they are thirsty and who have altered mental status, particularly older people, are at risk of these metabolic consequences.

Hypoglycaemia can occur if food is not absorbed, the calorie load is reduced and if there are blockages in the feeding tubes. Medicine interactions can also contribute to hyper and hypoglycaemia, see Chapters 5 and 19.

(3) Gastrointestinal problems, the most common is diarrhoea, which is usually osmotic in nature. Gastroparesis may be present.

Routes of administration

Enteral feeds

This route supplies nutrients and fluids via an enteral tube when the oral route is inadequate or obstructed. Feeds are administered via a nasogastric, duodenal, jejunal or gastrostomy tube.

Enteral feeding is preferred over parenteral feeding when the gut is functioning normally and oral feeds do not meet the patient's nutritional requirements (McClave *et al.* 1999). Nasogastric tubes may be used in the short term. Nasogastric feeds have a significant risk of pulmonary aspiration. The tubes are easily removed by confused patients and cause irritation to the nasal mucosa and external nares that can be uncomfortable and is an infection risk in immunocompromised patients and hyperglycaemia.

Duodenal and jejunal tubes do not carry the same risk of pulmonary aspiration but the feeds can contribute to gastric intolerance and bloating, especially in the presence of gastroparesis.

Gastroscopy tubes are used in the long term when the stomach is not affected by the primary disease. This may preclude their use in people with established autonomic neuropathy that involves the gastrointestinal tract. The tubes can be inserted through a surgical incision and the creation of a stoma. More commonly, percutaneous endoscopic techniques (PEG) are used (Thomas 2001). Inserting a PEG tube involves making an artificial tract between the stomach and the abdominal wall through which a tube is inserted. The tube can be a balloon tube or a button type that is more discrete and lies flat to the skin. An extension tube is inserted into the gastroscopy tube during feeding.

Gastrostomy (PEG) feeds

Feeds can usually be undertaken 12–24 hours after the tube is inserted but can be given as early as 4–6 hours after tube insertion in special circumstances. The initial feed may be water and or dextrose saline depending on the patient's condition.

Mode of administration

(1) Bolus instillation – may result in distension and delayed gastric emptying. Aspiration can occur. Diarrhoea may be a complication. *This method is not suitable for people with diabetes who have autonomic neuropathy, especially gastroparesis.*

(2) Continuous infusion – via gravity infusion or pump. This can lead to hyperinsulinaemia in Type 2 diabetes because glucose-mediated insulin production occurs. The effect on blood glucose can be minimised by using formulas with a low glycaemic index. Administering insulin via the IV route enables the caloric input to be balanced with the insulin requirements, but is not suitable for long-term use.

The strength of the feeds should be increased gradually to prevent a sudden overwhelming glucose load in the bloodstream. An IV insulin infusion is an ideal method to control blood glucose levels. Blood glucose monitoring is essential to gauge the impact of the feed on blood glucose and appropriately titrate medication doses.

The feeds usually contain protein, fat, and carbohydrate. The carbohydrate is in the form of dextrose, either 25% or 40%, and extra insulin may be needed to account for the glucose load. A balance must be achieved between caloric requirements and blood glucose levels. Patients who are controlled by OHAs usually need insulin while on enteral feeding.

Parenteral feeds

This is administration of nutrients and fluids by routes other than the alimentary canal, that is intravenously via a peripheral or central line.

Mode of administration

Parenteral supplements are either partial or total.

(1) Peripheral – used after gastrointestinal surgery and in malabsorption states. Peripheral access is usually reserved for people in whom central access is difficult or sometimes as a supplement to oral/enteral feeds. It is not suitable if a high dextrose supplement is needed because dextrose irritates the veins, causing considerable discomfort. It can cause significant tissue damage if extravasation occurs.
(2) Central – supplies maximum nutrition in the form of protein, carbohydrate, fats, trace elements, vitamins, and electrolytes. For example, in patients with cancer or burns, larger volumes can be given than via the peripheral route. In addition, it provides long-term access because silastic catheters can be left *in situ* indefinitely. If patients are at risk of sepsis, the site of the central line is rotated weekly using strict aseptic technique. Central lines enable the patient to remain mobile, which aids digestion and reduces the risk of pressure ulcers.

Choice of formula

The particular formula selected depends on the nutritional requirements and absorptive capacity of the patient. It is usual to begin with half strength formula and gradually increase to full strength as tolerated. The aim is to supply adequate:

- fluid
- protein
- carbohydrate
- vitamins and minerals
- essential fatty acids
- sodium spread evenly over the 24 hours.

Nutritional requirements can vary from week-to-week; thus, careful monitoring is essential to ensure the formula is adjusted proactively and appropriately.

Diabetes medication, insulin or oral agents, are adjusted according to the pattern that emerges in the blood glucose profile. The dose depends on the feeds used as well as other prescribed medicines, and the person's condition. Generally, the insulin/OHA doses are calculated according to the caloric intake.

Nursing responsibilities

Care of nasogastric tubes

(1) Explain purpose of tube to patient.
(2) Check position of the tube regularly to ensure it is in the stomach to prevent pulmonary aspiration.
(3) Confirm the position of the tube with an X-ray.
(4) Change the position of the tube in nose daily to avoid pressure areas.
(5) Flush regularly to ensure the tube remains patent.
(6) Check residual gastric volumes regularly to avoid gastric distension and reduce the possibility of aspiration, especially if gastroparesis is present.

Care of PEG tubes

The same care required for nasogastric tubes applies. Additional care:

(1) Monitor gastric aspirates at least daily.
(2) Elevate the head of the bed where there is a risk of pulmonary aspiration.
(3) Weigh the patient to ensure the desired weight outcome is achieved.
(4) Monitor nutritional status, see Chapter 4.
(5) Manage nausea and vomiting if they occur because they increase the risk of aspiration and are uncomfortable for the patient. Record the amount and type of any vomitus. Antinausea medication may be required. Warm herbal teas such as chamomile, peppermint or ginger may be non-medicine alternatives if oral intake is permitted.
(6) If the PEG tube blocks it can sometimes be cleared with a fizzy soft drink but local protocol should be followed because fizzy drinks can lead to electrolyte imbalances if they are used frequently.
(7) Ensure there is adequate fluid in the feeds to avoid dehydration and the consequent risk of hyperosmolar coma, see Chapter 7 (Thomas 2001).

Care of IV and central lines

(1) Dress the insertion site regularly using strict aseptic technique according to usual protocols.
(2) Check position of the central line with a chest X-ray.
(3) Maintain strict aseptic technique.
(4) Maintain patency, usually by intermittently installing heparinised saline (weekly or when line is changed).
(5) Patients should be supine when the central catheter is disconnected and IV giving sets should be carefully primed to minimise the risk of air embolism.

(6) Check catheter for signs of occlusion (e.g. resistance to infusion or difficulty withdrawing a blood sample). Reposition the patient: if the occlusion is still present, consult the doctor.
(7) Observe exit site for any tenderness, redness or swelling. If bleeding occurs around the suture or exit site apply pressure and notify the doctor.
(8) Monitor the patient for signs of infection, for example, fever. Note that elevated white cell count may not be a sign of infection in people with diabetes if hyperglycaemia is present.

General nursing care

(1) Ensure the person is referred to a dietitian.
(2) Maintain an accurate fluid balance chart, including loss from stomas, drain tubes, vomitus, and diarrhoea.
(3) Monitor serum albumin, urea and electrolytes to determine nutritional requirements, nitrogen balance, and energy requirements.
(4) Weigh regularly (weekly) at the same time, using the same scales with the person wearing similar clothing to ensure energy balance and sufficient calories are supplied. Excess calories leads to weight gain and hyperglycaemia. Insufficient calories leads to weight loss and increases the risk of hypoglycaemia.
(5) Monitor blood glucose regularly, at least 4-hourly, initially. If elevated, be aware of possibility of a hyperosmolar event (see Chapter 7). If stable, monitor less frequently.
(6) Record temperature, pulse and respiration and report if elevated (>38°C) or if any respiratory distress occurs.
(7) Check the date and appearance of all infusions before they are administered.
(8) Medications are given separately from the formula check with the pharmacist which medicines can be added to the formula. Follow pump instructions and local guidelines carefully. Be very careful with look alike and sound alike medicines.
(9) Skin fold thickness and mid-arm muscle circumference measurement can also be useful to ascertain weight loss/gain.
(10) Skin care around tube insertion sites and stoma care for gastrostomy tubes to prevent infection.

Care when recommencing oral feeds

(1) Monitor blood glucose very carefully. Long-acting insulin is usually commenced at this time so there is a risk of hypoglycaemia. Only rapid or short-acting insulin can be given by the IV route.
(2) Monitor and control nausea or vomiting, describe vomitus.
(3) Maintain accurate fluid balance chart, usually 2-hourly subtotals.

DIABETES AND CANCER

Diabetes has been linked to various forms of cancer but the relationship is not straightforward. There appears to be an increased risk of cancer of the pancreas, liver, and kidney (Wideroff *et al.* 1997). Endometrial cancer also appears to be associated with diabetes and obesity (Wideroff *et al.* 1997). Diabetes may be an early sign of pancreatic cancer (Vecchia *et al.* 1994). A recent study demonstrated a significant increased risk for all cancers at moderately elevated HbA_{1c} levels (6–6.9%) with a small increased risk at high levels (>7%) (Travier *et al.* 2007). These findings support the hypothesis that abnormal glucose metabolism is associated with an increased risk of some cancers but may not explain the mechanism.

Researchers have also suggested diabetes is an independent predictor of death from colon, pancreas, liver, and bladder cancer and breast cancer in men and women (Coughlin *et al.* 2004). Verlato *et al.* (2003) reported increased risk of death from breast cancer in women with Type 2 diabetes compared with non-diabetics and suggested controlling weight reduced the mortality rate. Likewise, median survival time is shorter (Bloomgarden 2001).

The management of the cancer itself is the same for people with diabetes as for other people; however, some extra considerations apply. Cancer cells trap amino acids for their own use, limiting the protein available for normal body functions. This sets the scene for weight loss, especially where the appetite is poor, and the senses of smell and taste are diminished. Weight loss is further exacerbated by malabsorption, nausea and vomiting, and radiation treatment. While weight loss may confer many health benefits it is often excessive in cancer and causes malnutrition, which reduces immunity and affects normal cellular functioning and wound healing. Glucose enters cancer cells down a concentration gradient rather than through insulin-mediated entry and metabolism favours lactate production that is transported to the liver, increasing gluconeogenesis. Hypoalbuminaemia also occurs.

For the person with diabetes this can contribute to hyperglycaemia and reduce insulin production, with consequent effects on blood glucose control. Hyperglycaemia is associated with higher infection rates and the risk is significantly increased in immuno-compromised patients and those on corticosteroid medications.

Diabetic management should be considered in relation to the prognosis and the cancer therapy. Preventing the long-term complications of diabetes may be irrelevant if the prognosis is poor, but controlling hyperglycaemia has benefits for comfort, quality of life, and functioning during the dying process (Quinn *et al.* 2006). However, many people have existing diabetes complications such as renal and cardiac disease that need to be considered. For example, the chemotherapeutic agent cisplatin causes renal insufficiency and can exacerbate existing renal disease; cisplatin, paclitaxel, and vincristine might exacerbate neuropathy. Side effects from chemotherapeutic agents are usually permanent. Where the prognosis is good, improving the complication status as much as possible and controlling blood glucose and lipids may help minimise the impact of chemotherapy.

Specific treatment depends on the type of cancer the patient has. Diagnosis of some types of cancer (e.g. endocrine tumours) can involve prolonged fasting and radiological imaging and/or other radiological procedures. The appropriate care should be given in these circumstances (see Chapter 9).

Corticosteroid therapy is frequently used in cancer treatment and can precipitate diabetes. Corticosteroids may be required for a prolonged time or given in large doses for a short period. Corticosteroids cause hyperglycaemia even in people without diabetes. Therefore, blood glucose needs to be monitored regularly in patients on corticosteroid medications, which are discussed later in this chapter.

Objectives of care

Primary prevention

People with chronic diseases such as diabetes often do not receive usual preventative health strategies such as cancer screening (Psarakis 2006). For example, Lipscombe *et al.* (2005) found Canadian women with chronic diseases were 32% less likely to receive routine cancer screening even though their doctors regularly monitored them. The discrepancy in screening rates could not be explained by other variables.

Proactive cancer screening and prevention programmes are important and should be promoted to people with diabetes, for example, mammograms, breast self-examination, and prostate checks. The findings also highlight another indication for normoglycaemia, controlling lipids, and weight management. Preventative health care also needs to encompass smoking cessation, reducing alcohol intake, and appropriate exercise and diet.

In addition to the specific management of the cancer indicated by the cancer type and prognosis, diabetes management aims are:

(1) To optimise cancer management to met the needs of the individual.
(2) To achieve as good a lifestyle as possible for as long as possible by optimising comfort, safety, quality of life, and enabling the person to make necessary life decisions by controlling symptoms and providing support and psychological care to the individual and their families.
(3) To achieve an acceptable blood glucose range in order to avoid the distressing symptoms associated with hyperglycaemia. Insulin may be required. The type of insulin and dose and dose regimen depends on individual needs and the effects of other treatment such as medicines and feeding. Insulin analogues such as levemir and glargine may provide adequate control in a simple regimen, see Chapter 5. The short-acting glitinides may be a useful OHA option if vomiting is not an issue.
(4) To prevent malnutrition, dehydration with possible consequent hypoglycaemia, delayed healing and decreased resistance to infection. Diet should be appropriate for the presenting cancer symptom and in some cases is part of the treatment of some cancers. Sufficient protein and carbohydrate are needed for hormone synthesis and to maintain stores that are being depleted by the cancer. Small frequent feeds; enteral or parenteral (TPN) feeds may be needed. Enteral and TPN feeding can lead to hyperglycaemia and be exacerbated by corticosteroid medicines, stress, and infection. Short or rapid acting insulin may be needed, usually 1 unit of insulin to 10 g of carbohydrate initially but higher doses may be needed. As indicated previously, selecting formulas developed for people with diabetes reduces the impact on blood glucose. High fibre diets can cause diarrhoea, vomiting, and bloating if the cancer involves the bowel.
(5) To adequately control pain.
(6) Control nausea and vomiting, which are common side effects of chemotherapeutic agents as well as some cancers. The possibility of ketoacidosis and hyperosmolar states must be considered. Other causes include bowel obstruction, gastroparesis, infection, lover disease, medicine interactions, and increased intracranial pressure such as cerebral oedema and radiation therapy. Nausea and vomiting can affect hydration status and physical comfort.

(7) To prevent trauma.
(8) To monitor renal and hepatic function during administration of cytotoxic drugs.
(9) To provide education and psychological support.

Nursing responsibilities

(1) To provide a safe environment.
(2) To consider the psychological aspects of having cancer and diabetes (fear of death, body image changes, denial, loss).
(3) To ensure appropriate diabetic education if diabetes develops as a consequence of the altered metabolism of cancer or medicines.
(4) To attend to pressure areas, including the feet and around nasogastric tubes.
(5) To provide oral care, manage stomatitis and mucositis, and ensure a dental consultation occurs.
(6) To control nausea, vomiting and pain, which contribute to fatigue and reduce quality of life.
(7) To manage radiotherapy. Fatigue often occurs as a consequence of radiotherapy; the rates vary between 14% and 90% of patients and can have a significant impact on quality of life and recovery (Faithful 1998). Radiotherapy is usually localised to a specific site and side effect are also usually localised but radiation-induced pneumonitis and fibrosis (late complication) can exacerbate fatigue and cause considerable discomfort, which compounds fatigue. The pattern of fatigue changes over the course of treatment and often declines on no-radiotherapy days. Ensuring the person understands and is given strategies to help them cope with fatigue is essential. Information should be oral and written. Stress management and relaxation techniques can be helpful as can providing an environment conducive to rest and sleep.
(8) To monitor blood glucose levels as frequently as necessary.
(9) To accurately chart fluid balance, blood glucose, TPR, weight.
(10) To ensure referral to the dietitian, psychologist, diabetes nurse specialist/educator.
(11) To be aware of the possibility of hypoglycaemia if the patient is not eating, is vomiting or has a poor appetite. Where the appetite is poor and food intake is inadequate hypoglycaemia is a significant risk. QID insulin regimes using rapid-acting insulin such as Novorapid or Humalog and/or long-acting insulin analogues may reduce the hypoglycaemia risk. Oral hypoglycaemic agents with long duration of action may need to be stopped because of the risk of hypoglycaemia. In addition, if hypoglycaemia does occur it can be more profound and the energy reserves may be insufficient to correct it. Short-acting sulphonylureas or insulin may be indicated in Type 2 diabetes. Biguanides may be contraindicated if renal or hepatic failure is present because of the risk of lactic acidosis. TZDs take some time to have an optimal effect, are difficult to adjust in the short term, and contribute to oedema, which might cause a decrease in haemoglobin and contribute to fatigue. They may be useful if prolonged low-dose steroids are required (Oyer *et al.* 2006). Incretin mimetics reduce post prandial hyperglycaemia but research into their benefit in corticosteroid use is limited. In addition, they cause significant nausea, vomiting, and weight loss, which can exacerbate malnutrition and increase morbidity in people with cancer.
(12) To be aware of the possibility of hyperglycaemia as a result of medications such as corticosteroids, pain and stress.

(13) To monitor biochemistry results and report abnormal results.

(14) To provide appropriate care during investigative and surgical procedures, see Chapter 9.

(15) To consider the possibility that people with cancer often try complementary therapies in an attempt to cure or manage their cancer. It is important to ask about the use of complementary therapies and provide or refer the person for appropriate information about the risks and benefits of such therapies (see Chapter 19).

(16) To maintain skin integrity by appropriate skin care especially where corticosteroid medications are used. They cause the skin to become thin and fragile and it is easily damaged during shaving and routine nursing care, brittle hair, which can exacerbate the effects of chemotherapy, and bone loss. Corticosteroids are also associated with mood changes, which can cause distress to the patient and their relatives. Careful explanations and reassurance are required.

Clinical observations

(1) Narcotic pain medication can mask the signs of hypoglycaemia.

(2) Insulin/oral agents may need to be adjusted frequently to meet the changing metabolic needs and prevailing appetite and food intake. In the terminal stages of cancer they may be withheld, so long as the patient is comfortable and not subject to excursions in blood glucose that can lead to symprims, dehydration, and discomfort.

Managing corticosteroids in people with cancer

People with cancer are often prescribed glucocorticoids as a component of chemotherapy to prevent or manage nausea, reduce inflammation or following neurological procedures. These medicines cause postprandial hyperglycaemia by downregulating GLUT-4 transporters in muscle, which impairs glucose entry into cells. They also promote gluconeogenesis. Not all glucocorticoids have the same effect on glucose. The effect depends on the dose, duration of action, and duration of treatment. Morning prednisolone doses usually cause elevated blood glucose after meals but the blood glucose usually drops overnight and is lower in the morning.

Complementary therapies and cancer

Many people with cancer use a variety of complementary therapies (CAM). Estimates vary from 7% to 83%: mean 31%. High usage occurs in children, older people, those with specific cancers such as prostate and breast cancer (Fernandez *et al.* 1998; Wyatt *et al.* 1999; Kao & Devine 2000; Boon *et al.* 2000). The type of CAM therapies used varies among countries and ethnic and cultural groups. Distinctive characteristics of CAM users with cancer include:

• Women.
• Younger age.

- Higher education.
- Higher socioeconomic group.
- Prior CAM use.
- Active coping and preventive health care behaviours and a desire to do everything possible to maintain or improve health and quality of life, as well as take an active part in management decisions.
- Participation in cancer support groups.
- Having a close friend or relative with cancer.
- Changed health beliefs as a consequence of developing cancer.

Many conventional practitioners are concerned that CAM holds out false hope of a cure, interferes with or delays conventional treatment, the risk of CAM medicine side effects and interactions, and because not all CAM is evidence based. Many of these concerns are well founded. Chapter 19 discusses CAM in more detail.

Where CAM is used it needs to be integrated into the care plan to optimise the benefits of both CAM and conventional management strategies. Some benefits include longer survival time and improved quality of life using mind body medicine (Spiegal *et al.* 1989; Wolker *et al.* 1999); and reduction in chemotherapy induced stomatitis (Oberbaum *et al.* 2001).

Useful CAM strategies include:

- Mind body therapies such as relaxation techniques, meditation, massage, and creative therapies such as music, art, and writing.
- Gentle exercise such as some forms of Tai Chi, walking that can include pet therapy (e.g. walking the dog).
- Essential oils can be used in psychological care as well as massage and education and some reduce stomatitis (Wilkinson 2008). The oils need to be chosen to suit the individual because some odours contribute to nausea or may provoke unpleasant memories. Alternatively they can recall happy memories.
- Nutritional medicine that focuses on a healthy well balanced diet, whole foods, low in fat and sugar and using vitamin and mineral supplements especially in immunocompromised patients if they are not contraindicated. Probiotics can help sustain normal gut flora. Soy products and vitamin D supplementation improve bone mineral density.
- Acupressure to acupuncture point P6 reduces nausea, and is a useful addition to conventional methods of controlling nausea (Dibble *et al.* 2007).
- Herbal medicines such as milk thistle complement the action of chemotherapy and reduce the toxic effects on the liver in animal models (Lipman 2003) and anti-inflammatory agents such as curcumin.

Practice point

Since the introduction of serotonin inhibitors, for example, Ondansetron, to control nausea and vomiting, these effects of chemotherapy have decreased. Consequently there is less disruption of normal eating patterns.

SMOKING, ALCOHOL, AND ILLEGAL DRUG USE

Substance use refers to intentionally using a pharmacological substance to achieve a desired effect: recreational or therapeutic. The term 'use' does not imply illegal use and is non-judgmental. However, the term 'substance abuse' is both negative and judgmental. Continued drug abuse can become an addiction. The American Psychiatric Association (2000) defined criteria for diagnosing psychiatric disease including drug abuse and drug addiction, see Table 10.1.

Smoking

Giving up smoking is the easiest thing in the world. I know because I've done it thousands of times.

(Mark Twain)

The prevalence of smoking has decreased in many countries but smoking continues to be the most common morbidity and mortality risk factor (Australian Institute of Health and Welfare 2006). Smoking is hazardous to health regardless of whether the individual has diabetes or not. In addition, constantly being in a smoke filled environment is a hazard for non-smokers causing ~50 000 death annually in the US (Surgeon General's Report 2006). Smoking during pregnancy has adverse effects on the fetus as well as the mother's health.

Nicotine is the primary alkaloid found in tobacco and is responsible for addiction to cigarettes. Tobacco also contains ~69 carcinogens in the tar, the particulate matter that remains when nicotine and water are removed, 11 of these are known carcinogens and a further 7 are probably carcinogens (Kroon 2007). Of these, polycyclic aromatic hydrocarbons (PAH) are the major lung carcinogens and are potent hepatic

Table 10.1 American Psychiatric Association criteria for drug abuse and drug addiction. Drug abuse is diagnosed when a person exhibits three of these criteria for 12 months.

Criteria for drug abuse	Criteria for drug dependence/addiction
Recurrent drug use and not fulfilling important/usual life roles. Using drugs in dangerous situations. Encountering legal problems from using drugs. Continuing to use drugs despite encountering problems.	Tolerance. Withdrawal symptoms when not using. Taking increasing amounts over time and for longer than intended (needing more drug to achieve and effect). Wanting to or unsuccessfully trying to reduce use or quit. Spending a considerable amount of time obtaining, using or recovering from drug use. Usual activities are affected by drug use. Continuing to use despite knowing it is harmful.

cytochrome P-450 inducers, particularly 1A1, 1A2 and possible 2E1. Thus smoking and quitting can interact with commonly prescribed medicines and foods. Smoking status is an important aspect of routine medication reviews and prescribing.

Interactions occur between tobacco smoke and many commonly prescribed medicines. With respect to diabetes these include:

- Subcutaneous and inhaled insulin. Absorption of subcutaneous insulin may be reduced due to insulin resistance, which is associated with smoking. Inhaled insulin is rarely used. Smoking enhances absorption rates and peak action time is faster and insulin blood levels are higher than in non-smokers.
- Propanolol and other beta blocking agents.
- Heparin: reduced half-life and increased clearance.
- Hormone contraceptives particularly combination formulations.
- Inhaled corticosteroids, which may have reduced efficacy in people with asthma.
- Tricyclic antidepressants.
- Other medicines such as olanzapine, clozapine, benzodiazepines, and opoids (Zevin & Benowitz 1999).

Other medicines and foods may also be affected leading to less than optional therapeutic effects and subtle malnutrition. Dose adjustments of many medicines may be required when people smoke and may need to be readjusted once they quit. The side effects of medicines may contribute to withdrawal symptoms.

People most likely to smoke:

- Are members of some ethnic groups such as Indigenous Australians, African American, and Hispanics.
- Have a mental health problem, 70% of people with a mental health problem smoke. In addition, people often commence smoking when they develop a mental health problem.
- Use illegal drugs and/or alcohol.

Quitting smoking reduces the risk of cardiovascular disease, respiratory disease, cancer and a range of other diseases, and dying before age 50 by 50% in the following 15 years. The risk of developing many of these conditions is increased in the presence of obesity and uncontrolled diabetes. Smoking in middle and old age is significantly associated with a reduction in healthy life years (Ostbye & Taylor 2004). A recent meta-analysis of observational studies suggests smoking increases the risk of developing Type 2 diabetes in a dose-dependent manner (Willi *et al.* 2007). Willi *et al.* found smoking was independently associated with glucose intolerance, impaired fasting glucose and Type 2 diabetes.

Quitting smoking is difficult and requires significant behaviour change on the part of the individual. In order to change, they must first recognise there is a problem and the scale of the problem. The desire to change may not be the same as wanting help to change. Almost 75% of smokers report they want to quit (Owen *et al.* 1992), but <7% remain smoke free after 12 months and the average smoker tries to quite 6–9 times in their lifetime (American Cancer Society 2007). Smoking at night appears to be a predictor of nicotine dependence and is a significant predictor of relapsing within 6 months of trying to quit (Bover *et al.* 2008). In addition, smoking at night is associated with poor treatment outcomes (Foulds *et al.* 2006). Bover *et al.* suggested health professionals should specifically ask about night smoking when assessing readiness to quit.

Research suggests timing smoking cessation interventions to coincide with the individual's readiness to change is important to success. In addition, sociologists highlight the importance of life course transitions in behaviour change and suggest the longer people live the more likely they are to make transitions in later life and the more likely such transitions are to be accompanied by changes in behaviour (George 1993). Thus targeting smoking cessation interventions to coincide with life transitions may be more likely to succeed.

For example, Lang *et al.* (2007) suggest individuals retiring from work are more likely to stop smoking than those who remain at work after controlling for retiring due to ill health. They recommended interventions be developed for those making the transition to retirement and employers should incorporate smoking cessation programmes into their retirement plans. Health events, particularly those that are disabling or affect work and lifestyle also affect smoking cessation rates (Falba 2005). These and other studies suggest several key transitions that could be used target smoking cessation in addition to regular prevention messages.

Nicotine addiction

Nicotine receptors, $\alpha_4\beta_2$ nicotinic acetylcholine receptors (nAChRs), are located throughout the central nervous system. Nicotine binds to these receptors, and acts as an agonist prolonging activation of these receptors and facilitating the release of neurotransmitters such as acetylcholine, dopamine, serotonin, and beta-endorphins, which engenders pleasurable feelings, arousal, reduced anxiety and relaxation. Nicotine action mode reinforces dependence in a cyclical manner: smoking stimulates dopamine, the dopamine level falls as the nicotine level falls producing withdrawal symptoms. Smoking again suppresses the cravings by restimulating the nAChRs receptors.

The area of the brain concerned with addiction appears to be the insula, a small structure within the cerebral cortex. People with damage to the insula from trauma or stroke often suddenly stop smoking and remain non-smoking (Naqvi *et al.* 2007). Five milligrams of nicotine per day is a large enough dose to cause addiction. Each cigarette contains between 0.13 and 2 mg of nicotine, thus even light smokers can be addicted. Nicotine is present in the blood stream within 15 seconds of smoking a cigarette, which provides immediate gratification (Watkins *et al.* 2000). Chronic nicotine use desensitises the receptors and increasing amounts of nicotine are required to achieve pleasurable effects.

Withdrawal symptoms usually occur within the first 24 hours and can be very stressful. Withdrawal symptoms include:

- Craving tobacco.
- Difficulty concentrating, which affects work and usual daily activities.
- Headache.
- Impaired motor performance.
- Fatigue.
- Irritability.
- Anxiety and restlessness.

• Sleep disturbances.
• Nausea.
• Hunger and weight gain. Concern about putting on weight can be a barrier to quitting.

All of these symptoms can lead to neglect of diabetes self-care. Smoking cessation programms need to help the individual manage these symptoms.

Assisting the person to stop smoking

Brief advice from general practitioners (GPs) and other health professionals has a limited effect: only 2–3% quit per year (Lancaster & Stead 2004) but the effect size can be increased if other strategies are also used. These include referral to Quitline, interested supportive follow up, setting achievable goals and pharmacotherapy. The 5As approach can be helpful. It consists of:

Ask about smoking habits and systematically document the information at each visit. Provide brief advice to quit in a clear supportive, non-judgmental manner regularly.

Assess interest in quitting so that advice can be appropriately targeted to the stage of change and to opportunistically support attempts to quit. Assess whether the individual has tried to quit in the past and the factors that prevented them from quitting and those that helped, as well as the level of nicotine dependence: ~70–80% of smokers are dependent on nicotine and will experience withdrawal symptoms when they try to quit. Nicotine addiction is a chronic relapsing condition (Wise *et al.* 2007). Repeated efforts to quit can be demoralising and set up learned helplessness. Helping the individual manage the symptoms can support their attempt. Sometimes mental health problems become apparent when a person stops smoking, thus mental health should be monitored.

Advise about the importance of quitting on a regular basis and provide new information as it arises. Advice can include information about smoking risks and quit programmes. Advice is more useful if it is tailored to the individual. In Australia some health insurance funds offer member discounts to quit programmes such as Allen Carr's EasyWay to Stop Smoking. This method consists of a combination of psychotherapy and hypnotherapy.

Assist those who indicate they want to quit by asking what assistance they feel would help them most, refer them for counselling, provide written information or recommend other therapies as indicated and follow up at the next visit. Relapsing after attempting to quit is common. Praise and support are essential as are exploring the reasons for relapsing and discussing strategies for continuing the quit process. Motivational interviewing can be a useful technique.

Arrange a follow-up visit preferably within the first week after the quit date (The US Public Health Service 2000). Some pharmaceutical companies offer support programmes through newsletters and Internet sites. Fu *et al.* (2006) showed 75% of relapsed smokers were interested in repeating the quit intervention (behavioural and medicines strategies) within 30 days of quitting, which highlights the importance of support and constant reminders. Advising and supporting partners may also be important.

Non-pharmacological strategies can be combined with the 5As. These include opportunistic and structured counselling that encourages the individual to think about the relevance of quitting to their life, helps them identify their personal health risks, and helps them determine the barriers and facilitators they are likely to encounter develop strategies to strengthen the facilitators and overcome the barriers.

Improving nutrition is important to health generally. Diets rich in tyrosine, tryptophane, and vitamins B_6, B_3, C, and magnesium, zinc, and iron may stimulate the dopamine pathway and help reduce the effects of nicotine withdrawal by increasing serotonin levels (Oisiecki 2006). Improving nutrition can also reduce oxidative damage, which is increased in smokers and help reduce weight gain.

CAM strategies may help manage withdrawal symptoms. These include acupuncture and acupressure to specific points to reduce the withdrawal symptoms (Mitchell 2008). Patients may be able to learn to self-stimulate specific acupressure points. Treatment consists of biweekly session for two weeks and then weekly for 2–6 weeks. Herbal preparations include green tea and lemon balm tea capsules, which improves focus and concentration and reduces anxiety without causing drowsiness; Ashwaganda capsules, an Ayurvedic medicine, which increases energy levels and wellbeing, *Silymarin* (milk thistle) before meals to control blood glucose and support the liver, flower remedies, melatonin and high-dose vitamin B. All of these interventions need to be combined with education, support, and counselling.

Self-help websites describe a time frame when symptoms resolve and people can expect to feel better, which gives them a goal to aim for. They also suggest some steps to stopping, which include:

- Make a firm decision to stop and ask for help without shame or guilt.
- Ask people who successfully quitted how they did it.
- Quit with a friend to support each other.
- Wash your clothes and air out the house to get rid of the smell and if possible avoid smoke filled environments.
- Write down the reasons you want to quit and the things that can help you succeed.
- Get information about all the quit options and decide which one/s is most likely to suit you.
- Set small achievable goals.

These strategies can be included in other strategies.

Medications to support smoking cessation

A number of medicines are available to assist smoking cessation but they are not a substitute for counselling and support, which need to continue if medications are indicated. Commonly used medicines to help people quit smoking are shown in Table 10.2. A combination of dose forms can be used, for example, patches and gums. In addition, nicotine replacement therapy can be prescribed for pregnant and lactating women but non-medicine options are preferred, people with cardiovascular disease, and young people aged 12–17 years (Tonstad *et al.* 2006).

Table 10.2 Medicines available to assist people to quit smoking. They should be combined with other counselling and support strategies and good nutrition and be considered as part of the medication record and their benefits and risks reviewed regularly while they are being used. The prescribing information should be consulted for specific information about each medicine.

Medicine	Dose	Duration of treatment	Side effects and precautions
Nicotine formulations: Gum (Nicorette)	2–4 mg: 1 piece of gum 1–2 hourly	Up to 12 weeks	Sore mouth, hiccups, dyspepsia Caution: unstable angina, 2 weeks post MI, serious cardiac arrhythmias Acidic drinks and caffeine affect absorption
Lozenge	2–4 mg: 1 lozenge 1–2 hourly for 6 weeks then 1 every 2–4 hours in weeks 7–9 and 1 every 4–8 hours in weeks 10–12 (9–20/day according to need).	Up to 12 weeks	Caution: uncontrolled hypertension, recent MI, arrhythmias, gastric ulcers, diabetes.
Transdermal patch (NicoDerm CQ, habitrol)	Available in 7, 14, and 21 mg doses. Patch applied every 16–24 hours	8–10 weeks	Localised skin reactions, headaches, disturbed sleep Caution: unstable angina, 2 weeks after MI, cardiac arrhythmias.
Inhaled	168 cartridges; 10 mg nicotine/cartridge but delivered dose is 4 mg; 1–2 doses/hour as required.	Up to 8 weeks dose needs to be reduced in the last 4–6 weeks.	Nasal irritation Caution: unstable angina, 2 weeks after MI, cardiac arrhythmias. Contraindicated if severe airways disease such as asthma and COPD is present.
Nasal spray	100 mg nicotine/10 mL bottle, dose delivered per spray is 0.5 mg; one dose is 1 mg in each nostril (1 spray).	Up to 6 months	Nasal irritation. May be contraindicated if severe airways disease such as asthma and COPD is present.
Bupropion SR (Zyban)	Starting dose 150 mg/day for 3 days then 150 mg BD.	Up to 24 weeks	Nausea, vomiting, constipation.
Varenicline (Chantix)	Starting dose 0.5 mg/day for 3 days then 0.5 mg BD for 3 days followed by 1 mg BD.	Up to 24 weeks	Nausea, vomiting, constipation.

MI = myocardial infarction.

Other medicines and an anti-nicotine vaccine are currently being developed to reduce the link between smoking and nicotine concentration in the brain to lower the related gratification. Transcranial magnetic stimulation (TMS) may be adapted in the future to specifically target the insula. Currently, TMS does not penetrate beyond peripheral tissues.

Alcohol addiction

Alcohol is also an addictive substance associated with significant morbidity and mortality. Between 15% and 20% of GP consultations relate to alcohol (Lee 2008). Short-term consequences include injury and domestic violence; longer term effects include other risk taking behaviours such as smoking, neglected self-care, driving while intoxicated, cognitive impairment, peripheral neuropathy, liver cirrhosis, and fetal damage in pregnant women. Approximately 10% of Australians and 20% of Indigenous Australians drink more than the recommended level (National Health and Medical Research Council (NHMRC) 2007). Young people are also likely to consume higher than recommended amounts of alcohol. Recommendations for alcohol intake were discussed in Chapter 1 and are defined in the draft NHMRC guidelines.

The criteria for alcohol dependence are three of the following seven features:

- Alcohol tolerance.
- Withdrawal symptoms.
- Drinking more than the recommended level or for longer than planned.
- Previous unsuccessful attempts to reduce consumption or stop drinking.
- Spending a significant amount of time procuring or drinking alcohol.
- Neglecting social interactions and work responsibilities because of alcohol.
- Continuing to drink despite the actual and potential health risks.

The strategies outlined for helping people quit smoking can be adapted to help people reduce alcohol consumption to the recommended levels or stop drinking. Screening for alcohol dependence can be accomplished using the World Health Organisation (WHO) Alcohol Use Disorders Identification Test (AUDIT) (Saunders *et al.* 1993). High AUDIT scores indicate the need for a comprehensive intervention and counselling. Support groups such as Alcoholics Anonymous have a well-recognised role in stopping drinking and preventing relapse.

Diabetes is difficult to manage because oral hypoglycaemic agents are often contraindicated because of the risk of lactic acidosis (metformin) and hypoglycaemia. Insulin is often indicated but adherence is often suboptimal and is compounded by erratic intake and malnutrition. Withdrawal processes for heavy drinkers need to be supervised and people require a significant amount of support.

Medicines to assist alcohol withdrawal include acamprosate and naltrexon, which are generally well tolerated and can be continued if the person drinks alcohol. They are effective at preventing relapse, delaying return to drinking and reducing drinking days. Disulfiram (Antabuse) causes acute illness if the person drinks alcohol while taking the medication. Supervision is required if Antabuse is used because life-threatening reactions can occur. It is not the ideal first-line treatment and probably should only be prescribed by doctors with experience using it or use it under the guidance of such experts (Shand *et al.* 2003).

Illegal drug use

The effect of marijuana, cocaine, and other illegal drugs on diabetes is unclear. These substances are associated with poor health outcomes and risk-taking behaviours in non-diabetics and people with diabetes. In addition, illegal drugs and the associated risks may compound or contribute to short- and long-term diabetes complications. The fact that they are illegal makes illegal drug use harder to detect. Generally, illegal drugs fall into three main categories:

- Uppers, for example, ecstasy, ice, crystal meth, cocaine, snow, speed.
- Opiates, for example, morphine, heroin, smack.
- Hallucinogens, for example, marijuana (cannabis, pot, weed), LSD, solvents such as petrol, glue, and paint. Table 10.3 outlines the effects of these substances and their impact on blood glucose.

In addition, many herbs have psychogenic properties. They may be stimulants, sedative, cognitive enhancing or analgesics as well as uppers, hallucinogens, or act in a similar way to opiates (Spinella 2005). Significantly, herbs may contain more than one chemical substance and are sometimes used to manufacture illegal drugs. Examples include but are not limited to:

- *Acorus calamus* (calamus). Ecstasy can be manufactured from calamus.
- *Salvia divinorum*
- Ephedra species
- *Amantia muscaria* (magic mushrooms)
- A herbal mixture called hoasia, yaje, or daime.

The effect of any drug depends on its pharmacokinetics and pharmacodynamics, bio-availability, and elimination. Thus, the effect depends on the administration route, how the individual metabolises drugs and is usually dose dependent. Common routes of illegal drug administration are:

- enteral
  - oral
  - sublingual
  - rectal
- parenteral
  - IV
- subcutaneous, for example, 'skin popping' heroin
- inhalation smoking, pipe, cigarettes, hookah.

Effects on diabetes

Illegal drugs appear to have two inter-related consequences for people with diabetes: physical effects, although the pharmacological effects on blood glucose appear to be minor (Glick 2008), effect on cognitive processes, which disrupt problem-solving, decision-making, and self-care. Cognitive effects are significant and contribute to erratic blood glucose control. They are also associated with other general health risks such as sexually transmitted disease, malnutrition, and reduced immunity, which impact on diabetes related well being.

As well as contributing to the development of long-term diabetes complication through inadequate self-care and hyperglycaemia, addiction to some illegal drugs exacerbate existing diabetes complications. Illegal drugs exert significant haemodynamic and electrophysiological effects. The specific effects depend on the dose, the degree of addiction (see Table 10.3), and the drug formulation. Marijuana, the most commonly used illegal drug, is associated with cerebrovascular events and peripheral vascular events (Moussouttas 2004) and atrial fibrillation and increased cardiovascular morbidity (Korantzopoulos *et al.* 2008). Smoking exacerbates the vascular effects and nerve damage may be exacerbated by excessive alcohol use.

Cardiovascular effects include:

- Slight increase in blood pressure especially in the supine position.
- Rapid tachycardia, most likely due to enhanced automaticity of the sinus node, which increases cardiac output and reduces oxygen carrying capacity due to increased carboxyhaemoglobin when smoking marijuana.
- Constriction of blood vessels increasing the risk of cardiovascular and cerebrovascular disease, for example, cocaine.
- Reduced peripheral vascular resistance but the extent varies in different peripheral sites.
- Angina and acute coronary syndromes especially in older people with postural or orthostatic hypotension.

Interactions with medicines

Information about interactions between illegal drugs and OHA and insulin is unclear but some drugs might affect OHA/insulin bioavailability. In addition, the different illegal drugs and the different dose forms (inhaled, smoked, intravenous, oral) are likely to have different pharmacodynamics and pharmacokinetics (Brown 1991). A significant problem is the fact that many such drugs are manufactured illegally and there are no quality control standard processes to ascertain purity, bioavailability, or the contents of the drug.

Management issues

Management is challenging and requires a great deal of tact and understanding. Referral to an appropriate 'drug and alcohol' service is advisable. Health professionals should be able to identify illegal drug use and refer early to reduce the likelihood of addiction developing, see Table 10.3. Strategies include:

- Providing an environment where patients feel safe and able to discuss difficult issues.
- Taking a thorough medical, work and social history, and monitoring changes.

Table 10.3 The effects of the drug or drug combination and duration of action depends on a number of factors including the dose and frequency of use and individual factors. Long-term use can contribute to psychiatric disorders and conversely psychiatric disorders can trigger illegal drug use. Illegal drugs can interact with conventional and/or complementary medicines and sometimes alcohol. All can lead to addiction, which has social, professional and financial implications and increases the risk of inadequate diabetes care, coma, and death.

Main class of illegal drug	Duration of action	Possible effect on blood glucose[a]	Some commonly reported effects
Uppers	Usually 4–6 but up to 24 hours	Hyperglycaemia from missing injections/OHA increasing the risk of ketoacidosis (DKA)/hyperosmolar states (HONK). Hypoglycaemia due to inadequate intake, nausea, and vomiting	Increased energy Tachycardia Weakness and lethargy Heightened sensations Ecstasy can cause boundless energy and the user might not want to rest or eat. Cocaine often reduces appetite. Sleep disturbances and/or lethargy and prolonged sleep due to 'come down' as the effects of the drug wear off. Dilated pupils. Nausea and/or vomiting Weight loss Impaired memory and cognition. These affect self-care and the ability to recognise hypoglycaemia.
Opiates	4–24 hours	Hypo or hyperglycaemia due to inadequate self-care such as OHA/insulin mismanagement and increased risk of DKA/HONK.	Euphoria Hallucinations. Relaxation. Slurred speech. Disinhibition Confusion and altered perception. Diminished libido Constricted pupils. Nausea/vomiting. Pain relief (therapeutic use).

(Continued)

Table 10.3 Continued.

Main class of illegal drug	Duration of action	Possible effect on blood glucose[a]	Some commonly reported effects
Hallucinogens	Often rapid onset, for example, Cannabis begins acting within 6–12 minutes and may be stored in fat deposits for weeks.	Hyperglycaemia due to increased intake and/or forgetting to take OHA/insulin. Increased possibility of DKA/HONK. Hypoglycaemia with some drugs such as large doses of marijuana.	Euphoria and disorientation Hallucinations Disinhibition Marijuana increases appetite. Difficulty with coordination, making judgement. Tiredness Can lead to psychiatric disorders including depression and paranoia.

[a]Note the effects on blood glucose may not be a direct effect of the drug but a consequence of cognitive impairment, effects on judgement, hypoglycaemia symptoms not recognised or confused with the effect of the drug, and inadequate self-care (Brink 2008 in Glick 2003). Frequent blood glucose testing is recommended if a person with diabetes uses illegal drugs but the cognitive effects of the drugs often means they do not test.

- Assess whether there are any existing mental health problems and their relationship to illegal drug use.
- Assess diabetes status and self-care capacity and provide information about ways to enhance safety that are consistent with the advice of the specific drug service if they continue to use illegal drugs. Having appropriate information about how drugs work and their potential effects can help the individual develop strategies to reduce the risk of immediate and long-term adverse events if they continue to use drugs. Diabetes-specific advice might include the:
  - Importance of frequent blood glucose testing.
  - Need to test for ketones if the blood glucose is high especially Type 1 diabetes.
  - Need to continue OHA/insulin but the fact that the doses may need to be adjusted according to blood glucose tests; advice about how to make such adjustments may be needed.
  - Importance of maintaining adequate fluid and food intake to avoid dehydration.
  - Importance of being able to recognise and treat hypoglycaemia and strategies for distinguishing hypoglycaemia from the effects of the drug.
  - Importance of seeking medical advice early if they are unwell, develop an infection, for example, at IV drug injection sites, have intractable nausea and/or vomiting, depression.
  - Ways to reduce personal risk such as:
    making sure they obtain drugs from a reputable source
    using sterile techniques and not sharing needles (e.g. risk of HIV and hepatitis C) or pipes/hookahs (e.g. risk of TB, influenza)
    not driving after using illegal drugs
    practicing safe sex
    using with a trusted person who can support their self-care and seek medical care if an adverse event occurs and using in a safe environment.
  - safe sharps disposal.

Practice points

(1) Although the risk of psychiatric disorders is high, not all illegal drug users have psychiatric disorders and not all people with psychiatric conditions use illegal drugs.

(2) The advice is easy to give but very difficult to follow because of the mental effects of most drugs on cognition, decision-making and judgement, which affect self-care capacity.

(3) Larger doses of drugs are often needed to achieve the desired effect as addiction worsens.

(4) Coffee, tea, and chocolate are also stimulants.

BRITTLE DIABETES

'Brittle diabetes' means different things to different people.

Introduction

There is no easy way to define brittle diabetes. Some experts consider it to be a psychological condition; others regard it as having a physical basis. Brittle diabetes usually refers to wide fluctuations in the blood glucose pattern despite optimal medical management. Whichever definition is used, brittle diabetes is difficult to manage and requires an holistic approach. Repeated admissions to hospital for bouts of DKA or severe hypoglycaemia are common.

The causes of brittle diabetes are multifactorial. It is easy to ascribe the problem to social/psychological factors alone but this is often not the case. However, there is a subset of people with diabetes, usually young women with Type 1 who have psychosocial problems, who manipulate their insulin and have frequent hospital admissions.

Management

Management is protracted and requires a great deal of patience and support for the person with diabetes and their family. Taking a careful holistic history and a thorough physical assessment can identify physical causes. Physical causes include:

- Impaired insulin response. This could be due to rare conditions such as degradation of insulin at the injection site. In these cases an insulin pump can improve insulin absorption. In other cases insulin absorption from specific injection sites can be reduced or delayed. Changing sites may help (Martin 1995).
- Communication problems such as dyslexia that can make education and therefore self-care difficult. People frequently hide their difficulty, and tactful questioning is needed to identify it.
- Drug addiction.
- Gastroparesis leading to erratic food absorption is discussed in Chapter 8. Other gastrointestinal problems can also be present, for example, coeliac disease, which is discussed in this chapter, and should be excluded.
- Seizure disorders.
- Inappropriate management regimen.
- Presence of other endocrine disorders, for example, thyrotoxicosis. Two to three per cent of people with Type 1 diabetes have Hashimoto's thyroiditis.
- Eating disorders, either under- or overeating.
- Unrecognised hypoglycaemia and inappropriate insulin dose increases that lead to further hypoglycaemia, rebound hyperglycaemia and DKA.

Psychological causes include:

- Anger and non-acceptance of diabetes.
- Difficult relationships where diabetes is used to escape from the situation or to manipulate it, or gain attention.
- Sexual abuse.

A long-term management strategy is required that involves an agreed coordinated care plan that is communicated to all relevant health professionals and the patient and their family/carers. Regular case conferencing with the relevant health professionals is important. Liaison with a psychiatrist is desirable if the underlying cause is psychological, and may help the individual come to terms with their diabetes by going back to the time of diagnosis and exploring the issues in operation at the time. The focus should be taken off 'diabetic control' and placed on quality of life, initially. If other issues are addressed metabolic control is easier to achieve. A basal bolus regimen using rapid-acting insulin can be commenced if it is not already being used.

Role of the nurse

Support and patience are required to manage people with brittle diabetes. Nurses need to be aware that it exists and that it can have a physiological basis as well as an underlying psychological component.

Nurses can play a key role in organising case conferences, supporting diabetes education and identifying barriers to learning. This might include inspecting injection sites and observing the person administering an injection and monitoring their blood glucose.

Follow agreed management protocols and/or identify strategies to enhance management and ensure the person has follow-up appointments with appropriate health professionals on discharge.

Regular blood glucose monitoring in hospital can help identify excursions in blood glucose levels and identify unrecognised hypoglycaemia, which will assist with appropriate care planning.

ORAL HEALTH AND DIABETES

Introduction

People with diabetes are at increased risk of periodontal disease, a deep infection that affects bone caused by bacteria (plaque), which destroys the fibrosis attachment that anchors the teeth to the jaw (Peridontal Position Paper 1996; Holmes & Alexander 1997). Increased glucose levels in saliva and reduced buffering power of saliva because of reduced saliva flow rates has been demonstrated (Connor *et al.* 1970). The pattern of dental decay and the decay rates vary between young and older people with diabetes but are largely unknown.

People with diabetes also have increased rates of oral candidiasis and a range of other oral cavity diseases, for example, lichen planus, painless swelling of the salivary glands (sialosis) that could be due to disordered fat metabolism, and changed taste sensation (Lamey *et al.* 1992).

Symptoms of oral cavity disease

- Bleeding gums.
- Halitosis.
- Inflamed receding gums.

- Loose teeth.
- Painful abscesses are a late symptom and indicate permanent damage.

Of people over 65, 67% have few or no natural teeth. This affects their overall food intake and the type of food selected. There is a propensity towards low fibre, low protein foods. This can represent a significant risk of hypoglycaemia and nutritional deficiencies, which in turn affect mental and physical functioning and quality of life, see Chapters 4, 15, and 12.

Ageing also leads to submucosal changes and increasing prevalence of gum disease due to hyperglycaemia and the resultant dry mouth as well as the effect on tissue and high sugar diets. Saliva production can be reduced (xerostomia) and is often exacerbated by medications that cause dry mouth (NHMRC 1999). The degree of metabolic control, duration, age, and dental hygiene influence the likelihood of gum disease occurring.

Younger people with diabetes are also at risk of tooth and gum disease primarily as a result of inappropriate diet and inadequate dental care.

Causal mechanisms

- Uncontrolled diabetes.
- Microangiopathy.
- Increased collagen breakdown.
- Defective neutrophil function such as reduced chemotaxis and phagocytosis during hyperglycaemia.
- Depressed immune response during hyperglycaemia.

Insulin resistance and deteriorating metabolic control can occur as a result of oral infection and requires adjustment to the diabetic medication regime.

Management

- Consider the possibility of oral problems where signs of infection or deteriorating control are present.
- Include dental assessment in nursing history and assessment.
- Provide opportunities for cleaning teeth during hospitalisation and in aged care facilities.
- Nurses have a responsibility to educate their patients about preventative oral hygiene. This includes:
  - the need to have regular dental checks and education about ways to maintain oral health
  - good blood glucose control
  - eating a healthy well-balanced diet
  - seek dental advice early for any pain, bleeding, redness, and persistent bad breath so infection can be treated early
  - correct method of brushing teeth, not gums, to reduce bleeding risk
- Refer for dental assessment if existing disease is identified.

- Check dentures regularly to ensure they fit.
- Educate dental practitioners about diabetes. Dental practitioners should also be aware of the possibility of hypoglycaemia occurring during dental procedures and how to manage it, see Chapters 6 and 9.

DIABETES AND LIVER DISEASE

Introduction

Research suggests liver disease is an important cause of death in people with Type 2 diabetes (Balkau *et al.* 1991; de Marco *et al.* 1999) and diabetes may be the most common cause of liver disease (US Organ Procurement and Transplantation Network 2005; Tolman *et al.* 2007). Some studies show cirrhosis accounts for 4.4% of diabetes-related deaths (Balkau *et al.* 1991). A range of liver diseases occur in Type 2 diabetes including:

- Abnormal liver enzymes. Elevated alanine transferase (ALT) is common in Type 2 diabetes and may be associated with liver disease. Some studies show elevated ALT is associated with liver disease in up to 98% of cases, commonly fatty liver (NAFLD) and chronic hepatitis. Alkaline phosphatase (AST) may also be elevated.
- Non-alcoholic fatty liver disease (NAFLD), the most common liver disease in Type 2 diabetes. NAFLD is defined as fatty liver disease with no alcohol intake or amounts <20 g/day (Caldwell *et al.* 1999). It is estimated to occur in 34–74% of people with Type 2 diabetes, up to ~100% of obese Type 2 patients (Tolman *et al.* 2007). NAFLD is characterised by a range of liver diseases such as steatosis and non-alcoholic steato-hepatitis (NASH). NASH is a similar condition that consists of steatosis, inflammation, necrosis, and fibrosis and can lead to cirrhosis. Fifty per cent of people with NAFLD have concomitant NASH and 19% have cirrhosis at diagnosis. These conditions rarely produce symptoms in the early stages. The exact cause is unknown. The associated lipid pattern, elevated triglycerides, low HDL, high LDL, and high cholesterol, also occur in Type 2 diabetes. Insulin resistance contributes to lipolysis and elevated free fatty acids (FFA), which overload the hepatic mitochrondrial β-oxygenation system and FFAs accumulate in the liver and affect normal liver function. NAFLD has been described as the hepatic manifestation of insulin resistance (Marchesini *et al.* 2003). Adipokines may play a role in the development of NASH.
- Cirrhosis, which is also associated with insulin resistance and reduced insulin secretion, which has implications for management.
- Hepatocellular carcinoma, which appears to be associated with insulin resistance, increased lipolysis, accumulation of lipids in liver cells, oxidative stress leading to cell damage, fibrosis, and proliferation of procarcinogenic cells (El Serag *et al.* 2002).
- Acute liver failure. The exact mechanism is unclear. Contributing factors include some medications, and/or diabetes-related abnormalities.
- Hepatitis C. People with hepatitis C are more likely to develop diabetes than those with hepatitis B. Cantly *et al.* (2002) suggested core hepatitis C proteins impair signalling in insulin receptor substrates, which leads to Type 2 diabetes. Different genetic manifestations have been described. There is an association between the hepatitis C medication α-interferon and Type 1 diabetes (Fabris *et al.* 2003).

Managing people with diabetes and liver disease

Managing people with diabetes and concomitant liver disease is complicated by changes in medicine metabolism, contraindication to medicines such as metformin and increased risk of medicine interactions. Screening for liver disease consists of:

- Liver function tests.
- Abdominal ultrasound.
- Computerised tomography.
- Magnet resonance imaging.
- Liver biopsy.

Management is essentially the same as for any patient with diabetes but the exact strategy depends on the severity of the liver disease and the blood glucose and lipid pattern. Identifying the presence of liver disease appears to be important.

Diet and exercise are important. Many people with liver disease are malnourished, which compromises their immune status and health outcomes. Nutrition and exercise are discussed in Chapter 4. Supplemental vitamins B_{12}, D, thiamine, and folic acid may be indicated. Alcohol and smoking should be avoided because of their toxic effects on the liver. Alcohol is a liver toxin and is high in calories. In addition, it contributes to vitamin deficiencies.

The usual contraindications to medicines should be considered. Liver failure, ascites, coagulopathy, and encephalophy is associated with altered medicine metabolism. The risk of lactic acidosis with metformin needs to be considered. TZDs appear to improve ALT and liver histology (Harrison *et al.* 2005) but are associated with weight gain, see Chapter 5. ALT levels should be ascertained before commencing TZDs and monitored regularly. Insulin is frequently required. Lipid lowering agents are usually also needed. Usual diabetes self-care and education is necessary, see Chapter 16.

CAM medicines

CAM medicine use should be monitored. People often take CAM medicines 'to support liver function'. These include milk thistle, alpha-lipoic acid, vitamins E, C, and B, cysteine, and omega-3 fatty acids. Health professionals should monitor usage of CAM medicines because some can worsen liver problems and may interact with conventional medicines. The liver damage caused by CAM medicines is the same as other forms of liver damage due to conventional medicines (Chitturi & Farrell 2000).

People with the various forms of hepatitis and HIV infections frequently use CAM. There is some preliminary evidence that one medicine, Jianpi Wenshen Recipe, might help reduce the viral load of hepatitis B surface and e-antigen. Some studies show beneficial effects of Chinese herbal medicine formula used with interferon on viral clearance but the research methods are often flawed (Lipman 2007).

Prolonged ingestion or repeated exposure may play a role in the development of chronic damage with some medicines, for example, Jin Bu Huan. The type of herbs likely to be used depends on geographical location, but migration and travel means they are often widespread. Significantly, many CAM medicines contain a mixture of herbs and sometimes supplements so it can be difficult to identify the specific liver toxin, which might actually be due to contaminants rather than the herb itself if CAM medicines are not obtained for a reputable source. CAM medicines should be taken under the direction of a qualified practitioner. Some commonly used CAM medicines that are reported to cause liver damage are shown in the following list. See also Chapter 19:

- Chaparral
- Dai-saiko to
- *Chelidonium majus* (greater celandine)
- *Lycopodium serratum* (Jin Bu Huan)
- *Ephedra* species such as Ma-Huang
- Oral ingestion of essential oils containing pulegone such as pennyroyal: pennyroyal is not usually used in aromatherapy
- *Serenoa* species (saw palmetto)
- *Valerian officinalis*.

Haemochromatosis

Haemochromatosis is an inherited disease and occurs secondary to thalassaemia, some types of anaemia, and excess alcohol consumption. It is characterised by increased iron absorption. The excess iron is deposited in the liver, pancreas, heart, and pituitary gland causing tissue damage that disrupts the normal function of these organs and glands. The liver is usually the first organ to be affected.

Sixty-five per cent of people with haemochromatosis have a family history of impaired glucose tolerance or a diagnosis of diabetes (Mender *et al.* 1999). Men are ten times more likely than women to develop haemochromatosis. This could be due, in part, to iron loss with menstruation in women. Haemochromatosis is rarely seen before the age of 20 and the peak incidence occurs in people aged between 40 and 60 years.

Other diabetic complications such as nephropathy, neuropathy, and peripheral vascular disease are often also present. Arthropathy occurs in two-thirds of patients with acute crystal synovitis, which can make self-care tasks, for example, insulin administration, difficult (Sherlock 1981).

Iron overload

Iron overload is associated with various metabolic conditions besides diabetes. Steatohepatitis is an iron overload condition distinct from haemochromatosis. It is characterised by hyperferritinaemia and transferrin saturation. Liver damage includes steatosis and non-alcoholic fatty liver disease (NASH). Type 2 diabetes is often associated with NASH (Mendler *et al.* 1999). Obesity and hyperlipidaemia that can lead to fibrosis and cirrhosis of the liver are common. The excess iron can increase the risk of cancer, and most probably stroke. Diagnosis is by MRI, liver biopsy, and blood glucose and lipid levels.

Management

Management consists of:

- Venesection to remove excess iron. Hypoglycaemia can occur after venesection and the nurse needs to be aware of the possibility and know how to prevent and manage hypoglycaemia. The patient should be informed of the possibility of hypoglycaemia and how to manage their diet and medications on venesection days to reduce the hypoglycaemia risk.

- Blood glucose can be easy to control or the patient might require large doses of insulin because of insulin resistance. Oral hypoglycaemic agents often do not lead to acceptable blood glucose control and insulin is needed.
- Blood glucose monitoring to enable changes to medication and diet to be made early.
- Regular blood tests to monitor ferritin, iron levels, and metabolic control.
- Counselling and medication to manage depression, if indicated.
- Care during tests and procedures such as liver biopsy (see Chapter 9).

DIABETIC MASTOPATHY

Diabetic mastopathy is a rare disease that usually occurs in women with long-standing Type 1 diabetes around the time of the menopause. Most women with diabetic mastopathy also have microvascular disease and often other concomitant diseases such as autoimmune thyroid disease and cheiroarthropathy. There is relatively little information available about the causes of the disease but it is likely that it occurs as a result of an immune reaction to deposits in the breast as a result of hyperglycaemia.

The breast masses are usually firm-to-hard, poorly defined, freely movable and not fixed to the skin. It is important to exclude cancer to allay fear and anxiety and avoid unnecessary surgical intervention (Wilmshurst 2002).

Diagnosis

Investigations include:

- Mammogram or ultrasound.
- Fine-needle aspiration biopsy. This is often difficult to perform in people with diabetic mastopathy because the fibrous tissue is difficult to aspirate into the needle. Frequently, core or excision biopsy is required. The tissue is usually fibrous with lymphocyte infiltration but no glandular changes.

Management

(1) Single lesions can be removed. However, 63% of lesions are bilateral and often recur after excision.
(2) Regular annual follow-up is necessary with repeat mammogram and ultrasound on a regular basis.
(3) Supportive bras may help relieve breast discomfort.
(4) Regular breast self-examination and early help-seeking should be routine practice.
(5) Counselling and reassurance is important.

DIABETES AND COELIAC DISEASE

Coeliac disease is a chronic disorder associated with many diseases in many body systems. The link among the various disorders and celiac disease is clear for some but not all disorders (Duggan 2004; Juvenile Diabetes Research Foundation (JDRF 2008). Coeliac disease can be present with few clinical signs and occurs in 0.5–1.0% of the population (Fasano *et al.* 2003).

Coeliac disease is caused by a complex immunological response to gliadin the main protein in wheat. Rye, barley, and oats have smaller quantities of gliadin. T cells associated with HLA-DQ2 or HLA-DQ-8 antigen become sensitised to gliadin and produce cytokines, which cause tissue damage in the mucosa and activate plasma cells to produce antibodies to gliadin. Not everybody with the particular HLA antigens develop coeliac disease but the reason is unclear. Interestingly, cigarette smoking reduces the risk of coeliac disease by 80% (Suman *et al.* 2003). Peak diagnostic times occur at 3–5 years and again in adulthood during the 40s and affects more women than men (Green & Jabri 2003).
Commonly associated diseases include:

- Liver disorders such as fatty liver, transaminitis, or hepatitis.
- Dermatitis herpetiformis, psoriasis.
- Type 1 diabetes. The prevalence of coeliac disease in Type 1 diabetes is between 1.3% and 6.4% (Farrell & Kelly 2002; Buysschaert & Tomasi 2005) and the prevalence of Type 1 diabetes in people with coeliac disease is 5% (Colin *et al.* 1994). There is limited information about whether a gluten-free diet relieves symptoms in people with Type 1 diabetes and coeliac disease (Duggan 2004). Cavallo (2004) suggests 1 in 20 people with Type 1 has coeliac disease and 1 in 10 tests positive for transglutaminase IgA antibodies.
- Irritable bowel syndrome.
- Anaemia, which is often a result of malabsorption of iron and/or folate and which responds to iron supplements.
- Bone loss.
- Various cancers.
- IgA nephropathy.
- Epilepsy.
- Neuropathies.
- Myelopathies.
- Ataxias.
- Male and female infertility.

Signs and symptoms

Common signs and symptoms include:

- Having a family history of coeliac disease.
- Chronic tiredness.
- Poor appetite.
- Weight loss, failure to thrive.
- Delayed growth in children.

- Abdominal symptoms such as bloating, discomfort, malabsorption syndromes, pot belly, diarrhoea if most of the intestine is involved.
- Irritability and depression.
- Discoloured tooth enamel.
- Skin disorders such as psoriasis.
- Unexplained hypo or hyperglycaemia.
- Elevated transglutaminase and endomysial antibody titres.
- Anaemia.
- Histological changes on endoscopy and duodenal biopsy such as flattened villi.

Management

Wheat, rye, barley, and oats need to be eliminated from the diet but the general principles of eating a healthy diet to manage blood glucose and lipids, applies. It is essential to ensure micronutrient intake is adequate to prevent anaemia and osteoporosis and other nutritional deficiencies such as vitamin B complex. Many gluten-free foods have a high GI and high fat content so referring the individual to a dietitian is essential. Grains such as buckwheat and millet may be acceptable alternative grains.

Managing intercurrent illness and optimal health to reduce the incidence and physiological impact of these illnesses is important. Regular screening for depression and quality of life might be indicated. Screening people with these symptoms and those with IgG antibodies and IgA deficiency may be useful because a gluten-free diet is likely to improve the symptoms and quality of life (Sjoberg *et al.* 1998; Green & Jabri 2003; Duggan 2004). Universal screening is not warranted and recommending a gluten-free diet when there are no symptoms may not be beneficial, may be socially restricting and reduce quality of life. However, Buysschaert & Tomasi (2005) advocated screening all people with Type 1 diabetes and to consider repeating the test every year for three years if the initial result is negative.

The causal association between Type 1 diabetes and coeliac disease are currently under investigation and possibly involve similar HLA genes, which are also associated with other autoimmune disorders such as Addison's disease and thyroid disease. The impact of environmental factors on the genetic predisposition is unclear. Current studies include the Disease Autoimmunity Research (CEDAR) study and the Diabetes Autoimmunity Study in the Young (DAISY).

Managing a gluten-free diet as well as balancing carbohydrate intake, insulin and activity can be challenging and stressful. However, the long-term consequences in people with diabetes include chronic hypoglycaemia (see Chapter 6) that can cause neurological deficits, osteoporosis and the development of potentially life threatening diseases such as non-Hodgkin's lymphoma and cancer of the mouth, pharynx, and oesophagus (JDRF 2008). Thus, routine screening for coeliac in people with Type 1 diabetes might be warranted.

DIABETES AND MUSCULOSKELETAL DISEASES

Musculoskeletal disorders associated with diabetes are often overlooked in usual clinical diabetes care. Diabetes is associated with several specific musculoskeletal disorders and others occur concomitantly. Diabetes-related musculoskeletal disease reflects the multisystem effects of defects in glucose homeostasis. Potential causal mechanisms include:

- Non-enzymatic glycosylation of proten resulting in advanced glycation end products (AGE) and stiffened connective tissue.
- Increased deposition of connective tissue as a result of myofibroblast proliferation.
- Neuropathy.
- Autoimmune diseases associated with Type 1 diabetes.
- Obesity-related changes and strain on joints.
- Hyperinsulinaemia and associated hormonal abnormalities such as elevated growth hormone (Browne *et al*. 2001; Smith *et al*. 2002).

Diabetes-related musculoskeletal conditions can significantly impact on quality of life, self-care, activities of daily living (ADL), quality of life, driving safety, and are often associated with stress and lowered mood. Some cause chronic pain. Thus they affect diabetes health outcomes. The prevalence of these conditions tends to increase with long duration of diabetes especially associated with chronic hyperglycaemia. These conditions include:

- Shoulder adhesive capsulitis, which is painful and limits movement.
- Shoulder–Hand Syndrome, which consists of painful shoulder capsulitis and swollen, tender hands.
- Cherioarthropathy (limited joint mobility) is specific to diabetes and causes stiffening of the small joints in the hands.
- Duputren's contracture, which is associated with vision threatening retinopathy, increased risk of foot ulceration, and other musculoskeletal disorders in Type 1 and Type 2 diabetes.
- Carpal tunnel syndrome, which is also associated with hypothyroidism. The causal process is usually not due to inflammation.
- Hyperostosis and Forestier's Disease, which commonly occurs in obese middle aged men with Type 2 diabetes. The thoracic spine most commonly affected.
- Gout, pseudogout and osteoarthritis.
- Osteopenia, usually in Type 1 diabetes may be associated with retinopathy. Bone density is usually normal or increased.
- Prayer sign.
- Flexor tenosynovitis (trigger finger).
- Diabetic foot diseases such as Charcot's foot, see Chapter 8.

Management

Specific management depends on the cause. Usually the diagnosis is made on clinical grounds but X-ray, MRI, and ultrasound may be required. Muscle biopsy, EMG testing may be useful. Improving metabolic control using an apprite diet and exercise is essential. Strength and flexibility training programmes such as progressive weight training and some forms of gentle Tai Chi, physiotherapy massage and appropriate pain management using non-medicine options where possible are helpful.

Some conditions such as carpel tunnel syndrome may require surgical management. The impact on quality of life, ADLs, and safety such as driving and falls risk need to be regularly assessed for example during annual complication screening programmes or driving license renewal assessment.

CORTICOSTEROID MEDICATIONS AND DIABETES

Key points

- Corticosteroid medications predispose the person to insulin resistance, dose-related hyperglycaemia, and hyperinsulinaemia.
- They are used to control disease processes or are given as hormone replacement therapy for some endocrine diseases, for example, pituitary tumours. In the latter case corticosteroid doses are usually small or physiological levels and are less likely to cause hyperglycaemia.
- Non-diabetics on high doses, long-term or intermittent corticosteroids should be monitored and should test their blood glucose. People with diabetes should test their diabetes and their medicines should be adjusted proactively.

Introduction

Steroids are naturally occurring hormones produced by the adrenal glands under the control of the pituitary hormone ACTH. There are three major classes of steroid hormones:

(1) Glucocorticoids
(2) Mineralocorticoids
(3) Androgens and oestrogen.

Glucocorticoid effects on blood glucose

Corticosteroid medicines are an essential part of the management of inflammatory disease processes, haematologic malignancies, allergic reactions, and shock. The long-term use, especially in high doses, predisposes the individual to steroid-induced diabetes or to hyperglycaemia in people with established diabetes.

Corticosteroids have the propensity to cause insulin resistance, increased hepatic glucose output, reduced glucose transport, and to inhibit insulin secretion resulting in hyperglycaemia.

Effect on blood glucose

The effect on blood glucose depends to some extent on the biological action of the particular preparation used and the length of time it is required. Hyperglycaemia usually occurs with doses of Prednisolone (or equivalent) >7.5 mg/day.

Specific short courses of corticosteroids usually only affect the blood glucose temporarily or not at all, but hyperglycaemia occurs if the dose is increased or the medication is needed intermittently or in the long term (Williams & Pickup 1992). If given for <1 week even large doses do not usually present problems, although impaired glucose tolerance can be present and can occur within 48 hours. IV steroids usually have a shorter duration of action than steroids given by other routes and do not increase the blood glucose if only 1–2 doses are given (Jackson & Bowman 1995).

Predisposing factors
People with existing risk factors for diabetes run the greatest risk of developing steroid-induced diabetes. These risks are described in Chapter 1. They include the following conditions:

- Old age.
- Existing impaired glucose tolerance.
- Current or previous GDM.
- Cardiac disease.
- Psychosis.

The presence of one or more of these risk factors may influence the decision to use steroids, the duration of the treatment, and the dose. In many cases steroids are the medicines of choice and management strategies should be implemented to minimise the impact on the blood glucose.

Management
- Screen for the risk factors for diabetes before commencing corticosteroids.
- Where diabetes is present, OHA and/or insulin need to be reviewed and may require adjustment according to the blood glucose profile. In many cases the postprandial blood glucose increases during the day but drops overnight and the fasting glucose may not be significantly elevated (Oyer *et al*. 2006).
- Over 50% of people with Type 2 diabetes treated with OHAs require insulin if they require corticosteroids, sometimes permanently (Williams & Pickup 1992). Shapiro (2008) suggested TZDs might be useful to overcome steroid-induced insulin resistance but recommending considering the individual characteristics before prescribing a TZD. TZD have a slow onset of action so they would not be beneficial when steroids are needed in the short term. When steroids are used in the long term they exacerbate cardiovascular risk factors and lead to weight gain. In such cases TZD may increase because they also cause oedema and exacerbate heart failure. Other OHA may be effective deepening on the individual cautions and contraindication. The American Diabetes Association (2007) suggested the GLP-1 agents might be effective in some patients. However, insulin is often required.
- Select the optimal route of administration for the particular problem: oral, IV, inhaled, topical cream.
- Use the lowest effective dose for the shortest possible time.
- Monitor blood glucose 4-hourly if the person has diabetes and at least weekly if they do not.
- Monitor for ketones, especially in Type 1 diabetes because steroids predispose them to DKA.

- Explain to the patient the reasons for the blood glucose monitoring, especially if they do not have diabetes. Reassure them that steroids are the medicine of choice for their condition and that hyperglycaemia can be controlled.
- Steroids required on a temporary basis must be withdrawn gradually to allow the pituitary–adrenal axis to return to normal activity (Jackson & Bowman 1995).
- If OHAs/insulin doses were commenced or increased they will need to be reduced as the steroid dose is reduced to avoid hypoglycaemia.
- Prolonged steroid use depresses the immune system. Aseptic technique is important if any invasive procedures are required and the immune system should be supported with a healthy diet and regular activity within the individual's tolerance level.

Steroids can mask some of the signs and symptoms of infection, as can diabetes. Common infection sites should be closely monitored, for example, injection sites, feet, mouth and gums, and the urinary tract.

- The skin can become thin and fragile and easily damaged if corticosteroids are required in the long term, predisposing the individual to bruising, skin tears, ulcers, and other trauma, especially older people. A protective skin care regimen is important.
- Protecting older people from falls that predispose them to trauma is essential where long-term corticosteroids are required because of the effects on bone and the increased risk of fractures if they fall.
- Alternate-day steroid regimens show greater effects on the blood glucose on the day steroid medications are taken. OHA/insulin regimes for steroid and non-steroid days may be needed.
- Insulin is often required for people on OHAs if long-term steroids are required or if hyperglycaemia persists despite compliance with their OHAs, and an appropriate diet.
- Where permanent steroid therapy is required, for example, after surgery for a pituitary tumour, the steroid dose usually needs to be increased during illness or surgery. Careful, *written* instructions detailing how to manage steroid dose reductions in these circumstances and close liaison with their endocrinologist is essential. OHAs/insulin will also need to be adjusted in these circumstances.
- Achieving acceptable growth and development in children on permanent steroids is important and should be closely monitored. Growth hormone may be required.
- Body changes can occur such as weight gain, moon face, thinning hair, and acne develop which can affect body image.
- Steroids can cause mental changes ranging from mild changes to psychosis, which can affect the person's self-care. If psychosis occurs it will need to be managed appropriately. The help of a psychiatrist may be necessary.

Corticosteroids and osteoporosis

Corticosteroids can also reduce bone formation and the viability of osteoblasts and osteocytes, reduce calcium absorption from the intestine and increase renal calcium excretion predisposing the individual to osteoporosis and fractures (Romas 2008). These negative effects can be managed with supplemental oral calcium and vitamin D or calcitriol. In some cases, gonadal hormone production can be affected, which exacerbates the other bone effects. Changes are noted even at low doses of corticosteroids and fractures can occur soon after commencing these medicines, especially in high-risk individuals. Risk factors include:

- age
- female gender
- post menopausal women who are at the highest risk
- low bone mineral density.

Bone mineral densitometry and dual energy X-ray absorptiometry of the lumbar spine and neck of the femur are warranted for all patients on corticosteroid therapy >3 months. Using a non-steroid medicine if possible and using these medicines in the lowest possible dose for the shortest time helps reduce the risk of adverse effects. Oral bisphosphonates with vitamin D are important primary prevention medicines for people in the high fracture risk category.

DIABETES AND DRIVING

The association among diabetes, diabetes complications, medications, coexisting comorbidities, intercurrent illness, alcohol intake, environmental conditions and driving accidents is complex and multifactorial. Individual driving risk needs to be assessed and monitored regularly, for example, when a complication is diagnosed, when the medication regimen is modified, as the person grows older, and following crash. In addition, the ability to operate other vehicles such as Go-Fors and farm vehicles also needs to be considered.

Diabetes can have a significant impact on driving safety, yet current management guidelines and diabetes complication screening programmes do not make provision for proactive structured assessment of driving ability, which usually occurs when the driving license needs to be renewed. Often license renewal may not be required for several years and the health status can change significantly between renewal periods. Statistically young men and older people are most at risk of road crash but people need to be assessed on an individual basis. Diabetes specific effects on driving are shown in Table 10.4.

Guidelines for assessing fitness to drive exist in most countries. For example, the Australian AUSTROADS (2003) standards, which is currently under review. Although the Australian standards are comprehensive, outline how health issues can impact on driving safety, and include standards for private and commercial licenses, they do not stress the cumulative impact of comorbidities on driving safety, even where the standards are cross referenced.

Prevalence of and risk factors for driving crashes

Evidence about driving crash rates in people with diabetes is confusing. Some researchers suggest the traffic crash rate is similar between diabetics and non-diabetics (MacLeod 1999). Others report a lower mileage-adjusted crash rate per million miles driven in people with diabetes than in the general population (Eadington & Frier 1989;

Table 10.4 Diabetes-related complications that can affect driving ability and safety. Frequently more than one factor is present, therefore, the cumulative effect on driving ability needs to be considered. MI= myocardial infarction; 'Hypo' = hypoglycaemia.

Complication	Effects	Possible consequences while driving
1. Short term Hypoglycaemia	Cognitive impairment Impaired decision making. Vision changes Symptoms may be distracting Hypoglycaemic unawareness. If nocturnal, daytime lethargy. Risk of falls. Risk of coma.	Can be distracting, for example, reaching for glucose to treat the hypo. May not be convenient to stop to treat the 'hypo' so mild hypoglycaemia progresses. Impaired decision-making, not recognising the need to stop or treat the hypo. Symptoms not recognised and episode not treated. Inability to control the vehicle due to cognitive and functional changes. Slow reaction time and erratic driving. Difficulty reading road signs. Loss of consciousness.
Hyperglycaemia	Increased rate of intercurrent infection and if severe risk of ketoacidosis and hyperosmolar states. Tiredness and lethargy. Changed cognitive functioning. Polyuria and polydipsia. Vision changes. Lowered mood. Compromised self-care. Risk of falls.	Distractions, for example, need to pass urine. Slowed reaction time. Inability to control the vehicle. Difficulty reading road signs. Impaired decision-making. Fall asleep while driving.

2. Long term

Microvascular disease:

(a) Retinopathy
- Vision impairment.
- Visual field defects.
- Self-care deficits.
- Risk of falls.

Distractions.
Slow reaction time as a consequence of the difficulty:
- gauging distance
- seeing oncoming vehicles
- reading road signs
- loss of peripheral vision
- Impact on night driving.
- Wearing appropriate glasses for driving and ID necessary.
- Effect of investigations such as retinal screening, angiograms and laser therapy.

(b) Nephropathy
- Changed medicine pharmacokinetics and pharmacodynamics.
- Hypotension especially if on dialysis.
- Increased hypo risk especially on dialysis days.
- Discomfort.
- Muscle weakness.
- Lethargy.
- Depression.
- Risk of falls.

Distractions.
Slow reaction time.
Inability to control the vehicle.
Difficulty reading road signs.
Impaired decision-making.

Macrovascular disease:

(a) Cardiac
- Cardiac dysrhythmias.
- Silent MI.
- Disorientation and confusion.
- Tiredness.
- Lightheadedness.
- Depression.
- Risk of falls.

Distractions.
MI during driving.
Sudden death while driving.
Impaired decision-making.
Daytime sleepiness.

(b) Cerebral
- TIAs, stroke.
- Not recognising hypos.
- Cognitive changes.
- Risk of falls.

Slow reaction time.
Impaired decision-making.
Reduces strength in affected limbs.

(c) Peripheral
- Intermittent claudication.

Difficulty operating pedals.
More likely to use a car because of difficulty walking.

(Continued)

Table 10.4 Continued.

Complication	Effects	Possible consequences while driving
Neuropathy: (a) Peripheral	Reduced sensation in feet and unstable gait. Pain. Risk of falls.	Difficulty operating pedals. Distraction
(b) Autonomic	Postural hypotension. Hypoglycaemic unawareness. Gastroparesis. Incontinence. Unstable blood glucose pattern. Depression. Silent MI. Silent UTI. Communication difficulties. Lethargy. Inadequate self-care. Depression. Suicide.	Distractions. Slow reaction time. Inability to control the vehicle. Erratic driving. Hypo not recognised and not treated. May not be convenient to stop to treat a hypo. Difficulty reading road signs. Impaired decision-making. Sudden death.
Musculoskeletal e.g. Carpel tunnel syndrome Dupuytren's contracture. Joint stiffness	Reduced fine motor skill affecting dexterity. Weakness. Pain Falls risk	Distractions. Slow reaction time. Difficulty controlling the vehicle. Difficulty turning the head.
Sleep apnoea usually occurs as a consequence of obesity.	Pain. Day time lethargy.	Distraction. Fall asleep while driving. Difficulty fitting seat belts.

Reproduced with permission from Odell (in press).

Mathiesen & Borch-Johnsen 1997). Older drivers generally appear to have a higher crash rate than any other age group except people <25 years (Williams *et al.* 1989; Guerrier *et al.* 1999; McGwin *et al.* 2000; Braver & Trempel 2004; The Foundation for Health and Aging 2007). Older women with heart disease, stroke, or arthritis are at high risk (McGwin *et al.* 2000). If they are in an accident, older people are more likely to suffer serious injury or die. The presence of diabetes was not reported in these studies. However, many older drivers voluntarily restrict their driving, for example, not driving at night or in peak hour traffic (Penckofer *et al.* 2007).

Falls in older people, especially a fall in the previous year, increases crash risk (Margolis *et al.* 2002). Falls are more likely to occur when the following factors are present. Almost all of these apply to diabetes:

- unstable balance
- neurological problems
- musculoskeletal problems
- cardiovascular disease
- vision deficits
- cognitive impairment
- insulin treatment
- significant postural hypotension
- female gender (Gregg *et al.* 2000).

Although insulin treatment is assumed to carry a higher crash risk, people managed by diet and exercise are also at significant risk (Sagberg 2006). Sagberg found a significant risk of road crashes and the presence of medical conditions, symptoms, and some medicines in drivers of all ages. In particular, Sagberg found significant associations among crash risk and diabetes, previous MI, wearing glasses while driving, myopia, difficulty getting to sleep, frequent tiredness, depression, and taking antidepressant medicines. Koepsell *et al.* (1994) also found increased crash risk when diabetes and heart disease were both present, people on insulin or OHA, and duration of diabetes >5 years. Experts suggest diabetes-related crashes involving insulin-treated people are often due to hypoglycaemia (Clark *et al.* 1980; Frier *et al.* 1980; Steel *et al.* 1981; Koepsell *et al.* 1994). However, McGwin *et al.* (1999) found no significant difference in crash rates according to diabetes treatment mode or in people with diabetes overall.

In some countries people on insulin are not permitted to drive articulated vehicles or other heavy vehicles such as passenger buses. However, there are no restrictions on driving other heavy vehicles such as tractors and farm vehicles in rural areas. Crashes involving these vehicles cause significant injury. Dionne *et al.* (1995) reported a higher crash rate associated with people with diabetes driving non-articulated but not articulated trucks. In contrast, Laberge-Nadeau *et al.* (2000) found no significant differences in crash rates between people with diabetes and non-diabetics driving either type of truck. Interestingly, non-insulin users and those with no diabetes complications were more likely to be involved in a crash while driving trucks.

Cox *et al.* (2000) used driving simulators to determine the effect of hypoglycaemia on driving ability in young people with diabetes. No effect was detected at blood glucose 3.6 mmol/L but significantly more swerving, driving over the line or off the road, and compensatory slow driving occurred at 2.6 mmol/L. Fifty per cent indicated they would not drive if their blood glucose were low. In a second simulator study,

Cox *et al.* progressively lowered blood glucose to <2.8 mmol/L. Most participants recognised they were hypoglycaemic but only a minority treated the hypoglycaemia or stopped driving despite impaired driving performance.

Lee *et al.* (2003) used a PC-simulator to assess older people's driving ability. Driving skill declined significantly with increasing age. Sommerfield *et al.* (2003) reported significant impairment in working memory, ability to make decisions under pressure, and less confidence driving at speed in a group of older people. It is not clear whether any of the participants in these studies had diabetes but the findings mostly likely also apply to older people with diabetes.

However, driving simulators, particularly in research settings, may not be an appropriate way to assess actual driving behaviour because of distractions such as intravenous lines, wearing an EEG cap and being asked questions while driving, as occurred in Cox *et al.*'s study. In addition, a different set off skills is needed to drive in simulators from driving on the road. Simulators can cause stress and anxiety as well as being distracting, all of which affect driving skill and compound the effects of medical conditions. Some people may enjoy 'playing the game'.

Driving can also be affected by weather and road conditions, level of vehicle maintenance, and the age and type of vehicle (Evans 2004). Some of these factors are significantly different from conditions operating when some older studies were undertaken. Likewise, many of the newer glucose lowering agents (OHA) and insulin analogues, and the trend towards using shorter acting OHA and insulin analogues have reduced the risk of hypoglycaemia.

Diabetes-related effects on driving

Diabetes-related factors that affect driving ability include:

- The duration of diabetes. Risk increases with increasing duration of diabetes largely because of the increasing risk of diabetes complications.
- Usual metabolic control. Hypoglycaemia is a recognised crash risk but hyperglycaemia also has short-term effects on driving ability and long-term consequences as a result of complications, see Table 10.4.
- Functional impairment and disability, for example, arthritis, and common diabetes complications; hypertension, stroke, and transient ischaemic attacks (TIA) are associated with functional decline (Stuck 1999). Diabetes-related musculoskeletal disease can make it difficult to grip the steering wheel or feel the pedals and affect the degree of control over the vehicle and/or make turning to view traffic and road signs difficult and may compound the effects of arthritis and vision deficits.
- Impaired cognitive functioning due to age-related changes, hypo or hyperglycaemia or other factors. Hyperglycaemia is linked to impaired cognitive functioning (Morley & Flood, 1990), slows recovery from injury following an accident (Scalea *et al.* 2007) and leads to tiredness and sleep disturbance, which affect concentration in the daytime.
- Long-term complications that cause functional and cognitive deficits such as cardiovascular disease, musculoskeletal problems, renal disease, retinopathy, and other vision deficits. Diabetic retinopathy is associated with a high rate of driving-related

fear, Coyne *et al.* (2004). Autonomic neuropathy causing hypoglycaemic unawareness represents significant crash risk in insulin-treated people.

- Medicines likely to affect physical and/or mental functioning such as insulin and OHA, antihypertensive agents, sedatives, antidepressive agents, some herbal medicines and illegal drugs. Polypharmacy is common in diabetes and medicine interactions and adverse events can occur that affect driving safety. Many people with diabetes use complementary medicines (CAM) and some CAM medicines can interact with conventional medicines, for example, glucose lowering herbal medicines.
- Self-care knowledge and behaviours, which encompasses diabetes-related and general self-care and safety considerations such as:
  - testing blood glucose before driving and not driving if it is low
  - carrying hypoglycaemia treatment
  - not consuming alcohol or taking illegal drugs before driving
  - maintaining the vehicle in a roadworthy condition
  - considering environmental factors such as the weather when planning a trip
  - stopping regularly on long drives
  - wearing seat belts
  - obeying road rules
  - knowing what to do if an accident occurs.

Hypoglycaemia effects on driving

Hypoglycaemia is the most significant side effect of insulin and most OHAs, see Chapter 5. Cox *et al.* undertook a simulator study and showed driving performance and decision-making were impaired during mild hypoglycaemia. Unless mild hypoglycaemia is treated the blood glucose usually continues to fall. However, Marrero & Edelman (2000) suggested the blood glucose range at which driving is impaired and the specific driving actions that are impaired vary among individuals. Generally, judgement is impaired during moderate-to-severe hypoglycaemia.

Low blood glucose triggers a counter-regulatory response: at about 3.5–3.7 mmol/L adrenergic symptoms such as sweating and trembling appear. Fine motor skills, coordination, mental processing, concentration, and some memory functions are impaired <3.0 mmol/L (Heller & Macdonald 1996; Sommerfield *et al.* 2003) and affect driving safety. Sommerfield *et al.* (2003) suggested decision-making ability is affected when blood glucose <3.0 mmol/L. However, McAulay *et al.* (2001) found no significant effect on problem-solving ability but significant effects on attentional ability.

The Edinburgh Hypoglycaemia Scale is often used to grade hypoglycaemia severity and could help define driving risk:

- Grade 1, mild: the person is aware of hypoglycaemia and responds and self-treats appropriately.
- Grade 2, moderate: the person cannot respond to hypoglycaemia and needs help. Oral treatment corrects the blood glucose level.
- Grade 3, severe: the person is semi- or unconscious and unable to self-treat. Glucagon or IV glucose may be required to correct the blood glucose.

Interpreting driving risk according to these grades suggests the person is at risk of an accident and should stop and treat hypoglycaemia immediately they recognise the symptoms. They are unlikely to manage alone and will be at greater risk if hypoglycaemia is moderate or severe. However, other factors that can affect judgement need to be considered. These include hypoglycaemic awareness, and alcohol and illegal drug use, which cloud judgement and may mask hypoglycaemic symptoms. If present, these factors significantly increase the risk of crash. Testing blood glucose before driving, not driving if the blood glucose is low and not drinking alcohol or using illegal drugs and driving reduce crash risk.

Most people recover from severe hypoglycaemia (Cryer 2007) without permanent effects on driving. The possibility of hypoglycaemia is increased with the trend towards stringent blood glucose targets but the effects on driving crashes is unknown and the overall rate of severe hypoglycaemia is difficult to establish. Severe hypoglycaemia occurred in 0.4–2.3% of insulin-treated Type 2 people per year compared with 0.4% on diet or sulphonylureas, in the UKPDS.

In a later UKPDS substudy, Wright *et al.* (2006) reported hypoglycaemia grades 1 and 2 occurred in 0.8% in the diet group and 1.7% in the metformin group per year; and grades 2–4 in 0.1% and 0.3% respectively, compared to 7.9%, and 1.2% in the sulphonylurea group. Hypoglycaemia increased significantly in the basal insulin group; 21.2% and 3.65; and 32%, and in those on basal bolus insulin, 5.5%. Hypoglycaemia frequency and severity in Type 2 diabetes is lower than Type 1 (Yki-Jarvinen *et al.* 1999).

The rate of OHA-induced hypoglycaemia may be lower than insulin-induced hypoglycaemia but when it does occur it is often prolonged and can recur within 24 hours despite treatment, and carries a mortality rate of 4–10% (Shorr *et al.* 1997; Stahl & Berger 1999). In addition 5% of survivors have permanent neurological damage (Salas & Caro 2002; Veitch & Clifton-Bligh 2004).

People on insulin have a higher crash risk than the general population but serious hypoglycaemia during driving is rare. Harsch *et al.* (2002) reported more hypoglycaemia in Type 1 diabetes; the accident rate was 0.19–8.26 or 0.02–0.63 per 100 000 kilometers per year per driver depending on the intensity of the insulin regimen. Harsch *et al.* also found fewer events in those on basal bolus therapy and insulin pumps 0.09–0.49 events per 100 000 kilometers or 0.007–0.01 per driver per year. Likewise, Ziemer *et al.* (2007) found lower hypoglycaemia risk in people on basal bolus insulin regimens and no increase in driving risk.

Lower accident risk with basal bolus regimens might be due to the fact that rapid-/ short-acting insulins have a shorter duration of action and smaller frequent doses significantly reduces the insulin depot. Long-acting insulin analogues also have a lower hypoglycaemic profile (see Chapter 5). Temporary driving restrictions usually apply if a person has severe hypoglycaemia. The license may not be renewed until blood glucose is stabilised and is in a safe range. Loss of their driving license can cause considerable hardship for the individual involved and sometimes their families and is a threat to independence and access to essential services including health professionals especially in outer suburban and rural areas.

If hypoglycaemic unawareness is a contributing factor, Blood Glucose Awareness Training (BGATT) may help the individual learn to recognise impending hypoglycaemia and improve their safety and confidence. Cox *et al.* (2001) reported 6.8 crashes in a group of people participating in a BGATT programme per million miles driven versus 29.8 in the control group in a four-year observational study. BGATT did not improve the decision not to drive when blood glucose levels were low. In contrast, Broers *et al.* (2005) found a significant improvement in deciding not to drive during hypoglycaemia in BGATT participants. They also had a lower crash rate compared to controls: 0.6 versus 0.2 per patient per year. These findings of the BGATT programmes may be a useful addition to driver rehabilitation/safety programmes for people with severe hypoglycaemia.

Strategies to enhance driving safety

Health professionals could adopt a more proactive, holistic education and risk management approach to diabetes and driving safety. Such an approach include:

- Conducting regular structured driving assessments as part of care planning and annual complication screening as well as during significant health and treatment changes would enable declining functional and cognitive ability and the potential effects on driving safety to be identified and remedial strategies implemented. If relevant, geriatric, mental health and/or driving assessments should be sought. Such an approach would enable a gradual, planned transition to stopping driving to occur and reduce the physical and mental impact on the individual.
- Undertaking opportunistic driving assessments instead of only at license renewal time or when a severe hypoglycaemic event or a driving accident occurs. For example, during an emergency department/hospital presentation, when medicines are changed, and during the annual complication assessment.
- Assessing the individual's level of risk and counselling them appropriately about how to reduce their risk. Circumstances and the level of risk sometimes change rapidly, thus forward planning for such contingencies is helpful especially for older people. This could include developing a proactive driving/transport plan and recognising when to suggest the individual implements their plan. The driving plan could include making plans to cope during temporary incapacity, for example, during acute illness, investigative procedures, or surgery as well as a long-term plan to eventually stop driving.
- Being aware of the general and diabetes-related risk factors that contribute to unsafe driving and ensure they are considered when undertaking education, health assessments, and formulating management plans.
- Knowing the relevant driving legislation and where/how to access information for themselves and patients. When providing information it needs to be relevant to the individual and in a format they are likely to use, for example, older people like and refer to written information, whereas Cox *et al.*'s (2000) simulator studies suggest computer programs that involve 'playing a game' may be appropriate to younger people.
- Knowing the commonly used classes of medicines that can impair driving skills such as:
  - Anticonvulsants
  - Antihistamines
  - Antipsychotics
  - Benzodiazepines
  - OHA and insulin

- ○ Muscle relaxants
- ○ Opioid analgesics
- ○ Serotonin reuptake inhibitors
- ○ Tricyclic and tetracyclic antidepressants
- ○ Sympathomimetics (Drummer 2008)
- Considering driving safety when managing medicines including when undertaking medicines reviews including home medicine reviews (HMRs) as a key aspect of the quality use of medicines (QUM). Ask about complementary therapy use, particularly herbal medicines and supplements.
- Ensuring diabetes and other relevant education programmes encompass driving responsibilities and safety.

Information for people with diabetes to help them drive safely

The following information can be included in patient education programmes and supportive information such as handouts. It could also be used as a framework for assessing driving knowledge:

- Be aware of your responsibilities as a driver. Make sure you comply with legislation such as informing traffic authorities that you have diabetes especially if you use insulin or glucose lowering tablets.
- Regularly think about your driving ability, to help you decide your level of risk and whether a formal driving assessment or attending a driving safety class would be useful. Advanced driving classes can be very helpful at improving driving safety for non-diabetics as well as people with diabetes and adapted for younger and older drivers in some countries. They can reduce the likelihood of an accident or improve the way you manage in high-risk driving situations. Formal driving assessment might be needed, for example, if you have a driving accident, a period of illness or your vision declines.
- Consider your own safety, that of your passengers, and other road users when you drive, for example, test your blood glucose before you drive if you are on insulin or diabetes tablets and do not drive if your blood glucose is low. Always carry glucose with you and wear a medical alert 'bracelet' containing relevant health information.
- Decide whether somebody should accompany you and/or whether you should inform relatives or friends where you are going.
- Discuss the factors likely to affect your driving safety with health professionals and your family on a regular basis, for example, when you have your annual diabetes complication check or winter influenza vaccinations. Make sure you have written advice about what to do when you are sick, have a hypo, need surgery, or an investigation such as an eye test. It may be advisable not to drive in these situations. Knowing before hand will enable you to make other arrangements.
- Develop a formal driving/transportation plan to ensure you have strategies in place when you can no longer drive safely and ease the transition to not driving.
- Consider factors likely to affect driving safety before you drive. These include your health at the time and other factors such as the weather, distance to cover, road

works, and the time of the day or night. Having a mobile phone enables you to call for help but should not be used while the vehicle is moving.

- Follow regulations such as wearing a seat belt, not speaking on a mobile phone while driving and not consuming alcohol or illegal drugs before or while driving. Make sure children and pets cannot move around in the car and place other objects such as groceries in the boot or secure them so they cannot move around and injure passengers if you have to stop suddenly.
- Stop regularly when driving long distances especially if you feel tired or have trouble concentrating. Test your blood glucose, walk around, have a powernap and a drink and some food.
- If you feel unwell, stop and pull over immediately. Check your blood glucose and treat a hypo if your blood glucose is low. If you have chest discomfort, feel dizzy or lightheaded call an ambulance.
- Make sure you know what to do if you have an accident.
- Be aware that motorised wheelchairs, Go-Fors, and farm machinery such as tractors can also cause 'traffic' accidents and result in significant injury. Safe driving advice also applies to these vehicles, particularly farm machinery.

References

Enteral and parenteral nutrition

McClave, S., Snider, H. & Spain, D. (1999) Use of residual volume as a marker for enteral feeding intolerance: prospective blinded comparison with physical examination and radiographic findings. *Journal of Parenteral and Enteral Nutrition*, 16, 64s–70s.
Middleton, M., Nazarenko, G., Nivison-Smith, I. & Smerdley, P. (2001) Prevalence of malnutrition and 12-month incidence of mortality in two Sydney teaching hospitals. *Medical Journal of Australia*, 31, 455–461.
Thomas, B. (2001) *A Manual of Dietetic Practice*. Blackwell Science, Oxford, pp. 86–87.

Diabetes and cancer

Bloomgarden, Z. (2001) Diabetes and cancer. *Diabetes Care*, 24, 780–781.
Coughlin, S., Calle, E., Teras, L., Petrelli, J. & Thun, M. (2004) Diabetes mellitus as a predictor of cancer mortality in a large cohort of US adults. *American Journal of Epidemiology*, 159, 1160–1167.
Dibble, S., Luce J. & Cooper, B. (2007) Acupressure for chemotherapy-induced nausea and vomiting: a randomized clinical trial. *Oncology Nursing Forum*, 34, 813–820.
Faithful, S. (1998) Fatigue in patients receiving radiotherapy. *Professional Nurse*, 13 (7), 459–458.
Fernandez, C., Stutzer, C., MacWilliam, I. & Fryer, C. (1998) Alternative and complementary use in pediatric oncology patients in British Columbia: prevalence, reasons for use and non-use. *Journal of Clinical Oncology*, 16 (4), 1279–1286.
Jung, R.T. & Sikora, K. (1984) *Endocrine Problems in Cancer*. Heinemann Medical Books, London.
Kao, G. & Devine, P. (2000) Use of complementary health practices by prostate carcinoma patients undergoing radiotherapy. *Cancer*, 88 (3), 615–619.
La vecchia, C., Negri, E., D'Avanzo, B. & Boyle, P. (1994) A case–control study of diabetes mellitus and cancer risk. *British Journal of Cancer*, 70 (5), 950–953.

Lipscombe, L., Hux, J. & Booth, G. (2005) Reduced screening mammography among women with chronic medical diseases. *Archives of Internal Medicine*, **165**, 2090–2095.

Lipman, T. (2007) The role of herbs and probiotics in GI wellness for older adults. *Geriatrics and Aging*, **10** (3), 182–191.

Oyer, D., Shah, A. & Bettenhausen, S. (2006) How to manage steroid diabetes in the patient with cancer. *Supportive Oncology*, **4** (9), 479–483.

Psarakis, H. (2006) Clinical challenges in caring for patients with diabetes and cancer. *Diabetes Spectrum*, **19**, 157–162.

Quinn, K., Hudson, P. & Dunning, T. (2006) Diabetes management in patients receiving palliative care. *Journal of Pain and Symptom Management*, **32** (3), 275–286.

Spiegel, D., Bloom, J., Kraemer, H. & Gottheil, E. (1989) Effect of psychosocial treatment on survival of patients with metastatic breast cancer. *Lancet*, **2** (8668), 888–891.

Travier, N., Jeffreys, M., Brewer, N., Wright, C., Cunningham, C., Hornell, J. & Pearce, N. (2007) Association between glycosylated hemoglobin and cancer risk: a New Zealand linkage study. *Annals of Oncology*, **18** (8), 1414–1419.

Verlato, G., Zoppini, G., Bonora, E. & Muggeo, M. (2003) Mortality form site specific malignancies in Type 2 diabetes patients form Verona. *Diabetes Care*, **26**, 1047–1051.

Wideroff, L., Gridley, G., Mellemkjaer, L., Chow, W., Linet, M., Keehn, S., Borch-Johnsen, K. & Olsen, J. (1997) Cancer incidence in a population-based cohort of patients hospitalised with diabetes mellitus in Denmark. *Journal of the National Cancer* Institute, **89** (18), 1360–1365.

Wilkinson, J. (2008) "Good gargling": evaluation of the use of an essential oil mouthwash in the management of radiation-induced mucositis of the oropharyngeal area. *Proceedings of the* 3rd *International Congress on Complementary Medicine*, Sydney, March 2008, p. 26.

Wyatt, G., Friedman, L., Given, C. & Beckrow, K. (1999) Complementary therapy use among older cancer therapy patients. *Cancer Practice*, **7** (3), 136–144.

Smoking, alcohol, and illegal drug use

American Cancer Society (2007) *Cancer Facts and Figures*. American Cancer Society, Atlanta.

American Psychiatric Association (APA) (2000) *Diagnostic and Statistical Manual of Mental Disorders* (4th edn.). Text Revision (DSM-1V-TR) APA, Washington.

Australian Institute of Health and Welfare (AIHW) (2006) *Australia's Health*. AIHW, Canberra; catalogue number AUS 73.

Bover, M., Foulds, J., Steinberg, M., Richardson, D. & Marcella, S. (2008) Waking at night to smoke as a marker for tobacco dependence: patient characteristics and relationship to treatment outcome. *International Journal of Clinical Practice*, **62** (2), 182–190.

Brink, S. (2008) in Glick D. (2003) Legal and illegal drugs: what every person with diabetes should know before they party. *Diabetes and Health* http://www.diabeteshealth.com/read/2003/11/0i/3163.html (accessed August 2008).

Brown, L. (1991) Clinical aspects of drug abuse in diabetes. *Diabetes Spectrum*, **4** (1), 45–47.

Department of Health and Human Services (DHSS) (2006) *The Health Consequences of Involuntary Exposure to Tobacco Smoke: A Report of the Surgeon General – Executive Summary*. Department of Health and Human Services (DHSS, Public Health Service, Center for Disease Control, Center for Chronic Disease Prevention and Health Promotion, Office of Smoking and Health, USA.

Falba, T. (2005) Health events and the smoking cessation of middle aged Americans. *Journal of Behavioural Medicine*, **28**, 21–33.

Foulds, J., Gandhi, K. & Steinberg, M. (2006) Factors associated with quitting smoking at a tobacco dependence treatment clinic. *American Journal health Behaviour*, **30**, 400–412.

Fu, S., Partin, M. & Snyder, A. (2006) Promoting repeat tobacco dependence treatment: are relapsed smokers interested? *American Journal of Managed Care*, **12**, 235–243.

Kroon, L. (2007) Drug interactions with smoking. *American Journal Health-Systems Pharmacy*, **64** (18), 1917–1921.

George, L. (1995) Sociological-perspectives on life transitions. *Annual Review Sociology*, **19**, 353–373.

Glick, D. (2003) Legal and illegal drugs: what every person with diabetes should know before they party. *Diabetes and Health* http://www.diabeteshealth.com/read/2003/11/0i/3163.html (accessed August 2008).

Korantzopoulos, P., Liu, T., Papaioannides, D., Li, G. & Goudevenos, J. (2008) Atril fibrillation and marijuana smoking. *International Journal Clinical Practice*, **62** (2), 308–313.

Lancaster, T. & Stead, L. (2004) Physician advice for smoking cessation. *Cochrane Database of Systematic Reviews*, Issue 4, Art. No. CD000165.

Lang, I., Rice, N., Wallace, R., Guralnik, J. & Melzer, D. (2007) Smoking cessation and transition into retirement: analysis from the English longitudinal study. *Age and Aging*, **36** (6), 638–643.

Lee, N. (2008) Alcohol intervention: what works? *Australian Family Physician*, **37** (1/2), 16–19.

Moussouttas, M. (2004) Cannabis use and cerebrovascular disease. *Neurologist*, **10**, 47–53.

Mitchell, D. (2008) Pushing the pin on smoking. *Journal of Complementary Medicine*, **7** (2), 55 and 63.

Naqvi, N., Rudrauf, D., Damasio, H. & Bechara, A. (2007) Damage to the insula disrupts addiction to cigarette smoking. *Science*, **315** (5811), 531–534.

National Health and Medical Research Council (NHMRC) (2007) *Draft Australian Drinking Guidelines for Low Risk Drinking*. www.nhmrc.gov.au/consult (accessed November 2007).

Osiecki, H. (2006) *The Physician's Handbook of Clinical Nutrition* (7th edition). AG Publishing, Australia.

Ostbye, T. & Taylor, D. (2004) The effect of smoking on years of healthy life (YHL) lost among middle-aged and older Americans. *Health Services Research*, **39**, 531–532.

Owen, N., Wakefield, M., Roberts, L. & Esterman, A. (1992) Stages of readiness to quit smoking; population prevalence and correlates. *Health Psychology*, **11**, 413–417.

Saunders, J., Aasland, O. & Babor, T. (1993) Development of Alcohol Use Disorders Identification Test (AUDIT). WHO collaborative project on early detection of persons with harmful alcohol consumption. Part 2 *Addiction*, **88**, 791–804.

Shand, F., Gates, J., Fawcett, J. & Mattick, R. (2003) *Guidelines for the Treatment of Alcohol Problems*. National Drug and Alcohol Research Center, Sydney.

Spinella, M. (2005) *Concise Handbook of Psychoactive Herbs*. Haworth Herbal Press, Oxford.

Surgeon General's Report (2004) *The Health Consequences of Smoking: Surgeon General's Report 2004*. Department of Health and Human Services (DHSS, Public Health Service, Centre for Disease Control, Center for Chronic Disease Prevention and Health Promotion, Office of Smoking and Health. DHSS publication number CDC 099- 7830.

Tonstad, S., Tonnesesn, P. & Hajek, P. (2006) Effect of maintanence therapy with varenicine. *Journal of American Medical Association*, **296**, 64–71.

Watkins, S., Koob, G. & Markou, A. (2000) *Nicotine Tobacco Research*, **2** (1), 19–37.

Wise, R., Sims, T. &Taylor, R. (2007) Smoking cessation – a practical guide fort eh primary care physician. *Primary Care Reports*, **13** (4), 49–60.

Zwar, N. (2008) Smoking cessation: what works? *Australian Family Physician*, **37** (1/2), 10–14.

Brittle diabetes

Martin, F. (1995) Brittle diabetes. *Diabetes Communication*, July, 7–8.

Oral health and diabetes

Connor, S., Iranpour, B. & Mills, J. (1970) Alteration in the parotid salivary flow in diabetes mellitus. *Oral Surgery*, **30**, 15.

Holmes, S. & Alexander, W. (1997) Diabetes in dentistry. *Practical Diabetes International*, **14** (4), 107–110.

Lamey, P., Darwazeh, A. & Frier, B. (1992) Oral disorders associated with diabetes mellitus. *Diabetic Medicine*, **9** (5), 410–416.

National Health Medical Research Council (NHMRC) (1999) *Dietary Guidelines for Older Australians*. Commonwealth of Australia, Canberra.

Position Paper (1996) Diabetes and periodontal disease. *Journal of Peridontology*, **67**, 166–176.

Diabetes and liver disease

Balkau, B., Eschwege, E., Ducimetiere, P., Richard, J. & Warnet, J. (1991) The high risk of death by alcohol-related diseases in subjects diagnosed as diabetic and impaired glucose tolerant: The Paris Prospective Study after 15 years follow-up. *Journal of Clinical Epidemiology*, **44**, 465–474.

Caldwell, S., Oelsner, D., Iezzoni, J., Hespenheide, E., Battle, E. & Driscoll, C. (1999) Cryptogenic cirrhosis: clinical characterisation and risk factors for underlying disease. *Hepatology*, **29**, 664–669.

Cantley, L. (2002) The phosphoinositide 3-kinase pathway. *Science*, **296**, 1655–1657.

Chitturi, S. & Farrell, G. (2000) Herbal hepatotoxicity: an expanding but poorly defined problem. *Journal of Gastroenterology and Hepatology*, **15**, 1093–1099.

De Marco, R., Locatelli, F., Zoppini, G., Verlato, G., Bonora, E. & Muggeo, M. (1999) Cause-specific mortality in type 2 diabetes: The Verona Diabetes Study. *Diabetes Care*, **22**, 756–761.

El-Serag, H. & Everhart, J. (2002) Diabetes increases the risky of acute liver failure. *Gasterenterology*, **122**, 1822–1828.

Harris, M., Flegal, K., Cowie, C., Eberhardt, M., Goldstein, D. & Little, R. (1998) Prevalence of diabetes, impaired fasting glucose, and impaired glucose tolerance in US adults: the Third National health and Nutrition Examination Survey 1988–1994. *Diabetes Care*, **21**, 518–524.

Harrison, S., Belfort, R., Brown, K., Darland, C., Finch, J., Fricke, J., Havranek, R., Hardies, J., Dwived, S., Berria, R., Tio, F., Schenker, S. & Cusi, K. (2005) A double-blind, placebo controlled trial of pioglitazone in the treatment of non-alcoholic steatohepatitis (NASH). *Gasterenterology*, **128** (Suppl. 2), A681.

Lipman, T. (2007) The role of herbs and probiotics in GI wellness for older adults. *Geriatrics and Aging*, **10** (3), 182–191.

Marchesini, G., Bugianesi, E., Forlani, G., Cerrelli, F., Lenzi, M., Manini, R., Natale, S., Vanni, E., Villanova, N., Melchionda, N. & Rizzeto, M. (2003) Nonalcoholic fatty liver, steatohepatitis and the metabolic syndrome. *Hepatology*, **37**, 917–923.

Mendler, M.-H., Turlin, B., Moirrand, R. *et al.* (1999) Insulin resistance-associated iron overload. *Gastroenterology*, **117**, 1155–1163.

Sherlock, S. (1981) *Diseases of the Liver and Biliary System*. Blackwell Science, Oxford.

The US Organ Procurement and Transplantation Network and Scientific Registry of Transplant Recipients (2004) Annual Report. http://www.optn.org/AR2005/904a_rec-dgn_li.htm (accessed January 2007).

Tolman, K., Fonseca, V., Dalpiaz, A. & Tan, M. (2007) Spectrum of liver disease in type 2 diabetes and management of patients with diabetes and liver diseases. *Diabetes Care*, **30**, 734–743.

Diabetic mastopathy

Wilmshurst, E. (2002) Facts about diabetic breast disease all women should know. *Diabetes Conquest*, **Autumn**, 13.

Diabetes and coeliac disease

Buysschaert, M. & Tomasi, J. (2005) Prospective screening for biopsy proven celiac disease, autoimmunity and malabsorption markers in Belgian subjects with type 1 diabetes. *Diabetic Medicine*, 22, 889–892.

Cavallo, J. (2004) Celiac disease: sometimes silent, often misleading, always serious. *JDRF Countdown,* Summer.

Colin, P., Reunala, T. & Pukkala, E. (1994) Coeliac disease – associated disorders and survival. *Gut*, 35, 1215–1218.

Duggan, J. (2004) Coeliac disease: the great imitator. *eMedical Journal of Australia* http://www.mja.com.au/public/issues/180_10_170504/dug10818_fm.html (accessed November 2007).

Fasano, A., Berti, I. & Gerarduzzi, T. (2003) Prevalence of celiac disease in at-risk and not-at-risk groups in the United States. *Archives of Internal Medicine*, 163, 286–292.

Green, P. & Jabri, B. (2003) Coeliac disease. *Lancet*, 362, 383–391.

Juvenile Diabetes research foundation (JDRF) (2008). Type 1 diabetes and celiac disease. http://. www.jdrf.org.au/living_w_diabetes/newsitem.asp?newsid=166 (accessed January 2008).

Sjoberg, K., Eriksson, K. & Bredberg, A. (1998) Screening for celiac disease in adult insulin-dependent diabetes mellitus. *Journal Internal Medicine*, 243, 133–140.

Suman, S., Williams, E. & Thomas, P. (2003) Is the risk of adult celiac disease causally related to cigarette exposure. *European Journal of Gastroenterology Hepatology*, 15, 995–1000.

Diabetes and musculoskeletal diseases

Brown, D., McRae, F. & Shaw, K. (2001) Musculoskeletal disease in diabetes. *Practical Diabetes International*, 18 (2), 62–64.

Smit, L., Burnet, S. & McNeil, J. (2002) Musculoskeletal manifestations of diabetes mellitus. www.bjsm.bmj (accessed March 2008).

Corticosteroids medications and diabetes

Dunning, T. (1996) Corticosteroids medications and diabetes mellitus. *Practical Diabetes International*, 13, 186–188.

Jackson, R. & Bowman, R. (1995) Corticosteroids. *Medical Journal of Australia*, 162, 663–665.

Romas, E. (2008) Corticosteroid-induced osteoporosis and fractures. *Australian Prescriber*, 21 (2), 45–49.

Williams, G. & Pickup, J. (1992) *Handbook of Diabetes*. Blackwell Science, Oxford.

Diabetes and driving

AUSTROADS (2003) *Assessing Fitness to Drive*. National Road Transport Commission, Sydney.

Braver, E. & Trempel, R. (2004) Are older drivers actually at higher risk of involvement in collisions resulting in deaths or non-fatal injuries among their passengers and other road users? *Injury Prevention*, 10, 27–32.

Broers, S., van Vliet, K., le Cessie, S., Spinhoven, P., van der Ven, N., Radder, J. (2005) Blood glucose awareness training in Dutch type 1 diabetes patients: one year follow up. *Netherlands Journal of Medicine*, 63, 164–169.

Clark, B., Ward, J. & Enoch, B. (1980) Hypoglycaemia in insulin dependent diabetic drivers. *British Medical Journal*, 281, 586.

Clark, D., Stump, T. & Wolinsky, F. (1998) Predictors of onset of and recovery from mobility difficulty among adults aged 51–61 years. *American Journal of Epidemiology*, **148** (1), 63–71.

Cox, D., Gonder-Frederick, L., Julian, D., Cryer P., Lee, J., Richards, F. & Clarke, W. (1991) Intensive versus standard blood glucose awareness training (BGAT) with insulin-dependent diabetes: mechanisms and ancillary effects. *Psychosomatic Medicine*, **53**, 453–462.

Cox, D., Gonder-Frederick, L., Kovatchev, B., Julian, D. & Clarke, W. (2000) Progressive hypoglycaemia's impact on driving simulation performance: occurrence, awareness and correction. *Diabetes Care*, **23**, 163–170.

Coyne, K., Margolis, M., Kennedy-Martin, T., Baker, T., Klein, R., Paul, M. & Revicki, D. (2004) The impact of diabetic retinopathy: perspectives from patient focus groups. *Family Practice*, **21**, 447–453.

Drummer, O. (2008) The role of drugs in road safety. *Australian Prescriber*, **31** (2), 33–35.

Eadington, D. & Frier, B. (1989) Type 1 diabetes driving experience: an eight year cohort study. *Diabetic Medicine*, **6**, 137–141.

Edinburgh Hypoglycaemia Scale http://www.datadictionaryadmin.scot.nhs.uk/isddd/15647. html (accessed December 2007).

Evans, L. (2004) Overview of traffic fatalities. *Traffic Safety*. Bloomfield Hills, MI, Science Serving Society, pp. 57–58.

Frier, B., Mathews, D., Steel, J. & Duncan, L. (1980) Driving and insulin-dependent diabetes. *Lancet*, **8180**, 1232–1234.

Harsch, I., Stocker, S., Radespiel-Troger, M., Hahn, E., Konturek, P., Ficker, P. & Lohmann, T. (2002) Traffic hypoglycaemias and accidents in patients with diabetes mellitus treated with different antidiabetic regimens. *Journal of Internal Medicine*, **252**, 352–360.

Heller, S. & Macdonald, I. (1996) The measurement of cognitive function during acute hypoglycaemia: experimental limitations and their effect on study of hypoglycaemic unawareness. *Diabetic Medicine*, **13**, 607–615.

Henderson, J., Allen, K., Deary, I. & Frier, H. (2003) Hypoglycaemia in insulin-treated type 2 diabetes: frequency, symptoms and impaired awareness. *Diabetic Medicine*, **20** (12), 1016–1021.

Lee, H., Lee, A., Cameron, D. & Li-Tsang, C. (2003) Using a driving simulator to identify older drivers at inflated risk of motor vehicle crashes. *Journal of Safety Research*, **34** (4), 453–459.

Margolis, K., Kerani, R., McGovern, T., Songer, J., Cauley, K. *et al.* (2002) Study of osteoporotic fractures research, risk factors for motor vehicle crashes in older women. *Journal of Gerontology. Series A, Biological Sciences and Medical Sciences*, **57**, M186–M191.

Marrero, D. & Edelman, S. (2000) Hypoglycaemia and driving performance: a flashing yellow light? *Diabetes Care*, **23** (2), 146–147.

MacLeod, K. (1999) Diabetes and driving: toward equitable evidence-based decision-making. *Diabetes Medicine*, **16**, 282–290.

McGwin, G., Sims, R., Pulley, L. & Roseman, J. (1999) Diabetes and automobile crashes in the elderly: a population-based case control study. *Diabetes Care*, **22**, 220–227.

McGwin, G., Sims, R., Pulley, L., Roseman, M. (2000) Relations among chronic medical conditions, medications, and automobile crashes in the elderly. *American Journal of Epidemiology*, **152** (5), 424–431.

Odell, M.S. (ed.) *Older Road Users: Myths and Realities* (in press).

Penckofer, S., Ferrans, C., Velsor-Fredrich, B. & Savoy, S. (2007) The psychological impact of living with diabetes: women's day-to-day experiences. *The Diabetes Educator*, **33** (4), 680–690.

Sagberg, F. (2006) Driver health and crash involvement: a case control study. *Accident Analysis and Prevention*, **38** (1), 28–34.

Salas, M. & Caro, J. (2002) Are hypoglycaemia and other adverse effects similar among sulphonylureas? *Adverse Drug Reactions Toxicology Review*, **21**, 205–217.

Scalea, T., Bochicchio, G. & Bochicchio, K. (2007) Tight glycaemic control in critically injured trauma patients. *Annals of Surgery*, 246, 605–610.

Shorr, R., Ray, W., Daugherty, J. & Griffin, M. (1997) Incidence and risk factors for serious hypoglycaemia in older persons using insulin or sulphonylureas. *Archives of Internal Medicine*, 157, 1681–1685.

Sommerfield, A., Deary, I., McAuley, V. & Frier, B. (2003) Short-term delayed, and working memory are impaired during hypoglycaemia in individuals with type 1 diabetes. *Diabetes Care*, 26, 390–396.

Stahl, M. & Berger, W. (1999) High incidence of severe hypoglycaemia leading to hospital admission in type 2 diabetic patients treated with long-acting sulphonylureas versus short-acting sulphonylureas. *Diabetic Medicine*, 16, 586–590.

Steel, J., Frier, B., Young, R. & Duncan, L. (1981) Driving and insulin dependent diabetics. *Lancet*, 8242, 354–356.

Stuck, A., Walthert, J., Nikolaus, T., Bula, C., Hohmann, C. & Beck, J. (1999) Risk factors for functional status decline in community living elderly people: a systematic review. *Social Science Medicine*, 48, 445–469.

The Diabetes Control and Complication Trial Research Group (DCCT) (1991) Epidemiology of severe hypoglycaemia in the Diabetes Control and Complications Trial. *American Journal of Medicine*, 90, 450–459.

The Diabetes Control and Complication Trial Research Group (DCCT) (1997) Hypoglycaemia in the diabetes control and complications trial. *Diabetes*, 46, 271–286.

UKPDS (1998) (United Kingdom Prospective Diabetes Study) Intensive blood glucose control with sulphonylureas or insulin compared with conventional treatment and risk of complications in patients with Type 2 diabetes (UKPDS 33). *Lancet*, 352, 837–853.

Yki-Jarvinen, H., Ryysy, L., Nikkila, K., Tulokas, T., Vanamo, R. & Heikkila, M. (1999) Comparison of bedtime insulin regimens in patients with type 2 diabetes mellitus. A randomised, controlled trial. *Archives of Internal Medicine*, 130, 399–396.

Chapter 11
Diabetes and Sexual Health

Key points

- Sexual problems are common in the general population but people with diabetes are at increased risk.
- The presence of a sexual problem and diabetes does not mean one led to the other.
- Physical, psychological, environmental, and social factors should be considered.
- The needs and perceptions of both partners are important.
- Sex education is part of preventative and holistic diabetes care.
- There is a fine line between taking a sexual history and voyeurism.
- Put the focus on what is normal and achievable for the individual/couple rather than dysfunction or 'performance'.
- Health professionals need to be comfortable with their own sexuality to advise effectively.

Rationale

Nurses are often the person's first point of contact. People with diabetes expect them to have some knowledge about the impact of diabetes on their sexual health. Sexuality is an integral component of health and sexual problems affect all aspects of health and well being. Sexual dysfunction in men with diabetes is well documented but sexual dysfunction among women with diabetes is not well understood. The sexual response is an interaction between two (usually) people. Sexual dysfunction is also likely to involve both partners in the relationship (Masters & Johnson 1970). Nurses are ideally placed to be able to emphasise the need for primary prevention and early identification of sexual difficulties and to dispel sexual mythology.

Sexual health

Sexual health is a core aspect of an individual's general wellbeing and is the result of an integration of many components into a unified complex system – endocrine hormonal regulators, and the vascular, nervous, and psychological systems. Diabetes can profoundly affect the individual's sexual identity and the physical ability to engage in sexual activity. Maximising sexual health should be an integral part of an holistic management plan for people with diabetes. Management should include education about, screening for where relevant, and managing general issues such as safe sex, contraception, sexually transmitted diseases, and the importance of planned pregnancies. Thus a life continuum approach may be required.

Contraception

Female contraception is described in Chapter 14. Contraception options for men include:

- Condoms.
- Withdrawal before ejaculation, which is not recommended and has a high failure rate for pregnancies and sexual satisfaction.
- Billing's method, which requires cooperation from female partners.
- Vasectomy.

Male contraceptive agents under study include depo-Provera, which stops spermatogenesis.

Sexual issues are highly sensitive and must be approached with tact and consideration of the person's culture, sexual beliefs, and their privacy and confidentiality. Thus, although partners can often provide important information about their partner's sexual functioning, they should not be included unless the individual agrees.

The World Health Organisation (WHO) (1975) stressed the importance of sexuality as an integral component of health and defined sexual health as:

> The capacity to control and enjoy sexual and reproductive behaviour, freedom from shame, guilt and false beliefs which inhibit sexual responsiveness and relationships. Freedom from medical disorders that interfere with sexual responsiveness and reproduction.
>
> (WHO 1975)

By the WHO definition, the majority of the general population as well as people with diabetes do not achieve sexual health!

Masters and Johnson first described the human sexual response in 1970. They described four phases: arousal, plateau, orgasm, and resolution (Masters & Johnson 1970). These phases blend into each other and sexual difficulties can occur in one or all of them. Kaplan (1979) described a biphasic response that involved parasympathic nerve activity – vasocongestion, vaginal lubrication and erection; and sympathetic nerve activity – reflex muscle contraction, orgasm, and ejaculation. Kaplan's description makes it easier to see how diabetes can affect physical sex given that autonomic neuropathy causes nerve damage, see Chapter 8.

Sex counsellors continue to utilise many of the sexual counselling techniques developed by Masters and Johnson. Sexual difficulties do not occur in isolation from other aspects of an individual's life and relationships and a thorough assessment and history is necessary to identify the causal factors. Masters and Johnson found that age and chronic disease processes do not affect female sexual responsiveness as severely as they affect male sexuality. In addition, the sexual response is more varied in women than in men. While these are old references, they are still relevant and widely cited in the relevant literature.

Sexual development

Sexual development occurs across the lifespan:

- Chromosomal sex is determined at fertilisation.
- 3–5 years – diffuse sexual pleasure, fantasies and sex play. Often form a close relationship with a parent of the opposite sex.
- 5–8 years – interest in sexual differences, sex play is common.
- 8–9 years – begin to evaluate attractiveness and are curious about sex.
- 10–12 years – preoccupation with changing body and puberty. Adolescents are often sexually active by this age, thus sex education should start early and information provided in accordance to the child's capacity to understand and using appropriate language.
- 13–20 years – puberty, development of self-image and sexual identity.
- Late 30–early 40 – peak sexual responsiveness.
- Menopause – variable onset and highly individual effect on sexuality.
- Old age – physical difficulties and limited opportunity.

Effective sex and diabetes education should be part of the diabetes management plan so that problems can be identified early and optimal sexual functioning maintained. Health professionals and people with diabetes often have limited information about the impact diabetes can have on their sexuality. Sex education, good metabolic control, early identification, and management of sexual problems are important, but often neglected, aspects of the diabetes care plan. When a sexual problem is identified the focus is often on dysfunction and performance rather than on what is normal, which can have a negative psychological impact on sexuality. Changing the focus to what can be achieved and focusing on feelings, intimacy, love, and warmth have a big impact on general and sexual well being.

Sexual problems

Sexual satisfaction is a combination of physical and emotional factors. Sexual problems can be:

- Primary – usually defined as never having an orgasm.
- Secondary – difficulties occur after a period of normal functioning. Most sexual difficulties fit into this category.
- Situational – where the situation itself inhibits sexual activity, other sexual problems may also be involved.

Possible causes of sexual difficulties and dysfunction

Sexual difficulties usually involve two people. It may be a shared problem or each person may have individual issues that need to be considered. Interpersonal factors, the relationship and environmental and disease factors need to be explored with the couple involved.

(1) Individual factors
   • Ignorance and misinformation, which are common, despite the sexually permissive society of today. A great deal of readily available literature in magazines and on television with an overemphasis on performance sets up unreal expectations.
   • Guilt, shame, and fear, which may be fear of getting pregnant, contracting a sexually transmitted disease, not pleasing their partner or being rejected by them.
   • Gender insecurity/uncertainty and sexual preference.
   • Non-sexual concerns, for example, about finances, children, job.
   • Past sexual abuse.
   • Physical condition, for example, presence of diabetes especially diabetes complications such as autonomic neuropathy and vascular disease.
(2) Interpersonal factors
   • Sexual relationships are one of the most complex undertakings people ever make; yet most people prepare for it casually.
   • Communication problems – the most common sexual difficulty.
   • Lack of trust.
   • Different sexual preferences and desires, for example, frequency of intercourse.
   • Relationship difficulties that can include difficulties associated with alcohol and violence or be related to disease process, including diabetes.
   • Changes in lifestyle, for example, having children, retrenchment, retirement, and illness.
(3) Chronic disease sequelae
   (a) Psychological.
      • Depression, anger, guilt, anxiety, fear, feelings of helplessness, changed body image and self-identification as a victim, lowered self-image and self-esteem may or may not accompany the disease. Loss of libido is one of the classic signs of depression.
   (b) Physical changes, for example, arthritis and diabetic neuropathy.
      • Pain, debilitation associated with changed mobility, for example, arthritis, bad odour associated with infections, cardiac and respiratory problems and sleep apnoea, and snoring. Some people worry about resuming sexual activity after an MI. Education can help allay such fears.
      • Disease processes and hormonal imbalance, including diabetes, as well as other endocrine and reproductive conditions.
      • Medications, for example, antihypertensive and antidepressive agents.
   (c) Diabetes-related.
      • Hypoglycaemia during intercourse can be frightening and off-putting, especially for the partner, and inhibit spontaneity and enjoyment in future encounters.
      • Tiredness and decreased arousal and libido are associated with hyperglycaemia.
      • Mood disorders such as depression and other psychological problems may be present but mood can change with hypo- and hyperglycaemia and can cause temporary sexual problems.

(d) Autonomic neuropathy leading to erectile dysfunction in men and possibly decreased vaginal lubrication in older women. Vaginal dryness is also associated with normal ageing, not being aroused and painful intercourse and has not been definitively linked to diabetes as a cause.

(e) Infections, for example, vaginal/penile thrush.

(f) Musculoskeletal diseases that limit mobility, dexterity and may cause pain, see Chapter 10.

(4) Environmental factors.
- Lack of privacy.
- Limited opportunity, for example, older people in aged care facilities.
- Uncomfortable, noisy surroundings.

Sexuality and older people

Older people are capable of having fulfilling sexual relationships but often lack the opportunity or are constrained by environmental factors, ageist attitudes, sexual stereotypes and disease processes (see Chapter 12). Sensory impairment can change the individual's response to sexual stimulation and the multiplicity of medications required by many older people can inhibit sexual functioning.

Touch is important throughout life and caring touch as distinct from providing nursing care is often lacking. Touch can provide a great deal of sexual pleasure when intercourse is not possible. Many older people are deprived of touch in aged care facilities or when a partner dies.

Women

The biological effect of diabetes on male sexual functioning has been well documented. The effects of diabetes on sexual function in women are poorly understood and the evidence for any effect is less conclusive than the evidence for the effects on male sexual functioning (Leedom *et al.* 1991). Physicians regularly ask men about their sexual functioning but not women (House & Pendleton 1986; Bernhard 1991). Although these are old studies there is no indication that things have changed. There is no real evidence that physical function in women is impaired by diabetes in the same way as it is in men, except decreased vaginal lubrication in older women with Type 2 diabetes. This could be due to normal ageing, related to diabetic neuropathy or other causes such as inadequate arousal. More women achieve orgasm from foreplay than from intercourse (Clarke & Clarke 1985) and this may also be a factor.

Women who have difficulty accepting that they have diabetes report higher levels of sexual dysfunction than those who accept their diabetes. Type 2 diabetes has a pervasively negative effect on women's sexuality (Schriener-Engel *et al.* 1991). There appears to be little or no effect in women with Type 1 diabetes but they often have concerns about pregnancy, childbirth, and hypoglycaemia during sex (Dunning 1994). There is a positive correlation between the degree of sexual dysfunction and the severity of depression that illustrates the connection between physical and psychological factors and the need for an holistic approach.

Changing blood glucose levels can have a negative transient effect on desire and sexual responsiveness and women often report slow arousal, decreased libido and inadequate lubrication during hyperglycaemia. Desire can fluctuate with stages of the menstrual cycle but this also occurs in women without diabetes. However, there is no correlation between the presence of complications and sexual difficulties in women with diabetes (Campbell *et al.* 1989; Dunning 1993). Polycystic Ovarian Disease and its effects could have adverse psychological effects (see Chapter 14).

The developmental stage of the individual should also be considered when assessing sexual health and the impact of diabetes when planning sex education and counselling.

- Children and adolescents – diabetes can affect normal growth and development if it is not well controlled and menarche and puberty can be delayed. This could impact negatively on body image and the development of sexual identity and self-esteem. Eating disorders and insulin manipulation can compound the problem.
- Young adulthood – attracting a partner, successful pregnancy and birth can be areas of fear and concern that affect sexual health (Dunning 1994). Hyperglycaemia can occur during menstruation resulting in tiredness, decreased arousal and libido. Vaginal thrush is common and causes itch and discomfort during sexual intercourse. It may be associated with taking oral contraceptives or antibiotics for intercurrent illness. Thrush and balanitis can inhibit male sexual activity.
- Older age group – hormonal changes due to menopause and associated fatigue and depression inhibit sexual enjoyment. Often a long-term partner's life course is different and this affects their sexual relationship. There are fewer partners and opportunities for sexual activity for older women especially those in care facilities.

Specific problems should be investigated depending on their presentation. Preventative sexual health care such as breast self-examination, mammograms, and cervical (pap) smears should be part of the care plan.

Men

Diabetes does have physical effects that cause erectile dysfunction (ED). Other ED causes include:

- Vascular damage, both systemic atherosclerosis and microvascular disease.
- Neurological diseases such as spinal cord damage, multiple sclerosis, and diabetic neuropathy.
- Psychological causes such as performance anxiety, depression and mood changes may be associated with hypo- or hyperglycaemia.
- Endocrine diseases that result in lowered sex hormones: testosterone, SHBG, prolactin, FSH, and LH. Hypogonadism can occur in chronic disease.
- Surgery and trauma to genitalia or its nerve and vascular supply.
- Anatomical abnormalities, for example, Peyronie's contracture, which is often associated with Dupuypten's contracture and other glycosylation diseases including diabetes, see Chapter 10.
- Medicines such as thiazide diuretics, beta blockers, lipid lowering agents, antidepressants, NSSRI, smoking, alcohol, and illicit drug use.
- Normal ageing.

ED is defined as the inability to achieve or maintain an erection sufficient for satisfactory sexual performance – penetration and ejaculation. It is common in men with diabetes especially if other diabetic complications are present. It occurs in 50% of men 10 years after the diagnosis of diabetes especially those who smoke. ED is gradual, insidious and progressive (Krane 1991). ED may be a predictor of cardiovascular risk and there is a higher incidence of undiagnosed coronary disease in men with ED. Elevated blood fats and hypertension and antihypertensive agents also play a part in the development of ED. Lowered sperm counts are associated with obesity, smoking and poor diet.

ED significantly reduces the man's quality of life especially in the emotional domain and has a negative effect on self-esteem. However, ED also has a significant effect on the man's partner. Partners play a key supportive role in the man's treatment and treatment success (Dean *et al.* 2008). When sexual functioning improves, improvement in mental and social status follows. Other sexual issues for men are fatigue, fear of performance failure, and concern about not satisfying their partners, but most men do not involve their partners when they seek advice about ED (Dean *et al.* 2008).

Investigation and management

A thorough history and physical examination are required. Some of the questions that need to be asked are very personal, which may be difficult and stressful, thus time, privacy, and tact are essential. The assessment includes diabetic complication status and blood glucose and lipid control, identifying the cause and determining the extent of the dysfunction, for example, using rigiscan and snap gauge to determine whether nocturnal erections occur, and sleep apnoea studies. There is an association between poor sleep, sleep apnoea and ED. Doppler studies are carried out to determine local blood flow. Testosterone, FSH, LH, SHBG, and prolactin levels are measured. Management consists of:

- Good metabolic control to prevent ED.
- Early intervention if ED occurs.
- Assessing fitness for sex and modifying risk factors, for example, losing weight, managing pain, smoking cessation, and reducing alcohol intake.
- Appropriate diet and exercise programme. Tai Chi and strength training can improve flexibility and strength and general well being in older men.
- Sex education that includes setting realistic expectations and planning for regular sexual health checks, for example, prostate disease.
- Diabetes education.
- Counselling, which should include partners and inform them about treatment options to help the couple find fulfilling sexual alternatives if the man cannot achieve erections.

Medication management

Oral medicines

Medication management includes oral phosphodiesterase type 5 (PDE-5) inhibitors Sildenafil (Viagra), Vardenafil (Levitra), and Cialis, which are vasodilators that enhance the natural sexual response. They can cause visual disturbances ('blue vision'), transient hypotension and can unmask cardiac ischaemia. PDE-5 medicines are contraindicated if nitrate medications are used and when cardiovascular disease is present. Cimetidine and Ketoconozale can increase Viagra levels and Rifampicin decreases them.

Other oral medicines currently under study include sublingual apomorphine (UPRIMA), which acts centrally and enhances the response to stimulation and oral phentolamine (VASOMAX), which improves penile blood flow (Endocare 2004).

Urethural and injected medicines

Urethurally introduced medicines such as MUSE have a success rate between 30% and 50% of men. Side effects include urethral pain and burning in 7–10% of men who use this medicine.

Intracavernosal therapy or penile injections such the vasoconstrictor agents papaverine, alprostadil (Caverject), VIP, and the vasodilator phentalamine. Men and/or their partners need to learn the technique of penile injections, which should be done under supervision. A rare but serious side effect is priapism, which requires urgent treatment to reverse the effects of the vasoconstricton. Other side effects include the formation of scar tissue, bruising, and rarely infection at injection sites. Caverject sometimes causes pain in high doses.

Non-pharmacological therapy

Non-pharmacological therapy includes external vacuum pumps. Vacuum devices are a simple effective method of achieving an erection. A man suffering from ED invented a device called ErecAid® in the 1960s. It consists of a clear plastic cylinder, which has either a manual pump or batteries and a special tension ring. The penis is placed into the cylinder and the man or his partner holds the device firmly against the body to form an airtight seal and then pumps the air out of the cylinder, which creates a vacuum and causes the penis to become erect. The special tension ring is inserted over the device around the base of the penis to maintain the erection, and the device is removed. The whole process takes about two minutes and the erection is maintained for about 30 minutes (longer than natural erections). The ring *must* be removed after intercourse.

Vacuum pumps have very few side effects. Sometimes, small red dots called petechiae and bruising can occur on the penis but these are not harmful. They are more likely to occur if the individual is on anticoagulant medicines. The temperature in the penis drops 1–2 degrees, which is caused by the tension ring. The device can be difficult to use, so learning how to use it, is important. It can reduce sexual spontaneity so it is very important that the man discusses sexual issues and their management options with his partner.

Hormone replacement therapy

Hormone replacement therapy (testosterone) might be indicated in 3–4% of men, but is contraindicated in men with liver disease, cardiovascular disease, renal disease, and prostate cancer. These contraindications probably apply to many men with diabetes. Testosterone comes in various dose forms including oral, injections, and implants.

Complementary medicines for sexual problems (CAM)

Men with sexual health problems commonly use CAM especially if they receive conflicting advice and worry a lot about the problem (Trutnovsky *et al.* 2001). CAM can be used to improve general health and well being and mange stress that can have benefits for sexual health, see Chapter 19. Likewise, recommendations about the importance of eating a healthy diet and exercise and adequate rest and sleep to sexual health are important. Often supplements such as flaxseed oil, vitamins E, and C and zinc are recommended. However, rigorous evidence for most is lacking and some are harmful. CAM therapies appear to target three main sexual issues: improving sexual 'stamina', aphrodisiacs, overcoming erection problems.

Commonly used CAM medicines include the following. They are often used in combination:

- Horney goat weed
- Passion treatment
- Damiana
- Yohimbe
- Asian Ginseng
- Goji berries, which are sometimes referred to as 'natural viagra' and also come chocolate coated.

Many so-called aphrodisiacs carry significant health risks (often for animals) and are not recommended. These include powdered rhino horn, crushed pearls, Spanish fly, and animal testicles.

The risks and benefits of these medicines are not known and they may interact with conventional medicines including those used to manage sexual problems. Therefore, it is important to ask men and women with sexual health problems about CAM use. The US FDA warned people about two unapproved dietary supplements sold online to treat ED: 'Blue Steel' and 'Hero', which contain active ingredients with similar actions sildenafil. These products could interact with conventional nitrate medicines and cause hypotension. People might unwittingly seek such alternatives if conventional ED medicines are contraindicated.

Involving partners in ED management

Partner may be able to contribute important information about the man's general health and sexual history but should only be involved if they are willing and the man agrees. The man, and ideally his partner, need to be involved in selecting the best management option. Partner's attitudes affect the man's uptake of and adherence to ED treatment and long-term management is more successful if the partner is involved (Fisher *et al.* 2005). The Index of Sexual Life (ISL) (Chevret *et al.* 2004) is a validated tool developed to assess women's sexual desire and satisfaction when their partner has ED.

Chevret *et al.* (2008) and Fisher *et al.* (2005) found partners of men with ED had significantly reduced sexual drive, orgasm, satisfaction, and frequency of sex compared with partners of men who did not have ED and prior to the onset of ED. In addition, partners of men with ED are more likely to have sexual dysfunction or avoid sexual activity.

A number of studies demonstrate significant improvements in sexual function, satisfaction, and quality of life for both partners following treatment, especially with PDE-5 medicines (Fisher *et al.* 2004) but discontinuation rates with these medicines appear to range between 10 and 45% (Madduri 2001).

Clinical observations

Improving sexual functioning can lead to changes in the relationship that result in conflict and disharmony.

Women have reported acute cystitis when their partners begin Viagra due to the increased sexual activity, so-called 'honeymoon cystitis'.

Sex education is part of the management for both men and women, and needs to include:

- Revision of diabetes knowledge and self-care and the importance of blood and lipid control.
- Knowledge about sex and sexuality and what 'normal' functioning is.

Sexual counselling

Good communication and trust is essential. Knowledge of the human sexual response, normal ageing, and the potential effects of diabetes is needed to counsel effectively. Sexual questions can be included when taking a nursing history. Including sexual questions in the nursing history can be simple and identify sexual problems that require specific questions to obtain a more detailed history or referral to a sex specialist. Respect and regard for the person and empathetic understanding and privacy are essential (Ross & Channon-Little 1991). The main areas to be covered when taking a sexual history are:

(1) Social aspects
- Childhood experiences.
- Marital status.
- Family relationships.
- Number and sex of any children.
- Interests, activities.
- Job demands/unemployment.
- Religious and cultural beliefs.
(2) Sexual aspects
- Sexual knowledge, education, fears, fantasies.
- Previous sexual experiences.
- Contraception method.
- If there is a current problem:
  - Whose problem does the person believe it to be?
  - Description of the problem in the person's own words.
  - Is the partner aware of the problem?
  - Does the problem follow a period of poor diabetic control or illness?
  - Have there been any previous sexual problems?
  - What were those problems?
  - How were they resolved?

(3) Psychological aspects
  • Acceptance of diabetes by self and partner.
  • Body-image concepts.
  • Presence of depression or other psychological problem.
(4) Diabetes knowledge
  • Self-care skills and knowledge of effects of poor diabetic control.

In addition questions to assess the level of communication among partners could include:

• Have you discussed your problem with your partner? Be specific about the problem after the man explains what the problem is and address each problem separately if there is more than one problem.
• Do you know what your partner thinks about the problem?
• Is your partner supportive of you seeking treatment to improve the problem?
• Does your partner have any question or concern about the treatment?
• Do you think your partner would come with you to discuss ways to improve your sex life?
• Does your partner have any concerns about his/her sexual function or general health?
• Is there anything else you would like to tell me to help me understand the problem?

The ISI questionnaire could also be useful to understand the woman's perspective.

The PLISSIT model

PLISSIT is an acronym for Permission–Limited Information–Specific Suggestions–Intensive Therapy. It is a model which uses four phases to address sexual problems and moves from simple to complex issues. It can be used in a variety of settings and adapted to the individual's needs (Anon 1975).

(1) Permission-giving
  Being open and non-judgemental allows the person to discuss their problem by offering:
  • reassurance.
  • acceptance of the person's concerns.
  • a non-judgemental attitude.
  • establishing acceptable terminology.
Questions about the person's sexuality can be asked or the nurse can respond to sexual questions the person asks. These actions establish that it is appropriate and acceptable to discuss sexual issues.
(2) Provision of limited information
  This involves giving limited information and general suggestions that might include practicing safe sex, diabetes, and sex education and giving:
  • accurate, limited information.
  • some reference information for home reading.

(3) Specific suggestions

These are usually made by a qualified sex therapist and often include sensate focus exercises and the squeeze technique for premature ejaculation (Clarke & Clarke 1985).

- involve the partner.
- provide sex education.

(4) Intensive therapy

Therapy at this stage requires referral to a sex psychologist/psychiatrist. Techniques include a range of counselling techniques based on Master's and Johnson's work, behavioural therapy and a range of other therapies.

Practice points

(1) The nurse must have adequate knowledge to undertake this and subsequent steps or refer the person appropriately.

(2) Examples of information to give at this stage is limited information about the differences between typical men and women, for example, women take longer to become aroused than men and need sufficient quality foreplay to be able to achieve orgasm; the effects of medications, smoking, alcohol, and diabetes on sexual responsiveness.

Role of the nurse

The nurse has an important role in the early identification of sexual problems and helping the individual or couple develop a health plan that includes sexual health. Some sexually transmitted diseases must be notified to government health authorities in some countries. Some specific nursing actions include:

- Being aware of the possibility that a sex problem may exist and allowing people to discuss their concerns.
- Debunking sexual myths, for example, old people who have sex are 'dirty old men/women'.
- Identifying sexual problems and addressing them or referring appropriately.
- Providing relevant care and information during investigative procedures and surgery.
- Medication advice and management.
- Advice about safe sex and contraception. People can be referred to family planning clinics, sexual health clinics, clinics that manage sexually transmitted disease if relevant. There is a great deal of useful information on the Internet but people need to be careful about the sites they access and the information provided. One useful booklet that can be downloaded free is *A Couple's Guide for the Treatment of Erectile Dysfunction* (Endocare 2004) available at www.osbonerecaid.com.
- Advice about monitoring quality sexual health.
- Advice about self-care and when it is safe to resume sex after hospitalisation, for example, after a myocardial infarct or cardiac surgery.

- In care homes for older people and rehabilitation settings, providing an appropriate environment and opportunities for couples to enjoy a sexual relationship might be possible.

References

Anon, J. (1975) *The Behavioural Treatment of Sexual Problems*. Enabling Systems, Honolulu.

Bernhard, L. (1991) Commentary. *Diabetes Spectrum*, **4** (1), 21–23.

Campbell, L., Redelman, M., Borkman, M., McLay, S. & Chisholm, D. (1989) Factors in sexual dysfunction in diabetic female volunteer subjects. *Medical Journal of Australia*, **151** (10), 550–552.

Chevret, M., Jaudinot, E. & Sullivan, K. (2004) Impact of erectile dysfunction (ED) on sexual life of female partners: assessment with the Index of Sexual Life (ISL) questionnaire. *Journal Sex and Marital Therapy*, **30**, 157–172.

Clarke, M. & Clarke, D. (1985) *Sexual Joy in Marriage. An Illustrated Guide to Sexual Communication*. Adis Health Science, Sydney.

Dean, J., Rubio-Aurioles, E., McCabe, M., Eardley, I., Speakman, M., Buvat, J., Saeenz de Tejada, I. & Fisher, W. (2008) Integrating partners into erectile dysfunction treatment: improving the sexual experience for the couple. *International Journal of Clinical Practice*, **62** (1), 127–133.

Dunning, P. (1993) Sexuality and women with diabetes. *Patient Education and Counselling*, **21**, 5–14.

Dunning, P. (1994) Having diabetes: young adult's perspectives. *The Diabetes Educator*, **21** (1), 58–65.

ED-Alliance Group (2000) *Practical Diabetes International*, **17** (5), 139–140.

Endocare (2004) *A Couple's Guide for the Treatment of Erectile Dysfunction* (available at www.osbonerecaid.com).

Fisher, W., Rosen, R. & Mollen, M. (2005) Improving the sexual quality of life of couples affected by erectile dysfuction: a double blind, randomized, placebo controlled trial of vardenafil. *Journal of Sex Medicine*, **2**, 699–708.

House, W. & Pendelton, L. (1986) Sexual dysfunction in diabetics. *Postgraduate Medicine*, **79**, 227–235.

Kaplan, H. (1979) *Making Sense of Sex*. Simon & Schuster, New York.

Krane, R. (1991) Commentary on erectile dysfunction. *Diabetes Spectrum*, **4** (1), 29–30.

Leedom, L., Feldman, M., Procci, W. & Zeidler, A. (1991) Severity of sexual dysfunction and depression in diabetic women. *Journal of Diabetic Complications*, **5** (1), 38–41.

Madduri, S. (2001) After 2 years, did Viagra live up to its expectations? *Mo Medicine*, **98**, 243–245.

Masters, W. & Johnson, V. (1970) *Human Sexual Inadequacy*. Little Brown Company, Boston.

Ross, M. & Channon-Little, L. (1991) *Discussing Sexuality. A Guide for Health Practitioners*. MacLennan & Pretty, Sydney.

Schriener-Engel, P., Schiavi, P., Vietorisz, D. & Smith, H. (1991) The differential impact of diabetes type on female sexuality. *Diabetes Spectrum*, **4** (1), 16–20.

Trutnovsky, G., Law, C., Simpson, J. & Mindel, A. (2001) Use of complementary therapies in a sexual health clinic setting. *International Journal of STD and AIDS*, **12** (5), 307–309.

World Health Organisation (1975) *Education and Treatment of Human Sexuality – The Training of Health Professionals*. Technical Report Series, 572, Geneva.

Chapter 12
Diabetes in Older People

Key points

- An holistic proactive and integrated approach is needed to achieve effective diabetes management, manage age-, and diabetes-related health risks and ensure management strategies are appropriate for the individual.
- Increasing age is associated with insulin resistance that predisposes older people to diabetes and diabetes is common in people over 65. Most have Type 2 diabetes but Type 1 and LADA also occur.
- The onset of diabetes is often insidious in older people with non-specific symptoms that can be mistaken for advancing age or other conditions.
- Long-term complications are often present at diagnosis.
- The individual should be encouraged to maintain independent, self-care within their capabilities for as long as possible but carer assistance is often needed especially during illnesses.
- There is limited evidence for metabolic targets in older people. Targets must be appropriate to the individual and limit the risk of adverse events such as hypoglycaemia, hyperglycaemia, and falls.

Where relevant, carers' wellbeing needs to be considered.

Rationale

Older people with diabetes are not a heterogeneous group. Some are healthy and active; others are frail and have multiple health problems. Managing diabetes in older people is complex and is an increasingly important aspect of nursing care as the population ages and the incidence and prevalence of diabetes increases with increasing age. Diabetes manifests differently in older people and their healthcare needs are different. Likewise, diabetes is likely to adversely affect many activities of daily living including, socialising and driving as well as physical and mental functioning all of which affect self-care ability.

Introduction

The ageing process is a progressive deterioration of bodily functions over the lifespan (US National Institute of Health (NIH) undated) whose characteristics are destructive, progressive, intrinsically determined and universal. Ageing occurs at different rates among individuals and among individual organs and tissues in the body. There are many theories but no consensus about what causes ageing. The two major schools of thought are: (1) Ageing is programmed and (2) Ageing is random, each accompanied by specific theories, see Table 12.1. These theories give rise to the question: Can ageing be cured (anti-ageing research) or should it be managed better to maintain wellness and a short decline to death because it is a natural process? Strategies to maintain wellness include:

- Reducing risk factors such as smoking, obesity, hypertension, and diabetes.
- Improving micronutrient deficiencies and using antioxidant supplements based on the Ames hypothesis that an adaptive triage process occurs in the body when micronutrients are scarce that favours short-term survival over long-term health-energy pathways are favoured over DNA repair (Ames 2006).
- Anti-ageing strategies such as:
  ○ diets, calorie restriction, and the Okinawa diet, mushrooms
  ○ anti-ageing nutrient supplements to reduce inflammation and oxidative stress such as SOD, CQ_{-10}, Gingko, Ginseng, Brahmi
  ○ hormones such as melatonin
  ○ medicines to improve insulin sensitivity, vasodilators, and mind stimulants.
- Under research: gene therapy, therapeutic cloning, cell therapy, nanotechnology (Grossman 2005).

Advancing age is associated with glucose intolerance, changes in renal function, which alters medicine pharmacodynamics and pharmacokinetics, reduced sense of smell, hearing, sight, mobility, reduced muscle mass, and changed cognitive functioning, all of which increase the individual's vulnerability to ill health. Significantly, chronological age is not the most important factor to consider when deciding management options. The functional status and biological age are more important determinants of care (National Health and Medical Research Council (NHMRC) 1994). Particular problems encountered in older people are shown in Table 12.2. It is important to realise that older people in hospital or living in residential aged care facilities do not represent the majority of older individuals living in the community (Australian Institute of Health and Welfare (AIHW) 2002).

The Victorian Department of Human Services (DHS) (2003) identified several specific care issues needed to maintain functional status:

(1) Improving nutrition
(2) Increasing functional mobility.
(3) Preserving skin integrity.
(4) Reducing incontinence.
(5) Avoiding and reducing the incidence of falls.
(6) Detecting and managing delirium and dementia.

Table 12.1 Theories of ageing. Currently there is no general agreement about the causes of ageing but most experts favour cellular damage theories. These seem to apply to uncontrolled diabetes where similar theories have been proposed for the development of diabetes complications. See Chapter 8.

Programmed theories	Damage theories
Ageing is a designed process (built in obsolescence)	Ageing is due to accumulated molecular damage especially to DNA and proteins that causes cell, organ, and system dysfunction
Disposable soma	Systematic damage theories:
Organisms exist to reproduce and then die	Immune system failure
	Failure of neuroendocrine regulation
	Failure to adapt
Antagonistic pleiotropy	Cellular damage theories caused by free radical
Genes that are essential and advantageous in young people cause damage in older people	damage by reactive oxygen species (ROS), hyperglycaemia causing advanced glycated end products (AGE) and binding of AGE receptors
Developmental programming	(RAGE) to AGE resulting in oxidative and
Ageing is regulated by genes and damage only begins to occur after development is complete	inflammatory effects (accelerated in diabetes), and/or chronic inflammation caused by inflammatory cytokines and eicosanoids, which
Neuroendocrine programming	with infection can induce oxidant-generating
Biological clock regulated by the hypothalamus. Hormone production eventually diminishes and causes changes associated with ageing	enzymes such as NADPH oxidase and nitric oxide synthase that produce ROS and reactive nitrogen species (RNS) that react with each other to form more potent reactive species
Rate of living (live fast die young)	that damage DNA and contribute to diseases
Every person has a fixed metabolic potential that can be affected by lifestyle also known as metabolic burnout	such as cancer by activating oncogenes and/or suppressing tumour suppressor proteins.
	Damage to cell membranes
Genetic programming	Somatic mutations
Ageing is preprogrammed in genes that might affect germ cell function, cell division, and cell death	Failure of repair processes

(7) Reducing medicine-related risks and maximising the benefits.

(8) Supporting and maintaining self-care.

(9) Detecting and managing depression.

DHS (2003) also noted the need to ensure relevant services are available and that they function optimally and to consider the health and well being of carers. The NHMRC series on clinical care of older people (number 3 1994) focuses on reducing hospital admissions and preventing complications in hospital encompasses most of these issues and highlights the need for multidisciplinary health professional care. In particular, The NHMRC emphasised the atypical presentation of many illnesses in older people.

Table 12.2 Particular problems encountered in the elderly person with diabetes and the resultant risks associated with the problem. Many of these conditions affect activities of daily living and extended activities of daily living. They represent a cumulative health burden and almost all represent a falls risk and contribute to the risk of driving accidents.

Problem	Associated risk
Hyperglycaemia leading to:	Constipation Postural hypotension Dehydration and electrolyte imbalance Polyuria and nocturia, which may present as urinary incontinence Hyperosmolar coma and ketoacidosis Impaired cognition Thrombosis Infection, for example, UTI Impaired wound healing Postural hypotension Decreased pain threshold Exacerbated neuropathic pain Lowered mood, lethargy, compromised self-care Driving deficits Falls
Chewing problems and swallowing difficulties	Hypoglycaemia Nutritional deficiencies: • Impaired immune response • Infection risk • Decreased plasma protein Impaired wound healing: • Higher fat intake • Dehydration • Muscle wasting and reduced strength in the lower limbs, which affect ADLs • Increased risk of systemic diseases such as cancer and cardiovascular diseases • Driving deficits • Difficulty swallowing medicines Energy deficits Increased morbidity and mortality Falls
Cerebral insufficiency	Stroke Non-recognition of hypoglycaemia Trauma Impaired cognition TIAs being confused with hypoglycaemia Increased prevalence of vascular dementia and Alzheimer's disease and other dementias Falls Driving deficits

Table 12.2 Continued.

Problem	Associated risk
Cardiac insufficiency	Myocardial infarction Confusion Poor wound healing Poor peripheral circulation Foot ulcers Driving deficits Falls
Autonomic neuropathy	Postural hypotension Gustatory sweating Urinary tract infections and incontinence Unrecognised hypoglycaemia Silent myocardial infarction Decreased/delayed food absorption Poor nutrition Infections, pain Decreased motor skills Erectile dysfunction Driving deficits Falls
Peripheral insufficiency	Trauma Foot/leg ulcers Claudication Falls
Peripheral neuropathy	Unstable gait Foot ulcers Depression Driving deficits Falls
Other neuropathies such as Bell's palsy	Reduced self-care Loss of independence Body image changes
Visual impairment Changed colour perception (blue, green, violet)	Self-care deficits Depression Loss of independence Social isolation Education difficulties with types of materials used and, differentiating medications Driving deficits
Skin atrophy	Pressure ulcers, skin tears Infection Progression of acute wounds to chronic wounds Stress and depression Oedema

(Continued)

Table 12.2 Continued.

Problem	Associated risk
Communication problems	Misunderstanding Confusion Inaccurate self-care Stress Social isolation
Stress and depression	Inadequate self-care Hypertension Hyperglycaemia Hypoglycaemia Impacts on wound healing Driving deficits Suicide risk Falls
Renal disease associated with diabetes and as a normal part of ageing	Decreased medicine clearance and prolonged activity End-stage renal disease requiring dialysis Difficulty interpreting investigative blood tests Malnutrition Reduced choice of OHA Dehydration Hyperosmolar coma Lactic acidosis Driving deficits Falls
Failure to recognise thirst (normal ageing process)	Dehydration Hyperglycaemia Confusion Driving deficits Falls
Cognitive impairment	Self-care deficits Education difficulties Reduced quality of life Falls Driving deficits
Musculoskeletal disorders such as Dupytren's contracture, cherioarthropathy, flexor tenosynovitis, carpel tunnel syndrome	Difficulty performing activities of daily living Pain and discomfort Driving deficits Falls

Many illnesses present with atypical symptoms, which can delay appropriate diagnosis and management and result in significant morbidity or death such as:

- Failure to thrive.
- Immobility.
- Postural instability.
- Incontinence.

- Confusion.
- Depression.
- Fatigue and lethargy.
- Weight loss.
- Undetected hyperglycaemia (IGT) can be present in non-diabetic older people and diabetes triggered by an intercurrent illness, a diabetes complication or emotional stress, and present as:
  - constipation
  - dehydration
  - postural hypotension
  - confusion
  - polyuria or urinary incontinence
  - infections such as UTI and URTI.

In addition, older people with diabetes usually have multiple health problems, some of which are the result of diabetes-related complications and are present at diagnosis in >20% of people (NHMRC 1992). Thus, actively screening older people in hospital and care facilities is warranted. Bayliss *et al.* (2007) found an average of 8.7 chronic diseases present per person in a cross-sectional survey of people aged >65 years. Compared with newly diagnosed non-diabetics, older people have a 9% mortality rate, 40% more lower leg complications (claudication, cellulitis), double the risk of cardiovascular disease including heart failure, double the risk of end-stage renal disease, and are 60% more likely to have vision problems (Bethel *et al.* 2007). They are also at great risk of falling, especially in hospital.

Managing diabetes, its complications, and other comorbid diseases requires multiple medicines, and often several doses per medicine per day. Many commonly used laboratory tests have lower specificity and sensitivity in older people, which can further complicate the clinical picture. For example, serum creatinine may not detect renal impairment especially in normal or underweight individuals (Gianelli *et al.* (2007) and contraindicated medicines may not be stopped.

Interestingly, despite the association among obesity and morbidity and mortality (Hu *et al.* 2005; Chen *et al.* 2006) being overweight is associated with longer life expectancy in men and women >80 years and underweight with shorter life expectancy even when other comorbidities are present (Takata *et al.* 2007). Weight loss is associated with total mortality in older people independently of low body weight (Keller *et al.* 2004). These findings suggest recommending older overweight people lose weight may actually put them at risk. Likewise, HbA_{1c} <7% increases the risk of hypoglycaemia and its consequences. HbA_{1c} >10% has immediate physiological effects as well as effects on neutrophil function and wound healing (Shekelle & Vijan 2007).

Evidence for ideal HbA_{1c} targets in older people is limited, apart from the UKPDS, which focused on preventing long-term complications rather than safety and maximising functioning. The Australian Diabetes Educators Association (ADEA) (2003) proposed targets based on a systematic review, but they are not intended for older people in aged care facilities. Brown *et al.* (2003) recommended HbA_{1c} <7% for most older people; and <8% in frail older people because preventing the short-term consequences of hypo and hyperglycaemia and their associated symptoms and risks to safety and quality of life, might be more important than preventing long-term complications. Management also depends on the individual's functional status.

Determining functional status

Older people in hospital and care facilities are a vulnerable group and the latter often receive suboptimal care (Kirkland 2000). Sinclair *et al.* (1997) found 40% of residents in elderly care facilities were on long-acting sulphonylureas, fewer than 1 in 10 had any regular diabetes follow-up, they had more hospital admissions than people without diabetes, stayed in hospital longer and had more complications. In addition, staff and resident knowledge about diabetes was deficient. Likewise, functional decline occurs in 30–50% of older people during hospitalisation and ~30% >70 years return home with ADL deficits (Royal Melbourne Hospital 2002). Functional decline is associated with long duration of hospitalisation and manifests gradually as malnutrition, reduced mobility, compromised skin integrity, incontinence, falls, delirium, depression, and inadequate self-care.

The degree of disability is likely to change over time, sometimes rapidly, and during illness, and affect the amount of assistance the individual needs, either on a temporary basis or in the longer term. Changing circumstances often have financial implications for the individual and the health system. Table 12.3 suggests some key questions that can help decide the level of assistance needed and appropriate management. In addition, geomaps and ecomaps can provide a great deal of information about the individual's social network and relationships, see Chapter 2. Annual diabetes complication screening should encompass screening for depression, comorbidities, falls risk, incontinence, pain and memory deficits, degree of frailty, functional status including driving ability, and a structured medicines review. The current Australian ANDIAB review does not encompass these issues and needs to be used in conjunction with other screening tools for older people.

Many of these activities depend on the ability to perform activities of daily living (ADL). There are two main types of ADL: physical (PADL) that encompasses essential daily activities such as bathing and dressing; and instrumental (IADL), which enable the individual to live independently in society and are more complex (Kock & Garratt 2001). IADL assessment must be based on activities relevant to the individual and take account of their physical surroundings, culture, and interests. For example, assessing an older person when they are in hospital and their blood glucose levels are in the optimal range may not accurately reflect their ADL and adverse event risk level at home (Dunning & Alford 1993).

Determining the frailty level (frailty index FI) might help identify older people likely to suffer adverse health effects (Kulminski *et al.* 2007). Frailty is a consequence of declining physical reserve and altered functioning in multiple physiological systems, which make the individual vulnerable to physical and mental stressors (Bortz 2002; Fried *et al.* 2004). Several definitions of frailty exist including the following:

The frailty state can be described using a cumulative index of health and well being deficiencies that is assessable for each individual . . . the fraction of deficits in a list of items that measure health and well being [constitutes the frailty index (FI)]

(Kulminski *et al.* 2007)

A number of methods of estimating the FI has been proposed. The most useful enable clinicians to use health information already being collected to predict those at risk of adverse health outcomes. Frailty could be calculated for older people with diabetes as part of the annual complication screening process and be monitored proactively and prospectively.

Table 12.3 Key issues that need to be considered when assessing disability in older people with diabetes. Repeat measures may be needed especially during acute illnesses when the physical and mental condition can change rapidly. These issues should be considered as part of the standard diabetes complication screening process. Reproduced with permission from Dunning, T. (2006) *Managing Diabetes in Older People*. Blackwell Publishing, Oxford.

Questions	Implications
(1) What activities are limited and to what degree?	A precise description of the disability is important in order to plan appropriate medical and nursing care and evaluate outcomes.
(2) Which disease processes are causing the disability?	Attributing disability to 'old age' is not an appropriate diagnosis. Common causes of disability include arthritis, cardiovascular disease, respiratory disease, stroke and visual impairment. One or more of these comorbidities often coexist with diabetes. Polypharmacy is likely. In some cases the medicine of choice for some comorbidities increases blood glucose levels.
(3) What is the person's mental state? Various assessment tools are used to assess mental status, for example the MiniMental, however their limitations need to be considered.	Evidence of memory loss, disorientation, confused behaviour and personality change may indicate diseases of the brain, dementia states or metabolic changes such as high or low blood glucose levels that impair mental processing. Consideration should also be given to the presence of anxiety, depression and the individual's general mental approach to life (positive or pessimistic) and hearing deficits.
(4) What is the person's social situation? See Figure 2.1	Disability implies dependence on others. It is important to identify the services and people likely to be able to support the individual if they do require help. In addition, it is important to ensure the person who takes on the care is supported and their personal health and wellbeing considered to prevent stress, sleep disturbance and ill health in the carer, especially if they are also elderly.

Cognitive impairment

Cognitive decline in older people with diabetes is multifactorial due to advancing age and vascular dementia but not other forms of dementia (Allen *et al.* 2004), hyperglycaemia (Morley & Flood 1990), and hypoglycaemia, and increasing duration of diabetes. Large community studies suggest older people with diabetes have worse cognitive functioning than non-diabetics (Croxon *et al.* 1995; Gregg *et al.* 2000; Logroscino *et al.* 2004), and the decline is more rapid in those with diabetes (Biessels *et al.* 2002). The Framingham Study suggests hypertension and diabetes are independent risk factors for poor performance on memory and visual organisation tests (Elias *et al.* 1997). In contrast, Asiakopoulou *et al.* (2002) demonstrated minimal effects on verbal and logical memory when blood glucose control is optimal.

In acute illness it is important to differentiate cognitive decline from hypoglycaemia, hyperglycaemia, and hyperosmolar states, delirium, MI, and other causes. Delirium is associated with:

- Prolonged hospitalisation, poor outcomes and admission to aged care facilities.
- Functional decline.
- Increased use of chemical and other restraints that increase the falls risk.
- Presence of infection, which can precipitate hyperosmolar states.
- Multiple comorbidities.
- Severe illness.
- Dehydration, which can precipitate hyperosmolar states and may lead to a diagnosis of diabetes in undiagnosed at risk individuals, see chapter 7.
- Alcohol abuse.
- Falls and fractures.
- Psychotropic medications.

Delirium, but not the severity, can be distinguished from non-reversible cognitive impairment using the Confusion Assessment Method (CAM) (Waszynski 2004). The CAM has concurrent validity with the MMSE but has not been tested in clinical settings and is associated with a 10% false-positive rate. The key aspects of the CAM are shown in the following list. A diagnosis of delirium is made if 1 and 2 and either 3 or 4 are present:

(1) Acute onset and fluctuating course during the day.
(2) Inattention such as being easily distracted and finding it difficult to recall what was said last.
(3) Disorganised thinking and unpredictable switching from topic-to-topic.
(4) Altered consciousness (Inouye *et al.* 1990; Waszynski 2004).

Fluid balance disturbances are common in older people largely as a result of changes in body water composition, declining renal function, and reduced thirst perception (Davies *et al.* 1995). Dehydration is common in community dwelling older people (Warren *et al.* 1996) occurring in ~6.7% of those >65 years in hospital and is the principal diagnosis in 1.4% (Warren *et al.* 1994). Dehydration is present in 50% of residents in aged care facilities with a febrile illness who are often referred to hospital due to dehydration (Bourdel-Marchasson *et al.* 2004). Dehydration should be preventable in hospital and aged care facilities. Management guidelines should encompass strategies to do so considering the following information.

Dehydration is associated with hyperglycaemia and DKA and HONK (see Chapter 7), thromboembolism, infections, renal calculi, falls and constipation, and causes up to 50% mortality if it is not adequately managed (Wilson *et al.* 2003), and poor mental functioning (Wilson *et al.* 2003; Faes *et al.* 2007). Early diagnosis is difficult because of the atypical presentation in older people and because there is no absolute definition of dehydration (Weinberg *et al.* 1995). A commonly used definition is:

'. . . a clinically relevant decrease of an individual's optimal Total Body water (TBW) amount and may occur with or without loss of electrolytes'.

(Faes *et al.* 2007)

Thus, the degree of dehydration depends on the relative rather than the actual total intracellular and extracellular water loss. People with low body weight show signs of dehydration after losing small amounts of water. Significantly, ~25% of older people drink <1 litre of fluid per day, especially those over 85 (Volkert *et al.* 2004). Risk factors for dehydration include:

- age over 85 years
- female
- having ≥chronic diseases
- using ≥5 medicines
- medicine-related factors such as high protein oral or enteral feeds, laxatives, anti-depressants, and diuretics
- fasting for surgery or investigative procedures
- fluid loss such as diarrhoea, vomiting, hyperglycaemia
- being confined to bed/chair
- poor mobility including manual dexterity
- poor eye-hand coordiantion
- communication difficulties
- inability to feed themselves
- social isolation
- hot weather
- having Alzheimer's disease and other cognitive disturbances (Lavizzo-Mourey *et al.* 1988).

The diagnosis is made on clinical signs such as recent weight loss >3% body weight, presence of an intercurrent illness, dry mucous membranes, coated tongue, sunken eyes, confusion, hypotension, muscle weakness in the upper body, and falls. Laboratory investigations such as serum osmolality, creatinine, blood urea nitrogen (BUN), BUN/creatinine ratio, and electrolytes as well as urine pH and output are useful. Three forms of dehydration occur:

- Hypertonic: sodium >150mmol/L or serum osmolality >300 mosmol/L.
- Isotonic dehydration occurs when water and electrolyte loss are balanced, for example, diarrhoea and vomiting.
- Hypotonic dehydration results when electrolyte loss is greater than water loss, for example, overuse of diuretics.

The prevalence of the isotonic and hypotonic dehydration has not been studied systematically and may be under-recognised. Having a high level of suspicion and care strategies to ensure optimal fluid intake such as prompting older people to drink are important preventative measure. Specific treatment depends on the clinical assessment and may include IV fluid replacement, preventing venous stasis, pressure ulcers and falls, as well as managing the underlying cause, and uncontrolled hyperglycaemia. Care must be taken not to over hydrate the individual and cause cerebral oedema or water intoxication.

Depression and older people with diabetes

Given the increasing prevalence of diabetes in older people, the fact that depression is a risk factor for diabetes, the 2-fold increased risk of depression in people with diabetes (Bogner 2007), it is likely that many older people have undetected diabetes as well as undetected depression. Undiagnosed depression contributes to physical and mental functional impairment.

Depression frequently precedes and may be the cause of placement in an aged care facility. Depression may be due to grief over loss of functional and self-care ability and independence (Fleming 2002) and is significantly correlated with quality of life (Goldney *et al.* 2004). Depression is often associated with diabetes-related complications such as cardiovascular disease (Fenton 2006) and is more likely to be recurrent in older people (Cluning 2001), and leads to inadequate self-care, unstable blood glucose patterns, and affects cognitive functioning. Treating depression in older people reduces mortality by 50% (Bogner *et al.* 2007).

Some clues to the presence of depression in older people are:

- Talking about physical symptoms and believing they have a serious illness (Cluning, 2001).
- Grief over lost opportunities, abilities, and self-determination.
- Withdrawing from communal activities.
- Experiencing chronic pain.
- Having had a stroke or MI.
- Not receiving any visitors at least once a week in hospital and aged care facilities.
- Difficulty establishing relationships with staff and other aged care residents in the first four weeks after admission.

Depression management is discussed in Chapter 15. When possible, non-pharmacological options should be used first.

Differentiating depression from dementia

The prevalence of dementia increases with age and ranges from 63% to 81% (Zimmerman 2007). Approximately one-in-4 Australians over age 85 have dementia (Gray *et al.* 2002). There are two main forms of dementia: Alzheimer's disease (AD) accounting for 70% of known dementias and Vascular Dementia (VD) accounting for the remaining 20%. Both AD and VD are present in ~20% of people especially those with diabetes (Stewart & Liolitsa, 1999).

The association between diabetes and dementia may be due to:

- Cardiovascular disease: TIAs and stroke that can cause multifocal brain damage.
- Hypoglycaemia, especially if it is frequent and recurrent, which may cause permanent neuronal destruction.
- Persistent hyperglycaemia increases protein glycosylation and contributes to the development of advanced contributes to AGE (see Chapter 8) found in AD plaques (Phillips & Popplewell, 2002).

Nay and Garratt (1999) outlined three main stages of AD. The first is characterised by absent-mindedness, emotional instability and poor concentration. These symptoms can include spatial disorientation, disturbed perception, changes in personal appearance and hygiene, a tendency to blame others for a range of occurrences, and an inability to successfully perform ADLs. Depression is often present in the early stages because the person is aware that something is 'not quite right' and they realise 'things are slipping away' from them (Katona, 1994).

Stage two can last up to 12 years. The person may withdraw and behaviour is often variable including anger, transient crying, poor sleep patterns, disorientation, and profound short-term memory loss. Gait often changes, people have difficulty recognising their own face in a mirror, and continence issues emerge as well as other behaviours such as exhibitionism. The person cannot live safely by themselves in the community.

Stage three is often the shortest, lasting up to 2 years. Profound physical and cognitive decline occurs, finally resulting in stupor and coma. Miller (1999) developed a useful process for distinguishing between depression and dementia.

Managing diabetes in older people

Age, life expectancy, other health problems and the person's social situation should be taken into account when planning care. Achieving near normal blood glucose levels and preventing long-term complications may not be priority management aims. It is important to control uncomfortable symptoms (polyuria, polydipsia, lethargy), maintain quality of life (QoL) and minimise the risk of hypoglycaemia and the attendant risk of falling.

Suboptimal metabolic control is associated with urinary incontinence, leg/foot ulcers, infections, nutritional deficiencies, exacerbation of neuropathic pain, affects the ability to communicate and cause confusion and aggression (Kirkland 2000). Strategies and priorities need to be implemented using a stepwise approach and non-pharmacological measures where possible.

Management aims

The issues outlined in the DHS, UK, and other policies and guidelines provide a useful framework for planning care. The main aims of care are to:

- Improve nutrition.
- Prevent hypo- and hyperglycaemia.
- Undertake a structured medication management programme using a quality use of medicine framework.
- Proactively screen for and prevent and/or manage diabetic complications, comorbidities, depression, and maintain independent self-care as long as possible.
- Undertake general preventative health measure such as vaccinations and health checks, for example, mammograms, prostate checks. Flu vaccine prevents respiratory illnesses, pneumonia, hospital admissions and death in older people (Gross *et al.* 1995). However, in years without influenza, booster vaccinations may not confer added benefits if routing trivalent vaccination does not produce seroprotection

(Gaughran *et al.* 2007). Research suggests people with chronic diseases are less likely to receive preventative care despite attending health professionals frequently (Beckman *et al.* 2001; Lipscombe *et al.* 2005).

- Manage coexisting illnesses to improve functional ability and improve quality of life.
- Maintain a positive attitude.
- Maintain a safe environment to limit adverse events such as falls.
- Have plan for regularly assessing driving safety and help the individual develop and maintain a transportation plan to make the transition to stop driving. Be aware that operating motorised wheelchairs, Go-Fors, and farm machinery may also constitute a driving risk.
- Ensure a comfortable and peaceful death at the end of life.

Factors that affect management decisions

- Age, but age alone may not give an accurate picture of an individual's ability to cope with self-care tasks and activities of daily living. Functional level should be assessed using appropriate tools in an appropriate familiar setting.
- Current diabetes control and complication status including the presence of liver and kidney disease.
- Presence and severity of comorbidities.
- Life expectancy.
- Mental and physical capacity to self-care.
- Nutritional status. Inadequate nutrition predisposes the person to hypoglycaemia, falls, decreased immunity, delayed wound healing and infections, and other diseases.
- Learning capacity, which is influenced by the individual's learning style, sight, hearing and cognitive ability, interest in the topic, and the way the individual presents the information, see Chapter 16.
- Social support from family and the community.
- Financial status and access to services.

Nutritional management

Elderly people are often malnourished. In hospital, malnourishment is associated with longer length of stay and increased mortality (Middleton *et al.* 2001). The causes of poor nutrition are shown in Table 12.4. Sometimes it is difficult to distinguish between the effects of malnutrition and disease processes, which are closely related (World Health Organisation 1999).

It is important to take a broad approach to nutritional management in older people with diabetes rather than the usual focus on reducing fat and sugar. In addition, older people need to be encouraged to:

- Incorporate omega-3 foods into the diet.
- Eat a variety of nutritious foods in at least three meals every day.
- Eat plenty of cereals, wholegrain bread and pasta especially those with a low Glycaemic Index; 50–60% of total intake.

Table 12.4   Risk factors for inadequate nutrition and malnutrition in older people.

Risk factor	Potential outcome
Living in an institution	Forced food choices, loss of control over environment, depression
Malabsorption	Bacterial infections, coeliac disease, medicines, disease processes and diabetes complications
Neurological deficits	Stroke, dementia
Medicines	Digitalis, alcohol, sedatives
Sensory deficits	Impaired sight and/or hearing, taste and smell
Dentition and swallowing difficulties	Ill-fitting dentures, caries, missing teeth, gum disease, malnutrition
Social circumstances	Isolation, poverty, inability to shop or prepare food, depression, malnutrition
Medical problems	Chronic disease, pneumonia, heart failure, chronic infection, thyroid disease, malnutrition

- Have adequate protein intake, consisting of at least 15% of the total intake.
- Eat plenty of fruit and vegetables to reduce the risk of cardiovascular and degenerative diseases and supply essential vitamins and minerals, such as calcium.
- Have an adequate fluid intake, including water (about 1500 millilitres per day) to reduce the likelihood of dehydration, especially in hot weather, unless fluid restriction is indicated.
- Drink alcohol in moderation. Because of the reduced muscle mass, the volume in which alcohol is distributed is reduced; therefore, the concentration of circulating alcohol is higher, putting the person at risk of cognitive impairment, hypoglycaemia, and falls. However, moderate consumption of alcohol might have health benefits.
- Use low salt food and only add small amounts of salt to food to help prevent hypertension (National Health and Medical Research Council 1999).

Practice points

(1) Many older people are malnourished even though they appear overweight. Malnutrition is common: 15% of homebound community dwelling, 35–65% of hospitalised people and 50% of residential aged care residents (Szony 2004). It is associated with longer length time in hospital and is a strong predictor of readmission and is associated with pressure ulcers, delirium, and depression.

(2) There is limited data about the nutritional needs of very old people.

(3) People over the age of 70 have special nutritional needs (Drewnowski & Warren-Mears 2001) especially if they have diabetes.

(4) Enteral feeding and supplements are often required.

Malnourishment can occur in hospital (McWhirter & Pennington 1994). In care facilities rates between 36% and 43% are reported (Friedman & Kalant 1998). Concomitant diseases that increase the risk of malnutrition in older people with diabetes include:

- Psychiatric disorders including depression, see Chapter 15.
- Parkinson's Disease.
- Chronic obstructive pulmonary disease.
- Polypharmacy, which is common in diabetes.
- Renal failure.
- Neurological dysfunction.
- Dental problems and chewing and swallowing difficulties. The latter also increases the likelihood that nasogastric or enteral feeding will be needed as well as the risk of coughing and choking during feeding and increases the risk of chest infections. Swallowing difficulties affect ~10% of hospitalised older people (Hudson *et al.* 2000).
- Disabled house-bound individuals.
- People with cancer or HIV/AIDS.

Specific nutritional deficits include vitamin D and calcium, which increases the risk of osteoporosis and fractures. Low intake of vitamin K-rich vegetables affects the stability of the INR in people on anticoagulant therapy (*Am J Med* 2004). Factors that help maintain optimal nutrition for people over 80 living in the community are supportive family and friends, having a microwave oven, transportation, and proximity to a grocery store (Callan & Wells 2003). The Australian Nutrition Screening Initiative was developed to highlight the importance of identifying older people at risk of malnutrition. The tool can help nurses decide when a comprehensive nutritional assessment is required and refer the individual to a dietitian.

The Hydration Assessment checklist detects hydration problems in older people (Zembrzuski 1997) and the Mini Nutritional assessment (MNA) detects actual and potential malnourishment in people over 65 (Reilly 1996) and may predict mortality in older people (Persson 2002). Other nutrition assessment tools are listed in Chapter 4.

Biochemical assessments include plasma proteins, recognising the concentration can be influenced by non-nutritional factors such as liver disease, some cancers, sepsis, and inflammatory bowel disease. Protein intake can be calculated using the blood urea nitrogen (BUN) with the serum creatinine. If the creatinine is low, protein intake is low. If both the creatinine and BUN are low, a state of tissue catabolism such as that associated with hyperglycaemia, exists. Low serum albumin indicates chronic protein deficiency. However, albumin has a long half-life (~20 days) thus it is not an accurate indicator of temporary protein lack (Baines & Roberts 2001). Specific tests for deficiencies such as zinc and vitamins may be indicated.

Nutritional supplements are a simple way of increasing the energy and nutrient content of the diet of older people. Even when the daily intake of vitamins and minerals is adequate these nutrients may not be bioavailable and supplements may be needed (Truswell 2003). For example, omega-3 supplementation may be beneficial to lower triglycerides of people with heart disease if the RDI cannot be consumed by eating oily fish. The American Heart Foundation (AHA) (Orford *et al.* 2002) recommended doctors supervise omega-3 supplementation in older people. Omega-3 supplements may cause gastrointestinal disturbances and hyperglycaemia and may interact with warfarin and cause bleeding.

Enteral therapy

An increasing number of older people, particularly those living in care facilities, require enteral feeding. Usually, OHAs/insulin should be administered and blood glucose tests performed before administering the enteral feed but other medications may need to be administered separately from feeds to ensure they are absorbed. Nasogastric tubes are usually used when temporary enteral feeds are needed. Gastroscopy, jejunostomy or PEG tubes are usually preferred when enteral feeding is required long term. Enteral therapy enables fluid and macronutrients to be provided to meet the individual's metabolic and nutritional requirements.

Feeds are administered slowly initially to prevent Refeeding Syndrome and to limit the metabolic and haemodynamic effects. For example, electrolyte shifts can precipitate congestive cardiac failure, cardiac arrhythmias, and neuromuscular and respiratory dysfunction (Cook *et al.* 2001).

The formula used depends on the indication, for example, the need to reduce CO_2 production in respiratory disease when CO_2 excretion is compromised. There are no specific guidelines for people with diabetes at risk of malnutrition who require nutritional support. General dietary recommendations for people with diabetes may not be appropriate for older malnourished people with diabetes (Elia *et al.* 2001). Formulas with less impact on blood glucose are available for people with diabetes. Types of formulas include:

- Standard, which are often used when commencing enteral feeding. These are high in carbohydrate and low in fat and fibre and can cause hyperglycaemia because of their rapid transit time and nutrient absorption and lead to post prandial hyperglycaemia due to impaired muscle and splanchic glucose uptake (Basu *et al.* 2001).
- Hypercaloric, used if fluid intake needs to be restricted, for example, end-stage renal disease.
- Fibre +, to reduce constipation.
- A range of specialty formulas exists for renal, hepatic, respiratory disease, wound management, and cancer. Specialty formulas for people with diabetes include, Nutrison low energy for diabetes, Nutrison diabetes, Resource diabetes, and Glucerna, which are all generally low GI. These formulas used as enteral feeds or supplements have less effect on blood glucose than standard feeds (Elia *et al.* 2005). Glucerna has less effect on blood glucose than Enrich, Ensure HN and Compleat Modified (Peters & Davidson 1992). Diabetes-specific formulas contain fructose, fibre monounsaturated fatty acids, protein and antioxidants. High GI feeds can precipitate osmotic diarrhoea, dehydration, and hyperosmolar states. If high GI foods are indicated they should be commenced slowly and increased slowly and oral hypoglycaemic agents/insulin adjusted according to the blood glucose pattern. Blood glucose should be monitored regularly.
- Elemental and sub-elemental formulas are easily digested and may be suitable for people with autonomic gastroparesis.
- Modular formulas, which contain a single nutrient enable feeds to be tailored to the individual.

The effects on the individual need to be considered when commencing enteral feeding: these include isolation, depression, and reduced QoL. In addition enteral feeds may not prevent malnutrition, even when they are carefully tailored. They may delay wound healing if they lead to hyperglycaemia, pressure sores and infection can develop around the tube insertion site and the nasogastric tubes can become dislodged and cause aspiration pneumonia. They can be a burden on carers, and incorrect administration of medicines occurs in home and aged care and hospital settings, for example crushing enteric-coated long-acting medicines.

Guidelines for administering diabetes medicines with enteral feeds

The policies and guidelines of the relevant facility should be followed. Generally:

(1) Liquid dose forms are the preferred formulations. If there are no contraindications to crushing tablets or opening capsules they should be crushed to a fine powder and mixed with 10–15 mL of water.
(2) The feed should be stopped 30 minutes before the scheduled medication administration time and flushed with 30 mL water before administering the medicines when medicines need to be administered on an empty stomach and recommenced 30 minutes after all the medicine is administered.
(3) If medicine/enteral formula incompatibilities are possible; alternative medicines or formulas should be prescribed if possible. It is not possible, the feed should be stopped 2 hours before medicine administered as a single daily dose and recommenced 2 hours after the medicine is administered. If more frequent doses are prescribed one hour should be allowed before and after the medicine/s are administered. However, this method does *not* guarantee complete bioavailability of the medicines but no incompatibility between commonly used diabetes medicines and enteral feeds were identified.
(4) Medicines should be remixed before they are administered using a syringe clearly labelled for oral dosing to avoid the possibility of a wrong route medication error. Allowed the medicines to flow in by gravity. If the mixture does not flow easily the plunger can be depressed very gently. Medicines should not be pushed through enteral tubes because they can obstruct the tube.

Different medicines should never be mixed together in a syringe

The syringe should be flushed with 5 mL of water between medicines when several medicines need to be administered at the same time. The tube should be flushed with 30 mL of water and clamped after all the medicines are administered. The feeding can then be recommenced. A feeding record should be maintained and the amount of water used to flush the tubing should be documented, especially when the person has oedema or renal disease. Medicines should be documented on the medication record.

It is advisable to consult a pharmacist before crushing medicines or opening capsules and administering them through enteral feeding tubes. Some medicines are more toxic if they are crushed, others have reduced efficacy, and the possibility of medicine interactions increases. If possible, liquid formulations should be used for enteral administration. Other dose formulations such as topical applications, intranasal sprays, patches, suppositories or injections should be used if applicable. Many lipid lowering agents and antihypertensive medicines should not be crushed.

The Product Information sheets and quality medicine handbooks detail specific information about administration medicines in relation to food, solubility, information about administration via enteral routes. For example, some medicines are absorbed from specific areas of the gastrointestinal tract and need to be enteric coated to reach the area before being absorbed.

Practice points

(1) During acute illness, surgical procedures and trauma blood glucose levels can be controlled more effectively with insulin.
(2) Insulin may be preferable and reduce the risk of adverse medicine events if enteral feeding is required temporarily and in the long term.
(3) OHA may be contradicted in some disease states, see Chapter 5.
(4) Diabetes medication management must relate to enteral therapy routines and not usual medication/meal administration times. For example, if the individual is scheduled for an enteral feed five times a day, for example, at 6 AM, 10 AM, 2 PM, 6 PM, and 10 PM, the diabetes medication must be administered and blood glucose tested considering these feed times. Thus, many diabetes medications need to be administered at 6 AM with the first feed and not at 8 AM when breakfast is served. Capillary blood glucose testing should be performed before an enteral feed and/or 2 hours after the feed to determine postprandial glucose clearance.

There is no specific information about compatibility between various enteral feeds and many medicines. Therefore, patients should be monitored according to the indication for the medicine and the enteral feed to ensure management aims are met. Enteral feeding may not be a contraindication to medicines but administering some medicines via enteral tubes can alter their bioavailability. For example, crushing may increase the absorption and affect the action profile of some medicines and increase the possibility of adverse events (Gilbar, 1999; Engle & Hannawa 1999; Young 2004).

Nutrition in dementia

Inadequate nutritional intake is common in people with dementia who accept or refuse meals erratically and may be anorexic. When a person refuses meals they can be encouraged to consume fluids and light foods such as hot chocolate, milkshakes, ice cream, fruit, yoghurt, and custard. Repeating favourite foods can sometimes help. For example, if the person likes breakfast foods, breakfast can be repeated at dinnertime. Nutritional supplements may also be useful, for example, 60 mL Two-Cal® administered with normal prescribed medications four times a day will increase protein intake.

Education approaches

Diabetes education is discussed in detail in Chapter 16. Factors that affect learning in older people include the environment, the time the education is delivered, the duration of the session, the type of education materials used and the person's physical and mental state. Where appropriate, people should have their glasses (spectacles) and hearing aid with them during diabetes education sessions (Jennings 1997; Rosenstock 2001).

Spouses and/or carers should be included in diabetes education sessions when appropriate especially when cognition is impaired for whatever reason. Support groups have long-term benefits for knowledge retention, psychosocial functioning and improved metabolic control and improve socialisation (Gilden *et al.* 1992). In the absence of dementia, the factor most likely to affect an older person's ability to learn, retain, and recall new information and skills and problem-solve depends on whether they are actively involved in their community. For example, an older person who participates social activities is more likely to want to learn about their diabetes management than socially isolated older people.

Many diabetes education programmers are not age-specific and often occur in groups, which makes it difficult for hearing and vision impaired people to participate. Computer-generated learning packages are also difficult to see, access and use for older people. In addition, many older people have low literacy skills. Small font sizes and/or text printed on shiny or coloured paper with insufficient contrast between the text and the background also compromises comprehension. Despite these limitations older people like to receive written information, are likely to refer to it and use it in their diabetes care.

Participating in education programmes can provide mental stimulus and help preserve mental functioning as well as reduce hospital admissions and improve QoL. Memory, learning, information retrieval and cognitive deficits have been demonstrated in people with Type 2 diabetes particularly when metabolic control is poor (Gilden *et al.* 1993). Several factors affect memory and learning besides cognitive function and vision changes. These include:

- Degree of wellness.
- Physical, psychological, and biological capacity.
- Social situation and available support.
- Degree of adjustment to being older and age-related changes, for example, wearing glasses.
- Sensory loss, tiredness, and incontinence can be barriers to effective education.

Poor blood glucose control is associated with reduced cognitive functioning and problem-solving and planning skills. Cognition sometimes improves when the blood glucose pattern improves (Gradman *et al.* 1993). Screen for cognitive impairment can be incorporated into the diabetes management plan using screening tools such as the Mini Mental State Examination (MMSE) and the results used to plan diabetes education strategies (Sinclair 1995).

Diabetes education strategies must include methods of increasing concentration and enhancing attention especially when vision and hearing are impaired. Incorporating relaxation techniques and other complementary therapies into the education session can relieve stress and enhance learning, see Chapter 19.

Self-care

Self-care is important and independent self-care should be maintained as long as possible. Older people may need help with some self-care tasks but not others. Health professionals need to realise that diabetes self-care is relentless and demanding. Support self-care can be an added burden to carers who may be old and have illnesses themselves. Self-care capacity should be assessed regularly as part of the annual complication assessment, following a hospital admission, and when medicine or medicine doses change. Barriers to self-care include declining physical and mental functioning, depression, intercurrent illness, comorbidities, and the effects of medications. Specific factors associated with inadequate self-care include:

- Lower levels of physical functioning.
- Inadequate knowledge about the medical condition/s.
- Limited participation in social activities.
- Depression.
- Financial constraints.
- Male gender.
- Low perceptions of health status.
- High number of concomitant conditions (Bayliss *et al.* 2007).

Potential barriers include high levels of morbidity, cumulative effects of comorbidities, inadequate health professional/patient communication, and health professional clinical inertia. In addition, self-perception, the desire to remain independent, health beliefs and attitudes play a role. For example, in general older people are reluctant to use walking aids. However, sudden changes in walking ability and positive cultural views about ageing make a difference to their willingness to accept a walking aid (Gooberman-Hill & Ebrahim 2007).

The person's home blood glucose testing record might provide important clues to self-care. For example, if it is smeared with blood it might indicate visual, eye-hand coordination, or manual dexterity deficits. Food-stained record books might indicate testing from contaminated fingers. If these deficits are suspected the issue needs to be approached with tact and in a non-judgmental manner. Record books can be used proactively and constructively to help people understand the effects of food, activity, medicines and stress on their blood glucose, help them find solutions to problems and involve them in planning their care. Wetzels *et al.* (2007) undertook a systematic review of the relevant literature that showed using a pre-visit record book in combination with an education session or consultation led to more questions and more self-reported health care.

Some older people find the print too small in commercial blood glucose record books and prefer to use 'exercise books'. Paper-based patient-held records are still popular with many people despite modern meters that automatically record blood glucose results and have the capacity to download the results directly onto computers (Davis 2003).

Factors that can affect metabolic control

'Barriers to good control are often in the minds of physicians rather than the capacity of the elderly person with diabetes' (Halter 2001). A current term is 'clinical inertia'. For example, many GPs are reluctant to commence insulin in older people when metabolic control deteriorates, even when the patient and their family/carers are willing. It is important to consider the health professional's influence on an individual's healthcare, especially when the individual is old. Health professionals often judge elderly people in general by the elderly people they manage in aged care facilities who may not accurately represent the majority of self-caring elderly people living in the community. Some of the factors that can affect diabetes control in the elderly are shown in Table 12.5.

Table 12.5 Factors that can affect diabetes control and management in older people.

Health professionals	Attitudes and beliefs Inadequate knowledge about diabetes Inappropriate advice, education materials Ageist approaches to services and diabetes management choices Clinical inertia Constraints on time and services
Altered senses	Communication difficulties Diminished vision, hearing and smell, altered taste, decreased proprioception Not understanding instructions
Food difficulties	Purchasing, preparing and consuming food, understanding nutritional requirements, poor appetite, early satiety, gastrointestinal problems Disease processes. Dental and oral problems
Disease processes/effects	Tremor, arthritis, poor dentition, gastrointestinal abnormalities, altered thirst sensation, altered renal and hepatic function, infection (acute and chronic)
Mobility	Limited ability to exercise Self-imposed driving restrictions or withdrawal of driving license
Medicines	Alcohol, medications such as glucocorticoids, interactions, self-prescribed medications
Complementary therapies	Hypo- or hyperglycaemia, medicine/herb interactions, herb/herb interactions
Malabsorption	Owing to diabetes medications, disease processes, medicine interactions, diabetes complications
Psychological issues	Bereavement, depression, cognitive deficits
Social factors	Social isolation, living alone or in care facilities, family expectations
Financial status	Purchasing recommended foods, monitoring equipment, diabetes complication screening, podiatry services

Access and equity to diabetes services

Elderly people are often unable to attend mainstream diabetes services especially where they are fragmented and essential services are offered on different days. Appointments scheduled to allow a 'one stop' approach to diabetes management enhance attendance rates. People are often required to attend different sites to have their eyes, kidneys, and feet checked for diabetic complications. Therefore, integrated care and careful transition care, discharge planning, and involving the GPs is essential. In Australia, the GP incentive schemes and integrated care planning and assessment strategies and the National Service Framework in the UK have significantly improved diabetes care in general practice.

Infection

The presence of infection can significantly affect the health status of older people. Any sudden increase in blood glucose that cannot be accounted for by dietary changes, inactivity, medicines, or stress should be investigated. The temperature should be recorded. Foot inspection is important to exclude occult infection. Reduced mobility and sitting with feet in the dependent position can cause lower leg oedema, which puts pressure on fragile, less flexible older skin causing small ruptures, weeping and increase the risk of infection and chronic ulcers. Mental stress associated with non-healing wounds delays wound healing.

Urinary tract infections are common in older people. A urine dipstick test for white cells and nitrate should be performed. There is growing evidence that consuming cranberry formulations on a daily basis can prevent UTI in older people with diabetes. Cranberry formulations can interact with warfarin so caution is needed in people on these medicines. As indicated, annual influenza vaccination should be part of the individual's routine health management plan.

An holistic approach to healing is needed that includes proactive screening for occult infections, optimal nutrition, education, and strategies that encompass physical, spiritual, and mental health. A single point of care coordination is desirable but the expertise of several health professional groups may be needed. For example, podiatrist, orthotist, endocrinologist, diabetes educator, dietitian, vascular surgeon, orthopedic specialist, infectious diseases physician and a wound consultant might all be required to manage an infected foot.

Quality of life

Quality of life refers to an individual's enjoyment of life and might or might not include prolonging life, see Chapter 15. QoL issues specific to the individual are more likely to accurately gauge life enjoyment than objective QoL tools even those well validated and frequently used tools. Such tools are essential if the objective is to compare individuals. However, they may be less relevant if the objective is to sequentially monitor individual QoL. For example, pets enhance QoL and are treasured companions for many older people, yet pets are not mentioned on any QoL tools. Older people identify QoL as being more important than length of life (Medical Research Council, 1993).

Many factors affect QoL in addition to personal QoL factors, these include:

- General health and medical issues such as diabetes type, treatment regimen, level of metabolic control and presence of complications. The greater the severity and effects of diabetes-related complications the greater the effect on QoL. Sexual health is often overlooked in older people. It is an important aspect of QoL often compromised by medical conditions, medications, the effects of age, and health professional and societal attitudes.
- Management strategies. The level of glycaemic control rarely relates to the level of well being (Testa *et al.* 1998) but diabetes symptoms of hypo or hyperglycaemia are more directly related to QoL (Van der Does *et al.* 1996). Maaravi *et al.* (2000) identified nutritional status as a major determinant of QoL in a community dwelling people over 70 years. There are conflicting about the effects of the different types of diabetes treatment on the QoL of older people. QoL is lower in people treated with insulin (Petterson *et al.* 1998; DAWN 2006). In contrast, Reza *et al.* (2002) reported better mental health, social functioning, and vitality and less carer strain associated with insulin.
- Cognitive functioning is affected by acute and chronic blood glucose fluctuations. The associated neuropsychological changes can reduce QoL of both the person with diabetes and their family.
- Health, diabetes, cultural, and general attitudes and beliefs, which influence factors such as self-efficacy and locus of control. Strategies that focus on understanding the individual's beliefs and attitudes, and encompass empowerment theories improve an individual's sense of well being and involvement in their care.
- Demographic factors such as gender, education level ethnicity, age, and social support. Men report better QoL than women and young people better than older people. Higher education is associated with a higher QoL. Individuals with good support generally have a better QoL and reduced risk of depression.

Various tools to measure QoL and other related factors are shown in Chapter 15.

Safety

In many respects diabetes management in older people encompasses managing risks regardless of whether the individual lives in the community or in a care facility, or is being cared for in acute, ambulatory, or primary care settings. There safety is multifactorial and cumulative issues affect safety as can be seen from Table 12.2. Many safety programmes focus on falls, but driving safety is also a significant concern.

Falls are the sixth leading cause of death in older people with and without diabetes, but having diabetes significantly increases the risk. People who fall do so repeatedly and falls are a common cause of placement in a home for the elderly. Falls are a result of a combination of accumulated effects of disease processes, impairment, and medications (Quayle 2001). It can be seen from Table 12.2 that a significant number of diabetes-related problems significantly increase the likelihood that an older person with diabetes will fall.

People at risk of falling:

- Fell in the last year.
- Have difficulty with mobility and sensory deficits.
- Are on four or more medications particularly oral agents, insulin, antihypotensives, antidepressive agents.

- Have an acute illness
- Were recently discharged from hospital.
- Have reduced strength and require a walking stick or frame.
- Wear inappropriate footwear.
- Are subject to environmental hazards.
- Have balance problems.
- Have diabetes complications such as autonomic neuropathy and visual loss.
- Are sedated, especially in an unfamiliar environment such as hospital or aged care facilities. They can become disorientated and fall going to the toilet at night.

Diabetes is associated with a two-fold increased risk of older people falling (Sinclair 2006) and older women are at increased risk of sustaining a fracture if they fall (Gregg *et al.* 2002). Ninety per cent of those who fall are likely to fracture a hip, shoulder, or foot (Schwartz *et al.* 2001). Women with diabetes aged 70–79 are more likely to fall if their HbA_{1c} is ≤6.8% and they are on insulin (Schwartz *et al.* 2003), which suggests hypoglycaemia may be implicated in many falls in older women with diabetes. Significantly, the presence of diabetes predicts failure to recover from mobility deficits, which increases the likelihood the individual will require supported care (Clark *et al.* 1998). Some diabetes-specific factors related to falls are shown in Table 12.2. Others include:

- Insulin treatment leading to hypoglycaemia. Sulphonylureas (OHA), particularly long-acting agents also cause hypoglycaemia but less frequently than insulin. The association between hypoglycaemia and OHA might be partly due to reduced renal clearance of active OHA metabolites of long-acting agents. Falls are associated with high levels of cystatin-c, an indicator of kidney function (Schwartz *et al.* 2008).
- Postural and postprandial hypotension. Hypertension is also associated with haemodialysis on dialysis days. See Chapter 10 and cardiovascular disease Chapter 8.
- Postural instability, and gait, and balance problems due to a wide range of health problems including erratic blood glucose pattern, muscle wasting and reduced lower limb strength, musculoskeletal problems, low vision and environmental factors.
- Weight loss and nutritional deficiencies.
- Neurological problems that may slow recognition of and response to falls risk situations.
- Cardiovascular disease: ~77% of presentations to emergency department due to unexplained falls have their basis in cardiovascular disease (van der Velde *et al.* 2007). Poon *et al.* (2006) suggested orthostatic hypotension might be contributory factor in up to 32% of falls associated with cardiovascular disease. Postprandial hypotension is also a falls risk. Postprandial hypotension is described as a blood pressure fall of 20 mmHg, an hour after eating. In aged care facilities postprandial hypotension is associated with an increased incidence of falls, syncope, stroke, and new coronary events (Aronow & Ahn 1997).
- Withdrawing medicines that contribute to orthostatic hypotension reduces the falls rate. Tilt table tests might be useful to detect hypotension (van der Velde *et al.* 2007). However, this equipment is unlikely to be readily available in most clinical situations.
- Cognitive impairment, which might be due to hyper or hypoglycaemia, hypotension, neurological problems, vascular disease, depression, dementia or a number of other causes.

Interestingly, Oates *et al.* (2007) showed older people, >80 years (*n* = 4071 from 10 US veteran's affairs sites) had lower 5-year survival rates if they had low blood pressure than those with higher blood pressure, which suggests current blood pressure targets might be harmful in very old people, particularly given the associated falls risk. Research in other populations also demonstrated better outcomes in older people with higher than recommended target blood pressure levels (Geuyffier *et al.* 1999; Goodwin 2003). However, blood pressure targets need to be considered in light of hypertension-associated risks such as stroke and cardiovascular events. All of these factors support the need for individualised, structured medicines reviews that are undertaken in the context of cumulative risk and QoL.

Multifactorial strategies are usually needed to prevent and manage falls. Interestingly, a meta-analysis of the literature about hospital falls prevention programmes demonstrated falls reduction between 30% and 49% but few studies used sound methodologies or represent strong evidence for their benefit (Coussement *et al.* 2008). After adjusting for falls risk Coussement *et al.* 2008 suggested current falls prevention programmes may only be useful in long stay care units. They suggested more research into primary falls prevention in hospitals is needed in which the number of fallers, the effect of the setting in which the fall occurred, and individual falls risk are examined to determine the effect of the separate components of falls reduction programmes.

Medications

Medications are discussed in detail in Chapter 5. Age-related medicine pharmacokinetic and pharmacodynamic changes must be considered when deciding which medicine, dose and dose interval, to use. As indicated declining renal function is a normal consequence of ageing, consequently long-acting medicines may be contraindicated if they have a prolonged half-life. Liver damage and inadequate or erratic food intake or food low in carbohydrate increase the risk of hypoglycaemia with insulin and many OHA.

When swallowing difficulties are present medication dose forms may need to be reviewed. Suggested strategies include:

- Identify medications that cannot be crushed and discuss these with the individual's doctor (hospital or GP) and pharmacist to determine whether the medicines are still required. If so, decide whether a non-medicine option could be used or whether there is an alternative dose form.
- Place a medication alert and a swallowing alert in the person's medical record.
- Communicate the alerts to the relevant carers and health professional carers especially when transferring among services.
- Provide education for people with diabetes and health professionals.
- Regularly review medications.

Practice point

The medicine dose forms that cannot be crushed are enteric coated, extended release, sublingual, medicines that irritate the oral mucous membranes, have a bitter taste, contain incipients and dyes that could stain the teeth, when specific protection is required when handling the medicine (Mitchell 1996; Simpson 2005).

Some medicines affect nutritional status by altering appetite, taste or sense of smell and affect food appreciation. Medicines such as antidepressants, sulphonylureas, and glucocorticoids contribute to weight gain. Others, such as anticholinergic medicines lead to dry mouth and difficulty in swallowing. Some medicines impair absorption, of vitamins and minerals, for example, antacids reduce iron and iron tablet absorption whereas vitamin C enhances iron absorption. There is increasing evidence that people with diabetic renal disease are at earlier risk of renal-associated anaemia but the exact mechanism and role of nutrition in this process is not known.

Phenytoin is sometimes used to manage painful diabetic peripheral neuropathy as well as seizures. It can inhibit absorption of vitamin D and folic acid. Some foods modify the absorption of some medicines, which explains why the timing medication doses in relation to food is important, especially in enteral feeding regimens.

Exercise/activity

Regular exercise has physical and mental benefits for people with and without diabetes of all ages. Exercise helps reduce the risk of developing diabetes and cardiovascular disease as well as improving mental wellbeing. Any movement of the body or limbs helps reduce cardiovascular fatalities by up to 50% and the chance of a second myocardial infarct by 25% as well as reducing hypertension and stroke risk (Vicfit 2004).

However, exercise is difficult for many older people because of the decline in muscle mass and general mobility, strength, and energy. These factors increase the risk of falls, injury, and fractures. Thus, exercise needs to be planned and individualised considering safety. At least 30 minutes of aerobic exercise per day and strength training exercises help maintain muscle mass and energy. In addition, adequate nutrition, especially protein, is important to preserving muscle mass and mobility, reduce falls, and improve well being (Viatkevicius *et al.* 2002; Stressman *et al.* 2002). It is not appropriate to merely recommend an older person to begin an exercise programme without assessing his/her physical status first. Assessment can be incorporated in usual care and includes assessing:

- Vascular status and detecting cardiac. Well older people in the community may require a graded exercise test. Blood pressure, lipid profile and assessment for autonomic neuropathy, which coud lead to silent MI is advisable (Flood & Constance 2002).
- The feet to detect peripheral neuropathy and any other foot pathology that could increase the risk of foot injury during exercise.
- The eyes to detect the presence and status of retinopathy.
- Gait and balance.
- Blood glucose pattern and do not encourage activity if the blood glucose is <6 mmol/L or >10 mmol/L.
- Self-care knowledge. Be aware of the signs of hypoglycaemia, such as sweating, faintness, weakness, and dizziness, can be missed or attributed to the effect of the exercise, especially if hypoglycaemic unawareness is present, or could have other causes such as angina, or silent MI. Important information includes:
  - Knowing some physical activity can lower blood glucose for up to 48 hours therefore, an adequate high GI intake is required when aerobic activities are planned and activity levels increased gradually.

○ The importance of wearing appropriate clothing and footwear that does not restrict blood flow and breathing or put the feet at risk.
○ The need to warm up and cool before and after exercise.
○ How to incorporate exercise/activity into the usual daily routine.
○ The need to consider their personal safety and be aware of risks such as being attacked when out walking, risk of falling on poorly maintained footpaths.

The Society of Geriatric Cardiology recommend older people to participate in physical activity programmes that include aerobic and strength training activities for example, Tai chi, which reduces blood pressure, blood glucose, and lipids, improves balance and wellbeing (Lan *et al.* 1998; Tsai *et al.* 2003). Resistance training reduces bone loss, improves strength, and makes routine activities such as carrying groceries and gardening easier (Meuleman *et al.* 2000; Simkin 2004). Walking 30 minutes/day or for 10 minutes three times per day is ideal. Swimming has the benefit of being non-weight bearing and might be easier for overweight people to manage. A great deal of incidental activity occurs during usual activities such as playing with grandchildren, housework, and gardening.

Hypoglycaemia

Hypoglycaemia is the most important side effect of insulin and OHAs, see Chapters 5 and 6. Hypoglycaemia occurring in older people managed with OHAs can be difficult to recognise. Usually the counter-regulatory response is triggered when the blood glucose drops below ~3.5–3.7 mmol/L, which triggers adrenergic symptoms such as sweating and trembling. Fine motor coordination, the speed of mental processing, concentration, and some memory functions are when blood glucose is <3 mmol/L (Sommerfield *et al.* 2003). The effects on decision-making are unclear. Some researchers suggest attentional ability is compromised but problem-solving ability remains intact (McAulay *et al.* 2001). Prolonged hypoglycaemia can result in neurological damage or death but these are rare (Cryer 2007).

The usual hypoglycaemia signs and symptoms can be masked or absent in older people and hypoglycaemia can present as chronic confusion, and not be recognised. The presentation of hypoglycaemia may resemble a cerebrovascular accident or mental confusion leading to an incorrect diagnosis of impaired mental function and delayed treatment or failure to treat the hypoglycaemia. The need to consider hypoglycaemia in older people with diabetes presenting to emergency departments has improved with education and since the introduction of capillary blood glucose testing on all unconscious patients presenting to emergency departments.

Hypoglycaemia caused by OHAs is often profound and prolonged and can become chronic or fatal. If it is prolonged it can cause brain damage or provoke a MI (Tiengo 1999). If a person on insulin and a sulphonylurea or Glitinide starts to feel unwell, test their blood glucose to exclude/confirm hypoglycaemia as a cause.

The risk of hypoglycaemia in the elderly is increased by:

• Treatment with oral hypoglycaemic agents, especially long-acting agents such as Glibenclamide (rarely used now in Australia) and Amaryl, see Chapter 5.
• Renal and/or hepatic disease that leads to impaired metabolism and excretion of medications and accumulation of medicines with long half-lives, and increased risk of medicine interactions (Jennings 1997; Howes 2001).

- Patients on multiple medicines where the risk of interactions is high.
- Impaired cognitive function where the individual fails to recognise hypoglycaemia and the signs can be confusing for family, carers, and health professionals.
- Patients who are sedated.
- Inadequate nutrition and malnutrition where glucose stores are inadequate to respond to the counter-regulatory hormone response to hypoglycaemia.
- Autonomic neuropathy, which can mask the symptoms of hypoglycaemia so the patient is unaware their blood glucose is low. These asymptomatic hypoglycaemic episodes are not recognised and therefore not treated early enough to avoid a severe episode. Alternatively, autonomic neuropathy can cause upper body sweating that can be mistaken for hypoglycaemia, see Chapter 6.
- Patients who are fasting for medical procedures or investigations.
- Excessive consumption of alcohol.
- Inadequate communication between health professionals caring for the patient and between health professionals and the patient, leading to confusion and management mistakes.

It is important to monitor the blood glucose of older patients and residents presenting with these risk factors and to be aware that usually more than one risk factor is operating. The more risk factors present the greater the likelihood of hypoglycaemia occurring.

Managing hypoglycaemia

The method of treating hypoglycaemia must reflect the functional level of the individual:

- People on a normal oral diet:
  - Treat with a high glycaemic index food such as 10 g of glucose powder dissolved in water *or* 1 glass glucozade *or* 5 glucose jelly beans.
- People having thickened fluids/vitamised diets:
  - 15 g tube glucose gel.
- People fed through a PEG tube:
  - 15 g tube glucose gel in the mouth.
- 10 g of glucose powder dissolved in water and inserted into the PEG tube.

Practice point

Hypoglycaemia leading to unconsciousness is rare in older people. However, such an event is very stressful and can precipitate an MI. An ECG should be performed.

Regular vaccinations against influenza and pneumonia are recommended for older people. A recent report recommended vaccinating infants as young as six months if they are in contact with frail elderly grandparents/relatives to reduce the spread of infection (Rouse 2004). Interestingly, researchers found that, although people's immune response depends on the vaccination they received, the side of their brain that is most active also had an effect on the degree of the response (Davidson 2003).

Davidson (2003), found people aged 57–60 with left-sided brain activity in the prefrontal cortex developed stronger immunity. This part of the brain is associated with a positive outlook on life. While the study is small, it demonstrates the effect of psychological parameters on physical status. Another earlier study (Lancet 1999), demonstrated that chronic stress reduces immune function in older people and impaired antibody responses to influenza vaccinations. These findings also apply to older carers. These studies suggest that chronically stress older people including carers may be vulnerable to infection and because they are not able to mount an adequate immune response. Therefore, infection control procedures and appropriate preventative measure must be in place.

Practice point

The drainage holes/slots in bath and shower seats can trap the genitalia of older people, especially males and lead to cuts, lacerations, bruising, pain and extreme distress. The UK Government drug and medical device safety department warned that the maximum weight should not be exceeded when using these seats because they bend under the weight and increase the risk of genital entrapment. Folded towels can be placed over the holes (Lowinger 2003). Bath seats are rarely used in Australia because of the safety risks.

Nursing care

- Careful assessment of the individual from an holistic approach that incorporates physical, psychological, social, spiritual and relationship functioning. The latter includes relationships with health professionals.
- Strategies need to be in place to assess and minimise the risk of falling. These include providing a safe environment, orientating the person to the ward, considering protective measures to avoid pressure ulcers such as hip protectors, careful discharge planning, and early referral to the social worker, domiciliary or aged care team for home assessment.
- Timing meals, PEG, and enteral feeds and medication rounds to reduce the risk of hypoglycaemia.
- Adequate preparation of the patient for surgical and investigative procedures, see Chapter 9.
- Reminding the person to drink, especially in hot weather.
- Monitoring blood glucose and taking steps to correct persistent levels outside the target range.
- Providing clear, careful explanations when relevant and checking the person understands what is required of them. Written information enhances verbal information.
- Identifying stress and depression and ensuring appropriate assessment and management ocurs.
- Identifying the barriers to self-care and recognising and changing those things that can be changed and those that cannot.

• Bed rest may be required initially, but it should not be prolonged because of the loss of muscle mass especially in the lower limbs, venous stasis, skin tears, pressure ulcers and falls risk. Thus, it is important to ensure timely assessment when an older person presents to the emergency department and to consult an aged care expert early in the admission to ensure appropriate management and reduce the likelihood of repeated presentations.

WHO (1983) emphasised the importance of helping older people live safe, dignified lives in society with their families and friends if possible. Similarly, the Victorian Department of Human Services (2003) recognised the important role carers play in supporting older people in the community. Carers should be included in assessment and health planning and outcome monitoring processes where appropriate. Carers are concerned when they are not consulted when their older relative is hospitalised from an aged care facility (Hong *et al.* 2004). Written action plans can support carers to manage older people at home but need to be relevant to the carer and the older person and revised regularly bearing in mind the burden of care.

Having such strategies in place for respite care can relieve the burden of care and improve outcomes for carers and older people (Berthold *et al.* 1991). Carers presenting with health problems:

• Have long standing health problems.
• Experienced health problems in the previous year.
• Are concerned about their health.
• Experience a high level of frustration.
• Perform personal tasks such as bathing and dressing the older person, which can be distressing for both parties. Many older people do not want 'physical help' from their family and friends (Connell 1991), even when they need it. Providing support when it is not wanted, even if it is needed, can result in negative outcomes and be perceived as interference. Carers often tread the fine line between support and 'interference' on a daily basis
• Have difficulty communicating with the older person (Idris 1989, pp. 167–169).
• Do not have adequate respite care/support services in place.
• Feel depressed and 'burnt out' (Tokaski 2004).

An education programme for caregivers that includes information about how to manage their relative's behaviour can foster closer relationships between the carer and their older relative, and fewer incidents of acute confusion and faecal incontinence during hospital admissions and fewer depressive symptoms (Hong *et al.* 2004).

References

Ames, B. (2006) Low micronutrient intake may accelerate degenerative diseases of aging through allocation of scarce micronutrients by triage. *Proceedings of National Academy of Science USA* **103** (47), 17589–17594.

Aronow, W. & Ahn, C. (1997) Association of post prandial hypotension with incidence of falls, syncope, coronary events, stroke, and total mortality at 29 months follow-up in 499 older nursing home residents. *Journal of the American Geriatrics Society*, **45**, 1051–1053.

Australian Quality Council (1998) *Accreditation Standards for Aged Care*. Australian Quality Council, Canberra.

Australian Diabetes Educators Association (ADEA) (2003) *Guidelines for the Management and Care of Diabetes in the Elderly*. ADEA, Canberra.

Basu, A., Basu, R., Sha, P., Vella, A., Johnson, C., Jensen, M., Sreekumaran, K., Schwenk, W. & Rizza, R. (2001) Type 2 diabetes impairs splanchnic uptake of glucose but does not alter intestinal glucose absorption during enteral glucose feeding. *Diabetes*, 50, 1351–1362.

Bayliss, E., Ellis, J. & Steiner, J. (2007) Barriers to self-management and quality of life outcomes in seniors with multimorbidities. *Annals of Family Medicine*, 5 (5), 395–402.

British Diabetic Association (1999) *Guidelines for Residents with Diabetes in Care Homes*. British Diabetic Association, London.

Department of Health (2001) *Care Homes for Older People: National Minimal Standards*. Care Standards Act 2000. HMSO, London.

Dunning, P. & Alford, F. (1993) Dilemmas in the management of the elderly diabetic. A community or medical problem? *Medical Journal of Australia*, 3, 158–164.

Egede, L., Xiaobou, Y., Zheng, D. & Silverstein, M. (2002) The prevalence and pattern of complementary and alternative medicine use in individuals with diabetes. *Diabetes Care*, 25, 324–329.

Elia, M., Ceriello, A., Laube, H., Sinclair, A., Engfer, M. & Stratton, R. (2005) Enteral nutrition support and use of diabetes-specific formulas for patients with diabetes. *Diabetes Care*, 28, 2267–2279.

Fleming, R. (2002) Report of Federal Department of Health survey into depression in the elderly. *Australian Doctor*, March 14.

Gaughram, F., Walwyn, R., Lambkin-Williams, R., Whelan, P., Chatterton, K., Oxford, J. & Macdonald, A. (2007) Flu: effect of vaccine in elderly care home residents: a randomized trial. *Journal of the American Geriatric Society*, 55 (12), 1912–1920.

Gilden, J., Hendryx, M., Clar, S., Casia, C. & Singh, S. (1992) Diabetes Support Groups improve health care of older diabetic patients. *Journal of the American Geriatric Society*, 40, 145–150.

Gradman, T., Laes, A., Thompson, L. & Reaven, G. (1993) Verbal learning and/or memory improves with glycaemic control in older subjects with non insulin-dependent diabetes mellitus. *Journal of the American Geriatrics Society*, 41, 1305–1312.

Gooberman-Hill, R. & Ebrahim, S. (2007) Making decisions about simple interventions: older people use of walking aids. *Age and Aging*, 36 (5), 569–573.

Halter, J. (2001) Report of the American Diabetes Association Meeting. *Practical Diabetes International*, 18 (7), 251–258.

Howes, L. (2001) Dosage alteration in the elderly – importance of mild renal impairment. *Current Therapeutics*, 42 (7), 33–35.

Jennings, P. (1997) Oral antihypoglycaemics: considerations in older patient with non insulin-dependent diabetes mellitus. *Drugs and Aging*, 10 (5), 323–331.

Katona, C. (1994). *Depression in Old Age*. John Wiley and Sons, New York.

Keller, H. *et al.* (2004) Nutritional risk predicts quality of life in elderly community-living Canadians. *Journal of Gerontological Association Biological Science Medical Science*, 59 (1), 68–74.

Kirkland, F. (2000) Improvements in diabetes care for elderly people in care homes. *Journal of Diabetes Nursing*, 4 (5), 150–155.

Kulminski, A., Ukrantseva, S., Akushevic, I., Arbeev, K. & Yashin, A. (2007) Cumulative index of health deficiencies as a characteristic of long life. *Journal American Geriatric Society*, 55 (6), 935–940.

Middleton, M., Nazarenko, G., Nivison-Smith, I. & Smerdely, P. (2001) Prevalance of malnutrition and 12-month incidence of mortality in two Sydney teaching hospitals. *International Medicine Journal*, 31, 455–461.

Mitchell, J. (1995) Oral dose forms that should not be crushed. *Hospital Pharmacy*, 31, 27–37.

Miller, C. (1999) *Nursing Care of Older Adults*, 3rd edition. Lippincott Williams and Wilkins, Philadelphia.

National Health and Medical Research Council (NHMRC) (1999).

Orford, J., Sesso, H., Stedman, M., Gagnon, D., Vokonas, P., Gaziano, L. (2002) A comparsion of the Framingham and European society of cardiology coronary heart disease risk prediction models in the normative aging study. *American Heart Journal*, 144 (1), 95–100.

Paolisso, G., Gambardella, A., Verza, M. D'Amora, A., Sgambato, S. & Varrichio, M. (1992) ACE-inhibition improves insulin-sensitivity in age insulin-resistant hypertensive patients. *Journal of Human Hypertension*, 6, 175–179.

Peters, A. & Davidson, M. (1992) Effects of various enteral feeding products on postprandial blood glucose response in patients with type 1 diabetes. *Journal Parenteral and Enteral Nutrition*, 16 (1), 69–74.

Quayle, S. (2001) Gains of minimising falls: managing the older patient. *Australian Doctor*, July, 43–44.

Rosenstock, J. (2001) Management of Type 2 diabetes in the elderly: special considerations. *Pulsebeat*, Oct–Nov, 5.

Schwartz, M., Woods, S., Porte, D., Seeley, R. & Baskin, D. (2000) Central nervous system control of food intake. *Nature*, 404, 661–671.

Simpson, C. (2005) Crushed medications: an emerging guideline. *Australian Nursing Journal*, 13 (1), Clinical Update 1–4.

Sinclair, A. (1995) Initial management of NIDDM in the elderly. In: *Diabetes in Old Age* (eds P. Funacane & A. Sinclair). John Wiley & Sons, pp. 181–201.

Sinclair, A., Allard, I. & Bayes, A. (1997) Observation of diabetes care in long-term institutional settings with measures of cognitive function and dependency. *Diabetes Care*, 20 (5), 778–786.

Tiengo, A. (1999) Burden of treatment in the elderly patient: reducing the burden of diabetes. *Diabetes Care*, 11, 6–8.

US National Institutes of Health (NIH) (undated) *Aging Under the Microscope: a Biological Quest*. http://www.nia.nih.gov/HealthInformationPublications/AgingUndertheMicroscope/ (accessed February 2008).

Wetzels, R., Harmsen, M., Van Weel, C., Grol, R. & Wensing, M. (2007) Interventions for improving older patients' involvement in primary care episodes. *Cochrane Database of Systematic Reviews*, Issue 1, Art. No.: CD004273. DOI 10. 1002/14651858. CD004273. pub2.

World Health Organisation (1999) *Guidelines for Older Australians*. Commonwealth of Australia, Canberra.

Zembrzuski, C. (1997) A three dimensional approach to hydration of elders: administration, clinical staff, and in service education. *Geriatric Nursing*, 18 (1), 20–26.

Zhao, W., Chen, H., Xu, H. *et al.* (1999) Brain insulin receptors and spatial memory. *Journal of Biological Chemistry*, 274, 34893–34901.

Chapter 13
Diabetes in Children and Adolescents

Key points

- A supportive family is an important aspect of diabetes management.
- Family stress and marital disharmony affect the child's metabolic control.
- Clinicians dealing with children with diabetes must spend time assessing the family structure and help the family to support their child.
- Management strategies must be applicable to the age and developmental stage of the individual.
- Most children have Type 1 diabetes and insulin should never be withheld in these children.
- There is an increasing incidence of Type 2 diabetes in children and complications are often evident at diagnosis or occur soon after.
- Management strategies are different for children with Type 1 and Type 2 diabetes.

Rationale

Diabetes management in children and adolescents changes during the various transitions that occur as the child grows and develops. Diabetes and its management impacts on the family dynamics and can affect quality of life and mental well being. Family support is essential if the child is to achieve euglycaemia and psychological well being. Thus, the family needs to be included in education and management decisions. Management plans need to make provision for normal growth and development and a gradual transition to independent self-care.

Introduction

The number of children diagnosed with Type 1 diabetes is increasing globally and Type 2 diabetes in children is an emerging global problem. The incidence varies but ~70 000 children <14 years are diagnosed annually and an estimated 440 000 children have diabetes worldwide (DIAMOND 1999; EURODIAB 2000; Soltesz 2006). Lee (2008) reported a 38% increase in the number of hospital admissions with diabetes aged

0–29 years between 1993 and 2004. The hospitalisation rate was higher in girls, 42% versus 29% for males.

In most countries girls and boys are equally affected but the rate is not the same among age groups. It tends to increase with age, peaking around puberty, usually slightly earlier in girls, which is consistent with the earlier onset of puberty. The global incidence is estimated to increase by ~50% in the next 15 years (Soltesz 2007). In Australia ~1 in 500 children <15 years have Type 1 diabetes.

A number of forms of diabetes occur in childhood but Type 1 is the most common especially in children <10 years:

- Type 1, which accounts for ~98% of diabetes in children.
- Type 2, which has an increasing prevalence.
- Other specific types:
  ○ Monogenic defects of beta cell function, for example, familial diabetes, neonatal diabetes. Neonatal diabetes presents in the first 6 months of life (Srinivasan & Donaghue 2007). About 50% have transient neonatal diabetes and insulin treatment is usually not required with ~3 months, but may recur in the second or third decade.
  ○ Diabetes as a consequence of diseases of the exocrine pancreas, for example, cystic fibrosis.
  ○ Diabetes associated with endocrine diseases such as Cushing's syndrome.
  ○ Medicine-induced diabetes, for example, chemotherapy, glucocorticoids.
  ○ Diabetes associated with genetic syndromes such as Trisomy and Turner's syndrome.

The reasons for the increased incidence of Type 1 diabetes in children are relatively unclear. Various explanations have been proposed; for example, genetic factors such as the 'thrifty gene' (Need 1962), the 'thrifty phenotype' (Hales & Barker 1992) theories. More recently, the focus has been on environmental changes that could overload the beta cells, which gave rise to the 'overload hypothesis' and the 'spring harvest hypothesis' in which genetically predisposed children have an accelerated growth rate and increased body fat. Likewise, puberty occurs at a younger age. Various environmental triggers such as the decline in breast feeding, age at which solids are introduced, exposure to foreign antigens early in life that impair the immune system, the 'hygiene hypothesis', have been implicated.

Diabetes is often misdiagnosed or the diagnosis is delayed in developing regions and under-resourced communities in developed countries, where the symptoms might be attributed to malnutrition or starvation because people do not know the signs and symptoms (Kaufman & Riley 2007). As a consequence, morbidity and mortality rates are high and is compounded by lack of equipment and essential medications. The International Diabetes Federation (IDF) insulin for life programme has had a significant impact on the lives of many children in underprivileged areas.

Type 2 diabetes, once rare in children, is increasing (IDF Consultative Section on Diabetes Education 2002; Sinha *et al.* 2002). Up to 45% of newly diagnosed diabetes in children and adolescents is Type 2 (Shaw 2007). Emerging epidemiological data indicate Type 2 diabetes mainly occurs in overweight children from specific ethnic groups particularly African Americans, Hispanics, Asians, Native Americans, Indigenous Australians, and Middle Eastern people (Shaw 2007). The increasing prevalence in

Asian countries is linked to the increase in western lifestyles with high fat diets and reduced exercise (Gill 2006).

A recent study points to a link between increasing obesity and high consumption of fructose (American Journal Public Health 2007). Fructose appears to affect fat degradation in the liver by inhibiting PPAR-alpha receptor activity, which is lower in humans than rats, and the leptin signalling system, which accelerates fat oxygenation in the liver and reduces fat synthesis (Hepatology 2007). Insulin resistance and impaired glucose tolerance and other features of the metabolic syndrome are present in 25% of obese children, which puts them at high risk of Type 2 diabetes (Sinha *et al.* 2002).

In addition, high rates of television viewing, an indicator of inactivity, are associated with increased risk of developing diabetes and higher HbA_{1c} (Margeirsdottir *et al.* 2007). Other possible causes include low birth weight (Wei *et al.* 2003) and low birth weight associated with 'catch up growth' (Bhargava *et al.* 2004), see Chapters 4 and 14. These findings led to the theory of the developmental origins of health and disease (DOHaD) (Yajnik 2007).

Although the onset of Type 2 diabetes may be less dramatic than Type 1, Type 2 diabetes in children is associated with significant risk of dyslipidaemia, hypertension, and polycystic ovarian syndrome, asthma, and obstructive sleep apnoea (Tait *et al.* 2008). Cardiovascular disease develops at an early age and is often present at diagnosis (Pinhas-Hamiel 2007) and progression to complications is faster than in children with Type 1 diabetes. Significantly, children and adolescents with Type 2 diabetes may be at higher risk of microvascular disease especially nephropathy than those with Type 1 (Shaw 2007).

Thus, early identification through comprehensive screening programmes and effective management of Type 2 diabetes in children is imperative to reduce the burden of the disease and the projects health care costs (Weiss & Caprio 2005; Zimmett *et al.* 2007). The IDF recently introduced diagnostic criteria for the metabolic syndrome in children, which is described in Chapter 1.

Managing children and adolescents with diabetes

The health care needs of children and adolescents change as they grow and develop regardless of diabetes type. Some aspects of care are common to both Type 1 and Type 2 but there are inherent differences in managing Type 1 and Type 2. Multidisciplinary team care involving a paediatric endocrinologist, diabetes educator, dietitian, psychologist, and other experts as indicated is essential to achieving optimal outcomes.

A number of management guidelines and position statements are in current use and should be referred to for specific detailed information. These include:

- Care of children and adolescents with Type 1 diabetes (American Diabetes Association (ADA) 2005).
- Standards of medical care in diabetes: special considerations for children and adolescents (ADA 2004).
- Australian Paediatric Endocrine Group (APEG).
- Position statements such as age-specific recommendations for screening for nephropathy (ADA 2004), retinopathy (ADA 2004), school and day care (ADA 2004), and camps (ADA 2004).

- Consensus guidelines for the management of Type 1 diabetes mellitus (ISPAD 2000).
- Type 2 diabetes in children and adolescents (ADA 2000).

Aspects of care that apply to both Type 1 and Type 2 diabetes in children and adolescents

Where possible, education and stabilisation at diagnosis should occur in an ambulatory setting. However, hospitalisation is necessary in ~30% of newly diagnosed Type 1 children (ADA 2005). If hospitalisation is necessary, for example, in the case of ketoacidosis, the time spent in the hospital should be kept to a minimum. The overall aims of management are to provide an individualised education and management plan to achieve:

- An accurate diagnosis.
- Prevent or delay the onset of diabetes-related complications including short-term complications such as hypoglycaemia and ketoacidosis. Long-term complications are rare before puberty but complication screening typically begins around the age of 10.
- A balanced nutritious diet suitable for the growth and development stage of the child.
- Acceptance of the diabetes by the child and the family.
- Assist the child to gradually take over the self-care tasks.
- Develop an holistic, integrated health plan that includes sexual health, responsible contraception and planned pregnancy as suitable to the age and development stage of the young person.
- Admission to acute care should the need arise.
- Smooth transfer to adult care.

The child should be involved in developing their diabetes management plan within their capabilities. Disagreements between the family and the child about who is responsible for management and poor adherence are predictors of high HbA_{1c} (Anderson *et al.* 1991). The child's involvement in their self-care gradually increases as they mature and their fine motor and problem-solving and coping skill develop.

Differentiating between Type 1 and Type 2 diabetes at diagnosis is not always straightforward due to the increasing prevalence of obesity, ketonuria, and diabetic ketoacidosis (DKA) (Svoren & Wolfsdorf 2006). About one third of adolescents with Type 2 diabetes are ketotic and 25% of newly diagnosed people present with DKA. If the diabetes type is not clear it may be advisable to measure islet cell autoantibodies and C-peptide. Table 1.2 in Chapter 1 depicts the main differences between Type 1 and Type 2 diabetes.

Regular assessment of general health and diabetes status and how the family is managing is essential because there are major physical, psychological, emotional, spiritual, and social differences among the growth and development stages. Assessing maturity, sensitive supervision and allowing the child to gradually take over specific diabetes self-care tasks according to their capability should be factored into an holistic diabetes plan. The family needs to be involved in developing the care plan and monitoring progress.

Educating teachers and other carers is also important and the child should be involved in these activities if appropriate. Diabetes should not preclude the child from attending school excursions and camps but extra precautions will need to be taken, for example, being able to eat on time. Diabetes camps provide an important learning experience and many children who attended camps when they were young help out on diabetic camps as they grow older. This kind of peer support contributes to psychological well being (ADA 2004).

Preventive care includes regular blood glucose monitoring, complication screening, immunisation according to immunisation schedules and influenza vaccinations during at-risk periods when the child is >6 months.

Managing Type 1 diabetes

Type 1 usually presents with a sudden onset of symptoms and insulin injections are needed for survival. A well balanced diet and adequate appropriate exercise are also essential. Insulin and dietary requirements can change rapidly, especially in children, due to rapid changes in activity levels and growth. Therefore, consistent acceptable blood glucose levels may be difficult to achieve.

ADA (2005) suggests the following insulin doses. The number of doses per day depends on a number of factors; increasingly basal bolus regimens are used for older children and adolescents:

- Newly diagnosed Type 1: initial dose ~0.5–1.0 units/kg/day. Lower doses may be required before puberty. Higher doses may be needed after puberty and in DKA. Infants and toddlers require very small doses. Insulin pens that can deliver 0.5 unit doses are available and should be used where possible. If these pens are not available the insulin may need to be diluted to achieve accurate 1 unit dose increments. Specific diluents are required for specific insulins and can be obtained from the relevant manufacturer. Great care and appropriate parental education is required for accurate dilutions.
- Newly diagnosed Type 1 is often followed by a honeymoon period once the acute metabolic disturbance is reversed. Endogenous insulin production increases for varying periods up to ~12 months. Insulin doses usually need to be reduced to prevent hypoglycaemia. Insulin requirements increase as the honeymoon phase ends and at the onset of puberty.
- During puberty 1.5 units/kg/day are often needed.

Screening for associated autoimmune diseases such as coeliac disease (Chapter 10), and thyroid disease may be required.

A supportive and encouraging family is important if the child is to accept diabetes and eventually take over diabetic self-management. The family in turn needs support, advice and encouragement. Good control is associated with a structured supportive family (Johnson *et al.* 1990; Thompson *et al.* 2001). Families need to provide appropriate supervision and discipline and maintain a family structure that meets the needs of the child and other family members.

Hypoglycaemia can be unpredictable in children whose activity level and intake and consequently insulin needs can vary enormously from day-to-day and within the day.

Insulin need also change with exercise and pubertal hormone changes. Hypoglycaemia can be difficult to deal with in young children and can manifest as:

- Unaccustomed naughtiness
- Noisy behaviour
- Aggression
- Crying
- Tremulousness

If it is not recognised and treated promptly the child can become unconscious, which is frightening for the child and those around them (see Chapter 6). Parents often feel safer if they have glucagon available and some also like it to be available at school if the teacher or school nurse is appropriately educated. Nocturnal hypoglycaemia can be particularly difficult to manage. There may not be any significant long-term effects associated with nocturnal hypoglycaemia but it can affect mood the following day. The child maybe irritable on waking and might impair recognition of daytime hypoglycaemia (Dunger & Hovorka 2007). If hypoglycaemia is severe and frequent diet, exercise, and medication regimen need to be revised and other contributing factors excluded. The parents may learn to use glucagon, see Chapter 6. Table 13.1 depicts the major management strategies according to developmental stage.

During adolescence the hormonal surge at puberty can make blood glucose control difficult. Dietary restrictions and the diabetic regimen can be seen as obstacles to fitting in with peer activities and may be neglected. Achieving independence from the family can be difficult if diabetes is diagnosed at this time.

Social pressure and the emphasis on food that is part of the diabetes management regimen can increase the likelihood of eating disorders. Young people with diabetes fear putting on weight and skip meals and run their blood glucose levels high to avoid weight gain (Dunning 1994). Eating disorders are widespread among adolescent girls and diabetic-specific concerns may contribute to their development. The full range of subclinical and clinical eating disorders may be more prevalent in women with diabetes (Levine & Marcus 1997; Colton 2007). Eating disorders in Type 1 diabetes often arises in adolescence and often persists into adulthood (Colton 2007). Colton distinguished between disturbed eating and eating disorders and found girls with an eating disorder had higher HbA_{1c} and BMI but that the HbA_{1c} was not necessarily higher in the presence of disturbed eating. Health professionals need to be sensitive to social pressures and body image issues and the possibility that an eating disturbance might be present. Screening for disturbed eating is essential and referral for specific counselling might be indicated to avoid long-term nutritional problems and other associated risks such as depression. Children with Type 2 diabetes may be at particular risk given the focus on weight loss.

The menarche affects control in girls and thereafter the blood glucose profile often reflects the stages of the menstrual cycle (see Chapter 11). When the child becomes an adolescent contraceptive and pregnancy counselling are vital. Metabolic control often deteriorates partly due to the increase in growth hormone and reduced insulin sensitivity at puberty. Psychosocial issues such as privacy, body image, and independence also have an impact. Negative feedback about the adolescent's metabolic control and 'nagging' about the risk of long-term complications is unlikely to be effective and may actually result in non-attendance.

Table 13.1 Self-management expectations according to age and stage. (a) Metabolic targets need to be appropriate to the age and stage and revised regularly as the child grows and develops; and (b) recommended HbA$_{1c}$ targets.

	Key milestones	*Management considerations*
(a) Developmental stage		
Babies <1 year	The parents are responsible for care Significant hypoglycaemia risk due to undeveloped catecholamine response	Family stress Unrecognised hypoglycaemia, coma, seizures Nocturnal hypoglycaemia
1–3 years	The parents are responsible for care Food refusal is common and increases the risk of hypoglycaemia Hypoglycaemia may manifest as temper tantrums	Consistent 'rules' and discipline are important Blood glucose testing is needed to distinguish normal toddler's behaviour from hypoglycaemia
3–7 years	Fine motor skills are developing and while the parents retain responsibility for providing care they should involve the child in their care	Involve the child in self-management
8–11 years	Children are capable of undertaking many diabetes self-management tasks but still require parental guidance and support They may enjoy diabetes camps and teaching their class about diabetes but care must be taken to ensure these activities do not negatively impact on their 'difference' from non-diabetic children	Diagnosis at this age often results in mild depression and depression increases with longer duration of diabetes but is different for girls and boys Depression may be precipitated when the 'honeymoon phase' ends.
Adolescence	Physical, cognitive, and emotional development occurs rapidly Puberty can affect metabolic control Diabetes self-care can inhibit independence Most adolescents should be responsible for their self-care but parental support and guidance are still needed	Poor metabolic control and non-adherence may indicate psychological problems or family conflict Parental support still needed but needs to be tactful
(b) HbA$_{1c}$ targets		
Age range	HbA$_{1c}$ targets	Blood glucose target range[a]
Children <6 years	7.5–8.5%	<6 months, 5–15 mmol/L
6–12 years	<8%	<6 years, 7–12 mmol/L (bedtime)
Adolescents	<7.5%	>12 years, 4–8 mmol/L, 7–10 mmol/L (bedtime)

[a]Australian Clinical Practice Guidelines (2005).

Polycystic Ovarian Disease (PCOS) is associated with insulin resistance and diabetes and often first manifests at menarche. The effects of unpredictable, heavy menstrual bleeding are disabling and place the young woman at risk of iron deficiency anaemia, and tiredness (Legro & Dunaif 1997). Chronic anovulation increases the risk of endometrial hyperplasia and endometrial cancer. Infertility is a consequence and has a negative impact on the young person's self-concept. Early diagnosis and management is important. PCOS often manifests as excess facial hair and irregular periods, see Chapter 14.

Generally, paediatric depression is serious, common, and persistent. It is the second leading contributor to the global disease burden between ages 15 and 44 and recurs in 70% of affected individuals (World Health Organisation (WHO)). It is more common in boys before puberty and in girls after puberty. Mood disorders are associated with high morbidity, concomitant diseases, and risk-taking behaviour such as excess alcohol consumption, smoking, and illegal drug use. Children with diabetes are at particular risk and higher rates of depression have been reported in young people with diabetes than the general population (Blanz 1993) thus regular mental health assessment is essential. Bryden *et al.* (2002) reported poor clinical outcomes in approximately one third of young people with diabetes, which highlights the need to identify problems early.

Children from single parent families and families with marital conflict are at increased risk of poor metabolic control (Thompson *et al.* 2001). Family dysfunction, inadequate treatment adherence and unacceptable glycaemic control often go hand-in-hand (Lorenz & Wysocki 1991). Unacceptable glycaemic control carries the risk of admissions to hospital with ketoacidosis and the development of long-term diabetic complications (see Chapter 10). Non-adherence is multifactorial and may be a sign of rebellion or forgetfulness. Aggressive antisocial conduct is more likely to result in poor metabolic control whereas emotional problems tend to lead to better glycaemic control (Bryden 2001).

Discrepancies between home blood glucose tests and HbA_{1c} might indicate underlying stress and coping problems. It represents an opportunity to explore factors operating in the young person's life, their feelings about diabetes and the management regimen and their coping mechanisms (Conrad *et al.* 206). This needs to be undertaken very tactfully using techniques suitable to the child. For example, inviting young children to write a story, poem, or draw a picture about their life with diabetes for the next visit, which can act as the basis for meaningful discussion and/or indicate whether referral for specialist counselling is needed.

An emerging issue that has both positive benefits and negative consequences for young people is their disclosure of personal information on the Internet. Internet support groups can enable young people to anonymously discuss diabetes with peers, access information, and reduce feelings of isolation. However, an analysis of information entered on MySpace revealed that most entries by 16 and 17 year olds included personally identifiable information, information about personal risk-taking behaviours such as sexual activity and drug and alcohol use, and often included a photograph/s (Moreno *et al.* 2007). Moreno *et al.* did not mention diabetes status but there is no reason to suspect the results would be different.

The transfer from paediatric care to adult specialist care can be very stressful. Neglecting the diabetes self-care, not attending appointments and poor metabolic control is common at this time (Court 1991). Tact and understanding are very important if these young people are not to be lost to adequate medical supervision (Court 1991; Dunning 1993).

Managing childhood Type 2 diabetes

The management goals and many of the issues discussed for children with Type 1 diabetes apply to children with Type 2 but the medication regimen and nutrition requirements are different. A comprehensive complication assessment should be undertaken at diagnosis and then as indicated, but at least annually.

Schwenk (2007) showed an intensive weight management programme consisting of intensive nutrition information, and a structured education programme led to improvements in blood pressure, HDL, and LDL cholesterol, weight loss, and lower BMI compared to controls. However, Schwenk noted the programme was intensive and time consuming. Cost–benefit analysis was not reported.

Medications are often needed to control fasting and postprandial blood glucose and blood lipids if they are not controlled using lifestyle interventions. Weight loss and exercise are central to management but symptoms, weight loss, and persistent hyperglycaemia indicates medications are needed. Insulin (~2 units/kg) may be required initially (Svoren & Wolfsdorf 2006).

The only glucose lowering medicines approved for use in Type 2 diabetes in children are insulin and metformin. The recommended starting dose of metformin for children 10–16 years is 500 mg/day, which can be increased to 500 mg DB with further weekly 500 mg increments to a maximum daily dose of 2000 mg provided there are no contraindications to its use or associated adverse events (Svoren & Wolfsdorf 2006). Alternatively, 500 mg metformin XR can be administered with the evening meal to reduce the gastrointestinal side effects. Bedtime basal insulin such as glargine can be commenced at bedtime if blood glucose is not controlled using metformin.

Medication self-management

Managing medicines is an important aspect of self-care that must gradually be assumed by the child. The transition to assuming responsibility for managing diabetes medicines is a key aspect of most diabetes education programmes. However, adolescents are likely to use a range of other medicines, thus medication management should include age appropriate information about other medicines including over-the-counter and complementary medicines (CAM) as well as diabetes medicines.

Self-initiated over-the-counter medicines use begins early in adolescence: by ~16 years the majority of adolescents have self-prescribed medicines such as analgesics and antipyretics, girls self-prescribe more frequently than boys (Buck 2007). However, adolescent's knowledge about these medicines is often inadequate and, significantly, parental education did not influence medication knowledge.

Medicine education programmes for adults are usually appropriate for children >11 years. A number of medicines education programmes have been developed for younger children (Curry *et al.* 2006; Gardiner & Dvorkin 2006; Federal Drug Administration (FDA) undated). Table 13.2 suggests important information to facilitate the transition to medication self-management.

Table 13.2 Important medicine-related information children need. Information should be provided using recognised education strategies and quality use of medicines. Quality use of medicines is discussed in Chapter 5.

(1) Children have a right to information about their medicines appropriate to their age, diabetes type, and developmental levels. The information should encompass over-the-counter and can medicines as well as conventional medicines be personalised.

(2) Children are innately curious and want to know about their medicines. Health professionals should provide relevant information to the child as well as their parents.

(3) Children should gradually assume responsibility for their medicines management including keeping a record of the medicines they are taking.

(4) Health professionals, family and carers should set a good example with respect to medicines use including safe use, appropriated storage and disposal, and sharps disposal.

(5) Children should be involved in discussions about participating in clinical trials and be given the opportunity to accept or decline participation.

Complementary therapy use in children

Complementary therapy (CAM) use in children is a complex issue. There are benefits and risks depending on the age of the child and the therapy used and their capacity to make an informed choice and understand the consequences of the choice to use or not use CAM. Young children with immature livers, developing central nervous systems and immune systems that increases their susceptibility to adverse medicine events: both conventional and CAM medicines.

CAM cathartic and diuretic medicines may cause electrolyte imbalance and dehydration rapidly in young children. Long-term use may increase the likelihood of acute, chronic, or cumulative adverse effects; others are contraindicated in children (Woolf 2003). However, therapies such as music, massage, yoga, and meditation have significant health benefits. Most parents/children who use CAM do not stop their conventional management regimen but only ~32% inform their conventional health professionals they use CAM. Thus, health professionals should ask about CAM use and the reasons for using specific therapies on a regular basis.

The reported prevalence of CAM use in children generally varies from 2% to 95% depending where the information was collected and the underlying condition being treated (Cranswick & Lim 2006; Picciano 2007; Tsao *et al.* 2007). In Germany, Dannemann *et al.* (2008) found 42% of a sample of children with Type 1 diabetes used at least one CAM modality. Significantly the children did not stop their insulin. Commonly used therapies include:

• Vitamin and mineral supplements.
• Echinacea for treating common childhood illnesses such as URTI or to boost the immune system.
• Massage, with and without essential oils. Massage reduces stress and improves quality in children with Type 1 diabetes and their parents providing the massage (Field *et al.*).
• Yoga.
• Meditation.
• Energy therapies.

- Music therapy.
- Hypnotherapy.

General reasons for using CAM include to improve well being, reduce stress and anxiety, the assumption that CAM have fewer side effects, and because the parents have an interest in self-care. Particularly risky therapies are:

- Ear candles.
- Aromatherapy candles.
- Essential oils in vapourisers within reach. Ingesting of even small doses of some essential oils, for example, *Eucalyptus* sp. from a vapouriser can cause oral burns and toxicity.
- Moxibustion.
- Case reports indicate Infacalm drops causing hypoglycaemia, drowsiness, and tachycardia in susceptible children.

More information about CAM can be found in Chapter 19.

Strategies for enhancing adherence during adolescence

Establishing a therapeutic relationship with the young person is essential so they feel comfortable about discussing issues with health professionals.

Young people with and without diabetes engage in risk-taking behaviour including not following medical advice, but no more so than adults (Johnson *et al.* 1990). A management approach that seeks concordance between health professional advice and the young person's behaviour is more likely to be successful (Fleming & Watson 2002).

A range of issues can impact on normal growth and development and some issues have a greater priority than health status for the young person. It is normal adolescent behaviour to think in the short-term, learn from their experience, and experiment. This means that short-term goals are more likely to be effective and can be modified progressively. Young people should be encouraged to discuss their experiences, which can be used as experiential teaching and learning strategies.

Many young people feel vulnerable and this can be exacerbated by diabetes and the need to take on the responsibility for adult roles and diabetes management. Exploring these concerns can help young people acknowledge and deal with them.

Many young people feel frustrated when they 'do all the right things' and their metabolic control is inadequate. This can lead to decreased motivation and feelings of helplessness and hopelessness especially if they do not have a supportive family (Kyngas 2000). Focusing on the positive aspects and small gains and not on 'good' and 'bad' control can take the focus off 'failure'. Striving for diabetes balance is more important than control. Metabolic control will be achieved if the individual's life is in balance.

The lack of a consistent and accessible health service and dealing with new health professionals when moving to adult care can be stressful. Collaboration between paediatric and adult services and a planned transition process can overcome some of these problems (Department of Health 2001; Dunning 1993).

Using multiple strategies and consultation techniques that encourage young people to ask questions is more likely to uncover accurate and meaningful information than the consultation where the young person tells the health professional 'what they want to hear' and the health professional does not pick up on relevant cues that things may not be 'all right'. Adherence issues should be discussed in the context of the young person's lifestyle and goals. Adherence can be enhanced by:

- Organising a youth appropriate service.
- Seeing the young person separately from their parents as they mature and begin to take responsibility for their diabetes management.
- Addressing the broader issues and life priorities and put diabetes into that context.
- Giving clear simple instructions and supporting verbal information with written instructions and the availability of telephone advice.
- Utilising family/carers as appropriate.
- Considering the type of questions likely to get honest answers, for example, instead of asking 'do you always take your correct dose of insulin?' try 'what dose of insulin suits you best?' (Fleming & Watson 2002).

Nursing responsibilities in hospital

In addition to those nursing tasks outlined in specific chapters it is important to:

- Document height and weight on percentile charts.
- Test blood glucose 4 times per day and when the child feels symptoms of hyper or hypoglycaemia. Vary testing times so that some tests are performed 2 hours after a meal or after activity. Test at night to detect nocturnal hypoglycaemia. Children managed using insulin pumps require more frequent monitoring.
- Test blood ketones if blood glucose is ~15 mmol/L or the child is acutely ill or has a fever.
- Encourage independence and encourage the child to administer their insulin injections and test their blood glucose. This can be an opportunity to assess technique or for the child to learn these techniques.
- Monitor dietary intake and ensure appropriate dietary review by dietitian.
- Ensure diabetic knowledge is assessed.
- Ensure privacy during procedures.
- Avoid admitting adolescents and children to wards with older people, if possible.

Clinical observations

Enuresis is an unusual presentation of diabetes in children.

Ketoacidosis in children

The management of ketoacidosis is described in Chapter 7. Additional issues specific to children are:

- Cerebral oedema is a very serious medical emergency in children. Monitoring mental status and strict fluid calculations are essential.

- Headache and/or altered behaviour may indicate impending cerebral oedema. Management includes bolus IV mannitol, nursing with the head of the bed elevated and fluid restriction.
- Sodium bicarbonate is not usually given in childhood DKA because of the risk of hypokalaemia, cerebral acidosis, and changed oxygen affinity of haemoglobin.
- Monitor sodium levels and adjust IV fluid appropriately as the blood glucose falls. Hyponatraemia can herald impending cerebral oedema.

References

Alberti, G., Zimmet, P. & Shaw, J. (2004) The International Diabetes Federation Consensus Workshop. Type 2 diabetes in the young: the evolving epidemic. *Diabetes Care*, **27**, 1798–1811.

American Diabetes Association (ADA) (2004) Standards of medical care in diabetes (position statement) *Diabetes Care*, **27** (Suppl. 1), S15–S35.

ADA (2004) Nephropathy in diabetes (position statement) *Diabetes Care*, **27** (Suppl. 1), S79–S83.

ADA (2004) Retinopathy in diabetes. Position statement. *Diabetes Care*, **27** (Suppl. 1), S84–S87.

ADA Diabetes care in the school and day care setting. Position statement. *Diabetes Care*, **27** (Suppl. 1), S122–S128.

ADEA (2000) Type 2 diabetes in children and adolescents. Consciences statement. *Diabetes Care*, **23**, 381–389.

ADA (2004) Diabetes care in camps. Position statement. *Diabetes Care*, **27** (Suppl. 1), S129–S131.

Anderson, B., Auslander, W., Jung, K., Miller, P. & Santiago, J. (1991) Assessing family sharing of diabetes responsibilities. *Diabetes Spectrum*, **4** (5), 263–268.

Australian Paediatric Endocrine Group (2005) The Australian Clinical Practice Guidelines on the Management of Type 1 Diabetes in Children and Adolescents (www.chw.edu.au/prof/services/endocrinology/APEG).

Bhargava, S., Sachdev, H. & Fall, C. (2004) Relation of serial changes in childhood body-mass index to impaired glucose tolerance in young adulthood. *New England Journal Medicine*, **350**, 865–875.

Bush, P., Ozias, J., Walson, P. & Ward, R. (1999) Ten guiding principles for teaching children about medicines. *Current Therapeutics*, **21**, 1280–1284.

Bryden, K. (2002) Turbulent time: the adolescent with type 1 diabetes. *Journal of Diabetes Nursing*, **6** (3), 83–87.

Bryden, K., Pevelr, R., Stein, A., Neil, A., Mayou, R. & Dunger, D. (2001) The clinical and psychological course of diabetes from adolescence to young adulthood: a longitudinal study. *Diabetes Care*, **24**, 1536–1540.

Buck, M. (2007) Self-medication by adolescents. *Paediatric Pharmacology*, **13** (5), 1–4.

Colton, P. (2007) Eating disturbance common and persistent in girls with type 1 diabetes. *Diabetes Care*, **30**, 2861–2862.

Conrad, S. & Gitelmand, S. (2006) If the numbers don't fit … discrepancies between meter glucose readings and haemoglobin A1c reveal stress of living with diabetes. *Clinical Diabetes*, **24**, 45–47.

Court, J. (1991) *Modern Living with Diabetes*. Diabetes Australia, Victoria.

Cranswick, N. & Lim, A. (2006) Use of over-the-counter and complementary medicine in children. *Australian Doctor*, 21st July, 25–32.

Curry, H., Schmer, C. & Ward-Smith, P. (2006) Kid Cards: teaching children about their medications. *Journal of Paediatric Health Care*, **20**, 414–418.

Dannemann, K., Hecker, W., Haberland, H., Herbst, A., Galler, A., Schafer, T., Brahler, E., Kiess, W. & Kapellen, T. (2008) Use of complementary and alternative medicine in children with type 1 diabetes mellitus – prevalence, patterns of use, costs. *Paediatric Diabetes on Line*, http://www.blackwell-synergy.com/doi/abs/10.111/j.1399–5448.2008.00377.x (accessed April 2008).

Department of Health (2001) *Diabetes National Service Framework: Standards for Diabetes Services*. Department of Health, London.

DIAMOND Project Group (2006) Incidence and trends of childhood type 1 diabetes worldwide 19901999. *Diabetic Medicine*, **23**, 857–866.

Dunning, P. (1993) Moving to adult care. *Practical Diabetes*, **10** (6), 226–228.

Dunning, P. (1994) Having diabetes: young adult perspectives. *The Diabetes Educator*, **21** (1), 58–65.

Federal Drug Administration (FDA) (undated) FDA Center for Drug Evaluation and Research. Medicines in my Home. www.fda.gov/medsinmyhome/MIMH_background.htm (accessed December 2007).

Field T., Morrow C., Valdeon C., Larsen S., Kuhn C., Schanberg S. (1997) Massage lowers blood glucose levels in children with diabetes. *Diabetes Spectrum*, **10**, 237–239.

Fleming, T. & Watson, P. (2002) Enhancing compliance in adolescents. *Current Therapeutics*, **43** (3), 14–18.

Gardiner, P. & Dvorkin, L. (2006) Promoting medication adherence in children. *American Family Physician*, **74**, 793–800.

Gill, T. (2007) Young people with diabetes and obesity in Asia: a growing epidemic. *Diabetes Voice*, **52**, 20–22.

Hales, C. & Barker, D. (1992) Type 2 (non-insulin dependent) diabetes mellitus: a thrifty phenotype hypothesis. *Diabetelogia*, **35**, 595–601.

International Diabetes Federation Consultative Section on Diabetes Education (2002) *International Diabetes Curriculum: Paediatric and Adolescent Module*. International Diabetes Federation, Brussels.

International Society for Pediatric and Adolescent Diabetes ISPAD (2000) *Consensus Guidelines for the Management of Type 1 Diabetes Mellitus*. Zeist, Medical Forum International.

Johnson, S., Freund, A. & Silverstein, J. (1990) Adherence–health status relationships in childhood diabetes. *Health Psychology*, **9**, 606–631.

Kaufman, F. & Riley, P. (2007) Protecting our children worldwide: the first UN-observed World Diabetes Day. *Diabetes Voice*, **52**, 9–12.

Kyngas, H. (2000) Compliance of adolescents with diabetes. *Journal of Paediatric Nursing*, **15** (4), 260–267.

Legro, R. & Dunaif, A. (1997) Menstrual disorders in insulin resistant states. *Diabetes Spectrum*, **10** (3), 185–190.

Levine, M. & Marcus, M. (1997) Women, diabetes and disordered eating. *Diabetes Spectrum*, **4** (5), 191–195.

Lorenz, R. & Wysocki, T. (1991) Conclusions: family and childhood diabetes. *Diabetes Spectrum*, **4** (5), 290–292.

Margeirsdottir, H. (2008) Time watching television linked to glucose control in pediatric type 1 diabetes. *Diabetes Care*, **30**, 1567–1570.

Moreno, M., Parks, M. & Richardson, L. (2007) What are adolescents showing the world about their health risk behaviours in MySpace? *Medscape General Medicine*, **9** (4), 9–15.

Need, J. (1962) Diabetes mellitus; a thrifty genotype rendered detrimental by 'progress.' *American Journal Human Genetics*, **14**, 353–362.

Picciano, M. (2007) Dietary supplement use among infants, children, and adolescents in the United States, 1999–2002. *Archives Pediatric Adolescent Medicine*, **161**, 978–985.

Pinhas-Hamiel, O. (2007) Complications of Type 2 diabetes in young people – a ticking bomb. *Medical News Today*, 30th May http://www.medicalnewstoday.com/medicalnews.php?newsid=72100&nfid=crss (accessed June 2007).

Schwenk, T. (2007) Weight management in overweight children. *Journal Watch*, **6** (6), 3.

Shaw, J. (2007) Childhood and adolescent obesity, diabetes and their consequences. *International Diabetes Monitor*, **13** (3),12–16.

Sinha, R., Fisch, G., Teague, B. *et al.* (2002) Prevalence of impaired glucose intolerance among children and adolescents with marked obesity. *New England Journal of Medicine*, **346**, 802–810.

Soltesz, G. (2007) Diabetes in children: changing trends in an emerging epidemic. *Diabetes Voice*, **52**, 13–15.

Srinivasan, S. & Donaghue, K. (2007) Paediatric diabetes – which children can gain insulin independence? *Medical Journal of Australia*, **186** (7), 436–437.

Svoren, B. & Wolfsdorf, J. (2005) Management of diabetes mellitus in children and adolescents. *International Diabetes Monitor*, **18** (95), 9–18.

Tait, A. (2008) Obese children at greater risk for perioperative adverse respiratory events. *Anesthesiology*, **108**, 375–380.

Thompson, S., Auslander, W. & White, N. (2001) Comparison of single-mother families on metabolic control of children with diabetes. *Diabetes Care*, **24** (2), 234–238.

Tsao, J., Meldrum, M., Kim, S., Jacob, M. & Zelter, L. (2007) Treatment preferences for CAM in children with chronic pain. *Evidence Based Complementary and Alternative Medicine*, **4** (3), 364–374.

Wei, J., Sung, F. & Li, C. (2003) Low birth weight and high birth weight infants are both at increased risk to have type 2 diabetes among schoolchildren in Taiwan. *Diabetes Care*, **26**, 343–348.

Weiss, R. & Caprio, S. (2005) The metabolic consequences of childhood obesity. *Best Practice & Research Clinical Endocrinology & Metabolism*, **19** (3), 405–419.

Woolf, A. (2003) Herbal remedies and children: do they work? Are they harmful? *Paediatrics*, **112**, 240–246.

World Health Organisation (2004) Mood (affective) disorders (F30–F39). *International Statistical Classification of Diseases and Health Related Problems* 2nd edn. World Health Organisation, Geneva.

Yajnik, C. (2007) Growth and nutrition in early life and risk of type 2 diabetes. *International Diabetes Monitor*, **19** (4), 1–8.

Zimmet, P., Alberti, G., Kaufman, F., Tajima, N., Silink, M., Arslanian, S., Wong, G., Bennett, P., Shaw, J. & Caprio, S. IDF Consensus Group (2007) The metabolic syndrome in children and adolescents – an IDF consensus report. *Paediatric Diabetes*, **8**, 299–306.

Chapter 14
Women, Pregnancy, and Gestational Diabetes

Key points

- Women with diabetes have particular health issues and care needs. These include pregnancy and childbirth, Polycystic Ovarian Syndrome (PCOS), and menopause.
- Good control before and during pregnancy reduces the risks to mother and baby.
- Better outcomes are achieved if the pregnancy is planned and normoglycaemia maintained before, during, and after pregnancy.
- Insulin is required in Type 2 diabetes during pregnancy and breastfeeding.
- Existing renal disease and retinopathy may deteriorate during pregnancy.
- PCOS is associated with obesity, insulin resistance, GDM, and infertility.

Rationale

Hormonal imbalance associated with PCOS and menopause affect glucose homeostasis and mental well being. Coordinated care and prepregnancy planning is necessary to ensure optimal outcomes for mother and baby. Planning for an optimal delivery begins in adolescence with diabetes education and sexual counselling.

Diabetes can develop during pregnancy, gestational diabetes. Most non-diabetic women are screened for diabetes during pregnancy so that blood glucose levels can be controlled to avoid the risks that having diabetes places on both mother and baby. Women particularly at risk are those with a history of diabetes in the family, diabetes during a previous pregnancy, or previous delivery of a large baby. There is increasing evidence that maternal hyperglycaemia has a lasting legacy for the child predisposing them to obesity in adolescence and Type 2 diabetes, and possibly memory deficits.

Polycystic Ovarian Syndrome

Polycystic Ovarian Syndrome (PCOS) is common, occurring in 6–10% of women in the reproductive age and 28% of obese women. Seventy five percent of women with PCOS are overweight or obese. PCOS has long term implications including menstrual irregularities, infertiliy, gestational diabetes (GDM), impaired glucose tolerance and insulin resistance, Type 2 diabetes, and emotional stress and body image concerns. Hyperinsulinaemia is associated with obesity and stimulates ovarian androgen production, insulin resistance, and cardiovascular disease.

Figure 14.1 Risk factors for Polycystic Ovarian Syndrome and the possible long-term effects. There is still controversy about the diagnostic criteria and several degrees of severity exist. There is no single diagnostic test: diagnosing PCOS is process of exclusion. Diagnostic criteria include National Institute of Health criteria, Rotterdam criteria, and International Androgen Excess Society criteria.

The risk factors for PCOS are shown in Figure 14.1. Making the diagnosis is a process of exclusion and consists of taking a careful family and individual history, hormone levels:

- Testosterone (normal <2.4 mmol/L in women).
- Sex hormone binding globulin (SHBG): likely to be low in PCOS (normal range 30–90) and is often secondary to insulin resistance and results in higher levels of free testosterone.
- Free androgen index (FAI): likely to be high in PCOS (normal range 1–5%).

FAI is more useful than testosterone unless the laboratory can test for free testosterone. Pelvic ultrasound to determine whether the ovaries are polycystic and whether the endometrium is thickened if oligo or amenorrhoea is present may be indicated (Zawazki *et al.* 1992; Rotterdam Concensus Workshop 2004; Teede *et al.* 2007). Determining follicle-stimulating hormone (FSH), thyroid stimulating hormone (TSH) and beta human chorionic gonadotrophin (HCG) and prolactin levels may be necessary to exclude other conditions.

Practice point

Hormone evaluation should be undertaken before prescribing oral contraceptives (OC) because OC can mask the hormonal changes associated with PCOS. Each woman should be individually assessed for cardiometabolic risk before commencing OCs (Yildiz 2008).

A multidiscipline supportive team approach is important to address the various underlying features of PCOS. Reassurance and education about diet and exercise and weight management aiming to lose 5–10% of weight at diagnosis, the need for regular follow up is important. The PCOS Association of Australia provides a useful website. In addition, counselling about fertility may be needed. Because PCOS is associated with insulin resistance and usually obesity, blood glucose and lipids should be checked regularly and an OGTT performed if indicated because fasting glucose is inadequate in PCOS (Teede *et al.* 2007) (see Chapter1). Cardiovascular assessment should be undertaken on a regular basis. Advice about diet and exercise are essential and psychological counselling may be required.

The dietary and exercise advice outlined in Chapter 4 is applicable to women with PCOS. Weight loss has been demonstrated in women with PCOS consuming the following diets: Atkins, Ornish, Weight Watchers, Zone, CSIRO Total Wellbeing Diet (Moran *et al.* 2003). The woman's food preferences should be considered and the diet should conform to dietary recommendations. If diet and exercise do not control blood glucose, metformin may be *added to* the diet and exercise regimen. The commencing dose is 500 mg of slow release metformin daily increasing to 2 g per day. Experts recommend giving metformin at night (Teede *et al.* 2007; Alberti *et al.* 2007) and there is evidence to support such a recommendation but metfromin is not currently approved for night dosing in Australia.

Metformin helps regulate the menstrual cycle and reduce hirsutism and the progression to diabetes by ~50 in high risk women (Alberti *et al.* 2007; Teede 2007). The role of metformin in improving fertility is unclear and it is not first-line fertility treatment. It may be more effective in lean women (De Maria 2007). Nevertheless, fertility should be discussed if metformin is commenced because of the chance of becoming pregnant. Obesity affects fertility independently of PCOS, thus loosing weight is essential if the woman wants to have a child. Age may also be a factor. Fertility declines from ~28 years and falls dramatically after age 35 and again after age 40.

Oral contraceptives (OC) may be indicated to help reduce hirsuitism and control menstrual irregularities. For example, low dose combined OCs such as Ethinyl Estradiol 20 µg increases SHBG and reduces free androgen levels. At higher doses OCP exacerbate insulin resistance (Meyer *et al.* 2007). Hair removal products or topical antiandrogens such as Vaniqua may be indicated, and cosmetic electrolysis or laser as a last resort. Obesity exacerbates hirsuitism so managing weight will help normalise androgen levels. The risks and benefits of all these options need to be carefully discussed with the woman considering her individual risk profile.

Antiandrogens such as spironolactone 50 mg BD or cyproterone acetate 25 mg daily for days 1–10 of the active OCP tablets may be prescribed to enhance fertility. These medicines must be taken with the OCP to prevent menstrual irregularities and adverse effects in pregnancy. The regimen takes ~6 months to be effective. Women who have more than four cycles of antiandrogens per year are at increased risk of endometrial hyperplasia and endometrial carcinoma. The woman should be monitored regularly for these conditions and plan to have a withdrawal bleed every 2–3 months to reduce these risks.

If endometrial hyperplasia is suspected a transvaginal ultrasound and endometrial biopsy are indicated to confirm the diagnosis especially if prolonged or irregular vaginal bleeding occurs. Hysteroscopy may be needed to determine whether fibroids or polyps are present. Endometrial hyperplasia sometimes resolves spontaneously. If endometrial hyperplasis atypia is present it may progress to endometrial carcinoma, which is induced by oestrogen and has a relatively good prognosis. Treatment depends on the woman. Intrauterine devices are appropriate if contraception is a goal and to control heavy bleeding. High-dose progestins may be indicated to limit endometrial thickening. The ultrasound and/or biopsy should be repeated after 6 months of treatment.

Partners and family need to be involved in explanations about PCOS and its effects as well as management discussions and education programes where relevant so they can support the woman and understand the associated risks. Achievable goals need to be set in consultation with the woman. The effect of having PCOS, its symptoms, and the impact on fertility can generate significant psychological distress, which exacerbates the physical issues, contributes to the diabetes and cardiovascular risk, and reduces quality of life (Coffey & Mason 2003; Wilhelm *et al.* 2003). Tools such as the K10 or HADs used on a regular basis can help identify the degree and progression of depression and are a helpful guide to treatment (see Chapter 15). Anxiety may be present in addition to depression. Depression needs to be treated, preferably with non-medicine options, because it affects the success of other treatment measures.

Exercise improves mood and fitness. Women with PCOS report significant body image issues, mood disturbances, depression, reduced emotional well being, low quality of life and life satisfaction and a negative impact of PCOS on their sexual self-worth and sexual satisfaction (Janssen *et al.* 2008). Managing symptoms such as hirsutism, obesity, menstrual irregularity and low fertility can significantly improve their emotional and sexual well being.

Tailored psychotherapy such as cognitive behavioural therapy or self-help programmes such as *Mood Gym*, and stress management can be beneficial. If medicines are indicated those that reduce PCOS symptoms may be useful. For example, SSRIs to control weight but the woman should be warned that these medicines could affect her sleep.

Pregnancy

Managing diabetes during pregnancy is challenging for the woman concerned and health professionals. Hormones released by the placenta predispose the mother to hyperglycaemia and increase the amount of glucose available to the fetus. Insulin sensitivity increases in the first trimester but insulin resistance develops in the second and third trimesters. The placental glucose transporter, GLUT-1, increases the transplacental glucose flux. The activity of GLUT-4 at the maternal cellular level decreases, which means glucose is not utilised by the mother and high levels cross the placenta where they are utilised by the fetus. This sets the scene for macrosomia and fetal abnormalities and makes vaginal delivery difficult (Hollingsworth 1992).

Prepregnancy counselling is essential to limit risks to mother and baby (Coustan 1997). Women who attend prepregnancy counselling have significantly lower risk of major fetal abnormalities (Ray *et al.* 2001). It should be provided to all women with diabetes of reproductive age, for example, at each annual review (Australian Diabetes in Pregnancy Society (ADIPS) 2005). Women with Type 2 diabetes and GDM are usually older than those with Type 1, are often overweight, higher parity, and belong to minority ethnic groups (Dornhurst *et al.* 1992). However, Type 2 diabetes is increasing in prevalence among adolescents and unwanted and unplanned pregnancy rates are high in this age group. In addition women are delaying childbirth, often until the mid-30s or 40s, which carries age-associated risks, and increases the likelihood that diabetes complications will be present and could affect the pregnancy. For example, age appears to be a significant factor in pregnancy-related MI although MI during pregnancy is rare (Karamermer & Ross-Hesselink 2007).

Coordinated multidisciplinary team care that includes as a minimum an obstetrician, endocrinologist, diabetes educator, dietitian, and paeditrician with experience managing diabetes is essential to optimal outcomes. Key management includes strategies to:

- Plan the pregnancy.
- Achieve and maintain HbA_{1c} as close as possible to normal before (<7%), during and after pregnancy.
- Commence folate supplements (5 mg daily).
- Undertake a comprehensive medication review (see Table 14.1). Stop OHA and commence insulin if the woman has Type 2 diabetes. Optimise the insulin regimen in women with Type 1 diabetes. Cease medicines likely to adversely affect the fetus. Commonly used medicines that *may* be contraindicated in pregnancy include:
- Ace inhibitors.
- B blockers
- Aspirin
- Coumarins
- Calcium channel blockers
- Statins
- NSAIDS
- Caution is required with antidepressants, corticosteroids, and opioids (Gardiner 2002).
- Ask about complementary medicine/therapy (CAM) use. Women frequently use CAM during pregnancy, particularly supplements such as raspberry leaf, ginger and chamomile tea (Foster *et al.* 2006). They also use massage and essential oils. Women who use CAM are generally well-informed and likely to take proactive self-care, be well educated, non-smokers and primiparous. The proportion of pregnant women with diabetes using CAM is unknown, but CAM use is high in the general diabetic population. While there are many benefits, there are also risks especially in the first trimester, and women with renal and liver disease, see Chapters 8 and 10. Some women elect to use complementary approaches (CAM) to pain management during labour or supplement conventional pain management strategies with CAM. Tournaire & Theau-Yonneau (2007). Undertook a systematic review of randomised controlled trials, which indicated pain was reduced and women receiving acupuncture and those receiving hydrotherapy required less analgesia. Women were not dissatisfied with conventional pain relief and had different expectations of pain management from health professionals. Strategies such as massage with or without essential oils, which reduce fear also have positive benefits

Table 14.1 Medication management during pregnancy. A comprehensive medication review should be undertaken regularly in all people with diabetes, when planning a pregnancy and when the woman becomes pregnant. See also Chapter 5.

Medication	Management	Potential adverse events
Insulin in Type 1 and Type 2 diabetes	Dose should be titrated regularly according to blood glucose monitoring to achieve targets and avoid hypoglycaemia. Insulin aspart has been shown to be safe to mother and fetus in Type 1 diabetes (Hod *et al.* 2007) and achieving postprandial blood glucose control (Pettitt *et al.* 2007). Glargine has been associated with mitogenic activity and should be used with caution in pregnancy (Hirsch 2005). Women with Type 2 diabetes will need education about managing insulin and hypoglycaemia as well as reassurance.	Hypoglycaemia, especially nocturnal hypoglycaemia during 6–18 weeks gestation. Significant repeated hypoglycaemia should be investigated to ensure there are no underlying disease processes and fetal growth and development monitored. Death, although rare, does occur (Ter Braak *et al.* 2002). Weight gain.
Oral glucose lowering agents (OHA) in Type 2 diabetes	Metformin The overall individual risks need to be considered just those associated with pregnancy. Metformin may be indicated in severe insulin resistance (Simmons *et al.* 2004). There is limited information about dose adjustment during pregnancy. Sulphonylureas Sulphonylureas cross the placenta, but second generation cross to a lesser extent: glipizide 6.6% and glyburide 3.9% (Feig *et al.* 2007). Thiazolidinediones (TZD) Rosiglitazone crosses the placenta especially after 10 weeks gestation	A number of studies suggest OHAs do not increase the risk of fetal malformation (Gutzin *et al.* 2003). Other researchers show metformin is not associated with fetal abnormalities and concentration in breast milk is low (Gilbert *et al.* 2006). Long-term data are not available thus, caution is recommended. The product prescribing recommends changing to insulin during pregnancy. Feig *et al.* (2007) found no evidence of fetal abnormalities in animal or human studies if the medicines were used in recommended doses. However, the studies were small and short term and these OHA cannot be recommended for use in pregnancy.

Table 14.1 Continued

Medication	Management	Potential adverse events
		However, when a woman with Type 2 diabetes becomes pregnant she should be referred urgently to an endocrinologist and OHAs continued until the transfer to insulin to avoid the risk of hyperglycaemia to the fetus (ADIPS 2005).
Antihypertensive agents	ACE inhibitors should be ceased during pregnancy. Methyldopa, oxprenolol, clonidine, labetolol, prazosin and nifedipine can be continued safely (Australasian Society for the Study of Hypertension in Pregnancy 2005). The effects of angiotensin 2 blocker is not known	ACE represent a threat to the fetus in the 3rd trimester and their safety is not established in the first trimester.
Lipid lowering agents		Statins have been associated with fetal abnormalities and are contraindicated in pregnancy (Edison *et al.* 2004).
Any other medicine	Check the prescribing information before using.	

including reducing lower back pain (Alaire 2001). Combination or single herbal medicines are sometimes used to manage pain, for example, motherwort. Women sometimes use herbal medicines during the last 4–5 weeks of pregnancy to prepare the cervix and facilitate delivery, for example raspberry leaf in tablet form and was found to shorten the second stage of labour and fewer women required forceps deliveries (Simpson *et al.* 2001). CAM use prior to and during labour should be discussed with the obstetrician and/or midwife. Thus, CAM use should be assessed at regular intervals.

- Blood glucose monitoring is essential: target levels are 4.0–5.5 mol/L fasting and <7.0 mmol/L two hours postprandial.
- Undertake a comprehensive diabetes complication and manage existing disease before pregnancy. For example, retinopathy requiring laser therapy, cardiovascular disease. The eyes should be examined through dilated pupils. Women should be aware that pre-existing retinopathy could progress during pregnancy. Pre-existing cardiovascular disease can be exacerbated by pregnancy due to haemodynamic changes and increased cardiac output. Delivery places extra demand on the heart (Karamermer & Ross-Hesselink 2007). Significant coronary artery stenosis should ideally be treated prior to pregnancy. The haemodynamic changes gradually return to normal in 3–6 months

(Karamermer & Ross-Hesselink 2007). Kidney function should be checked because women with microalbuminuria at risk of pre-eclampsia and microalbuminuria may progress during pregnancy if significant renal impairment is present and require dialysis (Biesenbach *et al.* 1992; Rossing *et al.* 2004), see Chapter 8. Some experts regard significant renal impairment to be a contraindication to pregnancy (ADIPS 2005) particularly given a third of women with severe renal impairment die within ~16 years (Rossing *et al.* 2004). Identify autonomic neuropathy-associated conditions such as gastroparesis, hypoglycaemic unawareness and orthostatic hypotension, which make management more difficult, are distressing for the woman and her family and may put her safety and/or life at risk. Autonomic neuropathy may predispose the mother to intractable vomiting and precipitate metabolic disturbances such as ketoacidosis.

- Assess general health and psychological wellbeing. For example detect the presence of comorbidities such as thyroid and coeliac disease in women with Type 1 diabetes, which could complicate the pregnancy.
- Undertake an education review of general diabetes knowledge and provide specific pregnancy and childbirth information. Revise home management of emergencies such as sick days/hyperglycaemia and morning sickness.
- Encourage women who smoke to quit and limit alcohol consumption.
- Perform an ultrasound at 18–20 weeks and if necessary the ultrasound should be repeated to check fetal cardiac status at 24 weeks and fetal growth at 28–30 weeks and again at 34–36 weeks.
- Encourage the woman to eat a healthy well balanced low GI diet to ensure optimal nutrition for herself and the developing fetus. The carbohydrates need to be spread over the day if problems occur. Foods likely to cause listeriosis should be avoided. Dietitian advice is advisable. Listeriosis can be transmitted from the mother to the fetus and cause miscarriage, stillbirth, premature delivery or a very ill baby at birth.
- Encourage participation in regular exercise such as 'Preggie Bellies' helps blood glucose control, general fitness, and well being and mental health.
- Encourage participation in childbirth classes.
- Develop and document a plan for managing insulin during delivery and in the immediate post partum period.
- Develop a plan for reviewing the mother's glycaemic control after discharge and ensuring the woman has adequate support at home.
- Foster mother–child bonding by providing woman-centred holistic care and supporting the woman and her family to adjust to parenthood. Monitoring for the 'three day blues' and postnatal depression is essential. For example, Rasmussen *et al.* (2007) found women with Type 1 diabetes were significantly stressed about the baby's safety if they had a 'hypo' and relied on their mothers and husbands for support. Mutual mother/daughter guilt feelings emerged (the guilt dynamic) where daughters felt guilty about the impact their diabetes had on their mother's lives and mothers felt guilty because their daughters developed diabetes and they could not prevent it. Chapter 15 describes psychological therapy. In addition, many small studies indicate massage, with and without essential oils, reduces stress, improves sleep for both the mother and baby, facilitates bonding and is safe (Bongaard 2007). Thus, massage may be a useful non-medicine option in high risk groups or could be used in combination with other therapies (Bongaard 2007).
- Specific care of the mother and baby during labour and delivery are specialty areas and outside the scope of this book. Most women should deliver at term and vaginally unless there are medical or obstetric reasons for earlier delivery/Caesarian section.

Usually blood glucose is measure every 1 2 hours and usual diet and insulin dose maintained. If a Caesarian section is needed, the procedure should be scheduled for the morning if possible. The dose of long-acting insulin on the evening prior to the surgery may need to be reduced to reduce the risk of hypoglycaemia after delivery. Women with Type 1 diabetes may need an insulin/glucose infusion.

- Women are encouraged to breast feed. Strategies to reduce hypoglycaemia during breastfeeding include having a snack before or while feeding, avoiding caffeine, drinking plenty of water, and having glucose close by to treat hypoglycaemia early if it occurs. Insulin is not contraindicated in breastfeeding.
- Discuss contraception plans prior to discharge.

Comprehensive assessment should be undertaken 1–4 weekly during the first 30 weeks of pregnancy and then weekly until delivery. Routine fetal monitoring should occur and an ultrasound performed to ensure the estimated date of delivery is accurate and develop the delivery plan. In most cases the women will be able to have a normal vaginal delivery unless there are obstetric complications.

Complications of pregnancy

Complications can be reduced by careful monitoring and proactively managing the pregnancy especially controlling blood glucose and other risk factors. The following maternal complications are associated with maternal hyperglycaemia:

- Early: miscarriage, fetal abnormalities, difficulty performing ultrasound.
- Antenatal: hypertension and pre-eclampsia, hypoglycaemia. During delivery: Increased possibility that labour will need to be induced or Caesarian section will be required because of conditions such as macrosomia, shoulder dystocia. Increased risk of perioperative complications if surgery is required. For example hypoglycaemia can have serious consequences in women having epidural anaesthesia because the usual counter-regulatory response is blocked and because pregnant women are more prone to hypoglycaemia. Hypoglycaemia can retard reversal of hypotension in these situations (Marx *et al.* 1987). However, maternal glucose is often higher during Caesarian section than vaginal delivery (Andersen *et al.* 1989).
- Postpartum: maternal haemorrhage, infection, thrombosis, hypoglycaemia.
- Deterioration in existing diabetes complication especially renal disease and retinopathy and cardiovascular status. Cardiovascular disease is encountered more frequently because women ore older when they begin their families, a family history of cardiac disease, and have often have diabetes for >10 years. In addition, obesity is more common and smoking increases the risk. An ECG should be performed if chest discomfort develops especially if the woman has known cardiovascular risk factors (Karamermer & Roos-Hesselink 2007). Indications of heart disease include:
  - Serious or progressive dyspnoea (mild dyspnoea is usual)
  - Syncope on exertion
  - Chest pain/discomfort associated with exertion.

The maternal death rate is comparable to non-diabetic women when care is delivered by a qualified, collaborative multidisciplinary team, ~0.5% of pregnancies in the UK (Chief Medical Officer's Report 2000).

Effects of diabetes on the baby

Consequences of maternal hyperglycaemia for the fetus include macrosomia, fetal distress, and birth injuries, which are largely preventable by good obstetric management and controlling maternal blood glucose levels. After delivery the baby may develop hypoglycaemia, hypothermia, hypocalcaemia, transient cardiomyopathy or other problems depending on the intrauterine conditions during pregnancy, delivery, and gestational age. The baby will need intensive monitoring initially, which might affect the bonding process.

Neonatal hypoglycaemia, defined as blood glucose <2.6 mmol/L up to 72 hours after birth, can cause significant morbidity and death if it is not recognised and treated effectively (Western Australian Center for Evidence Based Nursing and Midwifery 2006). The estimated incidence of newborn hypoglycaemia is between 1 and 5 per 1000 live births but may be up to 30% in at-risk infants (Hewitt *et al.* 2005). Hypoglycaemia is often present at birth and is usually transient in babies of non-diabetic mothers. Infants most at risk are:

- <2 kg or >4 kg at birth
- born before 37 weeks gestation
- <10th percentile for weight (small for gestational age)
- >90th percentile for weight (large for gestational age)
- retarded uterine growth
- born to mother with diabetes or GDM
- those with sepsis effectively (World Health Organisation (WHO 1997; Western Australian Center for Evidence Based Nursing and Midwifery 2006).

The maternal and baby's blood glucose levels correlate at birth. Thus, the maternal blood glucose level is the most significant determinant of neonatal hypoglycaemia (Andersen *et al.* 1989). The signs of hypoglycaemia in the neonate are often non-specific and include high pitched crying, hypothermia and poor temperature control, sweating, refusing to feed or poor sucking, exaggerated Moro reflex, irritability, hypotonia, tachyapnoea, tachycardia, cyanosis, and lethargy. All of these signs also occur in other conditions.

Traditionally, hypoglycaemia is diagnosed in the presence of Whipple's Triad: the presence of characteristic clinical signs of low blood glucose, low blood glucose, resolution of the signs once euglycaemia is re-established. However, the symptoms are unreliable in neonates, as can be seen from the preceding list. Having a high level of suspicion and performing a blood glucose test are essential. Once hypoglycaemia is corrected, babies are usually able to maintain blood glucose levels with normal breastfeeding on demand. Supplemental formula feeds may be required in the first 48 hours. Babies need to be kept warm and closely monitored in the neonatal nursery until they are stable.

Longer term effects of maternal hyperglycaemia on the child

Childhood obesity is increasing in many countries especially in ethnic minorities, see Chapter 1. The factors contributing to childhood obesity and associated consequences (insulin resistance, Type 2 diabetes, and diabetic complications) are debated. Genetic and environmental factors play a role (Dornhurst 2003) including the intrauterine environment during pregnancy, which has lasting effects on the child, the so-called Baker Hypothesis.

The fetus adapts structurally and functionally to reduced availability of essential nutrients. That is, under intrauterine 'famine' conditions available glucose is diverted to vital organs such as the brain and away from less immediately vital organs such as the pancreas. Insulin resistance develops in peripheral tissues to ensure a constant supply to vital organs and growth (birth weight) is retarded. The combination of reduced beta cell mass and pre-programming insulin-sensitive tissue to be insulin-resistant confers the risk of future diabetes on susceptible individuals (Baker *et al.* 1993). Low birth weight may be due to inadequate maternal intake and/or placental dysfunction. The association between Type 2 diabetes and low birth weight has been demonstrated in a number of population-based studies; however, the risk in developed countries with an adequate food supply is low (Boyko 2000) but may be higher in less affluent countries (Gray *et al.* 2002).

High birth weight is also associated with future risk of impaired glucose tolerance and Type 2 diabetes (Pettitt *et al.* 1996), which is likely to be a significant factor as the number of overweight women giving birth increases and they deliver higher birth weight babies. High birth weight is primarily due to maternal hyperglycaemia.

Memory deficits in childhood have also been attributed to poorly controlled maternal diabetes during pregnancy (De Boer 2007). De Boer suggested inadequate levels of iron and oxygen during development of the hippocampus (memory centre) *in utero* contributed to the deficits, which were significant by age three and a half. She suggested available iron was used to manufacture haemoglobin and diverted away from the hippocampus, which is a metabolically active part of the brain that requires a lot of iron during prenatal neuronal development. The longer term implications of De Boer's study are unknown and the research is ongoing. Significantly, the deficits were only noticeable on difficult memory tasks. The findings do underscore the importance of prenatal iron supplements and planning pregnancies.

Gestational diabetes

Gestational diabetes (GDM) refers to carbohydrate intolerance of variable severity that first appears during pregnancy (Metzger 1998). GDM is the most common metabolic complication of pregnancy. Insulin resistance and hyperglycaemia develop as a result of the hormones produced by the placenta and declining beta cell function. The hormones oestradiol, cortisol and human placental lactogen rise during pregnancy to ensure that the fetus receives sufficient glucose to grow and develop normally. As a consequence, the mother's cells become more resistant to insulin and the mother compensates by producing more insulin and using fat stores to produce energy for her own needs. GDM may in fact represent part of the continuum towards Type 2 diabetes.

It is recommended that all pregnant women be screened for diabetes between 24 and 28 weeks gestation, the time the placenta begins to produce large quantities of diabeto-genic hormones. The most frequently used screening test is a non-fasting morning glucose challenge using 50 g glucose load. Levels >7.8 mmol/L at 1 hour identify 80% of women with GDM (American Diabetes Association 2004) or ≥8 mmol/L at one hour if 75 g glucose load is used. If the screening test is positive, a diagnostic fasting OGTT is usually performed using 75 g glucose solution. Diagnostic levels are baseline ≥5.5 mmol/L and ≥8 mmol/L at 2 hours (Hoffman *et al.* 1998) (100 g is used in the US). Women who do not meet the diagnostic criteria for GDM may still have babies with glucose-related macrosomia, respiratory distress, hyperbiluribinaemia, hypoglycaemia and require admission to neonatal intensive care. Adverse pregnancy outcome such as stillbirth, Caesarian section, and pre-eclampsia can also occur.

Usually the blood glucose returns to normal after the baby is delivered. However, approximately 40% of women with gestational diabetes will develop diabetes in later life. In addition, the baby is at increased risk of Type 2 diabetes. In most cases the OGTT is repeated 6–8 weeks after delivery and then on regular basis, for example, yearly, although many women do not return for follow up. A recent study of women with GDM in Sweden between 1995 and 2005 (*n* = 385) were tested for beta cell autoantibody markers to determine their risk of developing Type 1 diabetes (Nilsson *et al.* 2007). Six per cent tested positive for at least one islet cell antibody: ICA, GAD or IA-2A. These women were followed and autoantibody levels reanalysed. On OGGT was performed in women who did not develop diabetes. Fifty per cent of the autoantibody positive women developed Type 1 diabetes and 21% had IFG or IGT but none had developed Type 2 diabetes. The overall numbers in the study were small, but autoantibody testing may be indicated in some women who develop GDM.

Who is at risk from gestational diabetes?

Gestational diabetes can occur in any pregnancy, however, those women at highest risk are categorised as:

- Older then 30 years.
- Having a family history of diabetes or previous gestational diabetes or having had a large baby previously.
- Belonging to an at-risk ethnic group, for example, Vietnamese, Asian Indians, Australian Aboriginals.
- Being obese >12% of ideal bodyweight and having other features of the metabolic syndrome, see Section 1.6.

Diet and exercise are first line treatment of GDM to control maternal blood glucose and supply essential nutrients for normal fetal growth and development. Generally low GI foods are recommended where 40–50% calories come from complex high fibre carbohydrate, 20% from protein and 30–40% from unsaturated fats distributed evenly throughout the day. Nutrition counselling by a dietitian is recommended. Blood glucose goals are fasting <5.5 mmol/L and 1 hour postprandial <8 mmol/L. Insulin is indicated if these targets cannot be met.

Calorie restriction can predispose the woman and the fetus to ketonaemia and reduce psychomotor development and IQ between the 3rd and 9th year of age in the child especially during the second and third trimesters (Rizzo *et al.* 1995). Pregnant women who remain active have a 56% lower risk of developing glucose intolerance and GDM than inactive women (Zhang *et al.* 2006) and lower risk of Type 2 diabetes in the longer term (Artal & O'Toole 2003; Ceysens *et al.* 2007). There are no data for optimal weight gain during pregnancy (Metzger *et al.* 2007). The Fifth International Workshop-Conference on GDM (2003) recommended a relatively small weigh increase during pregnancy: ~7 kg for obese women and up to 18 kg in underweight women.

Women at risk of GDM are advised to monitor their fasting and 2-hour postprandial blood glucose levels after each meal although there is no objective evidence to support the recommended frequency. CGM may be used to obtain a blood glucose pattern in some women, see Chapter 3. The aim of treatment is to keep blood glucose within the normal range (3–6.5 mmol/L), ensure the diet is appropriate, provide good obstetric care, and deliver the baby as close to term as possible.

Insulin will be required during pregnancy if blood glucose cannot be controlled using diet and exercise, generally when the fasting glucose is >7 mmol/L on three consecutive occasions but the duration of time on diet/exercise therapy before commencing insulin is unknown. Buchanan *et al.* (1994) recommended using insulin if the fetal abdominal circumference is >75th percentile for gestational age on ultrasound. However, a limitation of this method is that it provides a 'snapshop' rather monitoring continuous longitudinal fetal growth and should not be used alone especially given fetal macrosomia is related to maternal blood glucose levels. Insulin analogues are generally used, see Chapter 5 and the starting dose is calculated according to the woman's weight generally ~0.8 units/kg (non-obese), 0.9–1.0 units/kg (overweight and obese respectively).

Oral hypoglycaemic agents (OHAs) are contraindicated because they cross the placenta and cause neonatal hypoglycaemia and may have other unknown effects. However, metformin is used in Europe and South Africa and glibenclamide in South Africa without any reported fetal or maternal adverse outcomes. Although most other countries do not recommend OHA use during pregnancy (Metzger *et al.* 2007) the Metformin in Gestational Diabetes (MiG) (Rowan 2007) set up to compare metformin with insulin on perinatal outcomes suggests metformin is safe in the short term but may be contraindicated if the baby is small, or if the mother has pulmonary oedema or sepsis due to the risk of lactic acidosis, see Chapter 7. Metformin reduces absorption of vitamin B_{12} but this can be overcome by supplementing with calcium.

Insulin is given as required during labour. Some obstetric units use insulin infusions to control hyperglycaemia, which may be exacerbated by the pain and stress of labour. Frequent blood glucose monitoring is required because insulin requirements fall dramatically after delivery and maternal hypoglycaemia is possible. The baby is prone to hypoglycaemia after delivery and should be monitored closely for 24 hours as indicated in the preceding section.

Encourage breastfeeding. Breastfeeding provides essential nutrition and immunity for the baby. It decreases the risk of obesity and Type 2 diabetes in later life in babies of women who develop GDM.

Type 1 diabetes

As stated, planning the pregnancy and achieving optimal health before becoming pregnant significantly improves outcomes. Insulin requirements vary throughout the pregnancy and frequent blood glucose monitoring is essential so doses can be adjusted appropriately.

The specific insulin dose depends on individual characteristics. Overweight women may be less sensitive to insulin and may require larger doses than lean women. NovoRapid is approved for use in pregnancy. There do not appear to be any safety issues using the other insulin analogues in pregnancy but clinical experience with Apidra and Detemir is not as extensive with the other analogues (Nankervis 2008 oral presentation).

Blood glucose testing before and one hour after each meal is ideal to help titrate insulin doses as needed. Insulin requirements usually increases by ~20% in the first 5–6 weeks due to increased levels of progesterone and continues to rise slowly to weeks 9–11 at which time the placenta begins to produce progesterone and ovarian production ceases (Jovanovic 2004).

Progesterone levels may decline temporarily during the switch and consequently insulin requirements can drop especially in lean insulin-sensitive women. Hypoglycaemia risk increases. It may be necessary to perform 3 AM blood glucose tests to determine whether hypoglycaemia occurs during the night. Progesterone levels increase again after ~8–10 days and insulin requirements begin to increase and continue to do so during each trimester. At term when contractions begin insulin requirements drop because the available glucose is utilised to support uterine contractions. Three AM blood glucose testing may be required again at this time.

After delivery insulin requirements generally drop significantly and only very low doses may be needed in the first 24–48 hours and eventually return to prepregnancy requirements. However, breastfeeding women usually require less long acting insulin because blood glucose is used to produce milk, but they may need more short-acting insulin at mealtimes. Hyperglycaemia may mean extra lactose in breast milk and cause problems for the baby such as diarrhoea and putting on excess weight.

Women with Type 1 diabetes may have hypertension as a consequence of nephropathy or hypertension may develop as a consequence of the pregnancy (American Diabetes Association 2000). Blood pressure must be carefully monitored and controlled to reduce the risk of pre-eclampsia, progression of renal disease and retinopathy. Medicines management can be complication because ACE inhibitors, β blocking agents and diuretics are generally contraindicated.

Type 2 diabetes

Women with Type 2 diabetes and hyperglycaemia may be commenced on insulin prior to conceiving to optimise blood glucose levels and improve pregnancy outcomes.

Women with Type 2 diabetes are usually commenced on insulin during pregnancy. As with Type 1 diabetes insulin requirements slowly increase over the course of the pregnancy. However, the typical temporary drop seen ~9–11 weeks in women with Type 1 diabetes may not occur because women with Type 2 diabetes are generally insulin resistant. Insulin requirements are affected by hormone levels but also by arbohydrate intake and activity levels.

Women with Type 2 diabetes should monitor their blood glucose with the same frequency as those with Type 1 but are generally less prone to nocturnal hypoglycaemia.

After delivery women who were treated with diet and exercise may be able to resume that regimen but insulin is recommended if the woman decides to breast feed (ADIPS 2005). OHAs can be used but metformin is present in breast milk and the baby *may* develop hypoglycaemaia. Therefore, regular blood glucose testing may be needed, but could be stressful for the parents.

Practice points

(1) Some women worry about whether injecting into the abdomen can cause or exacerbate stretch marks. There is no evidence that any such effect occurs.

(2) It may be difficult to pinch up a fold of skin during late pregnancy as the skin stretches and tightens. It may be necessary to inject into other sites such as the side of the abdomen or thighs.

(3) The needles are not long enough to penetrate into the uterus and damage the baby.

Menopause and diabetes

Menopause is a normal life stage for all women as the ability to bear a child ends and levels of oestrogen and progesterone gradually decline. Small amounts of oestrogen are usually still produced. Menopause is complete when menstruation does not occur for 12 months around 51 years of age although women with Type 1 diabetes may experience menopause at an earlier age. However, overweight women with Type 2 diabetes may go through menopause later because oestrogen levels do not decline as rapidly in overweight women. Women are living longer, thus they spend a considerable proportion of their lives in the post menopausal stage. Older women may develop diabetes as discussed in Chapter 12.

Signs and symptoms of menopause

Some of the symptoms associated with menopause may be associated with normal ageing, others are due to hormonal fluctuations. These include:

- Mood swings, irritability, anxiety, and depression.
- Difficulty remembering things.
- Increased premenstrual tension.
- Heavier or lighter menstrual flow.
- Hot flushes.
- Changed sexual functioning such as lower libido, vaginal dryness, and recurrent candidia infections.
- Susceptibility to UTI.
- Fluctuating and unpredictable blood glucose levels, which adds to the distress associated with menopause. Some women with Type 1 diabetes experience more frequent hypoglycaemia. Unexplained hypoglycaemia may be one of the first signs of menopause.
- Sleep disturbance due to hot flushes and/or nocturnal hypoglycaemia.
- Weight gain, especially in Type 2 diabetes, which may be associated with reduced activity and may lead to hyperglycaemia.
- Chronic back and joint pain, which can be exacerbated by being overweight.

Managing the menopause

Maintaining a healthy active lifestyle is important for all women. A dietary review may be helpful to ensure adequate nutrition is maintained and limit the risk of common nutritional deficiencies such as calcium and vitamin D and the risk of osteoporosis and fractures. A diet rich in phytoestrogens such as soy products and legumes helps maintain hormonal balance. Limiting alcohol and caffeine helps control hot flushes. A healthy diet and regular exercise control weight and reduces strain on joints, which reduces back pain a well as improving blood glucose utilisation as well as reducing cardiovascular and osteoporosis risk, and improving mental wellbeing.

Regular blood glucose monitoring is important to distinguish menopausal symptoms such as sweating from hypoglycaemia and to guide OHA/insulin dose adjustment. Some overnight testing may be necessary.

A medication review is advisable. Medications, particularly OHA and insulin doses, may need to be adjusted. A through complication assessment is advisable. The risk of cardiovascular disease increases thus lipid lowering and antihypertensive agents may be needed, if they are not already prescribed.

Hormone replacement therapy (HRT) may improve glycaemic control and lipid levels, depending on the preparations used, and improve cardiovascular risk in younger postmenopausal women (Khoo & Mahesh 2005). Several cardiovascular events are reduced by 34–45% in women aged 50–59 on HRT and with longer use but not those >60 years (Hodis & Mack 2008). However, HRT should not be prescribed to prevent cardiovascular disease. Diet and exercise, lipid lowering medicines especially statins, and aspirin may be needed in women with cardiovascular risk factors, but fenofibrate may be contraindicated because of the risk of venous embolism. HRT is increasingly being known as menopausal hormone therapy (MHT) (National Center for Complementary and Alternative Medicine 2008).

The individual benefits and risks need to be considered and carefully explained to the woman. Younger recently menopausal women have fewer risks than older postmenopausal women. Possible adverse events include stroke, venous thrombosis, and breast cancer, but the relative risks are low if HRT is commenced within 5 years of menopause (WHI study 2002).

HRT may be useful in younger post menopausal women with Type 1 diabetes to prevent osteoporosis, but should be used at the lowest effective dose. Long-term HRT to prevent osteoporosis is not advisable but HRT does have a role in managing menopausal symptoms in the short term (Australian Drug Evaluation Committee 2003). Bisphosphonates may be an alternative if HRT is contraindicated (Khoo & Mahesh 2005).

Antibiotics and antifungal agents may be needed to manage UTIs and candida infections but general hygiene, passing urine after sexual intercourse, wearing cotton underwear, eating a healthy diet, and controlling hyperglycaemia are important preventative measures. Cranberry preparations prevent UTIs but may be contraindicated with some medications likely to cause bleeding.

Contraception options for women with diabetes

Planned pregnancy is vital in women with diabetes thus contraceptive advice is essential. Women with diabetes need specific advice about their contraception options from a qualified expert. The same range of contraceptive methods available to non-diabetic women is available to and suitable for women with diabetes and the same risks and benefits apply. However, extra precautions are needed, for example, women with hypertension, those at risk of embolism, and those with microvascular disease and cardiovascular disease. These risks may be greater in women with Type 2 diabetes (Damm *et al.* 2005). Thus, the benefits and risks need to be carefully considered for each individual woman.

Commonly used methods include:

- The Billing's method.
- Barrier methods such as condoms, diaphragms, and the recently released NuvaRing, which is placed in the vagina releases topical hormones.
- Intrauterine devices (IUD) including the mirena progesterone implant, which is used to control abnormal bleeding as well as contraception.
- Oral contraceptive agents (OCP), which may be progesterone only or combined oestrogen and progesterone preparations.
- Topical patches such as Ortho Evra.

Concerns have been raised about the effects of OCs on glucose and fat metabolism, which could exacerbate cardiovascular risks. However, several studies suggest OCs do not adversely affect blood glucose or lipid levels, or exacerbate retinopathy or hypertension (Klein *et al.* 1990; Kaunitz 2002). Other research suggests high-dose combined OC has a small beneficial effect on glucose homeostasis and lipid metabolism, whereas progesterone only OC improves lipid metabolism (Visser *et al.* 2006). The risks of vascular complications, retinopathy and rates of thrombolism appear to be low but progesterone only preparations cause more irregular bleeding. All methods were effective contraceptives. Thus, combination OCP and most likely recently introduced contraceptives such as monthly injections, for example, lunelle, the NuvaRing and OrthoEvra patch appear to be appropriate for women with diabetes <35 years (Kaunitz 2002). These methods might be contraindicated in older women and those with hypertension, micro and macrovascular disease. For these women IUD including progesterone-releasing mirena, progesterone only mini pills or depot progesterone, for example, depo provera injections or implanon implants (Kaunitz 2002).

Interestingly, Kim *et al.* (2002) reported lower blood glucose levels and lower odds of developing diabetes in young white and African-American women in the CARDIA study. Insulin levels were higher after adjusting for covariates but the clinical significance of this finding is unknown. Insulin sensitivity was found to decline in women with PCOS treated with triphasic OCs but there were no adverse effects on lipid metabolism (Korytkowski *et al.* 1995). The effects on insulin sensitivity and production might be a consideration in women with the metabolic syndrome, those at risk of GDM, or obese women with Type 2 diabetes, however, more research is needed to clarify the clinical implications.

Complementary approaches to managing the menopause

Many women began using CAM to manage menopausal symptoms in 2002 when the findings from the Women's Health Initiative study were released, which questioned the long-term safety of HRT use. At the time many women stopped using HRT and many tried CAM alternatives. The value of using CAM to manage menopausal symptoms is still debated and the long-term benefits of CAM hormone replacement medicines to prevent osteoporosis are unknown. Conventional hormone replacement medicines significantly reduce menopausal symptoms and osteoporotic fractures. Many research trials focus on managing hot flushes and preventing osteoporosis, however, CAM practitioners focus on managing the transition to and through menopause, rather then treating isolated symptoms.

For this and other reasons, CAM therapies continue to be popular with many menopausal women who fear the risks associated with conventional HRT. Australian women of menopausal age are high CAM users (MacLennan *et al.* 2002). Popular CAM menopausal treatments include phytoestrogens, herbal medicines, acupuncture, homeopathy, acupuncture, massage and essential oils, and wild yam cream.

Phytoestrogens

Phytoestrogens are naturally occurring plant compounds, which have a similar chemical composition to but lower potency than oestrogen. Phytoestrogens act at oestrogen receptor sites and may reduce menopausal symptoms but it is not clear whether the effects are due to phytoestrogens or other products in particular foods. Phytoestrogens reduce cholesterol and may have a place in managing cardiovascular risk. They may also improve cognition and increase bone mass. There are three main phytoestrogens:

(1) Isoflavones: found in soy products and beans, for example, lima beans and lentils.
(2) Lignans: found in fruit, vegetables, grains and seeds such as linseed and flaxseed.
(3) Coumestans: found in sprouted seeds such as alfalfa.

Phytoestrogen should be used with caution by women using medicines that contain oestrogen for example, OCs, HRT, and some cancer medicines, for example, selective oestrogen receptor modulators such as tamoxifen, and women at risk of breast, uterine or ovarian cancer, endometriosis or uterine fibroids. Women in these categories should seek expert advice rather than self-prescribing.

Herbal medicines

If women choose to use CAM medicines to manage the menopause they should be clear about their therapy goals and seek the advice of a qualified practitioner. CAM medicines are usually used to manage the symptoms of menopause such as hot flushes, to improve sleep, and maintain wellbeing. Commonly used medicines include:

• *Hypericum perforatum* (St John's Wort), which effectively reduces anxiety and mild to moderate depression (Ernst 1995).
• Evening primrose oil, which has limited evidence to support an effect.

- *Cimicifuga racemosa* (black cohosh), to reduce symptoms including hot flushes. It is a key ingredient in medicines such as remifemin, which has been shown to reduce LH without affecting FH (Duker 1991). Some studies have not shown any reduction in hot flushes (Newtown *et al.* 2006). There have been case reports of liver damage and hepatitis but no causal association has been proven. However, preparations containing black cohosh may be contraindicated in women at risk of these conditions. Generally it should not be used longer than 6 months or during pregnancy and lactation.
- *Angelica sinensis* (dong quai) there is limited evidence that dong quai reduces hot flushes. It interacts with warfarin and may be contraindicated in women using warfarin or the effects on the INR monitored carefully.
- *Panax ginseng or P. quinquefolius* (ginseng), which may be useful to improve mood, general well being, and sleep. It does not improve hot flushes. Ginseng has hypoglycaemic properties and may represent a hypoglycaemia risk. However, blood glucose levels are often higher during menopause and the glucose lowering effect may be a beneficial interaction.
- *Piper methysticum* (kava), reduces anxiety but has been linked to liver damage. Therefore, kava may be contraindicated in women with existing lover disease or those at risk of liver disease.
- *Trifolium pratense* (red clover) red clover contains phytoestrogens and is a key ingredient in CAM medicines such as promensil. Some women report overall benefits but there is limited evidence that it reduces hot flushing.
- Dehydroepiandrosterone (DHEA) occurs naturally in many foods and is often taken as a dietary supplement. DHEA is converted to oestrogen and testosterone in the body. It may reduce the frequency and intensity of hot flushes and improve sexual arousal. Significantly, endogenous DHEA levels decline with age and many people use DHEA supplements to reduce age-associated symptoms as well as menopause. It may increase the risk of breast and prostate cancer but evidence is lacking. DHEA is sometimes added to bioidentical hormonal compounds such as Biest and Triest, which increased in popularity after the release of the results of the WHI study, which suggested HRT was linked with increased risk of breast cancer (Rossouw *et al.* 2002).
- Progesterone creams are available on prescription, some formulations contain oestrogen and testosterone. Progesterone declines after menopause due to declining oestrogen levels. However there is little evidence that progesterone creams reduce menopausal symptoms or improve osteoporosis risk. Only a small amount of progesterone is absorbed form topically applied formulations. *Dioscorea villosa* (wild yam) cream does not contain progesterone although it was originally marketed in this way because it contains diosgenin, an oestrogen-like compound. Wild yam is an antispasmodic and gentle liver tonic and CAM practitioners prescribe it for these indications. Progesterone used in conventional pessaries, OCPs and suppositories is synthesised from diosgenin. However, specific enzymes are required to produce progesterone from diosgenin and these enzymes are not present in the human body. Traditionally, wild yam was taken orally rather than cream but the cream formulation is a popular self-prescribed menopausal treatment. Progesterone is mainly prescribed to protect the lining of the uterus in women who use oestrogen. Substituting progesterone creams especially wild yam for the progesterone component of combined HRT can increase the risk of endometrial cancer.

Practice points

(1) Women who elect to use CAM to manage menopausal symptoms should do so under the management of a suitably qualified practitioner.
(2) They should advise all their conventional health practitioners that if they use CAM.
(3) More research is needed into the benefits of most CAM for managing menopausal symptoms.
(4) CAM medicines used to manage menopausal symptoms can interact with conventional medicines.

References

Allaire, A. (2001) Complementary and alternative medicine in labour and delivery suite. *Clinical Obstetrics and Gynaecology*, **44**, 681–691.

Alberti, G., Zimmet, P. & Shaw, J. (2007) International Diabetes Federation Consensus on type 2 diabetes. *Diabetic Medicine*, **24**, 451–463.

Andersen, O., Hertel, J., Schmolker, L. & Kuhl, C. (1985) Influence of the maternal plasma glucose concentration at delivery on the risk of hypoglycaemia in infants of insulin-dependent diabetic mothers. *Acta Paediatrica*, **74**, 268–273.

Australian Drug Evaluation Committee (ADEC) (2003) Update to ADEC statement on use of hormone replacement therapy. ADEA 17th October http://www.tga.health.gov/au/docs/html/hrtadec2.htm (accessed December 2007).

Biesenbach, G., Stoger, H. & Zazgornik, J. (1992) Influence of pregnancy on progression of diabetic nephropathy and subsequent requirement for renal replacement therapy in female type I diabetic patients with impaired renal function. *Nephrology Dialysis Transplant*, **7**, 105–109.

Bongaard, B. (2007) Is massage beneficial for pregnant women? *Alternative Medicine Alert*, **10** (12), 133–136.

Buchanan, T., Kjos, S. & Montoro, M. (1994) Use of fetal ultrasounds to select metabolic therapy for pregnancies complicated by mild gestational diabetes. *Diabetes Care*, **17**, 275–283.

Ceysens, G., Rouiller, D. & Boulvain, M. (2006) Exercise for diabetic pregnant women. *Cochrane Database of Systematic Reviews*, Rev # CD004225.

Chief Medical Officer (2000) *The Report on the Confidential Enquiries into Maternal Deaths 1997–1999*. Her Majesty's Stationery Office, London.

Coustan, D. (1997) Is preconception counselling for women with diabetes cost-effective? *Diabetes Spectrum*, **10** (3), 1195–2000.

Damm, P., Mathiesen, E., Clausen, D. & Petersen, K. (2005) Metabolic syndrome and related disorders: contraception for women with diabetes mellitus. http://www.liebertonline.com/doi: 10. 1089/met.2005.3.244 (accessed February 2008).

DeBoer, T. (2007) Maternal diabetes linked to infant memory problems. *Child Neurology*, **47**, 525.

DeMaria, E. (2007) Bariatric surgery for morbid obesity. *New England Journal of Medicine*, **356**, 2176–2183.

Dornhorst, A. (2003) Maternal hyperglycaemia – food for thought. *Practical Diabetes International*, **20** (8), 283–289.

Dornhorst, A., Paterson, C. & Nicholls, J. (1992) High prevalence of gestational diabetes in women from ethnic minority groups. *Diabetec Medicine*, **9**, 820–825.

Dukes, E. (1991) Effects of extracts from *Cimicifuga racemosa* on gonadotropin release in menopausal women and ovariectomised rats. *Plana Medica*, 57, 420–424.

Ernst, E. (1995) St John's Wort, an antidepressant? A systematic criteria-based review. *Phytomedicine*, 2 (1), 67–71.

Feig, D., Briggs, G. & Koren, G. (2007) Oral antidiabetic agents in pregnancy and lactation: a paradigm shift? *Annals of Pharmacotherapy*, 41(7), 1174–1180.

Forster, D., Denning, A., Wills, G., Bolger, M. & McCarthy, E. (2006) Herbal medicine use during pregnancy in a group of Australian women. *BMC Pregnancy and Childbirth*, 6, 21.

Gardiner, S. (2002) Drugs in pregnancy. *Current Therapeutics*, October, 31–33.

Gilbert, C., Valois, M. & Koren, G. (2006) Pregnancy outcome after first-trimester exposure to metformin: a meta-analysis *Fertility and Sterility*, 86 (3), 658–663.

Gutzin, S., Kozer, E. & Mcgee, L. (2003) The safety of oral hypoglycaemic agents in the first trimester of pregnancy: a meta-analysis. *Canadian Journal of Clinical Pharmacology*, 10, 179–183.

Hewitt, V., Robertson, R. & Haddow, G. (2005) Nursing and midwifery management of hypoglycaemia in healthy term neonates: a systematic review. *Journal of Evidence Based Healthcare*, 3 (7), 169–205.

Hirsch, I. (2005) Insulin analogues. *New England Journal of Medicine*, 352, 174–183.

Hod, M., Damm, P., Kaaja, R., Visser, G., Dunne, F., Demidova, I., Hansen, A. & Mersebach, H. (2007) Fetal and perinatal outcomes in type 1 diabetes pregnancy: a randomized study comparing insulin as part with human insulin in 322 subjects. *American Journal of Obstetrics & Gynaecology*, 198 (2), 186 and 1–7.

Hodis, H. & Mack, W. (2008) The beneficial effect of hormone replacement therapy on mortality and coronary heart disease in younger versus older postmenopausal women. *Medscape Ob/Gyn 7 Womens' Health* http:www.medscape.com/viewarticle/569935?src=mp (accessed March 2008).

Hoffman, L., Nolan, C., Wilson, D., Oats, J. & Simmons, D. (1998) Gestational diabetes mellitus – management guidelines. *Medical Journal of Australia*, 169, 93–97.

Hollingsworth, D. (1992) *Pregnancy, Diabetes and Birth*. Williams & Wilkins, USA.

Janssen, O., Hahn, S., Tan, S., Benson, S. & Elsenbruch, S. (2008) Mood and sexual function in polycystic ovary syndrome. *Seminars in Reproductive Medicine*, 26 (1), 45–52.

Jovanovic, J. (2004) Answers to questions about pregnancy and diabetes. *Diabetic Mommy* http://www.diabeticmommy.com/sp-pregnancy-diabetes-bd-faq-answers.html (accessed November 2007).

Karamermer, Y. & Roos-Hesselink, J. (2007) Coronary heart disease and pregnancy. *Future Cardiology*, 3 (5), 559–567.

Kaunitz, A. (2002) Contraception for women with diabetes. *Medscape Obstetrics and Gynaecology & Women's Health*, 7 (2): (Posted 12. 9. 2002) (accessed February 2008).

Kim, C., Siscovick, D., Sidney, S., Lewis, C., Kiefe, C. & Koepsell, T. (2002) Oral contraceptive use and association with glucose, insulin and diabetes in young adult women: The CARDIA study. *Diabetes Care*, 25 (6), 1027–1032.

Klein, B., Moss, S. & Klein, R. (1990) Oral contraceptives in women with diabetes. *Diabetes Care*, 13 (8), 895–898.

Korytkowski, M., Mokan, M., Horowitz, M. & Berga, S. (1995) Metabolic effects of oral contraceptives in women with polycystic ovary syndrome. *Journal of Clinical Endocrinology and Metabolism*, 80, 3327–3334.

Khoo, C. & Mahesh, P. (2005) Diabetes and the menopause. *Journal British Menopause Society*, 11 (1), 6–11.

Marx, G., Domurat, M. & Costin, M. (1987) Potential hazard of hypoglycaemia in the parturient. *Canadian Journal of Anaesthiology*, 34 (4), 400–402.

Menato, G., Bo, S., Signorlie, A., Gallo, M., Cotrino, I., Botto, C. Massobrio, M. (2008) Current management of gestational diabetes mellitus. *Expert Review of Obstetrics and Gynaecology*, 3 (1), 73–91.

Metzger, B.E. (1998) International Hyperglycaemia and Adverse Pregnancy Outcomes (HAPO): temporary recommendations. Fourth International Workshop on GDM. *Diabetes*, **40** (Suppl. 2), 197–201.

Metzger, E., Buchanan, T. & Coulstan, D. (2007) Summary and recommendations of the fifth International Workshop – Conference on Gestational Diabetes Mellitus. *Diabetes Care*, **30**, S251–S260.

Meyer, C., McGrath, B. & Teede, H. (2007) Effects of medical therapy on insulin resistance and the cardiovascular system in polycystic ovarian syndrome. *Diabetes Care*, **30**, 471–478.

Moran, I., Noakes, M. & Clifton, P. (2003) Dietary composition in restoring reproductive and metabolic physiology in overweight women with polycystic ovarian syndrome. *Journal Clinical Endocrinology and Metabolism*, **88**, 812–819.

Nankervis, A. (2008) Practical management of diabetes in pregnancy. Sanofi-Aventis Seminar April, Melbourne.

National Women's Health Information Center (2006) Menopause and menopause treatments. http://nccam.nih.gov/health/menopauseandcam (accessed February 2008).

Newton, K., Reed, S. & Lacroix, A. (2006) Treatment of vasomotor symptoms of menopause with black cohosh, multibotanicals, soy, hormone therapy, or placebo. *Annals of Internal Medicine*, **145** (12), 869–879.

Oakley, C. (1992) Care of gestational diabetes mellitus. *Diabetes Care*, **1**, 6–8.

Pettitt, D., Ospina, P., Howard, C., Zisser, H. & Jovanovic, L. (2007) *Diabetic Medicine*, **24**, 1129–1135.

Polycystic Ovarian Syndrome Association of Australia. www.posa.asn.au (accessed March 2008).

Ray, J., O'Brien, T. & Chan, W. (2001) Preconception care and the risk of congenital abnormalities in the offspring of women with diabetes mellitus: a meta-analysis. *Quality Journal of Medicine*, **94**, 435–444.

Rizzo, T., Dooley, S., Metzger, B., Cho, N., Ogata, E. & Silverman, B. (1995) Prenatal and perinatal influences on long term psychomotor development in offspring of diabetic mothers. *American Journal of Obstetrics and Gynaecology*, **173** (6), 1753–1758.

Ross, G. (2002) How to plan a healthy pregnancy. *Diabetes Conquest*, **Autumn**, 28.

Rossouw, J., Anderson, G. & Prentice, R. (2002) Writing Group for the Women's health Initiative Investigators. Risks and benefits of oestrogen plus progestin in healthy menopausal women: principal results from the Women's health Initiative randomized controlled trial. *Journal American Medical Association*, **288** (3), 321–333.

Rotterdam ESHRE/ASRM Sponsored PCOS Consensus Workshop group. Revised 2003 consensus on diagnostic criteria and long term health risks related to Polycystic Ovarian Syndrome. *Fertility and Sterility*, **81**, 19–25.

Rowan, J. (2007) A trial in progress: treatment with metformin compared with insulin in the metformin in gestational diabetes study (MiG). *Diabetes Care*, **30**, S214–S219.

Simmons, D., Walters, J., Rowan, J. & McIntyre, D. (2004) Metformin therapy and diabetes in pregnancy. *Medical Journal of Australia*, **180**, 462–464.

Simpson, M., Parsons, M., Grenwood, J. & Wade, K. (2001) Raspberry leaf in pregnancy: its safety and efficacy in labour. *Journal of Midwifery and Women's Health*, **46**, 51–59.

Teede, H., Hutchison, S. & Zoungas, S. (2007) The management of insulin resistance in polycystic ovarian syndrome. *Trends in Endocrinology and Metabolism*, **18**, 273–279.

Ter Braak, E., Evers, I., Erkelens, W. & Visser G. (2002) Maternal hypoglycaemia during pregnancy in type 1 diabetes: maternal and fetal consequences. *Diabetes Metabolism Research Reviews*, **18**, 96–105.

The Australasian Diabetes in Pregnancy Society (2005) Consensus guidelines for the management of type 1 and type 2 diabetes in relation to pregnancy. *Medical Journal of Australia*, **183** (7), 373–377.

The Australasian Society for the Study of Hypertension in Pregnancy Consensus Statement. *The Detection, Investigation and Management of Hypertension in Pregnancy: Executive Summary.* http://www.racp.edu.au/asshp/asshp.pdf (accessed December 2007).

Tournaire, M. &, Theau-Yonneau, A. (2007) Complementary and alternative approaches to pain relief during labour. *Evidence Based Complementary and Alternative Medicine*, **4** (4), 409–417.

Visse, J., Snel, M. & Van Vilet, T. (2006) Hormonal versus non-hormonal contraceptive sin women with diabetes mellitus type 1 and 2. *Cochrane Database of Systematic Reviews*, **18** (4), cd003990.

Western Australian Center for Evidence Based Nursing and Midwifery (2006) Management of asymptomatic hypoglycaemia in health term neonates for nurses and midwives. *Best Practice*, **10** (1), 1–4.

World Health Organisation (WHO) (1997) *Hypoglycaemia in the Newborn.* WHO, Geneva.

Women Health Initiative (WHI) Writing Group for the WHI investigators (2002) Risks and benefits of HRT. *Journal American Medical Association*, **288**, 321–333.

Yildiz, B. (2008) Oral contraception in women with polycystic ovary syndrome. *Seminars in Reproductive Health*, **26** (1), 111–120.

Zhang, C., Solomon, C., Manson, J. & Hu, F. (2006) A prospective study of pregravid physical activity and sedentary behaviours in relation to the risk of gestational diabetes mellitus. *Archives of Internal Medicine*, **166**, 543–548.

Chapter 15

Psychological and Quality of Life Issues Related to Having Diabetes

Key points

- Focus on achieving a balanced life rather than control. Learning to achieve balance is a developmental process in which the individual gradually takes responsibility for their diabetes.
- Having support is essential to achieving optimal balance and diabetes and general health outcomes.
- Most quality of life research indicates people with diabetes have worse quality of life than those without diabetes.
- Quality of life is individual, complex, and multifactorial and encompasses life priorities, which might change according to life circumstances.
- Avoid using labels such as 'non-compliant' or 'a diabetic'.
- Offer support, respect and encouragement.

Rationale

Each person with diabetes is unique. People with diabetes focus on being well and living a normal life, thus, they strife for life balance. Achieving a balanced lifestyle and good quality of life is essential to the physical and psychological well being of people with diabetes. Depression is more common in people with diabetes and can impact on their self-care and long-term health outcomes. Health professionals are often preoccupied with metabolic control. Changing the focus to achieving balance is more likely to assist the person to achieve metabolic control. Health professionals' goal is to achieve optimal metabolic outcomes: a common goal of people with diabetes is to achieve a healthy life balance. Achieving such balance is a complex and changing process.

Introduction

People with diabetes are at increased risk of developing various degrees of psychological distress and psychological disorders including depression and eating disorders (Rubin & Peyrot 2001). Symptoms associated with hyperglycaemia, hypoglycaemia and the focus on diet can mask signs of psychological distress and disorders. If present, psychological disorders can interfere with self-care, medicine adherence and exacerbate hyperglycaemia, thus setting up a vicious cycle. Depression is often undetected in older people and is often considered to be part of normal ageing. Approximately 15% of older community dwelling older people experience depressive symptoms and at least 24% of people with diabetes of all ages are depressed (Goldney *et al.* 2004) the incidence rises sharply in older people living in residential facilities. In Australia, the second highest suicide rate occurs in men >85.

The decision to take control of diabetes and undertake self-care is vital Hernandez (1995). Hernandez found people with Type 1 diabetes were initially concerned with being normal and adopted a passive role in their care. The decision to assume control often occurred at a turning point in their lives. The impetus for assuming control include feeling betrayed by or not listened to by health professionals, realising that adhering to management regimens would not automatically prevent complications, and health professionals accusing them of 'cheating' when their blood glucose levels were unstable (Patterson & Sloan 1994). Life and other events may impact on an individual's willingness and ability to assume control because of work, religious, cultural, social, and health-related issues. These include:

- Knowing their body and being able to differentiate normal from abnormal. Currently, most diabetes education and management programmes focus on the abnormal or assume all people respond the same way, the way the 'average person' responds.
- Knowing how to manage diabetes and having the physical and mental capability to manage the self-care tasks and problem-solve in a range of situations.
- Having supportive, constructive relationships in place with family/carers/friends and health professionals.
- Positive attitudes, resilience and adaptive coping mechanisms.
- Health professionals knowing the person with diabetes in order to understand their feelings about diabetes, the lessons they learned for living with diabetes and the way they manage self-care.

Psychological adaptation and maintaining a good quality of life is dependent on the individual's degree of resilience. Resilience refers to the ability to overcome adversity and not only to rise above it, but also to thrive. It has its foundation in belonging, life meaning and expectations and happiness. Resilience is at the heart of spirituality, social cohesion, and empowerment.

Chronic conditions such as diabetes have a major impact on an individual's life plan, their partner, families, and other relationships. Acquiring coping skills and being resilient have positive effects on emotional well being and therefore on physical outcomes. Coping with diabetes is an issue for some people. Coping issues for young people with Type 1 diabetes centres around:

- being expected to cope
- being expected to cope all the time
- being seen to cope by others
- having to cope for the rest of their lives
- no respite from coping with diabetes (Dunning 1994).

These issues are important across the lifespan as people with diabetes face life's challenges.

This chapter presents a brief outline of the complex psychological and quality of life aspects of having diabetes. Reactions to the diagnosis of diabetes are unique to the individual concerned; however, several common reactions have been documented. They include: anger, guilt, fear, helplessness, confusion, relief and denial. Appreciating some of the issues involved will enable nursing staff to better understand the complexity of living with diabetes and help the individual plan appropriate care.

Many factors influence how a person reacts to and accepts the diagnosis of diabetes and assumes responsibility for self-care. These factors include:

- age
- gender
- existing knowledge about diabetes
- general and health beliefs
- locus of control
- spirituality
- family support
- social, cultural and religious attitudes.

A period of grief and denial is normal. Figure 15.1 is one model of the 'diabetic grief cycle' loosely based on Helen Kubler Ross' work, associated with death and dying. Lack of knowledge, or inaccurate knowledge about diabetes, produces stress and anxiety. The invisible nature of the condition – in Type 2 diabetes and most diabetic complications there are often no presenting symptoms e.g. MI, UTI and retinopathy are silent – can lead to disbelief and denial of the diagnosis. Denial is appropriate early in the course of the disease and enables people to maintain a positive attitude and cope with the altered health status.

Adequate time must be allowed for the person to grieve for their perceived losses, for example, loss of spontaneity, lifestyle, having to plan ahead, loss of the respect and love of the people they value (DAWN 2004) and a changed body image. However,

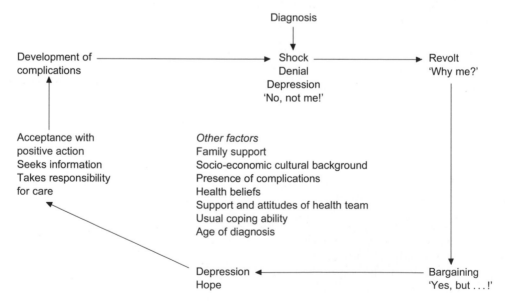

Acceptance of diabetes varies from months to year.
Some people never accepts diabetes.
The development of complications means another readjustment.

Figure 15.1   Model of the diabetic grief cycle.

prolonged denial can inhibit appropriate self-care, cause people to ignore warning signs of other problems and can lead to failure to attend medical appointments increasing the risk of diabetes complications. Denial can continue for longer than 5 years after the initial diagnosis in people with Type 1 diabetes (Gardiner 1997). Inadequate self-care could also indicate burnout from the unremitting demands of living with diabetes and lead to frequent use of health services by some people with diabetes.

Accepting diabetes involves dealing with some or all of the following:

- mental and physical pain
- hospitalisation or frequent outpatient or doctor visits
- the health system, including health professional's beliefs and attitudes, and often hospitals and emergency services
- lifelong treatment
- body image changes
- friends/family relationships
- fluctuating blood glucose levels
- emotional lability
- loss of independence
- societal attitudes and expectiations.

The tasks required to maintain acceptable blood glucose control are tedious and sometimes painful. There are financial costs involved, which can be a burden for some people (insulin, testing equipment, doctors' visits, increased insurance premiums). They add to the stress associated with having a disease they did not want in the first place.

Clinical observation

There is no holiday from diabetes for the patient. The individual has to live with diabetes 365 days a year 24-hours a day for the rest of their life.

Managing a chronic illness means straddling two paradigms – the biomedical and the psychosocial, neither adequately address spirituality, they all need to be integrated in order to achieve optimal health outcomes. An individual's path through life is influenced by life trajectories and turning points and these include the diagnosis of diabetes, expectations of treatment, and social support. Helping an individual define their life trajectory and identify turning points is part of holistic care.

In the context of this book, spirituality refers to the dimension of self that provides a framework for finding meaning and purpose in life and can be a motivating force that enables the individual to transcend life's trials such as the diagnosis of diabetes (Parsian & Dunning 2008). Hodges (2002) described four dimensions of spirituality, which each play a role in the incidence and degree of happiness or depression an individual experiences:

(1) meaning of and in life
(2) intrinsic values
(3) transcendence
(4) spiritual community.

Interestingly, Wolpert (2006) described depression as 'soul loss.' Parsian and Dunning (2008) found a significant association among spirituality, being female, higher education, duration of diabetes >10 years, lower HbA_{1c} and higher self-concept in young adults with diabetes. There was no significant association with religion. Spirituality may or may not encompass religion. Over the past 10 years research has demonstrated a link between being affiliated with a religious group and better physical and mental health outcomes although the association is not clear and may have a cultural element (UK Mental Health Foundation 2006; Gilbert 2007).

Diabetes has a 'bad reputation' in the community, with many associated myths, for example, 'eating sugar causes diabetes', and Type 2 diabetes is a mild form of the disease, which must be discussed and dispelled. Such myths can be associated with self-blame and guilt feelings. In addition, social pressures and ignorance often cause frustration and contribute to denial of the diabetes and failure to follow medical advice. For example, 'A little piece of cake won't hurt you' and is confusing for people with Type 1 and Type 2 diabetes.

Depression

The World Health Organisation predicts that depression will be the second major health issue by 2020. In Australia 5.8% of adults experience a depressive disorder (Andrews *et al.* 1999) and account for 8% of non-fatal disease burden. People with diabetes have a higher incidence of depression than the general public and the depression often precedes the diagnosis of diabetes. Depression may be an independent risk factor for diabetes (Rubin & Peyrot 2002). However, the mechanism linking diabetes and depression and whether depression precedes diabetes or diabetes leads to depression is unclear (Eaton *et al.* 1996; Peyrot 1997; Carnethon *et al.* 2003). Lustman (1997) suggested depression and hopelessness arise from having a chronic disease. Likewise, it is not clear whether depression increases the risk of diabetes *per se* or through the associated lifestyle risk factors such as poor diet, smoking and inactivity. Carnethon *et al.* (2003) found depression was associated with lower than high school education in a cohort from the NHANES 1 study (n = 6910): low education was independent of risk factors for developing diabetes. They proposed causal mechanisms could include genetic predisposition, inflammation and activation of the hypothalamic–pituitary–adrenal axis, similar to those proposed for the association among diabetes, cardiovascular diseases and depression, see Chapter 8.

Depression could be a component of the insulin resistance syndrome (see Chapter 1). People who are depressed are more likely to have inadequate self-care, present to the emergency department, require specialist intervention and exhibit lowered self-worth and physical functioning (Ciechanowski *et al.* 2000). The course of depression in people with diabetes is chronic and severe and depressive episodes may be particularly severe because of the metabolic effects (uncontrolled diabetes) and the neuroendocrine response (Rubin & Peyrot 2001). Thus, depression is associated with increased health care costs (Egede *et al.* 2002).

Cavan *et al.* (2001) suggested the reasons for depression in people with diabetes might be:

• The heavy disease burden.
• The strain diabetes places on relationships, especially family relationships.

- The stigma of diabetes in the family and the community.
- Shock and guilt at the diagnosis that are not adequately addressed and resolved.
- The uncertainty of the future.
- Loss of control.
- Past negative experiences with health professionals.

The perceived severity of diabetes affects the person's mental status. Type 2 diabetes has traditionally been considered to be less serious than Type 1 diabetes especially where it is treated without medications, even though Type 2 diabetes is a progressive disease of beta cell failure and complications are frequently present at diagnosis. Health professionals often convey these beliefs (Dunning & Martin 1997, 1999). Such messages convey false hope, and depression and stress occur when insulin is required. Considering the silent, insidious nature of Type 2 diabetes and the frequency with which complications are present at diagnosis, it is hardly a mild disease.

Symptoms of depression

The presence of five or more of the following signs every day for >2 weeks are suggestive of depression and should be formally assessed (US National Institute of Mental Health 2002):

- Persistent low mood, feeling sad, hopeless, anxious or empty
- Pessimism
- Feeling guilty, worthless or helpless, loss of interest in usual activities such as work, hobbies, and sexual relationships
- Low energy, fatigue
- Difficulty concentrating, remembering, making decisions
- Insomnia, waking early, oversleeping
- Appetite and/or weight changes
- Suicidal thoughts or attempts or dwelling on death
- Irritability.

In addition, depression is characterised by reduced confidence and neglect of self-care in people with diabetes. However, not all people who neglect their self-care are depressed and assumptions must always be checked (Lustman *et al.* 1996).

Maintaining mental health and managing depression

'The effectiveness of interventions depends on the context in which it is delivered' (Wilson 2001). The way the health professional interacts and delivers care may be more important than the care itself (Balint 1955). While this is an old study its message is still relevant today and many Balint Groups have been established especially in the US to help health professionals become more effective carers. Managing depression and diabetes is complex. Complexity theories suggest all the circumstances that influence behaviour must be considered (Lancaster 2000). This is certainly true of diabetes and depression where individuals:

- Operate within self-adjusting biochemical, cellular, physiological, social, cultural and religious systems. A change in one will result in a change in the others.
- Illness and wellness are part of a continuum, are dynamic and arise from an interaction among these factors.
- Physical and psychological health can only be maintained using an holistic model of care that incorporates all of these aspects.

Effective management strategies include:

- Counselling strategies such as cognitive behavioural therapy (CBT) (Lustman *et al.* 1998) and interpersonal therapy (Frank *et al.* 1991) have been shown to reduce self-defeating thought patterns and negative behaviours and improve adherence with management regimens. Clinicians can use counselling strategies in routine care. For example, Elley *et al.* (2003) showed counselling in general practice effectively increased physical activity and improved quality of life over 12 months. In a second study (Elley *et al.* 2007) found a personalised approach focusing on barriers and facilitators to physical activity, internal motivators, recognising time, physical and psychological limitations and spiritual benefits as well as the role of significant others, was important. CBT requires the individual to be able to think rationally and actively participate in their management. Usually, a close working relationship with the therapist is needed and it may take months for the individual to change unhealthy thought/behaviour patterns (Better Health Channel 2007).
- Coping strategies including problem-focused coping to deal with or prevent problems and emotion-focused coping to deal with negative emotions (Peyrot & Rubin 2007).
- Enhancing diabetes-specific self-efficacy, which involves encouraging realistic expectations and enhancing motivation by helping people identify their successes and encouraging optimism and realistic expectations. For example, motivational interviewing (Rollnick *et al.* 1999). High self-efficacy is associated with lower rates of depression (Steunenberg *et al.* 2007) and spirituality (Parsian & Dunning 2008).
- Improving metabolic control to relieve the effects of hyperglycaemia and fear of hypoglycaemia on mood and quality of life.
- Interactive behaviour change technology (IBCT), which includes PDAs, patient-centred Internet websites, coaching telephone calls, DVDs, audiotapes, touch screen kiosks designed to help maintain patient independence, can help people improve their diabetes self-care and monitor change (Piette 2007). They can also be useful in supporting informal caregivers and promoting activity, for example, pedometers. People search the Internet for information about depression more than any other condition (Taylor 1999). The Internet enables people to remain anonymous, which is important to some people (Rasmussen *et al.* 2007). People need advice about how to assess the veracity of websites because the information is often of low quality and may be misleading. Griffiths & Christensen (2002) undertook a cross-sectional study of 15 Australian depression Internet sites in November and December 2001 and found the quality of the content of many sites was poor. Sites receiving the highest rating were beyond Blue, BluePages, CRUIAD and InfraPsych. However,

information technologies do not take the place of human contact and are more effective when combined with human contact (Piette 2007).

- Complementary therapies (CAM) and self-help programmes. CAM with the best evidence for effectiveness are *Hypericum perforatum* for mild–to-moderate depression, exercise, bibliotherapy involving CBT and light therapy for winter depression. There is limited evidence to support acupuncture, light therapy for SAD syndrome, massage therapy, relaxation therapies, SAM-e, folate and yoga breathing exercises (Jorm *et al.* 2002). CAM medicines should be used under the supervision of a qualified practitioner.
- Identifying and treating underlying psychological/psychiatric disorders such as depression, and eating disorders and referring the individual to appropriate mental health services early. Counselling and/or antidepressant medicines may be needed. Antidepressant medicines such as serotonin reuptake inhibitors are commonly used and are effective in people with diabetes (Rubin & Peyrot 1994). The individual's previous experience with antidepressant medicines and the likely side effects need to be considered. As indicated, depression is a chronic condition and regular monitoring is essential and needs to be incorporated into routine care including in the acute care setting using screening tools such as:
  - Hospital Anxiety and Depression Scale (HADS).
  - Depression Anxiety Stress Scale (DASS).
  - Beck Depression Inventory (BDI (Beck 1974)).
  - Center for Epidemiological Studies Depression Scale (CES-D) (Radloff 1977).
  - Geriatric Depression Score.
  - K-10 Profile.
  - Patient Health Questionnaire (PHQ-9) (Spitzer *et al.* 1999).
  - Brief Case Finding for Depression (BCD) (Clarke).
  - Diabetes-Specific Quality of Life
  - Diabetes Health Profile
  - AddQoL
  - Diagnostic and Statistical Manual of Mental Disorders (DSM-1V 1994).
  - Wellbeing Enquirey for Diabetes.
  - World Health Organization Well Being Index (WHO-5) especially in older people (Bonsignore *et al.* 2001).

In order to achieve these goals health professionals need to ask good questions that aim to elicit a specific response, for example, ' what is the hardest thing about living with diabetes for you at the moment?' to identify the key issue to be addressed. Focus on successes and support the individual's problem-solving skills, for example, 'How do you think you can manage that?' Involve the family and significant others if relevant and with the individual's permission. Develop emotional resilience and optimism.

Antipsychotic medications and diabetes

Second generation antipsychotic medications effectively treat a range of psychiatric disorders and offer many benefits over older medications such as chlorpromazine and haloperidol (Wirshing *et al.* 2002; DeVane 2007). However, they do have significant side effects, namely rapid weight gain, hyperlipidaemia and insulin resistance, that can affect metabolic control and increase the cardiovascular risk in people with established diabetes and cause hyperglycaemia in non-diabetics, however, there is considerable variability in responses among individuals receiving the same medication.

A consensus panel of experts from the American Diabetes Association, American Psychiatric Association, the American Association of Clinical Endocrinologists and the North American Association for the study of Obesity (2004) recommended:

- Assessing weight, blood glucose, lipids and blood pressure before starting antipsychotic medicines or as soon as possible after.
- Actively managing these conditions, if present.
- If weight increases by >5%, consider changing to another antipsychotic less likely to cause metabolic effects.
- Antipsychotics listed in order of those with the most to the least metabolic effects are: olanzapine, quetiapine, risperidone, ziprasidone, aripiprazole. These medicines still cause weight gain.
- Institute lifestyle modification to mange weight if possible, which will involve helping the person adhere to advice.

Practice points

(1) Finding ways to help people cope with the diagnosis of diabetes could be as important as diet, medications and education.
(2) Monitoring the individual's mood and regular screening for depression should be part of complication screening.

Type 1 diabetes

Diabetes diagnosed in childhood can produce enormous guilt and anxiety for the child and the parents. Marital strife is not uncommon and is often exacerbated by the diabetes. The parents must learn how to care for the child at the same time as coping with their own feelings. Inflicting pain on a child (injections, blood tests) is very difficult to do, and such tasks often fall to the mother.

As the child matures and develops they need to take over the care of their diabetes. It can be extremely difficult for the parents to 'let go' and therefore for the child to achieve independence. Other children in the family may feel deprived of attention. Sweets, the traditional reward for good behaviour, are often withdrawn and this may be seen as a punishment.

Some childhood behaviour such as irritability and awkwardness can be difficult to distinguish from hypoglycaemia, making management difficult. Hypoglycaemia itself is feared and hated by children and parents and mostly underrated by healthcare staff. It is not unknown for people to deliberately run their blood glucose levels high to avoid hypoglycaemia (Dunning 1994).

Parents with diabetes may have concerns about passing diabetes to their own children in the future. Support, encouragement and referral for counselling, if necessary, are vital aspects of diabetes care.

Diabetes is the perfect disease for manipulating others and gaining attention. Withholding insulin can result in ketoacidosis, with the mobilisation of family, friends and health resources. Hypoglycaemia can have the same effect. Repeated admissions for hypoglycaemia or DKA need to be investigated carefully and diplomatically.

An individual's response to the diagnosis of diabetes depends on their overall psychological and social adjustment and the availability of structured family support (Johnson 1980) (see Chapter 20). Fitting diabetes into family life can be difficult and changes with duration of diabetes and the intensity of the treatment regimen (Gardiner 1997). Likewise, major life transitions such as leaving home, starting a new job, going to university and having a child require readaption (Rasmussen *et al.* 2007).

The *Australian National Diabetes Strategy and Implementation Plan* (Diabetes Australia 1998) identified some issues specific to people with Type 1 diabetes. They are:

- Dependency, for example, during severe hypoglycaemia and fears of being dependent should they develop complications such as blindness.
- Loss of control, either in the short term, e.g. during hypoglycaemia or in the long term.
- Public confusion about the difference between Type 1 and Type 2 diabetes. This confusion extends to health professionals as the following quote from a referral for diabetes education indicates: 'He used to have Type 2 but the doctor started him on insulin yesterday and he is now Type 1. Needs education.'
- Who to tell about their diabetes at work – workmates, friends.
- Restrictions, for example, some sporting activities and jobs, and hassles getting a driver's license.

Type 2 diabetes

The diagnosis of diabetes in later life means the person may need to change behaviours developed over years. Eating patterns often have to be modified. Restrictions are often resented with resultant anger, denial or neglect. Alternatively, the patient may meticulously follow the management plan.

Knowledge about possible diabetic complications or the development of complications leads to stress, which in turn contributes to elevated blood glucose levels. Relationships may be disrupted as in Type 1 diabetes, with families/spouses becoming overprotective, resulting in over dependence or rebelliousness. People tend to cope better and manage the self-care tasks more easily if the family is supportive yet allows independence.

Over half of the people with Type 2 diabetes on insulin report reduced quality of life. Insulin has a negative impact, which is greater in younger people with a long duration of diabetes from non-English-speaking backgrounds (Rubin 2000; Davis *et al.* 2001). Men with Type 2 diabetes self-report depression, disempowerment and perceived loss of control (Tun *et al.* 1990). This hopelessness and depression may well be the result of the mythology that insulin indicates severe disease. More support and early explanations of the likely progression to insulin are required.

However, Thoolen (2006) in the Netherlands found people with Type 2 diabetes experience little diabetes-related anxiety, do not regard diabetes as serious, have high self-efficacy, and low levels of self-care in the early years after diagnosis (*n* = 196).

People who had been diagnosed for >2–3 years were more likely to consider diabetes to be threatening to their health. Patients on intensive treatment reported higher levels of stress and lower self-efficacy. Like other studies, Thoolen's study emphasises the importance of taking a thorough history and considering individual factors and reactions.

The DAWN study (Funnell 2006) ($n = 3432$, Type 2 and 1672, Type 1) demonstrated that diabetes is associated with a number of physical and psychological symptoms such as shock and disbelief 35–55%, anxiety 38% Type 1 and 19% Type 2. Of these, 51% were concerned about hypoglycaemia, 48% about weight change especially Type 2, and the disease getting worse 34%. Despite these concerns many were relieved to have a diagnosis. In the Australian cohort 75% were optimistic about the future, ~25% said they felt burnt out by diabetes and <40% were tired of complying with diabetes self-care. Most agreed diabetes did not prevent them from doing what they wanted to do.

Fifty-two per cent of Type 2 not on insulin worried about having to commence insulin and only 10% thought insulin would help control their diabetes. Li *et al.* (2008) found a higher rate of major depression in people with Type 2 diabetes on insulin than those with Type 2 not using insulin and those with Type 1 diabetes. These studies suggest insulin has a negative impact on people with Type 2 diabetes despite the clinical observation that many report feeling better once they commence insulin and their control improves.

Compliance/adherence/concordance

These terms are judgmental, prejudiced and negative in nature. They are labels best avoided in relation to diabetic self-care tasks. Failure to comply with one aspect of care does not necessarily indicate complete neglect of the diabetes. In fact, forgetting and omitting aspects of care are probably 'normal' behaviours and obsessive attention to routine can indicate underlying fear and anxiety.

It is important to establish why a particular behaviour is neglected. Reasons include:

- Unreal expectations on the part of health professionals resulting from lack of knowledge about the person's goals, capabilities and social situation.
- Setting health professional rather than patient goals.
- Lack of knowledge of what is required.
- Lack of understanding as a result of poor communication, see Chapter 16.
- Inadequate support from family/friends and the healthcare team (see Chapter 20).
- Health beliefs and attitudes of the patient.
- Functional limitations such as low vision and diminished fine motor skills.
- Patient 'burnout'.
- Financial difficulties.

This is the human side of diabetes (Raymond 1992).

Psychological distress and cardiovascular disease

The effect of negative emotions on physical functioning is not new. William Harvey noted that mental distress affected the heart and impaired its function in 1628. Sound evidence for the link between emotions and cardiovascular disease, particularly myocardial infarction (MI) and stroke, has emerged in the last ten years and the risk appears to be comparable to those of other known risk factors such as smoking.

Although the course of chronic heart disease and depression fluctuate, negative emotions have cumulative pathophysiological effects. Diabetes is also linked to higher rates of depression than the general population and cardiovascular disease is a major long-term diabetes complication. The emotional impact people with diabetes attribute to MI and diabetes changes with the longer duration of time after the acute MI. In the initial stages surviving the MI is the major concern; by 3–4 months concerns about diabetes begin to re-emerge and predominate by 6 months (Gudjar & Dunning 2003).

Depression may contribute to physical damage by activating key neurohormonal systems as well as other mechanisms (Yusuf *et al.* 2004; Everson & Lewis 2005; Rozanski *et al.* 2005). Yusuf *et al.* (2004) showed psychological distress was associated with a 2.5-fold greater risk of acute MI than hypertension, abdominal obesity, diabetes (i.e. the metabolic syndrome, see Chapter 1), and other risk factors in the INTERHEART study (*n* = 29 972 in 52 countries). The association is evident in a number of other studies (Joost *et al.* 2004; Lett *et al.* 2004; Rozanski *et al.* 2004). Janszky *et al.* (2007) found admission for depression is associated with increased risk of MI, independent of other risk factors, but the mechanism remains unclear.

Lett *et al.* (2004) suggested depression could be a marker of a broader issue encompassing a range of factors such as:

- negative affect
- vital exhaustion
- limited social support
- personality factors
- anger
- hostility
- negative emotions
- anxiety.

Depression and negative affect appear to predict increased risk of cardiovascular disease (Frasure-Smith & Lesperance 2003). Significantly, optimistic individuals have lower risk of cardiovascular disease than pessimists when other risk factors were controlled for (Kubzansky *et al.* 2001; Giltay *et al.* 2006). Many researchers and clinicians note that people with heart disease have high rates of depression ranging between 40 and 65% (Januzzi *et al.* 2000). However, 53% of people have a history of depression prior to having an MI, which suggests depression precedes the MI (Rafinelli *et al.* 2005; Glassman *et al.* 2006).

The effect of negative emotions on cardiovascular disease is currently being explored, for example, specific biomarkers, genetic predisposition, and psychological resilience. They may have direct physiological effects by stimulating the hypothalamic-pituitary–adrenocortical axis, affecting the immune response, and contributing to inflammation. Psychological distress also affects self-care behaviours, in that highly stressed individuals often smoke, do not exercise or eat an appropriate diet and neglect self-care and do not adhere to health care regimens including medicines. Psychological distress occurs on a continuum ranging from normal to pathological.

However, the cognitive, behavioural and biological components of psychological distress are the same regardless of where the individual is on the continuum. Pathological psychological distress is characterised by intense emotions. There appears to be a dose-dependent relationship between the level of emotion and the degree of risk for cardiovascular disease (Kubzansky 2007).

Holistic diabetes assessment and successful depression management programmes encompass mental health and well being and may include using depression screening tools (Callahan *et al.* 1994). Despite the success of programmes such as Hospital Admission Risk Programs (HARP) in Australia, clinical practice guidelines for managing pre-event and psychosocial cardiac risk factors are lacking. Psychosocial and behavioural risk factors are not closely inter-related and structured integrated management systems are needed and are part of an emerging field of health care: behavioural cardiology (Rozanski *et al.* 2004).

What people with diabetes require from health professionals

- To be treated as normal.
- To be treated as a person, not 'a diabetic'.
- To be trusted, accepted and not judged.
- To be listened to and have their experience and knowledge of diabetes recognised.
- To know how and where to obtain advice.

Support, encouragement and focusing on positive achievements are far more helpful than 'shame and blame'.

Achievable goals should be negotiated with the patient. It is the patient's expectations that will be met rather than those of the health professional. It is important to recognise that diabetes is never easy. 'Good' and 'bad' when referring to blood glucose levels are judgemental terms. Substitute 'high' and 'low'. Some people resent being called 'a diabetic'. It is preferable to say 'a person with diabetes'.

Some patients express concern about being admitted to hospital, over and above the usual reactions to illness/hospitalisation. They feel abnormal by being singled out for special meals and having labels such as 'diabetic diet' attached to the bed. They are sometimes made to feel incompetent when they have often been caring for their diabetes for years. For example, when requesting sugar to avoid hypoglycaemia or not being allowed to test their blood glucose or give their own insulin injections.

Some people feel that they are blamed if they are admitted with a diabetic complication. They 'should have known better' and taken care of their diabetes better. Patients become frustrated when they are labelled 'non-compliant'. Continuous negative feedback only reinforces that the person is not coping and learned helplessness can result.

Quality of life

Quality of life (QOL) is a highly subjective and multidimensional concept concerned with cognitive status, satisfaction and emotional happiness (Cox & Gonder-Frederick 1992). It has become a major issue in behavioural diabetes research. Poor quality of life is associated with neglect of self-care and may predict an individual's capacity for self-care. According to life mission theory people lower their QOL when they are in crisis to survive and adapt. QOL can be increased when the person has the resources to heal (Ventegodt *et al.* 2003). Healing encompases 'salutogenesis' (Antonovsky 1987) where the individual develops a 'sense of coherence' and develops personally, or in modern terminology becomes empowered.

The person enters an holistic state of healing when:

- The individual and their health professionals have similar life perspectives and the intent of the health professional is to help the patient understand him/herself and take responsibility for their life, and in this case, diabetes.
- They are in a safe environment.
- They have the personal resources.
- They have the will to understand and overcome the crisis and let go of negative emotions and behaviours.
- The individual and their health professionals have healing intent. There is sufficient holding. Holding is a five-fold process that involves acknowledging the patient and giving them respect, trust, care, and acceptance (Ventegodt *et al.* 2003).

There are four categories of determinants of quality of life:

(1) Medical – diabetes type, treatment regime, level of metabolic control and presence of complications. The severity of complications reduces quality of life.
(2) Cognitive – acute and chronic blood glucose control and neuropsychological changes can reduce quality of life for the person with diabetes and their family. The effect of depression on quality of life is greater than the effect of diabetes and is additive to other factors (Goldney *et al.* 2004).
(3) Attitudinal – self-efficacy, locus of control and social support. People with good support have better quality of life and less depression. Empowerment strategies and improving an individual's sense of being in control improve their quality of life. This includes considering spirituality, an integral aspect of empowerment.
(4) Demographic – gender, education level, ethnicity and age. Men report better quality of life than women and young people better than old people. Higher education is associated with better quality of life.

Measuring quality of life

Most people understand what is meant by 'quality of life' but it is a difficult concept to measure. A number of tools have been developed that measure the general aspects of quality of life and are widely used. Diabetes-specific quality of life tools are now also available. These tools the include generic Health-Related Quality of Life, Short Form 36 (SF-36), the Diabetes Specific Quality of Life and the Symptoms Check List, and the DCCT tool (Bradley & Gamsu 1994), see the previous list. Sometimes a number of tools are used together.

Some are simple to use and could be incorporated into the routine diabetes assessment nurses undertake. However, it is important to realise that, although these tools are validated and widely used, they may not indicate an *individual's* specific quality of life issues. Patient-generated quality of life measures developed specifically by the individual may be useful in routine clinical care (Jenkinson & McGee 1998).

Measuring quality of life may be useful to plan holistic nursing care and address issues of empowerment. It is important to consider individual meaning of quality of life and to ask about these individual issues as well as global issues.

Guidelines to encourage mental and physical well being

- Recognise that psychological issues affect metabolic control and need to be addressed in order to maintain quality of life and effective diabetes self-care.
- Provide supportive education and advice, as it is required and tailor education to the individual's needs. An empowerment model of care and an holistic approach are more appropriate for chronic diseases such as diabetes where frequent visits to health professionals are required. Empowerment models seek to involve the individual in decisions about their management and to establish a therapeutic relationship with the individual, see Chapter 16.
- Improve communication. Provide an appropriate environment for consultations, plan for continuity of care, ask open questions and give the individual the opportunity to ask questions.
- Address complications honestly but optimistically. Foster self-esteem and coping skills. In hospital this may mean allowing the person with diabetes to perform their own blood glucose tests and administer their own medications.
- Offer options and help with goal setting.
- Give the message that diabetes is a serious disease and focus on the benefits of good control rather than what will happen if control is poor.
- Focus on the person not their diabetes or metabolic control.
- Acknowledge that it is difficult to live with diabetes.
- Monitor psychological well being as well as physical status (Bradley & Gamsu 1994).

References

American Diabetes Association, American Psychiatric Association, the American Association of Clinical Endocrinologists and the North American Association for the Study of Obesity (2004) Consensus development conference on antipsychotic drugs and obesity and diabetes. *Diabetes Care*, **27**, 596–601.

American Psychiatric Association (1994) *Diagnostic and Statistical Manual of Mental Disorders*, 4th edn. American Psychiatric Association, Washington, DC.

Andrews, G., Hall, W., Teeson, M. & Henderson, S. (1999) *The Mental Health of Australians*. Mental Health Branch, Commonwealth Department of Health and Aged Care, Canberra.

Antonovsky, A. (1987) *Unravelling the Mystery of Health: How People Manage Stress and Stay Well*. Jossey-Bass, San Francisco.

Balint, M. (1955) The doctor, his patient and the illness. *Lancet*, **1**, 683–688.

Beck, A. & Beamesderfer, A. (1974) Assessment of depression: the depression inventory. *Medical Problems in Psychopharmacotherapy*, **7**, 151–169.

Better Health Channel (2007) Cognitive behaviour therapy. http://www.betterhealth.vic.gov.au/bhcv2/bhcarticles.nsf/pages/Cognitive_Behaviour (accessed December 2007).

Bradley, C. & Gamsu, D. (1994) Guidelines for encouraging psychological wellbeing. *Diabetic Medicine*, **11**, 510–516.

Bonsignore, M., Barkow, K., Jessen, F. & Huen, R. (2001) Validity of the five-item WHO Well-Being Index (WHO-5) in an elderly population. *European Archives of Psychiatry Clinical Neuroscience*, **251**, (Suppl. 2), 1127–1131.

Callahan, C., Hendrie, H., Dittus, R., Brater, D., Hui, S. & Tierney, W. (1994) Improving treatment of late life depression in primary care: a randomized clinical trial. *Journal of the American Geriatric Society*, **42**, 839–846.

Carnethon, M., Kinder, L., Fair, J., Stafford, R. & Fortmann, S. (2003) Symptoms of depression as a risk factor for incident diabetes: findings from the National Health Nutrition Examination Epidemiologic Follow-up Study. *American Journal of Epidemiology*, **158**, 416–423.

Cavan, D., Fosbury, J. & Tigwell, P. (2001) Psychology in diabetes – why bother? *Practical Diabetes International*, **18** (7), 228–229.

Ciechanowski, P., Katon, W. & Russo, W. (2000) Impact of depressive symptoms on adherence, function and costs. *Archives of Internal Medicine*, **160**, 3278–3285.

Cox, D. & Gonder-Frederick, L. (1992) Major developments in behavioural diabetes research. *Journal of Consulting Clinical Psychologists*, **60**, 628–638.

Davis, T., Clifford, R. & Davis, W. (2001) Effect of insulin therapy on quality of life in Type 2 diabetes mellitus – The Fremantle diabetes study. *Diabetes Research and Clinical Practice*, **52**, 63–67.

DeVane, L. (2007) Antipsychotics and diabetes. http://www.medscape.com.viewarticle/ 558874?src=mp (posted 28.6. 2007, accessed August 2007).

Diabetes Australia (1998) *Australian National Diabetes Strategy and Implementation Plan.* Diabetes Australia, Canberra.

Diabetes Control and Complications Trial Research Group (1993) Influence of intensive diabetes treatment on quality of life outcomes in the DCCT. *Diabetes Care*, **19**, 195–203.

Dunning, P. (1994) Having diabetes: young adult perspectives. *The Diabetes Educator*, **21** (1), 58–65.

Dunning, P. & Martin, M. (1997) Using a focus group to explore perceptions of diabetes severity. *Practical Diabetes International*, **14** (7), 185–188.

Dunning, P. & Martin, M. (1999) Health professional's perceptions of the seriousness of diabetes. *Practical Diabetes International*, **16** (3), 73–77.

Eaton, W., Armenian, H. & Gallo, J. (1996) Depression and risk for onset type 11 diabetes; a prospective population based study. *Diabetes Care*, **19**, 1097–1102.

Elley, C., Kerse, N., Arroll, B. & Robinson, E. (2003) Effectiveness of counselling patients on physical activity in general practice: a cluster randomised trial. *British Medical Journal*, **326** (pp. 1–6 downloaded December 2007).

Elley, C., Dean, S. & Kerse, N. (2007) Physical activity promotion in general practice. *Australian Family Physician*, **38** (12), 1061–1064.

Egede, L., Zheng, D. & Simpson, K. (2002) Comorbid depression is associated with increased health care use and expenditure in individuals with diabetes. *Diabetes Care*, **25** (3), 464–470.

Everson-Rose, S. & Lewis, T. (2005) Psychosocial factors and cardiovascular diseases. *Annual Review of Public Health*, **26**, 469–500.

Frank, E., Kupfer, D., Wagner, E. & McEachran, A. (1991) Efficacy of interpersonal psychotherapy as maintanence treatment for recurrent depression. *Archives of General Psychiatry*, **48**, 1053–1059.

Frasure-Smith, N. & Lesperance, F. (2003) Depression and other psychological risks following myocardial infarction. *Archives of General Psychiatry*, **60**, 627–636.

Funnell, M. (2006) Diabetes attitudes and wishes and needs (DAWN) study. *Clinical Diabetes*, **24**, 154–155.

Gardiner, P. (1997) Social and psychological implications of diabetes mellitus for a group of adolescents. *Practical Diabetes International*, **14** (2), 43–46.

Gilbert, P. (2007) Spirituality and mental health: a very preliminary overview. *Current Opinions in Psychiatry*, **20** (6), 594–598.

Griffiths, K. & Christensen, H. (2002) The quality and accessibility of Australian depression sites on the World Wide Web. *Medical Journal of Australia*, **176**, S97–S104.

Goldney, R. & Phillips, P. (2004) Diabetes, depression and quality of life. *Diabetes Care*, **27** (5), 1066–1070.

Gujadhur, A., Dunning, T. & Alford, F. (2003) Metabolic and cardiac outcomes after acute myocardial infarction. *Journal of Diabetes Nursing*, **7** (6), 208–212.

Hodges, S. (2002) Mental health, depressions and dimensions of spirituality and religion. *Journal of Adult Development*, **9**, 109–115.

Jansky, I., Ahlbom, A., Hallqvist, J. & Ahnve, S. (2007) Hospitalisaton for depression is associated with an increased risk for myocardial infarction not explained by lifestyle, lipids, coagulation, and inflammation: The SHEEP Study. *Biological Psychiatry*, **62**, 24–32.

Jenkinson, C. & McGee, H. (1998) *Health Status Measurement*. Radcliff Medical Press, Oxford.

Johnson, S. (1980) Psychosocial factors in juvenile diabetes. *Journal of Health Psychology*, **9**, 737–749.

Joost, P., van Melle, M., Jonge, P., Spijkerman, T., Tussen, J. & Ormel, J. (2004) Prognostic association of depression following myocardial infarction with mortality and cardiovascular events: a meta-analysis. *Psychosomatic Medicine*, **66**, 814–822.

Jorm, A., Christensen, H., Griffiths, K. & Rodgers, B. (2002) Effectiveness of complementary and self-help treatments for depression. *Medical Journal of Australia*, **176**, S84–S96.

Kubzansky, L. (2007) Sick at heart: the pathophysiology of negative emotions. *Cleveland Clinic Journal of Medicine*, **74** (Suppl. 1), S67–S72.

Lancaster, T. (2000) Effectiveness of interventions to help people stop smoking. *British Medical Journal*, **321**, 355–358.

Lett, H., Blumenthal, J., Babyak, M., Sherwood, A., Strauman, T., Robins, C. & Newman, M. (2004) Depression as a risk factor for coronary artery disease: evidence, mechanisms, and treatment. *Psychosomatic Medicine*, **66**, 305–315.

Li, C. (2008) Depression common among adults with diabetes. *Diabetes Care*, **31**, 105–107.

Lustman, P., Griffith, L. & Clouse, R. (1996) Recognising and managing depression in patients with diabetes. In: *Practical Psychology for Clinicians* (eds B. Anderson & R. Rubin). American Diabetes Association, Alexandria, pp. 143–152.

Lustman, P. (1997) The course of major depression in diabetes. *Diabetes Care*, **59**, 24–31.

Lustman, P., Griffith, L., Freedland, K., Kissel, S. & Close, R. (1998) Cognitive behaviour therapy for depression in type 2 diabetes mellitus: a randomized controlled trial. *Annals of Internal Medicine*, **129**, 613–621.

National Institute of Mental Health (NIMH) (2002) *Depression and Diabetes*. NIMH, Bethesda, USA.

Parsian, N. & Dunning, T. (2008) Spirituality and coping in young adults with diabetes. *Diabetes Research and Clinical Practice*, **79** (S1), S121.

Paterson, B. & Sloan, J. (1994) A phenomenological study of the decision-making experience of individuals with long standing diabetes. *Canadian Journal of Diabetes Care*, **18**, 10–19.

Paterson, B., Thorn, S. & Dewis, M. (1998) Adapting to and managing diabetes. *Journal of Nursing Scholarship*, **30** (1), 57–61.

Piette, J. (2007) Interactive behaviour change technology to support diabetes self-management: where do we stand? *Diabetes Care*, **30** (10), 2425–2432.

Peyrot, M. (1997) Levels and risks of depression and anxiety symptomatology among diabetic adults. *Diabetes Care*, **20**, 585–590.

Peyrot, M. & Rubin, R. (2007). Behavioural and psychosocial interventions in diabetes. *Diabetes Care*, **30** (10), 2433–2440.

Rasmussen, B., O'Connell, B. & Dunning, T. (2007) Young women with diabetes: using Internet communication to create stability during life transitions. *Journal of Clinical Nursing*, **1365**, 17–24.

Rasmussen, B., O'Connell, B. & Dunning, T. (2007) Young women with type 1 diabetes' management of turning points and transition. *Qualitative Health Research*, **17** (3), 300–310.

Raymond, M. (1992) *The Human Side of Diabetes. Beyond Doctors, Diet, Drugs.* Noble Press, Chicago.

Radloff, S. (1977) The CES-D scale: a self-report depression scale for research in the general population. *Applied Psychiatric Measurement*, 3, 151–401.

Rafinelle, C. (2005) Depression, stress and the risk of heart disease. *Psychiatric Times*, 22, 11.

Rollnick, S., Mason, P. & Butler, C. (1999). *Health Behaviour Change: A Guide for Practitioners.* Churchill Livingstone, Edinburgh.

Rozanski, A., Blumenthal, J., Davidson, K., Saab, P. & Kubzansky, L. (2005) The epidemiology, pathophysiology, and management of psychosocial risk factors in cardiac practice: the emerging field of behavioural cardiology. *Journal of the American College of Cardiology*, 45 (5), 637–651.

Rubin, R. & Peyrot, M. (1994) Implications of the DCCT: looking beyond tight control. *Diabetes Care*, 17, 235–236.

Rubin, R. (2000) Diabetes and quality of life. From research to practice. *Diabetes Spectrum*, 13 (1).

Spitzer, R., Kroenke, K. & Williams, J. (1999) The Patient Health Questionnaire Primary Care Study Group; validation and utility of a self-report version of the PRIME-MD: the PHQ Primary Care Study. *Journal American Medical Association*, 282, 1737–1744.

Steunenberg, B., Beckman, A., Deeg, D., Bremmer, M. & Kerkhof, A. (2007) Mastery and neuroticism predict recovery from depression in later life. *American Journal Geriatric Psychiatry*, 15, 234–242.

Taylor, H. (2001) Explosive growth of 'cyberchrondriacs' continues (The Harris Poll #47), 5 August http://www.harrisinteractive.com/harris_poll/index.asp?PD=117 (accessed January 2007).

Thoolen, B. (2006) Early intensive treatment can negatively affect stress and outcome. *Diabetes Care*, 29, 2257–2262.

Tun, P., Nathan, D. & Perlminter, L. (1990) Cognitive and affective disorders in elderly diabetics. *Clinical Geriatric Medicine*, 6, 731–746.

Ventegodt, S., Andersen, N. & Merrick, J. (2003) Holistic medicine 111: the holistic process theory of healing. *The Scientific World Journal*, 3, 1138–1146.

Wilson, T. & Holt, T. (2001) Complexity science: complexity and clinical care. *British Medical Journal*, 323 (7314), 685–688.

Wirshing, D., Boyd, J., Meng, L., Ballon, J., Marder, S. & Wirshing, W. (2002) The effects of novel antipsychotics on glucose and lipid levels. *Journal of Clinical Psychiatary*, 63 (10), 856–865.

Wolpert, L. (2006) *Malignant Sadness: The Anatomy of Depression*, 3rd edn. Faber & Faber, London.

Yusef, S., Hawken, S. & Ounpuu, S. (2004) Effect of potentially modifiable risk factors associated with myocardial infarction in 52 countries (the INTERHEART study): case controlled study. *Lancet*, 364, 937–952.

Chapter 16
Diabetes Education

I never teach my students – I only try to provide the conditions in which they can learn.

Albert Einstein

Key points

- Teaching and learning is an interconnected process dependent on effective communication.
- Establishing a therapeutic partnership with the person with diabetes is very important. The focus of diabetes education should be on helping the person with diabetes become an empowered active participant in their care.
- Health literacy is an important consideration. Written information suitable to the individual's, age, culture, life stage and the current context should be provided to support verbal information.
- Diabetes self-care knowledge and capability should be assessed regularly.
- Information must be consistent among all health professionals caring for the person with diabetes.
- Establishing how a people learn is important in order to teach them appropriately and enhance their learning.
- Significant others should be included in the education where relevant.

Rationale

Diabetes education is the cornerstone of diabetes management and is a lifelong, ongoing process. Person-centred education that supports personal empowerment and autonomy and enhances self-care capacity is the most effective teaching method. A balanced therapeutic relationship between the person and their health professional carers is more likely to achieve person-centred education. Collaboration and communication are core elements of teaching and learning. Teaching and learning is an integrated process.

Introduction

Diabetes education is an integral part of the management of diabetes. The overall goal of diabetes education is to assist the person to integrate diabetes successfully into their concept of self and fit the management tasks into their lifestyle in order to achieve and maintain an integrated sense of self, appropriate self-care, a balanced lifestyle and optimum diabetic control. That is, to deliver holistic patient-centred diabetes care. As indicated in the preface, I prefer to use the term 'patient' as 'well as person with diabetes' in this book. Some people with diabetes object to being referred to as patients but in my experience the majority refer to themselves as patients and/or diabetics. Significantly, the International Alliance of Patient Organisations (IAPO 2005) uses the term 'patients'.

IAPO recognised that patients', families' and carers' needs and priorities differ among countries and diseases and described five key principles of patient-centred care:

(1) Respect for patients' unique needs, preferences, values, autonomy, and independence.
(2) Patients have a right and a responsibility to participate as equal partners in health care decisions that affect their lives to the level of their ability and choice.
(3) They have a right to be involved in developing health care policy at all levels to ensure policies are designed with the patient at the centre of care.
(4) Health care must consider emotional and non-health factors that affect health such as the social situation, education and employment, and patients must have access to healthcare services relevant to their condition.
(5) 'Accurate, relevant and comprehensive information is essential' to enable people to make informed decisions about their health care options and the benefits and risks of specific treatment to them. Information must be in a format suitable to the individual's age, literacy level, gender, culture, and health care needs (IAPO 2005).

Holistic patient-centred education and care is consistent with these principles and has a core aim of preventing disease and/or disease progression and promoting positive health to achieve the best possible outcomes (Bastable 1997). Patient education describes the theory and skills the individual needs to learn and encompasses establishing goals to be achieved and conditions in which learning can take place (Redman 2001). Thus, diabetes education is a planned, interactive process using a combination of methods to help people learn relevant information and develop appropriate health behaviours. Significantly, people who learn to and effectively manage their health and make appropriate lifestyle choices use fewer resources and make more effective use of available resources (Tankova *et al.* 2001).

Standardised patient education and self-management guidelines (a representative list is presented at the end of the chapter) act as important frameworks in which the IAPO principles can be met. However, some may be limited in their effectiveness because they rely on traditional teaching methods, primary and tertiary care is not well-integrated, and the programmes and services often only reach a small number of people (Wagner *et al.* 2002). Effective chronic disease management consists of:

- Delivering care according to evidence-based guidelines and protocols.
- Well designed service practices such as appointment systems, follow up procedures, referral processes, Alert systems, and education programmes suitable to the needs of the target population.
- A focus on prevention and supporting patients to self-manage and make relevant behaviour changes by using education methods that facilitate problem-solving and empowerment (Anderson *et al.* 2002; Anderson & Funnell 2005). Ideally this includes a process for identifying people who do not meet targets.
- Ensuring health care providers are educated, competent and supported to undertake their roles, that they function in a complementary, collaborative team, and there are clear links among service providers and resources. Health professionals may need training in health coaching methods.

- Education programmes that meet the needs of the relevant population and provide opportunities for continuing education for patients and health professionals. A recent review of >30 randomised controlled trials of diabetes education found only half the education interventions included behavioural components (setting goals, counselling techniques or problem-solving), only one third assessed psychosocial factors (beliefs, self-efficacy, mastery, or locus of control), and significant improvements in knowledge was only demonstrated in one-fifth of the studies (Knight & Donan 2006). These findings suggest most current diabetes education programmes are not holistic or patient-centred, despite the rhetoric.
- Accurate clinical and investigative procedures.
- Appropriate information is generated, documented and communicated including chronic disease registers, referral systems, patient reminders, outcome monitoring and care planning.
- Continuous quality improvement and audit processes that include patients in the design as well as the evaluation and not only as the subject of the evaluation.

Generally, the diabetes education literature focuses on the patient. However, to be an effective teacher, the educator needs to undertake reflective practice and consider their own learning style, teaching style, communication style, beliefs and attitudes, knowledge and competence, and how these affect the way they interact with patients. In addition, health professionals need to understand how the person's life environment and the teaching environment can facilitate or be a barrier to learning, behaviour change, and/or self-care. Thus, patient-centred education and care means really understanding people. Generally, peoples' teaching style reflects their preferred learning style. A learning style self-assessment tool can be found on http://www.idpride. net/learning-style-test.html.

Learning styles

Learning is 'a natural, evolving process originating within the learner and growing from the learner's need to interact with their environment' (Mackeracher 1996). Thus, the learner, not the teacher, is in control of what the learner learns. Learning can occur through experience (experiential) or as a planned process. People learning different ways (learning style). Learning style refers to the way an individual processes and uses information. Learning involves using the senses: sight, speech, hearing, and can be active or passive. Usually people use a mixture of learning styles and learn different things in different ways and children learn differently from adults. Table 16.1 is a composite overview of learning styles and teaching methods appropriate to each learning style. The table clearly shows that learning is a process not merely an outcome (Kolb 1984). Kolb described four learning styles:

(1) divergent – emphasises feeling rather than thinking
(2) assimulative – values facts and thinking over feeling
(3) convergent – like to apply information and hands-on activities
(4) accommodative – learn by trial and error/problem-solving.

A simple self-complete tool that can help health professionals identify an individual's learning style is shown in Table 16.2.

Table 16.1 Learning styles and some teaching strategies that can be used to facilitate learning. People participating in group education programmes are likely to learn in different ways. Therefore, a range of teaching strategies should be used. An individual's preference for one category may be mild, moderate of strong but generally a balance of styles results in more effective learning.

Learning style	Learning process	Teaching strategy
Active	Retain information by doing something active. Like learning in groups. Retain information better if they understand how to apply it.	Teach in group settings. Incorporate activities. Such as demonstrations and return demonstrations. Use problem-based learning.
Reflective	Prefer to think about things before they act. Prefer working alone.	Incorporate time for review and reflection. Provide short summaries of important information. Invite feedback.
Sensing	Like learning facts and solving problems using established methods. Like details and are good at memorising facts but may do this and not understand the information. Like hands on activities. Dislike complications and surprises. Do not like being asked about information that was not covered in education programmes. Practical and careful and like information to be connected to 'the real world'	Show how the information relates to their personal situation and the 'real world' in general. Use specific examples.
Intuitive	Like to discover possibilities and relationships Likes innovation. Are bored by repetition Are good at understanding new concepts Usually comfortable with abstract images and statistical information Are innovative and work quickly but may miss important details and make careless mistakes.	Link theories to facts
Visual	Remember best when they see pictures, diagrams, flow charts, films, and demonstrations.	Use visual and verbal information Incorporate concept and mid maps in the teaching. Colour code information for example, 'yellow insulin' or 'purple insulin' to refer to the package colour.

(Continued)

Table 16.1   Continued.

Learning style	Learning process	Teaching strategy
Verbal	Learn best by listening to words.	Use verbal teaching, tapes to take home. Group work.
Sequential	Learn best if a logical step wise or staged approach is used. May not fully understand the material unless they use it. May know a lot about specific topics but have trouble relating them to other aspects of the same subject or to different subjects,	Provide logical material where each piece of information follows the preceding information Do not move randomly from topic to topic. Give them 'homework' so they can use the information and develop their global learning skills. Explain how the information relates to other information.
Global	Learn large amounts of information without seeing connections and suddenly make the connection. May solve complex problems quickly or find innovative ways of doing things once they understand the information. May have problems explaining how they did it.	Paint the big picture first. Explain how topics relate to other topics. And to information the person already knows.

Note: other methods of describing learning styles include:
- Auditory, kinesthetic, and visual (Neurolinguistic programming (NLP).
- Multiple Intelligence model that consists of eight domains.

Table 16.2   A simple tool that can be used to estimate an individual's dominant learning style. It is not comprehensive but can be easily and quickly incorporated into routine education and care.

Please put a number in the circles in the order that best describes how you learn new important information from number 1 to 9. Number 1 is the way you learn best. If you choose the 'other' option please briefly describe what you do to learn new information.

- Read printed information such as books and pamphlets with a lot of words.
- Read printed information with lots of pictures and diagrams or see models of things.
- Watch videos.
- Listen to an audiotape or a lecture.
- Have somebody show you how to do a task such as testing blood glucose
- Talk with other people who have similar problems:
  - In a group
  - In an Internet chat room
  - Individual informal discussion
- Practice using equipment such as injecting insulin or cooking food.
- Other, please
  details: ....
  ....

Another method is to ask the individual how he or she became competent at a hobby or task they perform regularly.

Education theories

Key education and behaviour theories that can be applied to diabetes education include:

- The Health Belief Model, which can suggest best content, topics and information sequencing.
- Self-efficacy, the education should build confidence, for example, by ensuring people achieve successes however small and that these are acknowledged.
- Locus of control; if people feel they are not in control they may require more support, for example, coaching and carer/family support.
- Cognitive Dissonance Theory; design interventions that make people feel unhappy or dissatisfied with their current behaviour and reinforce to prevent relapse.
- Diffusion Theory; ensure the intervention is consistent with the individual's belief system and values.
- Stages of Change; design strategies that fit the individual stages and where the individual is at each stage.
- Adult education theories; use existing knowledge and problem-solving techniques.

Diabetes education is a lifelong process and information needs change as health status changes, new technology and medicines become available, and new models of service delivery emerge. Significantly, there is a poor correlation between knowledge and behaviour. Scare tactics and negative information lower mental and emotional well being and might lead to denial and/or non-adherence (Knight & Donan 2006).

On a practical level, diabetes education is often divided into:

- Survival skills – the initial information necessary to begin the self-care journey and be safe at home (described later in the chapter). Given the increasing prevalence of diabetes survival skills should actually commence before diagnosis and target at risk populations or the whole population. For example, programmes developed by the National Public Health Institute in Helsinki designed to be delivered in primary care achieved reductions in three key diabetes and cardiovascular risk factors: BMI, waist circumference, and diastolic blood pressure after one year. People who achieved reductions in four or more risk factors had a lower risk of developing diabetes. This suggests diabetes educators need to take a population based approach to diabetes education as well as providing individual education and management.
- Basic knowledge – information that builds on survival information and enables the individual to understand diabetes and its management and their role in diabetes management generally, and self-care in particular.
- Ongoing education – the continued acquisition of new information, including changes in technology and management practices as they emerge. A key aspect of delivering new information is helping the individual decide how it applies to them. That is, the information must be personalised to their particular life context.

Acquiring survival skills and undertaking relevant diabetes self-management usually requires changes in established behaviours. Understanding the individual's readiness to make relevant changes and identifying their personal barriers to change is central to behavioural change interventions. Several models have been developed that attempt to describe the behaviour change processes. These include:

- The Health Belief Model (HBM) (Becker & Maiman 1975).
- Social Learning Theory (SLT) (Bandura 1986).
- Theory of Reasoned Action and Planned Behaviour (TRA) (Ajzen & Fishbein 1980).
- The Transtheoretical Model of Change (Stages of Change) (SOC) (Prochaska & DiClemente 1983).
- Empowerment Model (Anderson & Funnell 2000).
- Coaching models such as the Health Care Australia Coaching Model (Linder *et al.* 2003; Gale 2007), which are based on positive psychology and focus on helping people form the intention to change and supporting them to make and sustain changes. This is different from telephone or Internet coaching models that aim to help individual's achieve management targets. For example, by prompting them to have various tests or recommending that they ask their doctor about treatment changes (Vale *et al.* 2003; Young *et al.* 2007).
- The Ecological Model, which focuses on identifying key resources and supporting self-management (RSSM) is an approach that grounds diabetes self-management in the context of the individual's social and environmental situation (Fisher *et al.* 2005). It enables the skills and choices of the individual to be integrated with the services and support they receive from their social environment, which includes family and friends, health services, and wider community services. The ecological approach determines the impact various factors in the individual's environment have on their self-care ability.
- Complementary medicine (CAM) models focus on finding the 'doctor within' and enhancing the individual's innate capacity for healing. CAM models suggests health professionals are most effective when '. . . we give the doctor who resides in each patient a chance to go to work'. (Schweitzer, in Cousins 2005, p. 78).

There are several common elements among these models: individual behaviours result from perceived benefit of and perceived barriers to change (HBM); expected outcomes and readiness to make changes (SOC); self-efficacy and perceived ability to control the behaviour (SCT); perceptions of social and cultural norms (TRA and CAM); individual innate capacity (doctor within) (CAM). Coaching involves helping people identify ways of changing (pathway thinking). In addition, these models all rely on understanding people with diabetes' explanatory models for diabetes, their lived experience of diabetes, and how they negotiate complicated health care systems with their contradictory language, focus on 'control', discipline, regular surveillance by a range of health professionals, and transferring a great deal of responsibility for diabetes care to the individual.

Health professionals need to understand the multiplicity of factors that influence people's explanatory models, including their own influence. For example, Type 2 diabetes is frequently described as a 'lifestyle disease,' which has a hidden subtext, for example, self-induced disease and blame, media advertising promotes foods such as 'guilt-free chocolate'. The 'voice' in which health professionals seek or deliver information as well as the actual words they use affect learning. Three health professional voices have been described:

- The 'doctor' voice used when the health professional is seeking information from the patient.
- The 'educator' voice used when imparting information to the patient.
- The 'fellow human' voice used when encouraging and supporting people.

People with diabetes are more likely to respond to the fellow human voice. They often try to reduce the judgmental connotations inherent within words by developing their own explanations for diabetes.

Communication – the central element of effective teaching and learning

Effective communication is central to teaching and learning and the patient's role in health-related decision-making. Communication means many things. In the context of diabetes education it is the art of asking good questions and *listening* to the answers.

Research consistently demonstrates low patient-health professional concordance about management decisions (Heisler *et al.* 2003; Parkin & Skinner 2003; Skinner *et al.* 2007), which health professionals frequently attributed to patients not recalling the content of the consultation. However, Skinner *et al.* (2007) demonstrated that both patient and health professional recall is poor. Significantly, Skinner *et al.* found some decisions patients and health professionals recalled were not evident in recordings of their conversations and there were discrepancies between the details even when both groups recalled the general topics discussed.

Parkin & Skinner (2003) found patients were more likely to recall talking about diet and less likely to recall discussing moods or emotions. Conversely, health professionals were more likely to recall discussing mood and emotions. They found complete disagreement between patients and health professionals in 19.6% of encounters and about decisions made 20.7% of the time. That is, the 'the two parties seem to recall different consultations'. Patients may forget a great deal of what they are told, but it appears health professionals forget a great deal about what they said.

Likewise, Rushford *et al.* (2007) found women hospitalised with a cardiac condition recalled receiving information about medication, smoking cessation, and exercise but very few recalled receiving information about resuming gardening, sexual activity, and driving. Obese inactive women only recalled a limited amount of information about diet and activity and only some women with diabetes recalled receiving information about medicines. Older women were least likely to recall advice.

The reasons for these discrepancies are not clear. However, the more people are told the more they forget and they tend to recall what they were told first or consider important to them, best. These findings suggest there are many barriers to effective communication, many of which are common to patients and health professionals, see Table 16.1.

Specific strategies to enhance education and promote behaviour change include:

- Having the individual write down their goals, a strategy used in health coaching, to encourage people to own the decision and to remind them of their behaviour change goals.
- Written or verbal contracts between patients and health professionals, patients and carers, or health professionals and carers where one or both parties commit to undertaking behaviours. There is little evidence that contracts improve adherence or achieve behaviour change (Bosch-Capblanch *et al.* 2007).
- Blood glucose awareness training (BGATT) has consistently demonstrated improved hypoglycaemia awareness (ability to detect hypoglycaemia) and fewer episodes of severe hypoglycaemia during driving (Cox *et al.* 2006). It was developed for people with Type 1 diabetes but there is no reason it should not be appropriate to Type 2. BGATT was recently made available on the Internet for health professionals and people with diabetes.
- Adopting a 'tell back-collaborative inquiry' approach (Kemp *et al.* 2008). Many people leave health professionals with limited understanding about what occurred in the encounter. Such misunderstanding is associated with high risk of adverse outcomes (Bittten *et al.* 2000). Kemp *et al.* used two video scenarios to assess how people like to receive information. One video showed a doctor explaining a medical condition and its management using three types of inquiry: yes–no (commonly used in health settings), tell back directive (health professional centred), and tell back collaborative (patient-centred and had elements to address patient's feelings). Not surprisingly, people preferred the tell back collaborative approach. Significantly, the Kalamazoo Consensus Statement developed by communication experts recommends checking for understanding as a core element of communication. Interestingly, Kemp *et al.* (2008) identified only one article, published long before the explosion of patient-centred models, in an extensive literature review that recommended checking for patient understanding (Bertakis 1977). Bertakis reported improved information retention and management satisfaction.

Thus, an empowering education model that encompasses a tell back collaborative approach enables the individual's explanatory model for diabetes and their personal health care needs and opportunities to negotiate and agree on compromises. Education encounters are often emotional as well as cognitive and rational, and involve reflection and action. Sometimes people have to make difficult management decisions several times a day, which can be stressful and emotionally exhausting. The ecomap and genomap shown in Chapter 2 could help health professionals understand the individual's social environment.

The following issues need to be considered when designing an empowering education encounter:

- Education alone will not change behaviour (World Health Organisation (WHO) (2003; Kinight & Donan 2006). For example, 28% of people with Type 1 diabetes do not have their insulin prescriptions filled or inject the prescribed doses (Morris *et al.* 1997); only one-third of people with Type 2 on monotherapy obtain at least 80% of their prescribed medicines (Donan *et al.* 2002), only follow dietary recommendations 50% of the time (Toobert *et al.* 2000); and only 30% who take out gym membership attend the gym.
- The individual's feelings, beliefs and diabetes explanatory models affect their health care behaviours.
- Psychosocial situation and key relationships.

- Education and literacy level.
- Coping style.
- Learning and teaching styles and methods.
- Goals for the session and the future life goals.
- Ability to undertake self-care behaviours.
- Satisfaction with the service.

Although current diabetes management and education care models focus on patients being active participants in their care and health outcomes are better if the patient actively participates, people's actual role in and preferences concerning health care decision-making is complex. Some people prefer to leave medical decisions to their doctors. Arora & McHorney (1998) found 58% of patients preferred their doctors to make medical decisions. There was a significant association between older age, lower education and income levels, and male gender and preference for doctor-driven decisions. People with severe cardiac disease and serious diabetes were more likely to adopt a passive role. In contrast, those with clinical or symptomatic depression were more likely to take an active role. People with the lowest coping skills and those who placed a higher value on their health were more likely to leave decisions to their health professionals.

Teaching: an art and a process

Teaching is a communication process involving planning, implementing and evaluating information to be learned. Teaching can be delivered individually or in groups and involves:

- Creating an environment in which learning can occur. This includes establishing a relationship with the person and finding their 'doctor within'.
- Assessing learning needs and learning style or styles. The learning needs are used to set goals and plan the teaching. Assessment is an essential first step because patients and health professionals have different ideas about what is important (Woodcock & Kinmouth 2001). Barriers and facilitators to learning and being able to use the information can be identified and the teaching can build on past experience, existing knowledge, and address misconceptions.
- Prioritising learning needs.
- Setting goals with the individual or group to be achieved that are agreed with the individual or group and are achievable and measurable.
- Identifying the teaching method most likely to enhance learning and the materials needed to deliver the teaching. This can be as simple as a stick to draw in the sand with or as complex as a sophisticated lecture room. In group settings a range of teaching strategies need to be used to accommodate different learning styles.
- Delivering the teaching using strategies most likely to facilitate learning.
- Having the insight to 'Seize the day' and teach at a teachable moments as the movie *The Dead Poet's Society* portrayed so poignantly.
- Evaluating the outcome. Evaluation is an essential aspect of quality improvement and should not only focus on patient outcomes (knowledge and behaviour). Teacher performance and the overall teaching programme should also be evaluated. There are different forms of evaluation depending on the purpose of the evaluation see recommended reading at the end of the chapter. When planning the evaluation, the data collection process and validity of any tools used need to be considered.

Thus, there is considerable overlap among teaching, storytelling, and counselling. In the context of diabetes education where the underlying goal is often to achieve and/or maintain behaviour change, the teacher must find the most effective way to invite the individual to see themselves and their role in a different way and find ways to help the individual help him or herself. Thus, education is a sophisticated form of marketing. It is a challenge selling the product 'diabetes', with all that entails and the meanings the word holds for individuals and society, to a usually reluctant buyer.

Health professional training in how to deliver patient-centred education and care may improve performance and patient satisfaction with and active engagement in their care (Lewin *et al.* 2001).

Diabetes education can be delivered individually and is equally effective delivered in groups including initiating insulin (Plank *et al.* 2004; Yki Jarvinen *et al.* 2007). However, people still need to be able to apply the information to their personal situation and have the opportunity to practice relevant behaviours. Group education provides a form of peer support and often helps people feel less alone in the problems they face and feelings about diabetes, which can have positive health benefits. Internet based education programmes are also effective for younger and older people especially when they are interactive and emphasise behavioural and motivational strategies (Bond *et al.* 2007).

Health professionals are often also patient advocates, in fact patient advocacy is listed as in *Role and Scope of Practice for the Credentialed Diabetes Educator in Australia* (Australian Diabetes Educators Association (ADEA) 2007). Specific advocacy actions for diabetes educators and nurses include helping people obtain relevant health care, advocating for services, and interceding with other health professionals on the individual's behalf. Health advocacy is a complex process and nurses are often hindered in their advocacy by issues such as a sense of powerlessness, lack of support form colleagues, lack of time, and insufficient knowledge and skills (Negarandeh *et al.* 2006).

Practice points

(1) Listening heals.
(2) Diabetes education is not about getting the patient to do what the health professional wants.
(3) Even if the health professional is not trying to control the individual's life it often feels that way to the patient. Most people's instinct is to resist. Core beliefs and values are held more strongly when people feel they have lost control over aspects of their life (Thomas 2001) and affect readiness and ability to make relevant behaviour changes.
(4) Emotions need to be acknowledged not solved. Health professionals' instinct is to try to solve the problem. The art of teaching is to help the individual find the solution.

Health literacy

Considering health literacy is essential to the success of patient focused interventions (Coulter & Ellins 2007). Health literacy refers to the ability to read, understand and use information to make appropriate decisions about health and management options

(Partnership for Clear Health Communication 2006; Weiss 2007). Health literacy is a complex skill involving reading, listening, speaking, conceptual knowledge and problem-solving. Low health literacy is a significant barrier to achieving optimal health outcomes and is a stronger predictor of health status than age, income, employment status, education level, or ethnic group. In addition, it is associated with significant hidden health care costs. The average reading level in the USA is 8th grade and 20% read at 5th grade level.

People with limited health literacy often feel ashamed and try to hide the fact from other people. For example, Parikh *et al.* (1996) found two thirds of patients had never disclosed their low health literacy to their spouses, more than half had never told their children, and one in five had never disclosed to anybody. Clues to low health literacy include the individual's response to written information, for example, 'I forgot my glasses, I will read it when I get home', responses to questions about health care behaviours, for example, inability to name medicines, actual behaviours, for example, missing appointments or not adhering to medicine regimens. However, these are clues to explore the issue: they are not diagnostic (Davis *et al.* 1993; Weiss 2007).

Methods of assessing health literacy include:

- Newest Vital Sign (NVS) (Weis *et al.* 2005) is used to screen for limited health literacy by answering questions about a nutrition label for ice cream.
- Rapid Estimate of Adult Literacy in Medicine (REALM) (Davis *et al.* 1993) is a word recognition test and is one of the oldest and most widely used health literacy assessment instruments. Variations on the original REAL include a version for adolescents (REALM-Teen), a shorter version than the original 66 questions (REALM-7). Other versions are under development, for example, for dentistry.
- Test of Functional Health Literacy in Adults (TOHLA) is more complex and is often used for research purposes (Parker & Baker 1995). It takes ~20 minutes to complete but a shorter version is available that can be completed in 12 minutes. It assesses numeracy as well as literacy.
- National Assessment of Adult Literacy (NAAL) can be used as a population screening tool and identifies four levels of health literacy from basic to proficient (Kutner *et al.* 2006).
- The eHealth Literacy Scale (eHEALS) is a measure of knowledge, comfort and skill at using information technology to obtain health information from electronic sources and has been validated with adolescents (Norman & Skinner 2006).
- Nutrition Literacy Scale, which is specific to nutrition.

It may be possible to incorporate health literacy assessments into routine clinical practice but it can be time consuming and patients may not be willing to undergo such testing. If time and resources permit, a health literacy point prevalence survey may provide a guide to the prevalence of the problem in a given target population. It may be more useful to ensure health information is at grade 8 or 9 level by undertaking various readability and usability tests on the information commonly provided such as:

- The Simple Measure of Gobbledegook (SMOG).
- CLOZE.
- DISCERN designed to evaluate the quality of written patient health information (Coulter *et al.* 1998).

- Material for Informed Choice-Evaluation (MICE) designed to assess the readability of scientific information for patients (Charnock 1998).

It is very likely that a great deal of information is not at an appropriate literacy level to promote informed health decision-making and may not suit all learning styles. Godolphin *et al.* (2001) found 50% of the pamphlets on display in doctor's consulting rooms was well below the required level on the DISCERN scale.

Generally people want health information and if their information needs are met in a form appropriate to their needs they are more likely to actively participate in their care (Larson *et al.* 1996; Coulter *et al.* 1999; McKenna *et al.* 2003) yet doctors often underestimate people's desire for information and are less likely to provide information for older people (McKenna *et al.* 2003).

Other design issues are also important such as colour contrast, font size, font type (sans serif fonts, e.g., Arial and all capital letters are harder to read them serif fonts, e.g., Times New Roman and sentence case), the amount of 'white space', and the graphics used.

Survival skills

While the preceding information largely addresses the need to consider the mental and social aspects of learning and teaching, there are some tasks that need to be mastered for safe, effective self-care. Survival skills are taught at diagnosis and throughout life as the need arises. The family should be involved whenever necessary if possible. Survival skills education refers to providing minimal information to enable the person to manage their medicines, eat an appropriate diet, monitor blood glucose and ketones, prevent and/or manage hypoglycaemia, safely dispose of used equipment and obtain relevant supplies. Written information can support verbal teaching and is more effective if the health professional gives the information to the individual and points out important information relevant to the individual. However, the individual's specific concerns/ questions must be addressed. The patient should be able to:

- Demonstrate correct insulin care and administration techniques (if appropriate).
- Know the effect of medications, exercise and food on their blood glucose levels.
- Know the names of their insulin/tablets (if relevant).
- Demonstrate correct monitoring techniques (blood and ketone testing) and appropriately document the results.
- Know the significance of ketones (Type 1).
- Recognise the signs and symptoms, causes and appropriate treatment of hypoglycaemia if on insulin or OHAs.
- Know that regular meals containing the appropriate amount of carbohydrate are important.
- Have an emergency contact telephone number if help is required.
- Demonstrate safe disposal of sharps.
- Enrol in the NDSS (in Australia).

A sample diabetes education record used to document 'survival information' and plan for further teaching is shown over the page.

Sample diabetes education record chart

DIABETES EDUCATION RECORD

Date of referral ....

Referred by Dr/RN ....

Language spoken ....

Literacy level ....

Other communication issues ....

Method used to address issues ....

Perceived level of skill and understanding attained ....

Follow-up requirements ....

Information supplied

(1) What is diabetes? ....

(2) How it is controlled:

    • diet ....

    • tablets/insulin ....

    • activity/exercise ....

(3) Ketone testing ....

(4) Home blood glucose monitoring ....

(5) Diet and nutrition ....

(6) Insulin and OHAs:

    • care of ....

    • insulin administration ....

    • when to take OHA/insulin ....

    • sharps disposal ....

(7) Hypos ....   (8) Sick days ....

(9) Foot care ....   (10) Sport & exercise ....

(11) Dentist ....   (12) Travel & Driving ....

Other information ....

Family support: good/fair/poor

Carer health status (especially older partners) ....

Follow-up care needed from practice, home care or community nurses or the GP ....

....

....

....

Discharge checklist

(1) Education material supplied – itemise ....

(2) List of medications that includes self-prescribed and complementary
medicines ....

(3) Record book ....

(4) Blood testing equipment – type ....

(5) Ketone testing .... (6) Specific diet advice ....

(7) Medic alert ....

(8) Starter pack: syringes/needles/lancets ....

(9) Medicines ....

(10) Discharged to: diabetic clinic/GP/specialist ....

(11) Referred for further education ....

Enrolment in Diabetes Association ....

Plan for next session ....

Signature .... Date ....

Ongoing education

Education can be continued on an individual basis or in group programmes. Education is a lifelong process, thus both methods are usually employed. Survival information should be reviewed and further information given. The patient should gradually be able to:

- Demonstrate appropriate insulin adjustment considering the effects of factors such as food, activity, medication and illness on blood glucose as relevant.
- Manage illnesses at home, especially continue insulin/diabetes tablets, continue to drink fluids and test for ketones, especially Type 1.
- Recognise the signs and symptoms of hypoglycaemia and treat appropriately.
- Cope in special situations, such as eating out, during travel and playing sports.
- Understand that appropriate complication screening such as foot care will help prevent long-term complications and hospital admissions.
- Know that normoglycaemia and regular examination of the eyes, feet, blood pressure, cardiovascular system and kidney function can prevent or delay the development of long-term diabetic complications.
- Understand that certain jobs and activities are unsuitable for people with diabetes on insulin, for example, scuba diving, driving heavy vehicles.
- Accept the wisdom of wearing some form of medical alert system identifying them as having diabetes.
- Understand that they should not neglect general health care such as mammograms, prostate checks, breast self-examination, regular dental checks, and preventative vaccinations.

- In order to recognise 'abnormal', for example, hypoglycaemia or signs of a complication, the individual needs to recognise what 'normal' is for them. This involves learning to listen to their bodies, interpret body cues, self-diagnose and make a decision about what to do. They may or may not seek assistance to interpret the body cues. They may test out their theories (legitimisation).

Practice points

(1) Education methods that incorporate behavioural strategies, experiential learning, goal setting and reinforcement are more likely to be effective.
(2) Patient satisfaction is a key element of adherence.
(3) Helping the person reflect on events and consider future strategies make education more personal.
(4) The therapeutic relationship between the patient and health professional is important to effective education and care.

Empowerment

There is no doubt that diabetes education is essential, but knowledge alone does not predict health behaviour. Beliefs, attitudes and satisfaction are some of the intervening variables between knowledge, behaviour, and disease status. These are not constants and they need to be assessed on a regular basis, for example deciding what is happening at the time, what could/will change and how will the change affect the individual and their significant others.

Empowerment models of diabetes education are based on shared governance considering the whole person and their life situation and personal environment. These issues are not a new concept. Hippocrates is credited with saying, 'In order to cure the human body it is necessary to have knowledge of the whole'. Likewise, the psychiatrist in T.S. Elliot's *The Cocktail Party* states that he needed to know a great deal more about the patient than the patient himself could always tell him.

Empowerment models recognise that people with diabetes must, and mostly want to be responsible for their own care. Empowerment is based on three characteristics of diabetes:

(1) The person with diabetes makes choices affecting their healthcare.
(2) The individual is in control of their care.
(3) The consequences of the choices affect the person with diabetes.

Empowerment then, is a collaborative approach to care where management is designed to help the individual make informed choices and maximise their knowledge, skills, and self-awareness. It requires the individual to make deliberate conscious choices on a daily basis.

Empowerment education requires health professionals to accept the legitimacy of an individual's goals even if they result in suboptimal control (Anderson *et al.* 1996) and the individual to accept responsibility for the consequences of their decisions. Not everybody is capable of taking control. Some people require specific instructions, for example, an individual who has an external locus of control. In addition, stress and anxiety at specific times can impair an individual's ability to take control.

An empowerment model of diabetes education seeks to determine what the person with diabetes wants, and to reach agreement between what should be done and what the individual wants or is capable of achieving in order to balance the burden of treatment and quality of life (see Chapter 15). Diabetes is only one aspect of people's lives and affects them on many levels:

- Observable, for example, signs and symptoms of hyper/hypoglycaemia.
- Not directly observable, for example, personhood, self-concept, body image.
- Insights into their disease.
- Relationships.

Special issues

The individual's questions should be addressed as they arise and planned into teaching programmes as appropriate to the individual. Questions may relate to:

- Pregnancy and diabetes.
- Sexuality and diabetes.
- Exercise.
- Weight control.
- A range of other issues such as diabetes information the person hears or reads in media reports.

It is not absolutely necessary for people with diabetes to have a detailed knowledge about the causes and pathophysiology of diabetes in order to achieve good control.

The nurses' role in diabetes education

Patient teaching is a recognised independent nursing function and education is a vital part of the diabetic treatment plan. Therefore, teaching patients in acute, elderly and extended care facilities is within the scope of professional nursing practice. Some key points should be kept in mind when educating people with diabetes:

(1) The aim of diabetes education is autonomy and empowerment.
(2) Consider the psychological and social aspects when discussing diabetes.
(3) Encourage questions and dialogue.
(4) Ask open questions and use active listening.
(5) Teach specific skills and allow the patient time to practice new skills (e.g. insulin administration).
(6) Allow time for patients to discuss difficulties and concerns about diabetes.
(7) Relate new information to the patient's experience.

Practice point

Although there are many disadvantages to bedside teaching, e.g. noise, distractions, illness, other priorities and concerns, and lack of privacy, it can allow teaching to occur at a 'teachable moment' and effectively reinforce information. The information must be consistent with hospital policies/procedures and the nurse must have the appropriate knowledge in order to teach effectively. Nurses make a substantial contribution to the health and wellbeing of the patient by allowing them to participate in decision making about their care in hospital and to make appropriate decisions at home.

Teaching in the ward effectively reinforces the information supplied by the diabetes nurse specialist/diabetes educator, doctor, podiatrist and dietitian. However, ward teaching *must* be consistent with that of the diabetes team and procedures such as insulin technique and blood glucose monitoring performed correctly according to the agreed protocols. Patients are quick to perceive inconsistencies and may become confused or loose faith in the staff if they perceive inconsistencies. Some examples of relevant instruction sheets can be found at the end of this chapter.

Learning is facilitated when the need/readiness to learn is perceived and immediately applied in a given situation: that is, 'teaching at a teachable moment'. Teachable moments often occur when the ward staff are performing routine nursing care, such as blood glucose tests, or giving injections.

Teaching is non-verbal as well as verbal. In fact >60% of communication is non-verbal. People learn by observation, therefore the nurse is a role model and care should be taken to perform procedures correctly and to refer questions to another person if they do not know the answer. In this way, formal and informal ongoing education in the ward is possible and desirable. The nurse's own knowledge about diabetes will influence their willingness and ability to participate in patient teaching. Theories of teaching and learning were not traditionally part of the nurse training. This is changing as empowerment in chronic disease management is recognised and accepted along with a focus on preventative healthcare.

Many factors can influence teaching and learning. Some of these are shown in Table 16.3. It is the responsibility of the teacher to ensure that the environment is not distracting. Noise in a busy ward can make conversation difficult and hinder learning. The patient should be as comfortable as possible and free from pain and other distractions.

The following basic principles need to be considered when planning a teaching session, whether it is for an individual or a group:

- The aim of the session.
- The patient's needs/goals and learning style.
- Objectives should be realistic and achievable.
- The environment must be conducive to learning.
- Ascertain and build on the patient's existing knowledge.
- Relate teaching to patient's own experience.

Table 16.3   Some common factors that influence teaching and learning.

Factor	Patient	Health professional
Health beliefs	✓	✓
Social support	✓	
Well being/illness	✓	✓
Environment	✓	✓
Knowledge	✓	✓
Skills	✓	✓
Time	✓	✓
Perceived responsibility	✓	✓
Work priority		✓
Perception of teaching role		✓
Learning style	✓	✓

- Demonstrate the skills to be acquired.
- Provide opportunities for the patient to practice the skill (return demonstration).
- Evaluate the skill and knowledge.
- Provide positive reinforcement.
- Review information before commencing the next teaching session.

It is usual to begin with the simple concepts and proceed to more complex ones.

The Instruction Sheets at the end of the chapter are examples of information material used in teaching, which is often available in several languages. In some cases the medical terms may need to be replaced with the patient's words. Blood glucose monitoring is discussed in Chapter 3. Specific patient instruction will depend on the testing system being used.

Insulin administration

Insulin can be administered using a range of insulin delivery systems, see Table 5.3. Syringes are not used as often as the other devices in some countries, because the devices offer greater flexibility, portability and are discreet, thus avoiding some of the stigma attached to syringes.

The person should be shown a range of options and helped to choose one that suits them. The short fine needles in use today mean injections are relatively painless – less painful than blood glucose testing.

Insulin should be given subcutaneously (see how to give an injection). IM injections, through incorrect technique, cause erratic blood glucose levels because the insulin is absorbed faster than via the subcutaneous route (Vaag *et al.* 1990).

Reusing needles and syringes causes local trauma, microscopic damage to the needle tip and increases the likelihood that the needle will bend and/or break off in the injection site; it should therefore be discouraged. Needles left on insulin pens form a conduit to the outside allowing air to enter the vial and dose inaccuracies (Ginsberg *et al.* 1994).

Guidelines for Instructing patients about insulin delivery systems

Patient learning requirements

The patient should be familiar with the structure and function of the particular insulin device chosen. They must be able to:

- Assemble the device in the correct sequence.
- Load the insulin correctly if necessary.
- Ensure insulin is expelled from the needle after loading the insulin.
- Know when to replace the insulin cartridge/device.
- Know how to inject the insulin according to the particular device chosen.
- Know how to store and transport the device.
- Know the appropriate method of cleaning and maintaining the device.
- Recognise signs that the device may be malfunctioning and know what action to take to remedy the situation.

It is important to discuss with and advise the patient about safe disposal of used equipment, especially sharps disposal at home. The guidelines for sharps disposal in the home can be found in Chapter 18.

Documenting diabetes education

Documentation was discussed in Chapter 2. Documentation is a legal requirement and a method of communication. Documenting diabetes education can be very time-consuming, thus using templates or teaching records that list standard education and make provision for individual differences to be recorded can save time.

Examples of patient instruction sheets appear on the following pages.

Examples Instruction Sheets

These Instruction Sheets were designed to be used with a practical demonstration of the procedure/s. They should not be handed out without adequate discussion. *They are examples only.*

Example Instruction Sheet 3: How to draw up insulin – one bottle only

Your insulin is called ....

It can be useful to indicate the particular insulin colour code especially if the person is not literate.

(1) Remove insulin bottle from fridge. Check expiry date – do not use if exceeded.

Cloudy insulin must be mixed before drawing up.

(2) Gently invert insulin bottle or roll between hands until well mixed (**do not shake**). Insulin should be 'milky'; there should be no lumps.

Clear insulin should be clear and colourless.

(3) Clean bottle top with spirit.

(4) Draw back plunger to ....   units of air.

(5) Inject air into insulin bottle, invert bottle and draw back ....   units of insulin, ensuring that all air bubbles are removed from the syringe.

(6) Administer insulin.

Example Instruction Sheet 4:
How to draw up insulin – two bottles

Your insulins are called .... (clear)

.... (cloudy)

(1) Remove insulin bottles from fridge. Check expiry date – do not use if exceeded.

(2) Gently invert or roll bottle of 'cloudy' insulin between hands, until 'milky' (**do not shake**).

(3) Clean bottle tops with spirit.

(4) Draw back plunger to .... units of air.

(5) Inject air into cloudy insulin and remove needle from the bottle.

(6) Draw back plunger to .... units of air.

(7) Inject air into clear insulin.

(8) Invert bottle and draw back .... units of clear insulin, ensuring that all air bubbles are removed from syringe.

(9) Put needle into cloudy bottle and withdraw .... units of cloudy insulin to the <u>exact</u> required dose of the syringe.

(10) If more cloudy insulin is accidently drawn up, discard contents of the syringe and start again.

(11) Total clear and cloudy insulin equals .... units.

Example Instruction Sheet 5:
How to give an insulin injection using syringes or insulin pens

(1) Insulin can be injected into the abdomen, thighs, buttock or upper arm. The abdomen is the preferred site.

(2) Inject into a different spot each time.

(3) Pinch up a fold of skin between two fingers.

(4) Quickly push the needle into the skin at right angles.

(5) Gently push the plunger all the way to inject your insulin.

(6) Pull the syringe/device out quickly and apply pressure to the injection site.

Insulin should be stored away from heat and light. The bottle/cartridge in use can be kept at room temperature.

Stores should be kept in the refrigerator.

The same injection technique applies to insulin pens.

Example Instruction Sheet 6a:
Managing your diabetes when you are ill:
patients with Type 1 diabetes

Illness (such as colds and flu) cause the body to make hormones which help the body fight the illness. These hormones usually also cause the blood glucose to go high. High blood glucose levels can lead to unpleasant symptoms like thirst, tiredness and passing a lot of urine.

By taking some simple precautions the minor illness can usually be treated at home.

What to Do

(1) Tell a family member or friend you are unwell.

(2) Continue to take your insulin. You may need to increase the dose during illness to control the blood glucose and prevent ketones from developing.

(3) Test your blood glucose every 2–4 hours. Write down the test results.

(4) Test your blood for ketones. If moderate to heavy ketones are detected consult your doctor.

(5) Continue to drink fluids or eat if possible (see recommended food list).

(6) Read the labels on any medication you take to treat the illness because it may contain sugar, sugar substitutes or other ingredients that cause the blood glucose to go high.

(7) Rest.

(8) Keep the phone number of your doctor, diabetes clinic or diabetes nurse specialist/ diabetes educator beside the telephone.

When to Call the Doctor

(1) If you have diarrhoea and/or vomiting.

(2) If ketones develop.

(3) If the blood glucose continues to rise.

(4) If you develop signs of dehydration (loss of skin tone, sunken eyes, dry mouth).

(5) If the illness does not get better in 2–3 days.

(6) If you feel you need advice.

What to Tell the Doctor When You Call

(1) How long you have been sick.

(2) What the blood glucose level is.

(3) How long the blood glucose has been high.

(4) The level of ketones in the blood.

(5) How frequently you are passing urine and how much.

(6) If you are thirsty, tired or have a temperature.

(7) What medications you have taken to treat the illness.

(8) If you have vomiting or diarrhoea, how frequently and how much.

Food for Days When You are Sick

It is important to continue to eat and drink. Small frequent meals may be easier to digest.

Suggested foods

- sweetened jelly (not low cal)
- ice cream (1/2 cup)
- custard with sugar (1/2 cup)
- honey (3 teaspoons)
- sugar (1 tablespoon)
- sweetened ice block (one small or 90 mL)
- egg flip – sweetened (similar to egg nog but less creamy 8 oz)
- milk (10 oz)
- Coke, lemonade or other sweetened soft drink (3/4 cup – not low cal)
- unsweetened tinned fruit (3/4 cup)
- orange juice (3/4 cup)
- apple juice (1/2 cup)
- pineapple juice (1/2 cup)
- orange (one medium)
- banana (one small)
- unflavoured yoghurt (100 g or 1/2 carton)
- flavoured (sweetened) yoghurt (200 g or one carton)
- broth or soup

Continuing Care

(1) If the doctor prescribes antibiotics to treat the illness it is important to complete the full course.

(2) Continue to test for ketones until they show clear for 24 hours.

(3) Continue to test your blood glucose 2–4 hourly and record the results until you recover and then go back to your usual routine.

(4) Go back to your usual food plan when you recover.

(5) If your insulin has been increased during the illness decrease it again when you recover to avoid hypoglycaemia.

(6) Develop a sick day management plan.

(7) Consider writing down a medical history for quick reference in times of illness or in an emergency.

List:

- all the medications you are taking

- past illnesses

- blood group

- date of last tetanus and flu injection

- illnesses that run in the family.

This can be worn in an identification tag or be kept with your diabetes record book.

Example Instruction Sheet 6b:
Managing your diabetes when you are ill:
patients with Type 2 diabetes

Illnesses (such as colds and flu) cause the body to make hormones which help the body fight the illness. These hormones usually also cause the blood glucose to go high. High blood glucose levels can lead to unpleasant symptoms like thirst, tiredness and passing a lot of urine.

By taking some simple precautions the minor illness can usually be treated at home.

What to Do

(1) Tell a family member or friend you are unwell.

(2) Continue to take your diabetes tablets. This is very important, because the blood glucose usually goes high. In severe illnesses or during an operation insulin injections may be needed until you recover.

(3) Test your blood glucose every 2–4 hours. Write down the test results.

(4) Continue to drink fluids or eat if possible (see recommended food list).

(5) Read the labels on any medication you take to treat the illness because it may contain sugar, sugar substitutes or other ingredients which cause the blood glucose to go high.

(6) Rest.

(7) Keep the phone number of your doctor, diabetes clinic or diabetes nurse specialist/ diabetes educator beside the telephone.

When to Call the Doctor

(1) If you have diarrhoea and/or vomiting.

(2) If the blood glucose continues to rise.

(3) If you develop signs of dehydration (loss of skin tone, sunken eyes, dry mouth).

(4) If the illness does not get better in 2–3 days.

(5) If you feel you need advice.

What to Tell the Doctor When You Call

(1) How long you have been sick.

(2) What the blood glucose level is.

(3) How long the blood glucose has been high.

(4) How frequently you are passing urine and how much.

(5) If you are thirsty, tired or have a temperature.

(6) What medications you have taken to treat the illness.

(7) If you have vomiting or diarrhoea, how frequently and how much.

Food for Days When You are Sick

It is important to continue to eat and drink. Small frequent meals may be easier to digest.

Suggested foods

- sweetened jelly (not low cal)
- ice cream (1/2 cup)
- custard with sugar (1/2 cup)
- honey (3 teaspoons)
- sugar (1 tablespoon)
- sweetened ice block (one small or 90 mL)
- egg flip – sweetened (8 oz)
- milk (10 oz)
- Coke, lemonade or other sweetened soft drink (3/4 cup – not low cal)
- unsweetened tinned fruit (3/4 cup)
- orange juice (3/4 cup)
- apple juice (1/2 cup)
- pineapple juice (1/2 cup)
- orange (one medium)
- banana (one small)
- unflavoured yoghurt (100 g or 1/2 carton)
- flavoured (sweetened) yoghurt (200 g or one carton)
- broth or soup

Continuing Care

(1) If the doctor prescribes antibiotics to treat the illness it is important to complete the full course.

(2) Continue to test your blood glucose 2–4 hourly and record the results until you recover and then go back to your usual routine.

(3) Go back to your usual food plan when you recover.

(4) Develop a sick day management plan.

(5) Consider writing down a medical history for quick reference in times of illness or in an emergency.

List:

- all the medications you are taking

- past illnesses

- blood group

- date of last tetanus and flu injection

- illnesses which run in the family.

This can be worn in an identification tag or be `kept with your diabetes record book.

References

Anderson, R., Funnell, M. & Arnold, M. (1996) Using the empowerment approach to help patients change behaviour. In: *Practical Psychology for Clinicians* (eds B. Anderson & R. Rubin). American Diabetes Association, Alexandria, pp. 163–172.

Anderson, B. & Funnell, M. (2005) *The Art of Empowerment*, 2nd edn. American Diabetes Association, Virginia.

Anderson, R., Funnell, M., Burkhart, N., Gillard, M. & Nwankwo, R. (2002) *101 Tips for Behaviour Change in Diabetes Education*. American Diabetes Association, Virginia.

Anderson, R., Funnell, M., Burkhart, N., Gillard, M. & Nwankwo, R. (2002) *101 Tips for Diabetes Self-Management Education*. American Diabetes Association, Virginia.

Arora, N., Mchorney, C. & Rao, S. (1998) Medical decision-making: do patients really want to participate? *Proceedings Health Services Review Annual Meeting*, 15, 252–253.

Australian Diabetes Educators Association (ADEA) (2007) *The Credentialled Diabetes Educator in Australia: Role and Scope of Practice*. ADEA, Canberra.

Barnstable, S. (1997) *Nurse as Educator*. Jones & Bartlett, Sudbury, Massachusetts.

Bertakiis, K. (1977) The communication of information from physician to patient: a method for increasing patient and physician satisfaction. *Journal of Family Practice*, 5, 217–222.

Bond, G., Burr, R., Wolf, F. & McCurry, S. & Teri, L. (2007) The effects of a web-based intervention on physical outcomes associated with diabetes among adults age 60 and older: a randomised trial. *Diabetes Technology Therapy*, 9 (1), 52–59.

Bosch-Capblanch, X., Abba, K., Prictor, M. & Garner, P. (2007) Contracts between patients and health care practitioners for improving adherence to treatment, prevention and health promotion activities. *Cochrane Database of Systematic Reviews*, Art. No. CD004808. Doi: 10.1002/1451858.CD004808.pub3.

Broom, D. & Whittaker, A. (2003) Controlling diabetes: moral language in the management of type 2 diabetes. *Social Science and Medicine*, 58, 2371–2382.

Charnock, D. (1998) *The DISCERN Handbook. Quality Criteria for Consumer Health Information on Treatment Choices*. Radcliff Medical Press, Oxford.

Coulter, A., Entwhistle, V. & Gilbert, D. (1998) *Informing Patients. Assessment of the Quality of Patient Information Materials*. King's College, London.

Coulter, A. & Ellins, J. (2007) Effectiveness of strategies for informing, educating and involving patients. *British Medical Journal*, 335 (7609), 24–27.

Cousins, N. (2005) *Anatomy of an Illness as Perceived by the Patient*. WW Norton, New York, p. 75.

Cox, D. & Gonder-Frederick, L. (1992) Major developments in behavioural diabetes research. *Journal of Consulting Clinical Psychologists*, 60, 628–638.

Cox, D., Goner-Frederick, L., Ritterband, L., Patel, K., Fehm-Wolfsdorf, G., Hermanns, N., Snoek, F., Schlundt, D., Kovatchev, B. & Clarke, W. (2006) Blood glucose awareness training: what is it, where is it, and where is it going? *Diabetes Spectrum*, 19, 43–49.

DAFNE Study Group (2002) Training in flexible, intensive insulin management to enable dietary freedom in people with Type 1 diabetes: Dosage Adjustment for Normal Eating (DAFNE) randomised controlled trial. *British Medical Journal*, 325, 746–751.

Davis, T., Long, S. & Jackson, R. (1993) Rapid estimate of adult literacy in medicine: a shortened screening instrument. *Family Medicine*, 25, 391–395.

Doak, C., Doak, L. & Root, J. (1996) *Teaching Patients with Low Literacy Skills*. JB Lippincott, Philadelphia.

Donan, P., MacDonald, T. & Morris, A. (2002) Adherence to prescribed oral hypoglycaemic medication in a population of patients with type 2 diabetes: a retrospective cohort study. *Diabetic Medicine*, 19, 279–284.

Fisher, E., Brownson, C., O'Toole, M., Shetty, G., Anwuri, V. & Glasgow, R. (2005) Ecological approaches to self-management: the care for diabetes. *American Journal of Public Health*, 95 (9), 1523–1535.

Gale, J. (2007) Health psychology meets coaching psychology in the practice of health coaching. http://www.psychology.org.au/publications/inpsych/health_coaching/ (accessed December 2007).

Ginsberg, B., Parkes, J. & Sparacina, C. (1994) The kinetics of insulin administration by insulin pens. *Hormone Metabolism Research*, 26, 584–587.

Godolphin, W., Towle, A. & McKendry, R. (2001) Evaluation of the quality of patient information to support informed shared decision-making. *Health Expectations*, 4, 325–242.

Felder, R.M. & Silverman, L.K. (1988) Learning and teaching styles in engineering education. *Engineering Education*, 78 (7), 674–681. (The article that originally defined the Felder–Silverman model and identified teaching practices that should meet the needs of students with the full spectrum of styles. The paper is preceded by a 2002 preface that states and explains changes in the model that have been made since 1988.)

Heisler, M., Vijan, S., Anderson, R., Ubel, P., Bernstein, S. & Hofer, T. (2003) When do patients and their physicians agree on diabetes treatment goals and strategies, and what difference does it make? *Journal of General Internal Medicine*, 18, 909–914.

International Alliance of Patients' Organisations (IAPO) (2005) *Declaration on Patient-Centred Care*. IAPO www.patientsorganisations.org/pchreview (accessed December 2007).

Kemp, E., Floyd, M., Mc-Cord-Duncan, E. & Lang, F. (2008) Patients prefer the method of 'tell back-collaborative inquiry' to asking for understanding of medical information. *Journal American Board Family Medicine*, 21 (1), 24–30.

Kolb, D. (1984) in Arndt, M. & Underwood, B. (1990) Learning style theory and patient education. *Journal of Continuing Education in Nursing*, 21 (1), 28–31.

Knight, K. & Donan, T. (2006) The diabetes educator: trying hard, but must concentrate more on behaviour. *Diabetic Medicine*, 23, 485–501.

Larson, C., Nelson, E., Gustafson, D. & Batalden, P. (1996) The relationship between meeting patients' information needs and their satisfaction with hospital care and general health status outcomes. *International Journal Quality Health Care*, 8, 447–456.

Lewin, S., Sea, Z., Entwhistl, V., Zwarenstein, M. & Dick, J. (2001) Interventions for providers to promote a patient-centred approach in clinical consultations. *Cochrane Database of Systematic Reviews*, (4), CD003267.

Linder, N., Menzies, D., Kelly, J., Taylor, S. & Shearer, M. (2003) Coaching for behaviour change in chronic disease: a review of the literature and the implications for coaching as a self-management intervention. *Australian Journal of Primary Health*, 9, 177–185.

Makoul, G. (2001) Essential elements of communication in medical encounters: the Kalamazoo consensus statement. *Academic Medicine*, 76, 390–393.

McKenna, K., Tooth, L., King, D., Clark, M., O'Rourke, P., Steinberg, M. & de Loose, F. (2003) Older patients request more information: a survey for use of written patient education materials in general practice. *Australian Journal on Aging*, 22 (1), 15–19.

Morris, A., Boyle, D., McMahon, A., Greene, S., MacDonald, T. & Newton, R. (1997) Adherence to insulin treatment, glycaemic control, and ketoacidosis in insulin-dependent diabetes mellitus. *Lancet*, 350, 1505–1510.

National Public Health Institute of Helsinki (2007) *The Goal Lifestyle Implementation Trial*. Helsinki, Finland.

Negarandeh, R., Oskouie, F., Ahmandi, F., Nikraves, M. & Rahmfallberg, I. (2006) Patient advocacy: barriers and facilitators. *BMC Nursing*, 5, 3. DOI: 10.1186/1472–6955-5-3.

Norman, C. & Skinner, H. (2006) The eHEALS: Health Literacy Scale. *International Medicine Internet Research*, 8, e27.

Page, P., Verstraete, D., Robb, J. & Etzwiler, D. (1981) Patient recall of self-care recommendations in diabetes. *Diabetes Care*, 4, 96–98.

Parikh, N., Parker, R., Nuss, J., Baker, D. & Williams, M. (1996) Shame and health literacy: the unspoken connection. *Patient Education and Counselling*, 17, 33–39.

Plank, J., Kohler, G., Rakovac, I., Semlitsch, B., Horvath, K., Bock, G., Kraly, B. & Pieber, T. (2004) Long term evaluation of a structured outpatient education programme for intensified

Insulin therapy in patients with type 1 diabetes a 12 year follow up *Diabeteologia*, 47, 1370–1375.

Parker, R., Baker, D., Williams, M. & Nuss, J. (1999) The test of functional health literacy in adults (TOFHLA): a new instrument for measuring patients' literacy skills. *Journal of General Internal Medicine*, 10, 537–545.

Parkin, T. & Skinner, T. (2003) Discrepancies between patient and professionals recall and perception of an outpatient consultation. *Diabetic Medicine*, 20, 909–914.

Partnership for Clear Health Communication (2006) What is health literacy? http://www.p4chc. org/health-literacy.aspx (accessed October 2007).

Redman, B. (2001) *The Practice of Patient Education*. Mosby, Toronto.

Rushford, N., Murphy, B., Worcester, M., Goble, A., Higgins, R., Le Grande, M., Rada, J. & Elliott, P. (2007) Recall of information received in hospital by female cardiac patients. *European Journal of Cardiovascular Prevention & Rehabilitation*, 14 (3), 463–469.

Skinner, T., Barnard, K., Craddock, S. & Parkin, T. (2007) Patient and health professional accuracy of recalled treatment decisions in out-patient consultations. *Diabetic Medicine*, 24, 557–550.

Tankova, T., Dakovska, G. & Koev, D. (2001) Education of diabetic patients – a one year experience. *Patient Education and Counselling*, 45, 139–145.

Thomas, N. (2001) The importance of culture throughout life and beyond. Holistic nursing practice. *The Science of Health and Healing*, 15 (2), 40–46.

Toobert, D., Hampson, S. & Glasgow, R. (2000) The summary of diabetes self-care activities measure: results from 7 studies and a revised scale. *Diabetes Care*, 23, 943–950.

Tope, R. (1998) The impact of interprofessional education in the south west region – a critical analysis. The literature review www.doh.gov.uk/swrp/tope.htm

Vaag, A., Handberg, M., Lauritzen, J., Pedersen, K. & Beck-Neilsen, H. (1990) Variation in absorption of NPH insulin due to intramuscular injection. *Diabetes Care*, 13 (1), 74–76.

Vale, M., Jelinek, M., Best, J., et al. (2003) Coaching patients On Achieving Cardiovascular Health (COACH): a multicenter randomized trial in patients with coronary heart disease. *Archives Internal Medicine*, 163, 2775–2783.

Wagner, E., Davis, C., Schaefer, J., Von Korff, M. & Austin, B. (2002) A survey of leading chronic disease management programs: are they consistent with the literature? *Journal Nursing Care Quality*, 16 (2), 67–80.

Weiss, B. (2007) Assessing health literacy in clinical practice. *Medscape*, http://www.medscape. com/viewprogram/802_pnt (accessed November 2007).

Yki-Jarvinen, H., Juurinen, L., Alvarsson, M., Bystedt, T., Caldwell, I., Davies, M., Lahdenpera, S., Nijpels, G. & Vahatalo, M. (2007) Initiate insulin by aggressive titration and educate (INITIATE). *Diabetes Care*, 30, 1364–1369.

Young, D., Furler, J., Vale, M., Walker, W., Segal, L., Best, J., Dunning, T., Blackberry, I., Audehm, R., Dunbar, J. & Chondros, P. (2007) Patient Engagement and Coaching for Health: the PEACH study – a cluster randomised controlled trial using the telephone to coach people with type 2 diabetes to engage with their GPs to improve diabetes care. *BMC Family Practice*, 8 (20), 8–13.

Chapter 17
Discharge Planning

Key points

- Commence early (on admission).
- Arrange follow-up care.
- Give relevant contact telephone numbers so people can seek advice after discharge if necessary.
- Ensure self-care knowledge is adequate.
- Ensure insulin and monitoring equipment are available.
- Ensure patient understands how and when to take medication.
- Communicate with appropriate health professionals/carers.

A discharge plan must be established and conducted in a proactive manner. It is important to incorporate discharge planning into the initial assessment and patient care plan, and to consider social and home needs, for example, prevent falls. It should look beyond the current episode of care in order to prevent readmission and relevant health professionals, family and carers should be informed of admission and discharge.

(1) Inform allied health professionals of admission on day one or two of admission (diabetes nurse specialist/diabetes educator, dietitian, podiatrist, social worker).
(2) Ensure self-care status has been assessed so that the patient is capable of caring for their own diabetes and will be safe at home.
(3) Refer for home assessment early if indicated.

On day of discharge

(1) Ensure patient has necessary medications and supplies, insulin delivery device, blood glucose testing equipment, fingerprick device and diabetic record book and understands their use, and where to obtain future supplies.
(2) Ensure relevant follow-up appointments have been made, and a discharge letter has been written to the GP.

(3) If further diagnostic investigations are to be performed on an outpatient basis ensure the patient has written instructions and understands what to do about medications and fasting and knows where to go for any investigations.
(4) Ensure the patient has a contact telephone number for assistance if necessary.
(5) Ensure the patient knows about the services offered by the Diabetes Association, and other relevant services, for example, meals-on-wheels, low vision clinic, rehabilitation services, community nurse for support especially when new to insulin and liaison with the diabetes nurse specialist/diabetes educator, counselling, and council services, for example, sharps disposal.

Transfer to another service, hospital or nursing home

In addition to the usual information provided relating to nursing and medical management the nursing letter accompanying the patient should contain information about:

- Diet.
- Progress of diabetes education.
  - Skills assessment for performing blood glucose testing and insulin administration.
  - Medication regimen.
  - Details of medical condition and nursing care.

Ensure transport has been arranged and that the family is aware of the discharge. Some nursing homes and special accommodation facilities may not have cared for people with diabetes in the past, or have done so on an infrequent basis. Diabetes education for the staff of the facility in this situation is desirable.

Chapter 18
Community, Practice Nursing, and Home-Based Care

Key points

- Practice nurses are playing an increasingly important role in diabetes care.
- Well established collaboration and referral procedures among health services and health service providers is essential.
- Community, practice and home care nurses are in an ideal position to deliver preventative health care education.

Introduction

Community care enables technical and professional care to be provided to acutely and chronically ill patients at home. The provision of specific services will be influenced by the home environment, the person's condition and capabilities, and available home support services. A nursing care plan should be prepared to complement the medical management plan.

Supporting people to enable them to remain at home is an important consideration of diabetic management. Practice nurses and community and home-care nurses play an important role in this respect.

These nurses also play and important role in supporting carers and identifying carer distress. A recent Australian study showed carers have lowest well being of any large societal group (Australian Unity 2008). Significantly, well being decreases as the number of hours spent providing care increases and women carers have lower levels of well being than male carers. The Australian Unity survey showed unpaid, largely family, carers provide ~$30.5 billion worth of care per year. Many carers have high levels of worry about their financial situations and their personal health that often results in depression. They often make significant lifestyle, family and work sacrifices in order to provide care. Many do not receive care for their own health issues, which include depression, chronic pain, injuries attributable to caring and many are overweight, which increases their risk of obesity-related diseases.

Diabetes-related care in the home includes:

- Preparing insulin doses.
- Administering insulin.
- Performing blood glucose tests.

- Assessing the general condition of the patient.
- Supporting the continuing education of the patient and of family/carers.
- Attending to wound dressings.
- Attending to personal hygiene.
- Assisting with medication management.
- Detecting deteriorating metabolic control, and functional and cognitive ability.

Making clinical decisions about the patient in the home situation without advice and support can be stressful and difficult. In addition, the home situation must be carefully assessed to ascertain how to obtain access to the home, and the correct address and telephone number. The safety of the nurse is an important consideration and issues such as the surrounding environment and household members should be assessed beforehand, if possible. The service base should have some idea of the route the nurse is likely to take. Other information (e.g. presence of dogs) should also be noted.

This chapter outlines the important diabetes-related information needed to gauge whether medical assessment is necessary.

How to obtain advice

It is important for home care and domiciliary nursing bodies to establish open communication links with the referring agency or practitioner.

The referring agency should be the first point of contact for advice.

General points

(1) Ensure diabetes teaching is consistent with that of the diabetes educator.
(2) Before recommending equipment, for example, meters, insulin delivery systems, ensure the person will be able to use it, can afford it and can obtain further supplies. This is particularly important if the person is visiting from another country or is travelling overseas where some brands of equipment may not be available. Assess:
    - vision
    - manual dexterity
    - comprehension.
    There may be costs associated with purchasing diabetes equipment and medications in some countries. It is important that the person understands the costs and any government initiatives to reduce/eliminate those costs.
(3) Ensure the patient is enrolled in the National Diabetes Services Scheme so that they can obtain syringes, lancets and test strips at the subsidised price (relevant only in Australia).

Diabetic problems commonly encountered in the home

(1) Finding an elevated blood glucose level.
(2) Hypoglycaemia.
(3) The patient has not taken their insulin/diabetes tablets.

(4) The patient does not follow the diabetes management plan.
(5) Management of wounds such as surgical wounds, trauma, and foot ulcers.
(6) Disposal of sharps (needles and lancets) in the home situation.
(7) How and where to obtain help/advice about specific patient problems.

Nursing actions

(1) Assess general clinical state (see Chapters 2 and 3).
(2) If the patient appears unwell, record:
  • temperature
  • pulse
  • respiration and presence of respiratory distress
  • blood pressure
  • colour.
(3) Assess presence, location, duration and severity of any pain and whether it is increasing or resolving.
(4) Note nausea, diarrhoea, and/or vomiting.
(5) Note presence of any symptoms of urinary tract infection but be aware there are often few, if any symptoms:
  • frequency
  • burning
  • scalding
  • itching.
(6) Assess state of hydration.
(7) Note time and dose of last diabetic medication.
(8) Note time and amount of last meal.
(9) Measure blood glucose level.

Interpreting the blood glucose level

To assess the diabetic status one must first ascertain whether the patient is in danger because of the blood glucose level. Ascertain:

• The present level.
• The usual blood glucose range.
• Why the blood glucose is outside the usual range. Whether the patient has suffered any illness, committed a dietary indiscretion, commenced on a new medication, missed a medication dose, or is using a complementary or self-prescribed medication.
• Whether it is likely to go up or down.

When ascertaining the blood glucose level check whether:

• The test was performed correctly.
• There was enough blood on the strip; if using a meter that the meter was calibrated and used correctly.
• The strips have exceeded the expiry date (see Chapter 4, Monitoring 1: blood glucose).
• The patient has commenced any new medication that could alter the blood glucose level (see Chapter 3).

The patient may require attention if the blood glucose level is:

- Low – hypoglycaemia <3 mmol/L.
- High – hyperglycaemia >17 mmol/L for a significant number of tests.

Hypoglycaemia

For more detailed information see Chapter 8.

(1) Treat according to the severity and time of occurrence of hypoglycaemia.
(2) Avoid over treatment.
(3) Give rapidly absorbed high GI glucose, if symptomatic, for example,:
    - glucose gel
    - orange juice
    - tea/coffee with sugar
    - jelly beans.
(4) Give more slowly absorbed low GI glucose, if the hypoglycaemia is asymptomatic and there is some time before the next meal is due.
(5) Suggest they have their meal if it is due in half an hour.
(6) Ensure patient has recovered before leaving the home. Check the blood glucose. Wash the person's hands before testing the blood glucose if they have been handling glucose to treat the hypoglycaemia.
(7) Record incident.

If severe follow the procedure for managing unconscious hypoglycaemia (Chapter 8). IM glucagon can be administered if it is available. If not, manage the airway and seek medical or ambulance assistance.

Practice point

The next dose of medication is not usually withheld.

Discuss recognition and treatment of hypoglycaemia with patient and family. Ensure that the person and/or their family and carers know how to manage hypoglycaemia, that there is appropriate food/fluids to manage hypoglycaemia and they know who to call in an emergency.

Hyperglycaemia

For more detailed information, see Chapter 7. Ascertain:

- How long the blood glucose level has been elevated.
- Whether the patient is unwell.
- Whether there are any symptoms of hyperglycaemia, for example, polyuria, polydipsia, thirst or lethargy.
- Whether there are ketones present in the urine.

If moderate/heavy ketones are detected seek medical advice (this usually only occurs in Type 1 people).

Check for any obvious source of infection:

- Urinary
- Foot ulcer wound
- Cold or flu.

Practice point

Infection can be present without any overt signs and symptoms.

Counsel the patient about managing at home when unwell. (Patient information guidelines are shown in Chapter 5.) The important points are that the patient should:

- Continue to take insulin or OHAs.
- Maintain fluid and carbohydrate intake.
- Test and record blood glucose regularly, for example, 2 to 4 hourly.

In addition:

(1) If the patient has Type 1 diabetes they should test their blood or urine for ketones every 4 hours.
(2) Maintain contact with the patient and liaise with the diabetes team.
(3) Advise them to seek medical advice if vomiting and/or diarrhoea occur, if the blood glucose continues to increase, if ketones develop in the urine or their conscious state changes.

The patient with chest pain

(1) Reassure the patient and family.
(2) Instruct the patient to stop current activity and to sit or lie down. Loosen tight clothing.
(3) Instruct patient to take anginine if prescribed by doctor.
(4) Assess the severity of the discomfort and the frequency of attacks.
(5) People with long-standing diabetes may have 'silent myocardial infarcts'. Complaints of vague chest discomfort should be investigated. The classic pain radiating into the jaw, arm, and chest may be absent.
(6) Seek medical advice/ambulance service.
(7) Record BP.
(8) Discuss decreasing risk factors for cardiac disease (see Chapter 8).

The patient who has not taken their prebreakfast insulin or diabetes tablets and it is '11 AM' or later

More than 80% of people miss medication doses (Morris *et al.* 2001; Gilbert *et al.* 2002). If medication is missed frequently, self-care capability, cognitive functioning and mental status (e.g. depression), beliefs about medications should be assessed. Often medications are missed or taken incorrectly because the person is given inaccurate, hurried or conflicting information or the information is presented in a format the person cannot read or does not understand.

Stopping medications without consulting a doctor and inappropriately altering doses is common (Kriev *et al.* 1999). Older people in particular make more mistakes including incorrect doses when drawing insulin up in a syringe (DeBrew *et al.* 1998). Home-based nursing services play a vital role in assisting elderly people to manage their medicines safely.

Medications that have long duration of action are less of a problem if a dose is missed than medications with short duration of action. Missing several consecutive doses of medicines with a narrow therapeutic index may lead to a loss of efficacy, for example, the effect of aspirin on platelet stickiness might be diminished. Time will be required to re-establish therapeutic blood concentrations if consecutive doses of medicines with a long half-life are missed.

(1) Check blood glucose level.
(2) Ascertain why the medication was omitted. Did the person omit other medicines due to prebreakfast?
(3) Ascertain whether this is a regular occurrence.
(4) Ascertain whether they have eaten breakfast, and what they ate.

In general, medication may need to be modified and the dose reduced. The amount will depend on the dose and types of insulin and the blood glucose level:

(1) If it is not appropriate to administer medicines, seek advice from the referring agency or the person's general practitioner.
(2) Document any medication adjustment.
(3) Have the order signed by the appropriate doctor within the specified time period, for example, 24 hours.
(4) Plan strategies with the individual that set out what to do if a dose is missed in future and set up cues to minimise the number of missed doses, for example, a reminder on the refrigerator door. Medical information leaflets are provided with medications when they are dispensed as part of the Quality Use of Medicines Program in Australia, but this may not be the case in other parts of the world, including the UK. These information leaflets often contain advice about what to do if a dose of the medicine is missed.

Readings <6.0 mmol/L may indicate good control and the usual dose should be taken. If non-diabetic medications have been missed the person should take their normal dose at the usual time.

If it is before 11 AM counsel the patient to check their blood glucose; if it is 6 mmol/L or above the patient should:

- Take usual medication dose and eat breakfast.
- Eat lunch within 3 to 4 hours then tea 3 to 4 hours after that.
- Have medication and breakfast at normal time the next day.

Follow-up visit
Ascertain whether:

- The patient followed advice.
- The management strategy was effective.
- Hypo/hyperglycaemia occurred as a result of missed medication and modified dose.
- Further dietary counselling is necessary.

Managing diabetic foot ulcers at home

Diabetic foot ulcers are a common complication of diabetes and occur as a result of peripheral neuropathy and vascular changes (see Chapter 8).

On first visit
(1) Ascertain the extent to which the individual can be involved in their care, for example, cleanliness, knowledge of foot care.
(2) Check treatment plan and medication prescriptions.
(3) Assess ulcer to obtain a baseline for future comparison:
   - dimensions: width:depth
   - type and quantity of discharge
   - colour of surrounding tissue
   - presence of oedema.
(4) Counsel patient to:
   (a) rest with foot elevated as much as possible.
   (b) protect foot:
      - bed cradle (stiff cardboard or polystyrene box)
      - appropriate footwear
      - regular inspection.
   (c) complete full course of antibiotics.
(5) Monitor blood glucose tests.

Subsequent visits
(1) Perform the dressing according to the prescription. The dressing may be:
   - dry
   - occlusive
   - or the wound may be cleaned and left open.
(2) Assess progress of the wound using objective documentation such as measuring the depth and width and amount and type of exudate.
(3) If the wound deteriorates:
   - note odour and amount and type of discharge
   - take a swab for culture and sensitivity

- record TPR
- record blood glucose level
- refer for assessment.

Practice points

If bandages are used ensure they are correctly applied and do not constrict the blood supply. People with neuropathy may not be able to tell if the bandage is too tight.

(1) Bandage from the foot upwards, even if the ulcer is on the leg.
(2) Do not put bandages or tape in a circular fashion around the toes.
(3) Never prick the toes to obtain a blood glucose test.
(4) Small wounds can hide deep infection including bone involvement.
(5) Swabs need to be taken from deep in the wound, not from the surface of the wound because mixed anaerobic and aerobic organisims are often present. Superficial swabs may not detect anaerobic organisms and delay appropriate treatment.

The patient who does not follow the management plan ('non-adherence'; see Chapters 15 and 16)

'Non-compliant' is a derogatory and negative term. There may well be good reasons why people do not follow prescribed treatment, including:

- A complicated regimen that the patient does not understand.
- Treatment goals are those of the management team and not the patient.
- Inability to comply (patient may not have a refrigerator, may suffer from low vision, or loss of fine motor skills).
- Cultural and language differences.
- Economic factors – cost of supplies.
- Non-acceptance of diabetes and constraints imposed on lifestyle.
- Other concerns may outweigh those about diabetes.
- 'Burnout'.
- Learned helplessness.

Counselling, education and appropriate modification of health professional expectations may help. Behavioural changes may take years; patient, supportive health professionals and family can assist the patient to eventually make some changes.

Disposing of sharps in the home situation

In the community the person with diabetes is responsible for the safe disposal of used needles and lancets. Thousands of diabetes needles are discarded every week, outside hospitals. All health professionals have a responsibility to promote the safe disposal of used sharps. The safe disposal of used needles, syringes and lancets should be an integral part of teaching injection technique and blood glucose monitoring.

Practice point

Ensure the patient understands what you mean by a 'sharp'.

Guidelines for handling and disposing of sharps at home

(1) Take care with sharps at all times.
(2) Store needles and lancets out of reach of children.
(3) Use a 'standards approved' container if possible (check with the local council about how to obtain one).
(4) Only recap your own syringe and lancet.
(5) Recapping of syringes and lancets is a good idea if an approved container is not available, for example, at a restaurant.
(6) If testing blood glucose for family/friends always use a new lancet.
(7) Check arrangements for disposal of full containers with:
  • your local diabetes association
  • your local council.
(8) If an approved container is not available it is advisable to:
  • recap needles and lancets
  • place immediately into a puncture-proof, unbreakable container, clearly labelled 'used sharps'
  • keep the container out of the reach of children
  • keep the lid tightly closed (Diabetes Australia 1999).

In the UK people are advised to use a safe-clip device to remove needles and to dispose of lancets in an opaque container.

Storing insulin

Insulin should be stored in the refrigerator if possible; *it should not be frozen*. The vial in use can be stored at room temperature if it is protected from heat and light and should be used within one month of opening. Any unused insulin stored at room temperature should be discarded after one month.

Practice point

If there is any change in appearance or consistency of the insulin, or if the expiry date is exceeded, discard the insulin.

Guidelines for premixing and storing insulin doses for home and district nursing services

General recommendations

Mixing and storing insulin for periods of 24 hours or more may be necessary for older people, those with poor vision and of those with limited hand mobility who live alone and where no other assistance is available.

The correct method of mixing short- and long-acting insulins is included in the Example Instruction Sheets at the end of Chapter 16 but other insulin administration devices may be more suitable, see Chapter 5.

The proportions to be mixed are prescribed by the doctor to suit individual patient requirements. In practice, biphasic insulin is frequently used in these situations.

Recommended guidelines

(1) Only use insulin syringes for drawing up insulin.
(2) The filled syringe should be stored:
   • in the refrigerator if possible or in a cool dark place
   • vertically or horizontally; they should not be stored with the needle pointing downwards which may cause clogging in the needle, preventing insulin being injected.
(3) Syringes should be rolled between the palms of the hands before administration to mix the contents.
(4) If the patient is on more than one injection per day the doses should be clearly understood by the patient. The doses should be clearly marked and stored separately from each other, for example, in plastic food storage containers marked 'morning' and 'evening' or with the administration times.
(5) Injection technique should be assessed periodically to ensure insulin administration is accurate, especially in people with low vision and those with unexplained hyperglycaemia.
(6) One extra dose could be drawn up in case of emergencies provided the patient understands that it is not an additional dose of insulin.
(7) Monitor blood glucose when visiting the patient.
(8) Any concerns about control, mental state or accuracy of technique should be discussed with the relevant doctor.
(9) Signed and dated records of all advance doses of insulin (type, dose, frequency of administration) should be maintained. All blood glucose results and insulin doses should be recorded and accompany the patient to medical appointments.
(10) Ensure there are enough supplies to last until the next visit.

Practice point

If the patient has required a period in hospital, unused previously drawn up doses of insulin should be discarded. A new batch should be drawn up when the patient is discharged.

Practice nurses

Practice nurses (PN) are nurses who provide nursing services in general practice. They have a broad and collaborative role with general practitioners (GP) and other health professionals. In Australia their role in diabetes education and management is expanding and enhances the range of services available to patients of the practice and collaboration with other service providers. Changes to the Medicare Benefits schedule has enabled funding for nurses to provide services such as wound care and managing chronic illness such as diabetes under GP management plans and team care arrangements, which can improve patient outcomes, deliver cost effective care (Raftery *et al.* 2005), increase the practice income (Australian Divisions of General Practice, undated) and is acceptable to patients (Cheek *et al.* 2002).

GP management plans are developed in collaboration with the patient with a chronic disease and encompass:

- Ensuring the individual does not already have a care plan and that they are eligible under the Medicare benefits Schedule.
- Discussing the process, benefits and costs with the individual and if relevant their carer.
- Undertaking a thorough assessment to identify current and predict future care needs.
- Develop a plan that is agreed with the patient and that identifies relevant management targets to be met and the self-care the patient needs to undertake in order to meet agreed management targets and the actions the GP needs to undertake.
- Document the management in the relevant places and communicate the plan to other relevant health professionals.
- Document a date to review the outcomes.

The individual may be eligible for a team care arrangement if they have complex care needs or are at significant risk of complications. Team care arrangement provide for interventions from a multidisciplinary team. The arrangements must involve the GP and at least two other health or community care providers. The process is essentially similar to the care plan process. The patient must have a GP management plan and a team care arrangement in place, or a current enhanced primary care plan, or the GP must make a contribution to a care plan developed for an older person in a residential aged care facility to be eligible to access Medicare for allied health and dental services.

Both PNs and GPs have unparralled access to a large proportion of the population and are in an ideal position to provide structured and opportunistic health promotion and illness prevention messages (Sim 2006). These include general and diabetes-specific primary prevention programmes as well as secondary prevention programmes such as complication screening and early initiation of medicines such as insulin in Type 2 diabetes, antihypertensive and lipid lowering agents when they are indicated.

References

Australian Divisions of General Practice (undated). Nursing in general practice business case models. www.adgp.com.au/site/index.cfm?display=4002.

Australian Unity (2008) Carers wellbeing lowest on record. *Australian Unity Journal*, August, 10–11.

Cheek, J., Price, K., Dawson, A., Mott, K., Beilby, J. & Wilkinson, D. (2002) Consumer perceptions of nursing and nurses in general practice. *University of South Australia*. November.

DeBrew, K., Barba, B. & Tesh, S. (1998) Assessing medication knowledge and practices of older adults. *Home Healthcare Nurse*, **16** (10), 688–691.

Gilbert, A., Roughead, L. & Sanson, L. (2002) I've missed a dose; what should I do? *Australian Prescriber*, **25** (1), 16–18.

Kriev, B., Parker, R., Grayson, D. & Byrd, G. (1999) Effect of diabetes education on glucose control. *Journal of the Louisiana State Medical Society*, **151** (2), 86–92.

Morris, A., Brennan, G., Macdonald, T. & Donnan, P. (2000) Population-based adherence to prescribed medication in Type 2 diabetes: a cause for concern. *Diabetes*, **40**, A76.

Raftery, J., Yao, G., Murchie, P., Campbell, N. & Ritchie, L. (2005) Cost effectiveness of nurse led secondary prevention clinics for coronary heart disease in primary care: follow up of a randomized controlled trial. *British Medical Journal*, **330**, 707–710.

Sim, M. (2006) Prevention: building on routine clinical practice. *Australian Family Physician*, **35** (1/2), 12–15.

St Vincent's Hospital (2001) Drawing up insulin doses for patients who are unable to draw up their own doses. Department of Endocrinology and Diabetes Policy Manual, Melbourne.

United Kingdom Royal College of Nursing Guidelines (1999a) Guidelines on premixing and preloading of insulin for patients to give at a later date.

United Kingdom Royal College of Nursing Guidelines (1999b) Guidelines on preparing and preloading of insulin for patients to give at a later date.

Chapter 19
Complementary and Alternative Therapies and Diabetes

Key points

Modern diabetes management philosophy is consistent with complementary therapy (CAM) philosophy, specifically, prevention, the central role of the individual in their care and empowerment.

- People with diabetes are high users of complementary therapies and are entitled to unbiased information about the benefits and risks CAM.
- Complementary therapies can work synergistically with conventional medicine to improve diabetes balance and quality of life provided the benefits and risks are considered in the context of the individual.
- Many herbal medicines have hypoglycaemic effects but do not assume people with diabetes use CAM to control blood glucose. Thus herb/medicine and herb/herb interactions and other adverse events can occur.
- Health professionals should ask about complementary therapy use during routine diabetes assessments especially when medicines are initiated or the dose is adjusted and prior to surgical and investigative procedures.

Rationale

Complementary therapy (CAM) use is increasing, as is the interest in integrative medicine. If used appropriately within a quality use of medicines (QUM) framework some CAM can help people with diabetes heal and become proactive and empowered participants in their diabetes management. CAM use is associated with both benefits and risks. An essential aspect of any management strategy is making informed decisions about the individual's level of risk and tailoring treatment to meet their needs.

CAM has both risks and benefits for people with diabetes undergoing surgery and having investigations. Not all CAM people use is medicines and not all CAM carry the same level of risk or confer equal benefits. Adopting an holistic QUM approach can optimise the benefits and reduce the risks. A key aspect of QUM is asking about and documenting CAM use. People with diabetes who use CAM need written advice about how to manage their CAM during the surgical/investigative period. People with diabetes and renal disease and those on anticoagulants are at particular risk if they use some CAM medicines.

Introduction

CAM use is increasing, possibly as part of the evolution of a new health paradigm as people try to solve modern health problems: chronic lifestyle diseases and depression. When people consider their therapeutic options they are likely to make choices that are congruent with their life philosophy, knowledge, experience, societal norms, and culture. Depending on these factors they may or may not choose to be actively involved in their care. Understanding these associations is important to understanding an individual's self-care, adherence, and empowerment potential. For example, there is a high correlation among health beliefs, spirituality and CAM use (Hildreth & Elman 2007). In addition, there is good evidence that CAM users adopt health-promoting self-care strategies, undertake preventative health care (Kelner & Welman 1997; Garrow *et al.* 2006), and believe responsibility for their health ultimately rests with them.

CAM is used by >50% of the general population and the rate of use is increasing in most western countries, particularly by people with chronic diseases, especially women educated to high school level or higher, those with poor health who often have a chronic disease, are employed, and are interested in self-care (Lloyd *et al.* 1993; MacLennan *et al.* 1996; Eisenberg 1998; Egede *et al.* 2002; MacLennan *et al.* 2002). The true prevalence of CAM use by people with diabetes is largely unknown. Old studies (Leese *et al.* 1997; Ryan *et al.* 1999) found approximately 17% of people with diabetes in diabetic outpatient settings used a range of CAM, particularly herbs, massage, and vitamin and mineral supplements such as zinc. People using CAM were satisfied with their chosen therapy even if it 'did not work'. Satisfaction with treatment improves well being (see Chapters 15 and 16). The researchers appeared to assume people used CAM to 'control their diabetes', however, the individuals concerned may have had different goals for using CAM from those assumed by conventional health professionals. Controlling blood glucose may not have been their primary aim. The author's experience in a diabetes service suggests that, in many cases, people use CAM to maintain health (prevention) as well as to manage conditions such as arthritis, stress, and the unpleasant symptoms of intercurrent illness and diabetes complications, for example, nausea, pain, anxiety, and depression.

More recently, Egede *et al.* (2002) found people with diabetes were more likely to use CAM than non-diabetics, as were people with other chronic conditions, in a national study in the USA. In particular, people with diabetes over 65 years were the most likely group to use CAM. The most commonly used CAM was nutritional advice, spiritual healing, herbal medicine, massage, and meditation. The high usage rates in people with diabetes are hardly surprising and accord with the established demographics of CAM users.

Many health professionals, especially nurses and general practitioners (GPs), are incorporating CAM into their practice to enrich and extend their practice and provide holistic care. Many nurses and GPs who use CAM in their practices do not have formal

Table 19.1   Commonly used complementary therapies.

Acupuncture	Meditation
Aromatherapy using essential oils for therapeutic purposes	Music
	Naturopathy
Ayurveda (traditional Indian medicine system uses several techniques such as herbal medicines, massage, diet, and exercise)	Nutritional therapies
	Pet therapy
	Reflexology
	Reiki
Chiropractic	Therapeutic Touch
Counselling (a range of techniques)	Traditional Chinese Medicine (uses several techniques such as herbs, cupping,
Herbal medicine (from several traditions – Indian, Chinese, North American, Australian Aboriginal, Japanese)	moxibustion, diet and exercise)[a]
Homeopathy	

[a]Often referred to as Chinese medicine in Australia. Many therapies are combined, for example, aromatherapy and massage. Likewise, traditional medical systems use a range of strategies in combination (CAM within CAM) and different diagnostic techniques instead of or in addition to conventional diagnostic processes, for example, tongue and pulse diagnosis. Often they are also combined with conventional care, formally and often informally, in self-prescribed regimens.

CAM qualifications and do not effectively document or monitor the outcomes of CAM usage. In addition, they often use CAM in their own healthcare. Dunning (1998) found that 50% of a sample of 37 diabetes nurse specialists/diabetes educators used CAM in their practice and none had a CAM qualification.

There are a great many CAMs ranging from well-accepted therapies with a research basis to 'fringe' therapies with little or no scientific evidence to support their use. Commonly used CAMs are shown in Table 19.1. The public interprets the term 'CAM' differently from health professionals and CAM and conventional practitioners and researchers use different definitions, which makes it difficult to compare studies. Several definitions and categories exist. The Cochrane collaboration defined CAM as:

> All health systems, modalities and practices and their accompanying theories and beliefs, other than those intrinsic to the politically dominant health system of a particular society or culture in a given historical period. They include all such practices and ideas self-defined by their users as preventing or treating illness or promoting health and well being. *The boundaries within and between* complementary therapies are not always sharp or fixed.
>
> (Cochrane Collaboration 2000)

Likewise, several terms are used to refer to CAM including complementary and alternative medicine (CAM), traditional medicine and non-scientific therapies. These terms are generally understood to mean therapies that are not part of conventional medicine. As the Cochrane definition indicates, the status of CAM is not fixed and some CAMs become part of conventional medicine as the evidence base for their safety and efficacy accumulates, for example, acupuncture.

CAM philosophy

The various CAM have a common underlying philosophy. Current diabetes person-centred empowerment strategies that focus on effective professional–patient partnerships, good communication, and preventative healthcare are consistent with this philosophy. CAM philosophy embodies the notion that:

- Each individual is unique, thus there is no single 'right' way to manage their health problems.
- Balance is important.
- The body has the capacity to heal itself. Healing is not synonymous with treating, managing or curing. The word is derived from the Anglo Saxon 'haelen', to make whole. Likewise, health is derived from the Anglo Saxon 'haelth' from 'hal', which also means to make whole. To achieve healing all parts and polarities need to be integrated – mind, body, and spirit within the individual's social environment.
- Healing occurs by intent.
- A positive attitude is important to health and well being. Positivity encompasses resilience, the capacity to overcome adversity and find meaning and purpose in life (transcendence). Thus, resilience is an essential aspect of healing, particularly in chronic diseases (Lloyd 2006).
- The client–therapist relationship is a key aspect of the healing process.
- The therapist's role is to support the innate healing potential of the individual.
- The mind, body, and spirit cannot be separated – what affects one affects the others (mind–body medicine). The mind-body-spirit model is embodied in eastern medical philosophy and 'encompasses fundamental and universal elements of well being' (Chan *et al.* 2006).
- Illness represents an opportunity for positive change (transcendence).

The following core Hippocratic tenets underpin CAM philosophy, particularly naturopathy, but they apply to all health care:

(1) *Vis medicatrix naturae* – the healing power of nature.
(2) *Primum non nocere* – first do no harm.
(3) *Tolle causam* – treat the cause.
(4) Treat the whole person.
(5) *Docere* – the doctor is a teacher.
(6) Prevention is the best cure.

Practice point

Healing does not mean curing. It refers to a process of bringing the physical, mental, emotional, spiritual, and relationship aspects of an individual's self together to achieve an integrated balance where each part is of equal importance and value (Dossey *et al.* 1998). Disruption to any aspect affects the others.

Understanding CAM philosophy is important to understanding why people use CAM. They seek answers to their health problems that match their existing beliefs and explanatory models and their health choices are part of their larger orientation on life and are not made in isolation from their beliefs and attitudes. They frequently mix and match CAM with CAM and CAM with conventional therapies to suit their needs. Adverse events can arise when due consideration is not given to the potential effects of such combinations, for example, potentially damaging medicine/herb interactions. Alternatively, CAM can enhance the effects of conventional medicines, allow lower doses of medicines to be used, reduce unwanted side effects and improve healing rates (Braun 2001).

Integrating complementary and conventional care

Quality use of medicines (QUM) is a useful framework for safely integrating health options including the broad categories of CAM and conventional care (see Chapter 5). QUM is congruent with CAM philosophy. QUM is essentially a decision-making framework to achieve optimal heath care including medicines if they are indicated, that encompasses, prevention, lifestyle strategies, and risk management. QUM is an holistic, integrated framework that recognises not everybody requires medicines to maintain health.

Integrative medicine (IM) is becoming increasingly popular among health professionals, although it was originally consumer-driven. CAM and integrative medicine (IM) are not synonymous terms. IM focuses on providing best practice conventional medicine, prevention, and emotional wellbeing, thus it might encompass CAM. Likewise, QUM is not concerned with either/or choices but with providing holistic care by helping the individual make informed choices about the best way to maintain optional health. IM is defined as:

> The blending of conventional medicine and complementary medicines and/or therapies with the aim of using the most appropriate of either or both modalities to care for the patient as a whole.
>
> (Australian Integrative Medicine Association)

IM is concerned with wellness and is a flexible approach to responding to the individual and societal factors impacting on health care. The specific therapies used in IM depend on the individual, objective evidence for benefit and risk, consideration of alternative choices (QUM), cost/benefit, practitioner experience and knowledge, and/or the need to refer to other practitioners.

Significantly, ~80% of the global population depends on herbal medicines and traditional medical systems (WHO 2002) although the medicines and systems may be different among countries and cultures. Migration and refugee displacement through war and natural disasters mean the types of CAM available outside the country of origin is increasing. Individuals import some in their new countries and these products may not be subject to good manufacturing practice or other relevant regulations that control many of the systems-related risks.

Many health institutions are concerned with regulatory and supply issues as well as benefits and risks as part of the safe use of CAM. The degree and processes for regulating CAM therapies, products and practitioners varies from country-to-country and from therapy-to-therapy. Frequently there are no formal regulatory processes in place but some CAM professional associations have stringent training and ongoing professional development requirements as part of self-regulation. Some require competence in first aid, for example, the International Federation of Aromatherapists.

The safe, effective combination of conventional and CAM care involves considering the following issues:

- The safety of the client, allowing for their personal choices.
- Facilitating people to make informed choices based on understanding the risks and benefits involved when using CAM, especially combining CAM and conventional care. When the patient is not competent to consent, guardianship issues may arise.
- The knowledge and competence of health professionals to give advice about CAM and how to refer to a suitably qualified practitioner if necessary. CAM needs to be appropriate to the individual's physical, mental, and spiritual status and selected after considering all the options, after a thorough assessment considering potential interactions with conventional therapies. The continued suitability of CAM, like all management strategies, should be reviewed regularly because diabetes is a progressive disease and continued use may be dangerous, e.g. in people with renal and liver disease (see Chapters 8 and 10). Conventional medicine doses should be monitored and may need to be changed.
- Guidelines should be followed where they exist and consent is required in some settings. Policies and guidelines need to include processes for communication between CAM and conventional practitioners and for collaboration and referral mechanisms to prevent fragmented care (Dunning 2001). Where possible, guidelines should be evidence-based to support best practice. They should not be prescriptive and inflexible.
- Processes for monitoring outcomes and accurately documenting the effects of the therapy should be in place and objective data relevant to the aims of the therapy, should be collected.
- Ensuring that safe quality products are used is important. Dose variations, contamination and/or adulteration with potentially toxic substances such as heavy metals, and unsubstantiated claims made about the product can lead to serious adverse events including irreversible kidney failure (Ko 1998; Bjelakovic *et al.* 2007).
- Safety data information should be available where possible and could be included with research papers or medication reference books in a portfolio on the ward.
- It is important that an accurate diagnosis is made and a thorough health history and assessment have been carried out prior to using any therapy. These considerations are often overlooked, especially when the person with diabetes self-diagnoses and self-treats. Such practices can result in delays in instituting appropriate management and deteriorating metabolic control.

These considerations apply equally to the selection and use of conventional therapies.

Practice points

(1) There is an increasing body of scientific evidence as well as a large body of traditional evidence for many CAM. However, evidence about the *combination* of CAM and conventional medicines is not well documented.
(2) Many, but not all, CAM have a strong evidence base of traditional use but this is not the same as 'scientific evidence'. In addition, modern technology has changed the traditional method of manufacturing, administering, and monitoring some CAM therapies. Therefore, the traditional evidence base needs to be considered in the light of any such changes.
(3) There are methodological flaws in a great deal of CAM research. However, the same is true of a great deal of conventional research.

Can complementary therapies benefit people with diabetes?

Managing diabetes effectively is about achieving balance. To achieve balance a range of therapies used holistically, is needed. For example Type 2 diabetes is a progressive, multifactorial disease, thus a single strategy is unlikely to address the underlying metabolic abnormalities or the consequent effects on mental health and well being. From a general perspective CAM can assist people with diabetes to:

- Incorporate diabetes into the framework of their lives, which encompasses two key aspects of spirituality: transformation and connectedness.
- Accept and manage their diabetes to achieve balance in their lives by reducing stress and depression, which can help them achieve management targets (balance) and reduce hepatic glucose output and insulin resistance. That is address spirituality, resilience and coping.
- Develop strategies to recognise the factors that cause stress and methods to prevent stress from occurring.
- Take part in decision-making, increase their self-esteem, self-efficacy and sense of being in control by improving their quality of life and enabling personal growth and transformation.
- Increase insulin production and reduce insulin resistance, either by the direct effects of the therapy, by reducing stress, or by enhancing the effects of conventional medications.
- Manage the unpleasant symptoms of diabetic complications such as pain and nausea.
- Preventative health care, for example, foot care to maintain skin integrity and prevent problems such as cracks that increase the potential for infection and its consequences.
- Teaching and learning situations to enhance learning, retention and recall.

Some specific benefits for people with diabetes have also been reported. They include:

(1) A reduction in blood glucose levels in children being given regular massage by their parents. The parents reported reduced anxiety levels in themselves (Field *et al.* 1997). Massage has also been shown to reduce pain intensity, unpleasantness, and anxiety in postoperative patients in the short term, especially in the first four days (Mitchison 2007). Likewise, yoga and meditation reduce features of the metabolic syndrome such as waist circumference, systolic blood pressure, fasting blood glucose and triglycerides, as well as improve mental health (Agrawal *et al.* 2007; Kjellgren *et al.* 2007).

(2) Many herbs have been shown to lower blood glucose by various mechanisms, HbA_{1c} and lipids, for example, American ginseng (*Panex quinquefolius*) (Vuksan *et al.* 2000); Gymnema/gurmar (*Gymnema sylvestre*) (Baskaran *et al.* 1990), fenugreek (*Trigonella foenum-graecum*) (Sharma *et al.* 1990, 1996), chromium picolinate (Finney *et al.* 1997). These herbs and supplements have primarily been used in Type 2 diabetes, but fenugreek has also been shown to lower blood glucose in Type 1 diabetes (Sharma *et al.* 1990). Chromium possibly has a role in reducing insulin resistance. It is excreted in urine at a faster rate in people with diabetes than non-diabetics, thus a relative chromium deficiency may contribute to insulin resistance (Udani *et al.* 2006). The evidence for a glucose lowering effect of chromium is confusing and may depend on the formulation used and the dosage. People who use chromium report improved blood glucose levels but the required dose may be higher than that usually used (400 μg): at least ~5000 μg chromium picolinate is probably required (Udani *et al.* 2006). Martin *et al.* (2006) compared chromium picolinate 1000 μg plus either glipizide or placebo for 24 weeks and reported lower fasting and post prandial glucose, HbA_{1c} less weight gain and less body fat measured using DEXA. Herbal medicines are also used in diabetes-related conditions such as heart failure *Crataegus species* (hawthorn) (Pittler & Ernst (2007); gastrointestinal reflux (peppermint) (Chaudhary 2007).

(3) Manage weight. Some CAM weight loss medicines and dietary strategies are beneficial, others are associated with significant risks and they should not be self-prescribed or used indiscriminately. Both the FDA in the US and the AMA in Australia have warned the public about the safety of many weight loss preparations. Weight loss requires and integrated approach that encompasses diet and exercise (see Chapter 4). The Diet-Pill-Study group regularly monitors conventional and complementary 'diet pills' and evaluates them according to set criteria for safety and efficacy and also evaluates the company marketing the product. Three products recently met the criteria: (*Hoodia gordonii* plus, Dietrine, and herbal Phentermine. In particular, products containing ephedra may lead to adverse events. Einerhand (2006) found conjugated linoleic acid (CLA) led to weight loss from the abdomen in men and women and women also lost weight from the thighs. Insulin sensitivity was not affected. The clinical significance of this finding is not clear. CAM therapies frequently used with CAM weight loss medicines include yoga, meditation, acupuncture, massage and Eastern martial arts (Sharpe *et al.* 2007). There is good pooled data to support small weight loss associated with Chromium picolinate but it is not a replacement for diet and exercise.

(4) Remain active. The benefits if Tai Chi in improving strength, balance, and mood in older people is well documented (Chou *et al.* 2004). Muscle wasting and

reduced strength in the lower limbs is associated with advancing age and can lead to inactivity and contribute to falls. Tai Chi can be combined with a healthy diet, resistance training, correcting malnutrition, and controlling blood glucose and lipids. Recent research suggests creatine supplementation may enhance the effects of resistance training but the clinical relevance has yet to be determined (O'Mathuna 2007).

(5) Acupuncture can improve the pain of diabetic peripheral neuropathy (Abuaisha *et al.* 1998). Acupuncture has also been shown to be equivalent to monotherapy at reducing mild to moderate hypertension if it is performed by expert practitioners (Flachskampf 2007). Glucosamine and chondroitin are widely used to manage arthritic and joint pain. There is no evidence that oral dosing contributes significantly to hyperglycaemia.

(6) There is a range of biofeedback, relaxation and counselling therapies that can reduce stress by attenuating the effects of increased autonomic activity and catecholamine production. Improved mood and reduced blood glucose levels have been reported with biofeedback (McGrady *et al.* 1991). Exercise also plays a key role. There is good evidence that St John's Wort (*Hypericum perforatum*) effectively improves mild-to-moderate depression and is better tolerated than conventional antidepressants. Recent research suggests it is as effective as paroxetine in moderate to severe depression (Szegede *et al.* 2005). However, St John's Wort interacts with many conventional medicines, thus a medication review before commencing the medicine and its use should be monitored.

(7) Antioxidant therapies receive significant press coverage. There is accumulating evidence that oxidation plays a role in the development of many diseases including vascular disease due to the development of oxidative stress and free radicals (see Chapter 8). For example, O'Brien & Timmins (1999) and Verdejo *et al.* (1999) suggested antioxidants may delay the progression of retinopathy by increasing blood flow to eyes and kidneys (vitamin E) and/or replenishing vitamin E (vitamin C), and/or improving nerve function (the B group vitamins). Other researchers suggest free radicals might be markers of disease rather than the cause, and that eliminating them may interfere with normal defense mechanisms (Bjelakovic *et al.* 2007). Antioxidants are also associated with adverse events and medicine interactions especially in the high doses often used. However, consensus has not been reached about the benefits of using antioxidants, the dose needed and when in the course of diabetes they should be used.

(8) Prevent illness. For example cranberry preparations, which prevents bacteria sticking to the bladder wall can reduce UTIs over a 12-month period particularly in women who suffer recurrent UTIs (Jepson *et al.* 2008). Cranberry juice may also effectively control *Helicobacter pylori* (Zhange *et al.* 2005).

(9) In 2000 the media reported that baths could help reduce blood glucose levels. The claims have not been substantiated and there could be risks such as postural hypotension, falls, and burns to neuropathic feet if the water is too hot. Faster uptake of injected insulin or reduced stress levels could be methods whereby blood glucose is reduced.

(10) Aromatherapy can be used to enhance well being and relaxation and to reduce stress, which benefits metabolic control. It can also be used for physical conditions such as alleviating pain, reducing hypertension, improving sleep, and foot care. Aromatherapy may also alleviate stress during procedures such as CAT scans, and

post-cardiac surgery (Stevenson 1994, Buckle 1997). Managing stress improves the individual's quality of life and psychological wellbeing. Aromatherapy is beneficial for fragrancing the environment to increase work performance, reduce absenteeism and reduce keyboard errors. In this respect the benefit is for the health professionals and organisations rather than an individual but it can have a role in diabetes education sessions. Aromatherapy is often combined with music and massage. There is a strong link between touch and aroma and wellbeing. In aged care settings aromatherapy is used to reduce pain, improve sleep, maintain skin integrity and manage behavioural problems (Thompson 2001). Significantly, difficulty identifying odours may be an early sign of Alzheimer's disease and precedes signs of cognitive dysfunction (Wilson *et al.* 2007). Wilson *et al.* showed that every 1 point decrease in the odour identification score represents an 18% risk of mild cognitive impairment progressing to Alzheimer's disease.

Clinical observation

The powerful effect of odour on physical and mental well being is often overlooked. On a practical level, several media reports about dogs being able to recognise when their owners with diabetes were hypoglycaemic and alert them early enough to enable the people to manage the episode themselves, or to alert another person occurred in late 2001. Guide dogs for visually impaired people are standard therapy and help visually impaired people to lead independent lives. Are 'hypo dogs' the way of the future?

Spirituality

Spirituality is a neglected aspect of conventional health care and is often confused with religion. The two are quite different although spirituality may encompass religion and prayer and religion may encompass spirituality. Information already presented in this chapter demonstrates that spirituality is central to optimal self-care. There are many definitions of spirituality. Most encompass the following core aspects:

- Positive empowering aspect of being human
- Quest for meaning, purpose
- Transcendence
- Holistic perspective
- Connectedness
- Resilience and confidence to turn crises into opportunities for personal growth.
- Synergy – all components work together and small changes in one component can positively or negatively affect all other components

These are essential to effective diabetes management. Recently Parsian & Dunning (2008 a,b) validated a tool for assessing spirituality and coping in young people with diabetes and demonstrated a significant association among spirituality, coping, and lower HbA_{1c}. Females were more spiritual than males and there was no significant association between religion and spirituality.

CAM and surgery

CAM usage is high among surgical patients, >51%; especially women aged 40–60 years, and is often used on the advice of friends (Tsen *et al.* 2000; Norred *et al.* 2000) (see Chapter 9). There are some well-documented benefits of using CAM to improve the health outcomes of people undergoing surgery. For example, foot massage using essential oils reduced stress and anxiety post CAGS (Stevenson 1994) and MRI-associated claustrophobia and stress. Massage reduced postoperative pain intensity, pain unpleasantness, and anxiety during the first four post operative days (Mitchinson 2007). Acupuncture and peppermint or ginger tea reduces nausea, and a range of strategies can relieve pain and improve sleep. Early research suggests prophylactic CQ_{10} prior to cardiac surgery improves postoperative cardiac outcomes (Rosenfeldt *et al.* 2005).

However, the risks also need to be considered in the context of the individual, the type of procedure and the overall management plan. Significant risks include bleeding, hypo or hypertension, sedation, cardiac dysrhythmias, renal damage, and electrolyte disturbances (Norred *et al.* 2000, 2002). Many conventional medicines need to be adjusted or ceased prior to surgery. There is less information about managing CAM medicines in surgical settings but there is a growing body of evidence to suggest that many CAM medicines may also need to be stopped or adjusted before surgery. Thus, it is important for conventional practitioners to ask about CAM use, although most do not (Braun *et al.* 2006).

The following general information is relevant to people already using CAM medicines and those considering using them before or after surgery. People are advised to consult a qualified CAM practitioner for specific advice. Self-prescribing is not recommended because many CAM medicines require supervised use especially in the context of the complex metabolic and neuroendocrine response to surgery.

Before surgery

People need written information about how to manage CAM medicines in the operative period. Conventional health professionals can provide such information if they are qualified to do so. They should refer the person to a qualified CAM practitioner if they do not have the relevant information. People also require written instructions about how to manage their conventional medicines as well as any special preparation needed for the surgery or investigation.

Great care is needed if the surgery is major or high risk such as heart, orthopaedic, or neurosurgery, if the person has renal or liver disease, or is very young or elderly. The conventional medication list is unlikely to include CAM medicines or supplements, although it should, thus health professionals should discuss CAM use with people during a structured medicines preoperative health assessment.

Some CAM medicines such as evening primrose oil, bilberry, cranberry, fish oils, ginger, Gingko, liquorice, guarana, willow bark, meadowsweet, and ginseng need to be stopped at least one week before surgery. St John's Wort and supplements such as vitamin E should be stopped two weeks before surgery, primarily because of the risk of bleeding. Some, such as St John's Wort, need to be stopped gradually (like conventional antidepressants). However, where CAM medicines are the main form of treatment, alternative management may be required to prevent the condition deteriorating and affecting the surgical outcome, for example, glucose lowering herbal medicines.

Some commonly used CAM medicines might/do interact with some anaesthetic agents and prolong their sedative effects, others increase the risk of bleeding, some affect blood pressure and the heart rate, others cause changes in the major electrolytes, potassium, calcium and sodium, levels in the blood. Grapefruit juice interferes with the action of some antibiotics such as cyclosporine, which may be needed pre or postoperatively. Not everybody experiences such problems and it is sometimes difficult to predict who will or will not have problems. General safety issues also need to be considered.

Some hospitals have policies about using CAM although they may not address surgery, investigations or diabetes specifically. People who wish to continue using CAM in hospital should clarify with the relevant hospital before they are admitted. Most do not prescribe or supply CAM.

In addition to managing medicines, achieving the best possible health status before surgery improves recovery afterwards. The preoperative assessment is an ideal time to revise the importance of eating a healthy balanced diet and exercise within the individual's capability to control blood glucose and lipids as well as to support the immune system and enhance wound healing. Most people should continue their usual physical activity unless it is contraindicated to maintain strength and flexibility. Stress management strategies such as meditation, guided imagery, essential oil massage or inhalations, and music help reduce anxiety and fear about the surgery. Ginger capsules or tablets taken one hour before surgery reduces postoperative nausea (Gupta & Sharma 2001).

The preoperative assessment is also an ideal time to discuss postoperative recovery including pain and sleep management. CAM may be a useful alternative to some conventional medicines provided a quality use of medicines framework is adopted.

After surgery

A range of CAM strategies can be used to manage pain and most are less likely to cause constipation and drowsiness than pethidine and morphine-based medicines. Alternatively, if these medicines are the best method of managing pain, high fibre CAM medicines such as *Aloe vera* juice, probiotics, and psyllium can reduce constipation once oral feeding is allowed. Probiotics also increase bowel health and support natural bowel flora. Peppermint or ginger tea reduces mild-to-moderate nausea. Lymphatic drainage massage is very effective after some surgery to reduce swelling and relieve pain. Valerian, hops and lavender in a vapourised essential oil blend or massage promote restful sleep without the side effects of some conventional sedatives.

Some CAM products promote wound healing, for example, *Aloe vera*, Medihoney, and calendula and could be used depending on the wound. Arnica ointment reduces bruising but should not be used on open wounds. Comfrey poultices are very effective at reducing local oedema and local pain but should not be used on open wounds or taken internally.

After surgery the person needs information about whether and when it is safe to start using CAM again. New conventional medicines might be prescribed or dose and or dose intervals of medicines taken preoperatively might change, for example, anticoagulants, which could influence the choice of CAM medicines or the dose. Likewise, some non-medicine CAM might need to be used with care such as needle acupuncture and deep tissue massage because they can cause bruising and/or bleeding.

Adverse events

Adverse events encompass safety, which is a complex multifactorial issue, see Table 19.2. Using QUM strategies significantly reduces the risk of adverse events. These may be

Table 19.2 Medicine-related safety and quality use of CAM and conventional medicines involves considering all of the inter-related issues outlined in the table.

Issue	Considerations for practitioners
Health system at global, national and local levels	Degree of product regulation including manufacture and marketing. Affordability and accessibility of medicines. Support for research. Evidence based guidelines to support use. Adverse event monitoring systems. Pre- and post-market surveillance systems including adverse event reporting systems. Medicine scheduling systems. Marketing processes. Methods of communicating important medicine-related information to the public.
Practitioner	Education and competence including ongoing professional development. Regulation and self-regulatory processes, which includes scope of practice. Licences to practice Professional liability insurance. Communication, documentation, and referral processes. Attitudes towards and beliefs about medicines and CAM.
Herbal medicines	Research and development. Pre- and post-market testing surveillance. Manufacturing practices including herb identification, handling, storing, and infection control procedures, and whether the herb is prepared according to the traditional method. Adulteration and contamination. Labels. Adverse event monitoring including interactions. Inappropriate dose and/or dose interval. Prescribing to at risk groups. Contraindicated.
Person with diabetes	Age. Physical and mental health status. Knowledge. Not disclosing herbal medicine use. Self-diagnosis and self-treatment, which can delay treating serious problems. Storage and handling of medicines. Inappropriate use of medicines and CAM. Monitoring defined outcomes False hope of cure or control. Polypharmacy. Cost.

general or diabetes specific. Diabetes-specific adverse events associated with CAM reported in the literature include:

- Stopping insulin in a person with Type 1 diabetes leading to ketoacidosis (Gill *et al.* 1994).
- Trauma and burns to neuropathic feet and legs from cupping and moxibustion (Ewins *et al.* 1993)
- Allergies, drug/herb interactions and hospital admissions, largely from adulterated traditional Chinese medicine (Beigel & Schoenfeld 1998; Ko 1998).
- Hypoglycaemia following prolonged massage and using herbal therapies.
- Bleeding from herb/anticoagulant interactions, see Table 19.3.
- Kidney and liver damage, see Chapter 8.
- Heavy metal poisoning (Keen *et al.* 1994).

A number of initiatives have been taken to limit some of these problems, for example, in 1991 the World Health Organisation developed guidelines for the safe use, manufacturing and labelling of plant medicines, the Chinese Government introduced strategies for identifying the content of Chinese herbal medicines and global strategies are in place to protect endangered animal and plant species as well as to improve the quality of CAM research.

Herb/medicine interactions

There are four main potential mechanisms for herb/medicine interactions. Herbs can:

(1) Induce production of liver enzymes, especially the cytochrome P450 system, which reduces medicine availability.
(2) Induce intestinal D-glycoprotein, which inhibits medicine absorption and metabolism.
(3) Stimulate neurotransmitter production especially serotonin enhancing the effects of some medicines, i.e. they both do the same thing. Others decrease the effects of serotonin-inhibiting medicines (Braun 2001).
(4) Compete with medicines for binding sites on serum protein increasing the amount of free medicine available. People with low serum albumin are especially at risk, for example, the older people and those with malnutrition.

Herb/medicine interactions are a two-way street – alone neither the medicine nor the herb might be a problem, but when used together, the *combination* can be potentially dangerous. However, the other ingredients in the medicine might also be responsible for the adverse effects, for example, incipients, preservatives, and contaminants. It should also be noted that liver failure (20–30%) and kidney damage (30%) are recognised serious side effects of readily available conventional medicines, but the benefits are considered to outweigh the risks.

Table 19.3   Commonly used herbs and supplements, their potential interactions, reported adverse events and some management strategies to use should an adverse event occur. Many of these interactions are theoretical, others are well documented. When considering the likelihood of an interaction, the total individual situation and medication regimen must be considered. In addition, although 'medicine interactions' is usually used to denote negative interactions, the term itself is objective and non-judgmental. Many interactions may actually be beneficial and it is just as important to document these.

Herb	Potential interactions	Reported adverse events	Management strategies
Echinacea	Hepatoxic medicines, for example, anabolic steroids, amiodarone, methotrexate, ketaconazole	Allergic reactions especially in atopic people	Do not use continuously for >8 weeks at a time
	Immunosuppressants, for example, corticosteroids, cyclosporin	Impairs the action of immunosuppressive drugs	
		Can cause immunosuppression if taken long-term	
		In acute surgery impairs wound healing	
Garlic	Aspirin	Risk of bleeding especially when taken with anticoagulants	Discontinue 7 days before surgery
	Warfarin	Increased GIT activity	Do not use concomitantly with antacids
	Cholesterol lowering agents	Decreased effectiveness of antacids	
		Inhibits platelet aggregation	
		Additive effects	
Gingko biloba	Aspirin	Bleeding risk if used with anticoagulants	Stop 36 hours before surgery
	Warfarin		Do not use concurrently
	SSRI		
	MAO inhibitors		
Fenugreek	Anticoagulants	Bleeding	Do not use concurrently
	Oral hypoglycaemic agents	Hypoglycaemia	Monitor
			Adjust dose of OHA or the herb

Complementary therapy	Interacts with	Effects	Action
Ginseng *Note:* there are several species in common use	Corticosteroids Oral contraceptives Warfarin Digoxin Oral hypoglycaemic agents MAO inhibitors and tricyclic antidepressants	Increased risk of bleeding with anticoagulants Suppresses immune system – infections risk Hypoglycaemia Headache Additive effects	Stop 7 days before surgery Do not use concomitantly
Ginger	Antacids Warfarin	Decreased effectiveness of antacids	Do not use at the same time
Guar and bulking agents	Antibiotics Alpha-glucosidase inhibitors	Decreased food absorption – hypoglycaemia risk	Do not administer at the same time
Glucosamine		GIT complaints Allergy if allergic to seafoods Nausea, vomiting abdominal pain Sleepiness Hyperglycaemia	Avoid with seafoods
Zinc	Increased HbA$_{1c}$ in Type 1 diabetes		
Valerian, hops	Anaesthetic agents Barbiturates Hypnotics Antidepressive medicines	Enhance/potentiate the effects of sedatives With long-term use the amount of anaesthetic needed is increased	Withdrawal – symptoms resemble valium addiction Taper dose preoperatively
St John's Wort	MAO inhibitors SSRI Decreases effect of HIV medications Warfarin Anticonvulsants Activates liver enzyme, hastening drug metabolism and reducing their effectiveness	Alters metabolism of some medicines, for example, cyclosporin, warfarin, steroids Interacts with psychotrophic drugs and can increase their effect Skin allergies	Stop 5 days before operation Do not use concomitantly

(*Continued*)

Table 19.3 Continued.

Herb	Potential interactions	Reported adverse events	Management strategies
Slippery elm		Decrease GIT absorption Hypoglycaemia	
Vitamin supplements C & E, B group; often as antioxidants	Vitamin toxicity Niacin	Decreases the beneficial effects of statins on HDL levels	
Feverfew	NSAIDS, warfarin, offset the herb's effect for migraine and might alter bleeding time	Changed bleeding time	
Hawthorn	Antihypertensive agents Digoxin Alcohol, Antipsychotics	Hypotension Dizziness Falls	
Kelp (contains iodine)	Thyroid hormones Antithyroid hormones	Altered thyroid function	
Liquorices	Corticosteroids Antihypertensive agents Oral contraceptives Digoxin	Fluid retention Electrolyte imbalance Block oestrogen in contraception Digoxin toxicity	

People most at risk of herb/medicine interactions are those who.

- are taking medicines with a narrow therapeutic window such as lithium, phenytoin, barbiturates, warfarin and digoxin and high risk medicines such as insulin
- are at risk of, or have, renal and/or liver damage and therefore, have altered ability to metabolise and excrete medicine
- have atopic conditions such as allergies, asthma or dermatitis
- are elderly
- are children
- are taking >5 medicines (polypharmacy)
- take alcohol or drugs of addiction
- lack knowledge or consult practitioners who lack knowledge about appropriate therapies to use. This includes CAM and conventional practitioners
- self-diagnose, delay seeking medical advice, do not tell conventional or CAM practitioners about the therapies/medicines they are using
- import products or use products when travelling that are not subject to regulations governing good manufacturing practices. The danger of contamination of products from some countries is significant.

People with diabetes are at increased risk because they usually have more than one risk factor present and risk factors may be additive.

How can complementary therapies be used safely?

Giving people appropriate advice so they can make informed decisions is an important aspect of nursing care (see Table 19.4). The following information could help nurses assist people with diabetes to use CAM safely and choose therapies appropriate for the problem they want to treat. Patients need to know there could be risks if they do not follow conventional evidence-based diabetes management practices. They should not be made to feel guilty or lacking in judgment if they choose to use CAM. People can be advised to:

- Develop an holistic health plan and decide what they hope to achieve by using CAM and use a therapy that is best suited to achieve these goals, for example, to reduce stress: use massage, counselling or time-line therapy.
- Find out as much about the therapy as they can before using it. Seek information from unbiased sources and be wary of information they find in chat rooms on the Internet and advertising material.
- Consult a reputable practitioner, for example, a member of the relevant professional association, and buy products from reputable sources that are approved and have relevant safety data available.
- Store and maintain products appropriately and consider safety issues if children and confused elderly people are part of the household. This also applies to storage of products in healthcare settings.
- Ensure the condition for which they want to use CAM is correctly diagnosed before they treat it, otherwise appropriate treatment could be delayed and the condition deteriorate.

Table 19.4 Advice health professionals can provide to people with diabetes to help them use CAM safely.

- Consider what you want to achieve by using CAM.
- Decide on your general life and health goals and your diabetes goals.
- Select a therapy that is likely to achieve these goals.
- Learn all there is about it/then so you can use the therapy from an informed perspective.
- Consult reputable practitioners for example a member of a professional association that has training standards and requires practitioners to keep up-to-date.
- Buy products from reputable sources that comply with good manufacturing and regulatory processes and are stored appropriately before purchase. Be wary of importing other medicines or buying on the Internet.
- Read labels carefully and look for Aust L or Aust R on the label.
- Have a correct diagnosis before using any therapy. Inform conventional and complementary practitioners about all the therapies you are using and understand there may be risks associated with not following evidence based conventional care.
- Monitor the effects against the health goals you set.
- Keep a list of all the CAM medicines and therapies you use, update it regularly and make sure your CAM and conventional health professionals have a copy.
- Realise that some CAM may take longer to show an effect than conventional medicines.
- Do not stop conventional medicines without consulting your doctor or diabetes educator. CAM medicines may need to be adjusted or stopped temporarily before surgery, illness, investigations, and changes in conventional medicines. You should seek advice in these circumstances.
- Seek advice quickly if any of the following occur: hypo or hyperglycaemia, mental changes, abdominal pain, skin rashes, nausea, vomiting, diarrhoea, falls.

- Be aware that there are risks if they do not follow conventional evidence-based diabetes management recommendations.
- Be aware that they should not stop or change recommended conventional treatments without the advice of their doctor.
- Inform all practitioners, conventional and complementary, about the therapies they are using so the health plan can be coordinated.
- Some CAM should not be used continuously for long periods.
- Take extra care if they are old, very young, pregnant, breastfeeding, have kidney or liver damage or are using a lot of other treatments, because these people are at increased risk of adverse events.
- Seek advice about how to manage the therapy if they need surgery or an investigative procedure especially if radio contrast media are required (see Chapters 3 and 8), or starting any new conventional treatment.
- Seek advice quickly if any of the following occur:
  - hypo/hyperglycaemia
  - mental changes
  - abdominal pain

○ skin rashes
○ nausea, vomiting, diarrhoea
- Monitor the effects on their diabetes, for example, blood glucose, lipids and HbA_{1c} as well as their response with respect to the reason they chose the therapy, for example, to manage pain.

Nursing responsibilities

Nurses have a responsibility to respect people's choices and not to be judgmental about the choices they make. They also have responsibilities to their employer, other patients, visitors and staff. Nurses can use CAM as part of holistic nursing care but they have a duty of care to practice at the level of their education and competence and use safe therapies. The following general advice applies. Specific information about individual CAMs should be sought before using it or giving advice about it.

- Be sensitive to the philosophical and cultural views of people with diabetes and be aware that they may perceive risks and benefits differently from health professionals.
- Follow guidelines for using CAM where they exist, for example, those of the NMC in the UK. In Australia the state nurse registering authorities, the Australian Nursing Federation and Royal College of Nursing, Australia, all have produced guidelines for nurses using CAM (McCabe 2001).
- Ensure you are appropriately qualified and competent if you decide to use, recommend or offer advice about CAM to a person with diabetes.
- Look for evidence of safety and efficiency but do not be too quick to accept or reject 'evidence'.
- Communicate the risks and benefits to people with diabetes and their families/carers. If the person chooses not to follow advice, documentation should outline the information that was given.
- Develop a portfolio of evidence for reference in clinical areas.
- Use herbs and essential oils within the philosophy of QUM and prescribe, administer, document and monitor within that philosophy. Nursing assessment should ask about CAM. People are not always willing to disclose such information and skilful questioning is required. Questions should be asked in a framework of acceptance. The patient has a responsibility to disclose. Nurses can make it easier for them to do so.
- Value the nurse–patient relationship as an essential aspect of the healing process.
- Consider the effect of CAM on other staff, visitors and patients, for example, vaporising aromatherapy, playing music.
- Know how to contact the Poisons Advisory Service in the area.
- Have mechanisms in place to clean and maintain any equipment needed, for example, aromatherapy vaporisers. Processes should be in place to deal with any CAM products the patient brings with them.
- Document appropriately, in the same manner as conventional treatment, the type, dose and duration of the therapy, condition it is used for, advice given, expected outcome, actual outcome and report any adverse events.
- Reliably report suspected or actual CAM adverse events, see Table 19.5.

Table 19.5 Scale for assessing the likelihood of a CAM-conventional interaction and information that should be included in the report. One point is allocated to each of the following criteria.

Interpreting the score:

0–3: Insufficient information to be able to assessed/attribute the event to CAM use.

4–7: Interaction is possible but other explanations for the event need to be excluded.

8–10: Interaction is likely.

(1) The health history is well documented.

(2) The person has:

    (a) renal disease

    (b) liver disease

    (c) atopic conditions

    (d) significant alcohol or illegal drug use

    (e) is very young or elderly.

(3) The AE[a] was associated with using a CAM medicine or therapy.

(4) The medication regimen is documented and includes conventional medicines, CAM medicines, and over-the-counter medicines and doses and dose frequency.

(5) Alternative explanations for the event are excluded.

(6) The AE is adequately described, for example, time of onset of symptoms in relation to taking the medicine, what actually happened, what else was occurring at the time the event occurred.

(7) The time between taking the medicine and the onset of the event is reasonable considering the medicine usual action profile.

(8) The reaction resolves when the CAM medicine is stopped.

(9) The sequence of events is consistent with an AE.

(10) The event recurs when the medicine is used again.

---

[a]AE: adverse event. The event should be noted in the individual's health history and an adverse event report forwarded through the relevant process in the country of origin. In Australia reports go to the Adverse Drug Reactions Advisory Committee (ADRAC) on the 'blue' reporting form (www.tga.gov.au/addr/bluecard.pdf). In the US suspected interactions can be reported via the MedWatch program (www.fda.gov/medwatch/how.htm). In the UK reports can be submitted on the yellow card to the MHRA and the Commission Human Medicine (CHM) (www.yellowcard.gov.au). The information is based on Fugh-Berman & Ernst (2001) and the websites cited above.

Identifying quality health information on the internet

Many people gain information about CAM from the media. Generally, the media and pharmaceutical bodies are careful to only make medium to general level claims consistent with regulations. They often rely on information published in quality peer-reviewed conventional journals often as meta-analysis or systematic reviews or presented at conferences and frequently use 'experts' to promote their message. These experts should declare any conflict of interest, which is increasingly required in publications but is not common in other media. However, the media also specialises in telling stories and sensationalising information, therefore, you may need to verify the source of the information and be wary of sites that quote 'experts' to gain credibility. In addition, the media often reports 'exciting breakthroughs' but the product may not actually be available for many years.

When accessing Internet information carefully scrutinise the site – the quality and reliability varies a great deal. Non-sponsored sites are likely to be more objective. Questions to ask include:

- What is the name of the individual or organisation that produced the site? Information produced by reputable organisations is likely to be more reliable than that produced by individuals.
- What are their credentials?
- Are their links to other sources I can use to verify the information?
- Is the information presented in an objective way and does it discuss a range of options and their benefits and risks?
- Is the discussion comprehensive or does it only discuss one or two options all available from one manufacturer; i.e. is the information actually advertising/marketing?
- Is the site clearly selling products? As a general rule of thumb, if the site is selling or promoting a product and has a number of glowing testimonials from 'happy, satisfied customers', be wary, and check the information in another source.
- Is there evidence the information has been verified in any way e.g. there is a list of peer-reviewed references or links to other reputable sites.
- Is any conflict of interest declared?

Various guidelines have also been developed to evaluate Internet health information but some may not be applicable to CAM (Cooke & Gray 2002). The following are examples that might be useful when assessing the reliability of Internet information:

- Biome Evaluation Guidelines.
- Sandvik Score.
- European Commission Guidelines.
- Discern instrument, which was developed for use by the general public.
- eHealth Code of Ethics.

The following processes are commonly used to grade evidence into a hierarchy according to the quality of the science:

- JADAD score (formulated for CAM).
- National Health and Medical Research Council levels of evidence.
- Cochrane Data base process.
- Joanna Briggs Center for Evidence Based Nursing.

Other factors to consider are advertising codes.

Self-reflection

(1) How will you respond to a person with diabetes who asks you about taking a Chinese herbal medicine to control their blood glucose?

(2) What will you do when a person with diabetes and end stage renal failure elects to use herbal medicine?

(3) How would you advise a person with diabetes who asks you can she use aromatherapy to help her sleep?

Clinical observation

A young Aboriginal man from Central Australia was studying research methods at a University. At the same time he was being educated about traditional tribal practices. He fractured his tibia and fibula playing football. It was a simple fracture but he became depressed and the bones were not mending as well as expected.

The young man's mother took him to consult with the Tribal Elders. On his return the doctor said to the mother, 'That won't cure him you know'. The mother replied, 'No, but it will put him in a frame of mind to accept your medicine. That will work now'.

References

Abuaisha, B., Boulton, A. & Costanz, J. (1998) Acupuncture for the treatment of chronic painful diabetic peripheral neuropathy: a long-term study. *Diabetes Research and Clinical Practice*, **39** (2), 115–121.

Australian Integrative Medicine Association. www.aima.net.au

Agrawal, R. (2007) Yoga improves sense of well-being, reverses changes in metabolic syndrome. *Diabetes Research and Clinical Practice*, **78**, e9–e10.

Baskaran, K., Kizar, A., Radha, K. & Shanmugasundaram, E. (1990) Antidiabetic effect of leaf extract from *Gymnema sylvestre* in non insulin-dependant diabetes mellitus patients. *Journal of Ethnopharmacology*, **30** (3), 295–300.

Biegel, Y. & Schoenfeld, N. (1998) A leading question. *New England Journal of Medicine*, **339**, 827–830.

Braun, L. (2001) Herb–drug interactions: a danger or an advantage? *Diversity*, **2** (6), 31–34.

Braun, L. *et al.* (2006) Use of complementary medicines by surgical patients. Undetected and unsupervised. In: *Proceedings of the Fourth Australasian Conference on Safety and Quality in Health Care*, Melbourne.

Buckle, J. (1997) *Clinical Aromatherapy in Nursing*. Arnold, London.

Bjelakovic, G. & Nikolova, D. (2007) Mortality in randomized controlled trials of antioxidant supplements for primary and secondary prevention: systematic review and meta-analysis. *Journal American Medical Association*, **297**, 842–857.

Chan, C., Ng, S., Rainbow, T. & Chow, A. (2006) Making sense of spirituality. *Journal of Clinical Nursing*, **15**, 822–834.

Chaudhary, S. (2007) Peppermint oil may relieve digestive symptoms, headaches. *American Family Physician*, **75**, 1027–1030.

Chou, K., Lee, P. & Yu, E. (2004) Tai Chi on depressive symptoms amongst Chinese older patients with depressive disorders: a randomized clinical trial. *International Journal of Geriatric Psychiatry*, **19** (11), 1105–1107.

Cochrane Collaboration (2001) *The Cochrane Library Complementary Medicine Field*. Oxford.

Cooke, A. & Gray, L. (2002) Evaluating the quality of internet base information about alternative therapies: development of the BIOME guidelines. *Journal of Public Health Medicine*, **24**, 261–267.

Diet-Pill-Study http://www.diet-pill-study.com/product-reviews.htm (accessed December 2007).

Department of Health and Aging (2002) *National Strategy for the Quality Use of Medicines.* Canberra http://www.health.gov.au/haf/nmp/advisory/pharm.htm

Dossey, B., Keegan, L., Guzzetta, C. & Kolkmeier, L. (1998) *Holistic Nursing: A Handbook for Practice.* Aspen Publications, Gaithersburg.

Dunning, T. (1998) Use of complementary therapies by diabetes educators. Unpublished data, St Vincent's Hospital, Melbourne.

Dunning, T. (2001) Developing clinical practice guidelines. In: *Complementary Therapies in Nursing and Midwifery* (ed. P. McCabe). Ausmed Publications, Melbourne, pp. 37–48.

Dunning, T., Chan, S.P., Hew, F.L., Pendek, R., Mohd, M. & Ward, G. (2001) A cautionary tale on the use of complementary therapies. *Diabetes in Primary Care*, 3 (2), 58–63.

Egede, L., Xiaobou, Y., Zheng, D. & Silverstein, M. (2002) The prevalence and pattern of complementary and alternative medicine use in individuals with diabetes. *Diabetes Care*, 25, 324–329.

Einerhand, S. (2006) CLA weight loss debate continues. *WebMD Health News* 2006.

Eisenberg, D. (1998) Advising patients who seek alternative medical therapies. *American Journal of Health Medicine*, 127 (1), 61–69.

Ewins, D., Bakker, K., Youn, M. & Boulton, A. (1993) Alternative medicine: potential dangers for the diabetic foot. *Diabetic Medicine*, 10, 980–982.

Fetrow, C. & Avila, J. (1999) *Professional's Handbook of Complementary and Alternative Medicines.* Springhouse Corporation, Pennsylvania.

Field, T., Hernandez-Reif, M., LaGreca, A., Shaw, K., Schanberg, S. & Kuhn, C. (1997) Massage lowers blood glucose levels in children with diabetes. *Diabetes Spectrum*, 10, 237–239.

Finney, L. & Gonzalez-Campoy, J. (1997) Dietary chromium and diabetes: is there a relationship? *Clinical Diabetes*, Jan/Feb, 6–8.

Flachskampf, F. (2007) Blood pressure changes with acupuncture comparable to those with ACE inhibitor monotherapy. *Circulation*, online June 4, 2007.

Fugh-Berman, A. & Ernst, E. (2001) Herb–drug interactions: review and assessment of report reliability. *British Journal Clinical Pharmacology*, 52, 587–595.

Garrow, D. & Egede, L. (2006) Association between complementary and alternative medicine use, preventative care practices, and use of conventional medical services among adults with diabetes. *Diabetes Care*, 29, 15–19.

Gill, G., Redmond, S., Garratt, F. & Paisley, R. (1994) Diabetes and alternative medicine: cause for concern. *Diabetic Medicine*, 11, 210–213.

Gupta, Y. & Sharma, M. (2001) Reversal of pyrogallol-induced gastric emptying in rats by ginger (*Zingiber officinalis*). *Experimental Clinical Pharmacology*, 23 (9), 501–503.

Hildreth, K. & Elman, C. (2007) Alternative worldviews and the utilization of conventional and complementary medicine. *Sociological Inquiry*, 77 (1), 76–103.

Jepson, R. & Craig, J. (2008) Cranberries for preventing urinary tract infections. *Cochrane Database of Systematic Reviews*, Issue 1, ART. No. CD001321. DOI: 10: 1002/14651858. CD001321. pub4.

Keen, R., Deacon, A., Delves, H., Morton, J. & Frost, P. (1994) Indian herbal remedies for diabetes as a cause of lead poisoning. *Postgraduate Medicine Journal*, 70, 113–114.

Kelner, M. & Wellman, B. (1997) Health care and consumer choices: medical and alternative therapies. *Social Science and Medicine*, 45, 203–212.

Ko, R. (1998) Adulterants in Asian patent medicines. *New England Journal of Medicine*, 339, 847.

Leese, G., Gill, G. & Houghton, G. (1997) Prevalence of complementary medicine usage within a diabetic clinic. *Practical Diabetes International*, 14 (7), 207–208.

Lloyd, P., Lupton, D., Wiesner, D. & Hasleton, S. (1993) Choosing on alternative therapy: an exploratory study of sociodemographic characteristics and motives of patients resident in Sydney. *Australian Journal of Public Health*, 17 (2), 135–144.

Martin, J., Wang, Z., Zhang, X., Wachtel, D., Volaufova, J., Matthews, D. & Cefalu, W. (2006) Chromium picolinate supplementation attenuates body weight gain and increases insulin sensitivity in subjects with type 2 diabetes. *Diabetes Care*, 29 (8), 1826–1832.

McCabe, P. (ed.) (2001) *Complementary Therapies in Nursing and Midwifery*. Ausmed Publications, Melbourne.

McGrady, A., Bailey, B. & Good, M. (1991) Controlled study of biofeedback assisted relaxation in Type 1 diabetes. *Diabetes Care*, 14 (5), 360–365.

MacLennan, A., Wilson, D. & Taylor, A. (1996) Prevalence and cost of alternative medicine in Australia. *The Lancet*, 347, 569–573.

MacLennan, A., Wilson, D. & Taylor, A. (2002) The escalating cost and prevalence of alternative medicine. *Preventative Medicine*, 35 (2), 166–173.

Michinson, A. (2007) Massage may help relieve acute postoperative pain. *Archives of Surgery* http://www.medscape.com/viewarticle/567550 (accessed December 2007).

O'Brien, R. & Timmins, K. (1999) Trends. *Endocrinology and Metabolism*, 5, 329–334.

O'Mathuna, D. (2007) Creatinine and resistance training for older adults. *Alternative Medicine Alert*, 10 (11), 121–124.

Parsian, N. & Dunning, T. (2008a) Validation tool to assess spirituality and coping in young adults with diabetes. *Proceedings of the 3rd International Congress of Complementary Medicine Research*, Sydney, Australia.

Parsian, N. & Dunning, T. (2008b) Spirituality and coping in young adults with diabetes. *Proceedings of the 7th International Diabetes Federation Western Pacific Region Congress*, Wellington, New Zealand.

Pittler, M., Guo, R. & Ernst, E. (2008) Hawthorn extract for treating chronic heart failure. *Cochrane Database of Systematic Reviews*, Issue 1, ART. No. CD005312. DOI.

Ryan, E., Pick, M. & Marceau, C. (1999) Use of alternative therapies in diabetes mellitus. *Proceedings of the American Diabetes Association Conference*, San Diego, USA.

Sharma, R., Raghuram, T. & Rao, N. (1990) Effect of fenugreek seeds on blood glucose and serum lipids in Type 1 diabetes. *European Journal of Clinical Nutrition*, 44, 301–306.

Sharma, R., Sarkar, A. & Hazra, D. (1996) Use of fenugreek seeds powder in the management of non insulin-dependent diabetes mellitus. *Nutritional Research*, 16, 1331–1339.

Sharpe, P., Blanck, H., Williams, J., Ainsworth, B. & Conway, J. (2007) Use of complementary and alternative medicine for weight control in the United States. *The Journal of Complementary and Alternative Medicine*, 13 (2), 217–222.

Szegede, A., Kohnen, R. & Dienel, A. (2005) Acute treatment of moderate to severe depression with hypericum extract WS 5570 (St John's Wort): randomized controlled double blind non-inferiority trial versus paroxetine. *British Medical Journal*, 330 (7490), 503.

Thomson, S. (2001) Complementary therapies in aged care. In: *Complementary Therapies in Nursing and Midwifery* (ed. P. McCabe). Ausmed Publications, Melbourne, pp. 257–275.

Udani, J., Kavoussi, B. & Hardy, M. (2006) Chromium for type 2 diabetes mellitus and weight loss. *Alternative Medicine Alert*, 9 (7), 78–82.

Verdejo, C., Marco, P., Renau-Piqueras, J. & Pinazo-Duran, M. (1999) Lipid peroxidation in proliferative vitreoretinopathies. *EYE*, 13 (Part 2), 183–188.

Vuksan, V., Stavro, M., Seivenpiper, J. *et al.* (2000) Similar postprandial glycaemic reductions with escalation of dose and administration time of American ginseng in Type 2 diabetes. *Diabetes Care*, 23, 1221–1226.

Wilson, R. (2007) Difficulty identifying odours may herald mild cognitive impairment. *Archives of General Psychiatry*, 64, 802–808.

World Health Organisation (WHO) (2002) *Traditional Medicine Strategy 2002–2005*. WHO, Geneva.

Zhang, L., Ma, J. & Pan, K. (2005) Efficacy of Cranberry juice on *Helicobacter pylori* infection: a double-blind randomized placebo-controlled trial. *Helicobacter*, 10, 139–145.

Chapter 20
Nursing Care in the Emergency and Outpatient Departments

Rationale

Diabetes accounts for a great many presentations to outpatient clinics and emergency departments every year. In addition, people present to community centres and general practitioners with potential emergency situations, for example, silent myocardial infarction, see Chapter 8. People are also being managed in general practice settings and practice nurses are playing increasingly important roles in diabetes ambulatory care. These nurses provide important care planning, education, monitoring, and assessment care that complements that of the GP and specialist diabetes services. They often act as the link between the specialist and primary care services.

This chapter outlines important issues. The other chapters in the book should be cross-referenced for specific information about the conditions patients present to these areas. It is important that diabetes is identified as soon as the individual presents for treatment and their metabolic status is assessed to limit the morbidity and mortality associated with diabetic emergencies.

It is important to be aware that conditions such as myocardial infarction and urinary tract infections can be present with few of the classical signs and symptoms.

The emergency department

Medical emergencies are a major source of morbidity and mortality for people with diabetes. The particular presenting problem may be unrelated to diabetes; however, the existence of diabetes usually affects metabolic control and complicates the management of the presenting problem such as trauma and other medical or surgical emergencies. Extra vigilance is needed to reverse or limit the abnormalities arising as a consequence of altered glucose metabolism due to stress, illness, or trauma.

Diabetes-related abnormalities frequently presenting to the emergency department are:

- myocardial infarction
- cerebrovascular accident
- severe hypoglycaemia
- infected/gangrenous feet
- hyperglycaemia
- ketoacidosis
- hyperosmolar coma.

Rapid effective therapy and effective nursing care increase the chance of a good recovery.

Practice point

In serious emergency situations clear rapid or short-acting insulin is preferred as an IV infusion for ketoacidosis, hyperosmolar coma and myocardial infarction.

Nursing responsibilities

(1) Carry out assessment and observations appropriate to the presenting complaint.
(2) Note medic alert/identification tags.
(3) Enquire whether the patient has diabetes.
(4) Record blood glucose.
(5) Record blood ketones.
(6) Ascertain time and dose of last diabetes medication.
(7) Ascertain time and amounts of last meal, especially the amount of carbohydrate consumed.
(8) Assess usual day-to-day diabetic control and the period of deteriorating control.
(9) Record any other medication, those prescribed by a doctor and anything taken to treat the present complaint including complementary therapies.
(10) Seek evidence of any underlying infection.
(11) Assess pain, severity, site, cause, and relieve appropriately.
(12) Consider the psychological aspects of the illness. Give a full explanation to the patient and family about the findings of the examination, treatment, and likely outcomes.
(13) Avoid long delays in assessing the patient if possible, and be aware of the possibility of a hypoglycaemic episode in people with diabetes on medication.
(14) Have appropriate carbohydrate available to treat promptly if hypoglycaemia does occur.
(15) Assess diabetic knowledge and refer for further education if necessary.
(16) Ensure that the patient knows when to take their next diabetes medication if discharged from the emergency department, especially if the medication regimen or the dose/s have been adjusted, and that the patient understands the new dose.
(17) Arrange appropriate follow-up care.

Clinical observations

(1) Blood glucose can be elevated by infection, pain, and anxiety.
(2) TPR and BP can also be affected by emotional stress.
(3) Reassure, rest the patient, repeat the TPR and BP.

Practice points

(1) Hypoglycaemia may be masked by coma from other causes, some medications, and autonomic neuropathy.
(2) Prolonged hypoglycaemia can result in hypothermia especially in cold weather.
(3) UTI and myocardial infarction can be present with few, if any, of the usual presenting signs due to autonomic neuropathy.
(4) Repeated visits to the emergency department especially for hypoglycaemia or ketoacidosis can indicate an underlying psychosocial problem (see Chapters 7 and 15).

The outpatient department

People with diabetes may present to the outpatient department for routine appointments or for minor surgical or radiological procedures. They are usually basically well and mobile, although some may require a wheelchair, interpreter and/ or guide dog assistance. Water should be provided for guide dogs especially in hot weather.

Nursing responsibilities

(1) Avoid long delays in seeing the doctor if possible.
(2) Be aware of the possibility of hypoglycaemia and know how to recognise and treat it effectively. Know where glucagon and other hypoglycaemic treatments are kept and be sure to restock after use. Have available at least one of the following:
 • dry biscuits
 • sandwiches
 • tea/coffee, sugar
 • glucose gel
 • orange juice
 • glucose.
(3) Have blood glucose monitoring equipment available.
(4) Test blood of Type 1 diabetics for ketones if blood glucose is elevated.
(5) Ensure test results are available in the medical record.
(6) Ensure appropriate examination equipment is available, including:
 • tendon hammer
 • sterile pins
 • Semmens–Weinstein filaments
 • ophthalmoscope
 • tuning fork
 • biothesiometer
 • stethoscope

- eye chart
- midriatic drops if still used.

(7) Ensure patient knows the location of toilets, other clinics, pharmacy.

Nurses and other health professionals should ensure that they are up-to-date with emergency procedures such as cardiopulmonary resuscitation especially when they are working in community settings.

Appendix A
Associations Providing Services for People with Diabetes

Diabetes associations

Diabetes associations have been established in most countries, including the UK (Diabetes UK), The USA (American Diabetes Association), and Australia (Diabetes Australia). Membership of these associations consists of lay people and health professionals who work together to develop management policies and educational material/programmes for the care of people with diabetes.

Diabetes Australia

Diabetes Australia (DA) is the national diabetes organisation in Australia. It has branches in all states. A magazine, *Diabetes Conquest*, is produced quarterly. A national diabetes supply scheme (NDSS) is administered through Diabetes Australia and allows diabetic equipment (blood and urine test strips, syringes, meters) to be purchased from DA selected outlets at subsidised prices. People must enroll in the scheme, and a doctor's or Credentialled Diabetes Educator's (CDE) signature is required on the enrolment form. There is no cost to enroll. Supplies can be ordered and received by mail under this scheme. Insulin is not available through the NDSS scheme.

> Diabetes Australia
> 5th Floor, 39 London Circuit
> Canberra City ACT 2600
> Australia
> www.diabetesaustralia.com.au

Diabetes UK

Diabetes UK is the national diabetes organisation in the UK, with 400 branches and groups. Diabetes UK provides education, develops educational material and trains volunteers. A magazine, *Balance*, is produced six times each year. Diabetes UK also produces a quarterly publication for professionals working in diabetes healthcare and research, *Diabetes Update*.

Diabetes UK
10 Parkway
London NW1 7AA
UK
www.diabetes.org.uk/

Both associations can provide information about specific services available and whom to contact for advice or additional information. Both are active in promoting research into diabetes and fund-raising activities to help finance diabetic research. Most of the reading material suitable for people with diabetes listed in Appendix C can be obtained from these associations.

USA

Similar services are provided in the USA by the American Diabetes Association. Enquiries can be directed to:

American Diabetes Association
ATTN: National Call Center
1701 North Beauregard Street
Alexandria, VA 22311
USA
www.diabetes.org

Professional diabetes associations

Health professional groups with a particular interest in diabetes also work to ensure uniformity of diabetic information, a high standard of care and the professional development of their members. Such associations include:

- American Association of Diabetes Educators www.diabeteseducator.org/
- Australian Diabetes Educators' Association www\\adea.com.au
- Australian Diabetes Society www.racp.edu.au/ads/
- Diabetes UK www.diabetes.org.uk/
- Canadian Diabetes Association (CDA) www.diabetes.ca/ - 14k
- European Association for the Study of Diabetes www.easd.org/
- Federation of European Nurses in Diabetes (FEND) www.fend.org
- Juvenile Diabetes Research Foundation www.jdrf.org/ (or www.jdrf.org.au/ in Australia)

International Diabetes Federation (IDF)

The IDF is an international federation of the national diabetes associations. An International Diabetes Federation Congress is held every three years in a different part of the world. It has two consultative sections:

- IDF Consultative Section on Diabetes Education
- IDF Consultative Section Pediatric and Adolescent Diabetes

It produces a number of publications including the IDF Diabetes Atlas, which provides a very helpful overview of global diabetes organisations and data.

International Diabetes Federation
Avenue Emile De Mot 19
B-1000 Brussels
Belgium
www.idf.org

Other professional associations

Other professional associations have diabetic interest groups within their membership. They include:

- National heart foundations
- Kidney foundations
- Dietetics associations
- Podiatry associations

Pharmaceutical companies

Many of the pharmaceutical companies produce diabetic products and supply patient information material. They also provide research and education grants and continuing education opportunities for doctors, diabetes educators, and other health professionals.

Addresses and telephone numbers can be found in the telephone directory, or from the diabetic association in your country.

Appendix B
Diabetes Reference Material for Nursing Staff

Guidelines and policy statements

Australian Diabetes Educators Association (ADEA) and the Dietitians Association of Australia (DAA) (2005). Joint statement on the role of accredited practising dietitians and diabetes educators in the delivery of nutrition and diabetes self-management education services for people with diabetes. ADEA and DAA, Canberra.

ADEA (2006) *Guidelines for Sick Day Management for People with Diabetes*. ADEA, Canberra.

ADEA, Australian Association for Exercise and Sports Science, Dietitians Association of Australia (2007) *Type 2 Diabetes Medicare Groups Information Pack*. ADEA, Canberra.

ADEA (2006) *Guidelines for Sick Day Management for People with Diabetes*. ADEA, Canberra.

ADEA and the Dietitians Association of Australia (DAA) (2005) *Joint Statement on the Role of Accredited Practising Dietitians and Diabetes Educators in the Delivery of Nutrition and Diabetes Self-management Education Services for People with Diabetes*. ADEA and DAA, Canberra.

ADEA (2008) Position statement: client centred care. *Australian Diabetes Educator*, **11** (1), 26–28.

American Diabetes Association (2005) Care of children and adolescents with Type 1 diabetes. *Diabetes Care*, **28**, 186–212.

American Diabetes Association (ADA) (2002) Position statement: preconception care of women with diabetes. *Diabetes Care*, **25**, S82–S84.

Asia-Pacific Type 2 Diabetes Policy Group (2002) *Type 2 Diabetes Practical Targets and Treatments*. International Diabetes federation, Western Pacific Region (3rd Edition).

Barr, E., Magliano, D., Zimmet, P., Polkinghorne, K., Atkins, R., Dunstan, D., Murray, S. & Shaw, J. (2006) *AusDiab 2005: The Australian Diabetes, Obesity and Lifestyle Study: Tracking the Accelerating Epidemic: Its Causes and Outcomes*. International Diabetes Institute, Melbourne.

Commonwealth of Australia (2004) *Alcohol and Other Drugs: A Handbook for Health Professionals*. Commonwealth of Australia, Canberra.

Cameron, A., Welborn, T., Zimmet, P., Dunstan, D., Own, N., Salmon, J. *et al.* (2003). Overweight and obesity in Australia – the 1999–2000 Australian Diabetes, Lifestyle and Obesity Study (AusDiab). *Medical Journal of Australia*, **178**, 427–432.

Department of Health and Ageing (2006) *What the Australian Government is Doing About Diabetes*. Retrieved November 15, 2006, from www.aodgp.gov.au

Department of Health (DOH) (2001) *National Service Framework for Diabetes*. DOH, London.

Diabetes Australia (DA) (2002) *Diabetes Facts*. www.diabetesaustralia.com.au (accessed January 2007).

DA (2004) *Diabetes Australia's Plan for a Better Life for People with Diabetes*. www.diabetesaustralia.com.au (accessed February 2007).

Diabetes Australia (DA) *National Priorities for Turning Around the Diabetes Epidemic 2007– 2008*. Diabetes Australia, Canberra.

Diabetes Self-Management Guidelines: Guidelines for Providing Services to Newly Diagnosed people with Type 2 Diabetes (2007). Department of Human Services, Victoria.

Diabetes Education Study Group of the European Association for the Study of Diabetes (DESG) (2001) *Basic Curriculum for Health Professionals on Diabetes Therapeutic Education*. DESG. Available at www.desg.org.

Funnell, M. *et al.* (2007) National standards for diabetes self-management education. *Diabetes Care*, **30** (6), 1630–1637.

International Diabetes Federation (IDF) (2006) *IDF Atlas*. IDF, Brussels (www.eatlas.idf.org).

IDF (2007) *Guideline for the Management of Postmeal Glucose*. IDF, Brussels.

IDF (1997) *International Consensus Standards of Practice for Diabetes Education*. IDF, Brussels.

Mensing, C., Boucher, J., Cypress, M., Weinger, K., Mulcahy, K., Barta, K. *et al.* (2000). National standards for diabetes self-management education. *Diabetes Care*, **23** (5), 628–629, 644–651.

Morrissey, J., Shaikh, J. & Patel, V. (2005) Multifactorial intervention and cardiovascular disease in patients with type 2 diabetes. *New England Journal of Medicine*, **348**, 383–393.

National Institute for Health and Clinical Excellence (NICE) (2003) *Guidance on the Use of Patient Education Models for Diabetes*. Technology Appraisal 60. NICE, London.

National Health and Medical Research Council (NHMRC) (2006) *National Evidence Based Guidelines for the Management of Type 2 Diabetes Mellitus*. NHMRC, Canberra.

Reece, E., Coustan, D. & Gabbe, S. (2004) *Diabetes in Women: Adolescence, Pregnancy and Menopause*. Lippincott Williams & Wilkins, Philadelphia.

St Vincent Declaration Primary Care Diabetes Group (SVDPCDG) Guidelines Working Group (1999) *Approved Guidelines for Type 2 Diabetes*. SVDPCDG, UK.

United Nations General Assembly Resolution (UN) December (2006) World Diabetes Day. A/Res/61/225, UN, Geneva.

Victorian Government Department of Human Services (DHS) (2003) *Improving Care for Older People: A Policy for Health Services*. DHS, Melbourne.

World Health Organisation (WHO) (2003) *Adherence to Long Term Therapies: Evidence for Action*. WHO, Geneva.

Useful reading in addition to the texts listed in the preliminary pages and reference list following each chapter

Chiasson, J., Aris-Jilwan, N., Belander, R., Bertrand, S., Beauregard, H., Ekoe, J., Fournier, H. & Havrankova, J. (2003) Diagnosis and treatment of diabetic ketoacidosis and the hyperglycaemic hyperosmolar state. *CMAJ*, **168**, 859–866.

Commonwealth of Australia (2004) *Alcohol and Other Drugs: A Handbook for Health Professionals*. Commonwealth of Australia, Canberra.

Daneman, D. (2002) Eating disorders in adolescent girls and young adult women with type I diabetes. *Diabetes Spectrum*, **2** (15), 83–105.

Glastras, S. & Donaghue, K. (2005) Management of the neonate after gestational diabetes. *Diabetes Management Journal*, **12**, 4.

Malmberg, K., Ryden, L., Wedel, H., Birkeland, K., Bootsma, A., Dickstein, K., Efendic, S., Fisher, M., Hamstem, A., Herlitz, J., Hildebrandt, P., MacLeod, K., Laakso, M., Torp-Pederson, C. & Waldenstrom, A. (2005) Intense metabolic control by means of insulin in patients with diabetes mellitus and acute myocardial infarction (DIGAMI 2): effects on mortality and morbidity. *European Heart Journal*, **26**, 650–661.

Ng, R., Darko, D. & Hillson, R. (2003) Street drug use among young patients with type 1 diabetes in the UK. *Diabetic Medicine*, **21**, 295–296.

Sakurai, T. & Yokono, K. (2006) Comprehensive studies of cognitive impairment of the elderly with type 2 diabetes. *Geriatrics and Gerontology International*, **6**, 159–164.

The Diabetes Prevention Program Research Group (2004) Strategies to identify adults at high risk for type 2 diabetes: the Diabetes Prevention Program. *Diabetes Care*, **28**, 138–144.

Recommended journals

The following diabetes-specific journals are easy to read, contain clinically relevant articles, and are available in most hospital libraries.

Diabetes Care (USA)
Diabetic Medicine (UK)
Diabetologia (Europe)
Practical Diabetes International (UK)
The Diabetes Educator (USA)
International Diabetes Monitor
Journal of Diabetes Nursing (UK)
Diabetes Spectrum (USA)

Appendix C
Reading Material for People with Diabetes

Diabetes Conquest, Diabetes Forecast, Diabetes Voice, and *Balance* are magazines for people with diabetes produced by the diabetic associations of Australia, the USA, and the UK, respectively. They are available to people who become members of the relevant association.

Index

Note: Page numbers in *italics* refer to figures; **bold** refer to tables.

acceptance, of diabetes, 421
acetone, 63
adolescents (diabetes mellitus in), 6–7,
    339, 380–92
advanced glycated end products (AGE),
    16–17
age-related macular degeneration, 218, 219
alcohol, 56, 72, 96–7, 116, 171, 298,
    308, 309, 339
alcoholic ketosis, 190
alitame, 95
allergic reactions, 314
allergies
    corticosteroid therapy, 314
alpha-glucosidase inhibitors, 106,
    109, 114
angiotensin converting enzyme (ACE)
    inhibitors, 151–2
anorexia
    lactic acidosis, 110
    renal disease, 228
antibiotics, 237
antidiabetic agents *see* oral
    hypoglycaemic agents (OHAs)
antihypertensive agents, 151–2
antiplatelet agents, 152, 154
antipsychotic medications, 425–6
Apple Report, 90
aromatherapy, 490–91
    renal disease, 234
aspirin, 148, 217, 273
atherosclerosis, 208
autonomic neuropathy, 208, **209**,
    248–50, 253, 338, **351**, 371,
    402, 506, 509

complications
    brain, **251**
    cardiovascular system, **251**
    gastrointestinal tract, 250,
        251, 252
    gastroparesis, **251**, 266, 282, 283
    genitals, **251**
    lower limbs, **251**
    urinary tract, **251**

Baker Hypothesis, 405
beta blockers, 116, 210, 213, 339
beta-hydroxybutyrate (B-OHB), 63
biguanides, 106–11, **108**, 289
biofeedback techniques, 490
Blood Glucose Awareness Training
    (BGATT) programme, 324–5
blood glucose levels, 23, 55–6, 144,
    168, 186, 189, 213, 263, 338,
    366, 369, 385, 401, 403,
    472–3, 489
blood glucose monitoring, 49, 53–64, 69,
    142, 267, 272, 284, 472–3
    brittle diabetes, 54
    cardiovascular disease, 209
    continuous ambulatory peritoneal
        dialysis, 230
    continuous blood glucose
        monitoring, 135
    corticosteroids/glucocorticoid,
        57–8, 314
    HbA1c/glycosylated haemoglobin, 70
    insulin infusion, 57, 134
    meters, 58–9
    oral hypoglycaemic agents, 106

blood glucose monitoring (*contd.*)
  pregnancy, 54
  self-monitoring, 53
  sharps disposal, 477–8
  total parenteral nutrition, 58
  visual impairment aids, 223
blood ketone monitoring, 57, 62–3,
      64–5
  acetoacetate, 63, 189
  acetone, 63, 189
  beta-hydroxybuterate (B-OHB), 63,
      65, 189
blood urea nitrogen (BUN), 73
Body Mass Index (BMI), 80–81
brittle diabetes, 54, 136, 196, 303–5
bypass surgery, 261

cancer, 286–90
candidiasis, oral, 305
carbohydrate modified food, 95
carbohydrates, 84, 172
cardiac failure, thiazolidinediones
      adverse effects, 113
cardiovascular disease, 207–17,
      428–30
  complementary medicines, 210–11
  in elderly, **350**
  epidemiology, 208–9
  medical tests/procedures, 215
  medicines, 209–10
  mental health, 212
  mortality, 208
  myocardial infarction, 28, 138, 196,
      208, 209, 506–9
  nursing responsibilities, 213–14
  objectives, 212–13
  procedures, 260
  rehabilitation, 215
  risk factor modification, 215–16
  therapy, 213–14
care models, 37–8
care pathways, 47
care plan, 40–41
carpal tunnel syndrome, 313
cataracts, 219
caverject, 341
cerebral oedema, 195, 391
cerebrovascular accident, 28, 507

cerebrovascular disease, 217–18
  management, 218
  signs and symptoms, 218
Charcot's deformity, 235, 236, 237
cherioarthropathy, 313
children (diabetes mellitus in), 6–7, 339,
      380–92
cholesterol monitoring, 72
cholestyramine, 252
cialis, 340
cimetidine, 341
cirrhosis, 307
cisapride, 250
classification
  of diabetes, 2–3
  of foot ulcers, 245
Clinical Management Guidelines
      for Diabetes in General
      Practice, 21
coeliac disease, 311–12
colonoscopy, 273
communication, 145, 304, 443–5, **352**
complementary/CAM therapies, 56, 175,
      210–11, 276–8, 290, 291,
      389–90, 411–12, 482–9, 501–3
  acupuncture, 490
  antioxidant therapy, 490
  aromatherapy, 490–91
  biofeedback techniques, 490
  herb/medicine interactions, 495–9
  Internet information, 502–3
  manage weight, 489
  medicines, 308–9
  relaxation techniques, 490
  safe use, 499–501
  spirituality, 491
  surgery, 492–3
complementary weight loss
      programmes, 91–2
compliance/non-compliance, 55, 179,
      428, 430, 475–6, 477
complications, of diabetes mellitus, 24,
      27–9, 30, 196–7, 205–7, **251**,
      262, 282–3, 313, 403, 476–7
continuous ambulatory peritoneal
      dialysis (CAPD), 230
continuous glucose monitoring system
      (CGMS), 60, 173

continuous subcutaneous insulin infusion (CSII), 133–5
contraception, 410–11
corticosteroid, 287, 290, 314–17
    prednisolone, 290, 314
cost of diabetes, 29
C-peptide, 72–3
creatinine, 73, 85

dawn phenomenon, 174
dehydration, 353
    in elderly, 356–7
        diagnosis, 357
        prevalence, 357
        risk factors, 357
    investigative procedures, 272–3
    ketoacidosis, 189
denial, 420
depression, 228, 358, 422–5
Diabetes Control and Complications Trial (DCCT), 28, 146
    quality of life, 431
    renal disease, 224–5
diabetic foot disease, 235–6, 237
diabetic ketoacidosis *see* ketoacidosis
diagnosis (of diabetes mellitus), 14–17, *16*
    autonomic neuropathy, 250–52
    during cardiac surgery, 209
    dehydration, in elderly, 357
    foot infection, 237
    gestational diabetes mellitus, 406
    mastopathy, 310
    psychological issues, 420–21
dialysis *see* renal disease
diet and nutrition, 79–80
    advice, 483
    blood glucose levels, 56
    deficiencies, 85
    in dementia, 365
    diabetes mellitus, 82–4
    dietary changes, factors associated, 92
    dietary management, principles, 85–9
    drug absorption, **93**
    elderly *see* elderly (diabetes mellitus in)
    enteral nutrition
        complications, 282–3
        elderly, 363–4
    exchanges and portions, 86

exercise, 97–8
food types
    additives, 96
    carbohydrate, 86, 87
    drug interactions, **94**
    fat, 86
    sugar, 87
    sugar-free foods, 93–5
glycaemic index, 86
importance, 76–7
management, in elderly, 360–62
micronutrients, deficiency, 76
mineral deficiencies, 76
nursing responsibilities, 92–3
obesity, 90–91
parenteral nutrition, 282–4
principles, 85–9
renal disease, 227–8
screening, 85
status, 85
support, 282–6
    administration routes, 283
    aims, 282–3
    blood glucose monitoring, 282
    complications, 282–3
    formula choice, 284–5
    malnourishment, 282
    nursing responsibilities, 285–6
    recommencing oral feeding, 286
DIGAMI protocol, 213
discharge planning, 468–9
documentation, 47–50
    clinical observation, 48
    diabetes specific, 49
    education, 455
    flow charts, 48
    in health record, 47
    nursing care plans, 47–8
    nursing notes, 48
    nursing responsibilities, 49
    by patient, 49–50
    patient confidentiality, 48
    preoperative care, 263
driving, 317, 321–7
drug dependence/addiction, **292**
duodenal tubes, 283
Duputren's contracture, 313
dyslipidaemia, 79

eating disorders, 83, 178, 304, 339, 385, 418, 425
ecograms, 47
ecomaps, 47, 444
education (diabetes), 27, 69, 84, 145, 215, 436–7, 441, 448, 449–51, 452–4, 455–6, 456–64
  basic knowledge, 441
  behaviour theories, 441
  children/adolescents, 383
  communication, 443–5
  elderly, 366–7
  empowerment, 444, 451–2
  health literacy, 446–8
    assessment, 447
  learning styles, 438–40
  patient-centred care, 437
  renal disease therapy, 229–30
  sexual problems, 337
  teaching, 445–6
elderly (diabetes mellitus in), 347–9, **350–52**, 359–60, 368, 369, 370–73, 376–7
  activities of daily living, 354
  ageing process, **349**
  assessing disability, **355**
  blood glucose control, 369
  cerebral insufficiency, in elderly, **350**
  cognitive impairment, 355–7
  comorbidities, 353
  corticosteroid effects, 316
  dehydration, 356–7
  delirium, 356
  dementia, 358–9
  depression, 358
  education, 366–7
  exercise/activity, 373–4
  falls, 370–72
  foot care, 369
  frailty index, 354
  functional status, 354–5
  hypoglycaemia, 374–6
  nutrition, 360–62
    dementia, 365
    enteral, 363–4
    malnutrition, **361**
  peripheral insufficiency, **351**
  quality of life, 369–70

  self-care, 367
  sexual problems, 338
  urinary tract infections, 369
empowerment, 431, 432, 444, 451–2
endocrine disorders
  blood glucose levels, 56
  brittle diabetes, 304
erectile dysfunction *see* sexual health
exercise, 24–7, 373–4
eye diseases/disorders, 218–22
  aids/resources for, 222
  associated with diabetes, 221
  detection, 221
  in elderly, **351**
  epidemiology, 218–19
  fluorescein angiography, 221
  insulin therapy commencement, 275
  nursing care, 223
  retinopathy, 28, 219
    aetiology, 219
    cardiovascular disease, 215
    epidemiology, 219
    investigation, 273
    photography, 221, 273
    prevention, 218, 221
    renal disease, 219
    risk factors, 219–20

falls, 370–71, 372
fasting
  blood glucose, 12, 14
  colonoscopy, 273
  hypoglycaemia, 375
  investigative procedures, 272
  ketones, 63
  preoperative care, 263
fibrates, **150**
FlexPen, **129**
foot care, 235, 239, 369
  infected/gangrenous, 507
foot disorders/diseases, 235–48, 476–7
  aetiology, 235
  assessment, 242
  bed rest, 237
  care objectives, 243
  dressing, 246
  in elderly, 369
  infection, 236–8

management, 237–8
morbidity/mortality, 235
prevention, 243
ulcer classification, 245
wound management, 246–8

gastrostomy feeds
administration mode, 283–4
nursing responsibilities, 285
genograms, 47
genomaps, 47, 444
gestational diabetes mellitus (GDM), 3,
    11–12, 14, 399, 405–7
classification, 3
definition, 11–12
diagnosis, 406
ethnicity, 12
risk factors, 406–7
Type 2 diabetes development, 11
glaucoma, 219
glucosamine, **497**
glucose
homeostasis, overview of, 3–6
meters, 58–9
    control testing, 58, 59
    light reflectance meters, 58
monitoring *see* blood glucose monitoring
Glucowatch® G2 Biographer, 59–60
glutamic acid carboxylase (GAD)
    antibodies, 73
glycaemic index (GI), 86
glycaemic load (GL), 87
glycosuria, 14, 66
glycosylated haemoglobin (HbA1c), 16,
    70–71, 106, 206, 353
assay methods, 70
blood glucose monitoring, 53–4
false results, **72**
outpatient stabilisation, 144
recommendations, 70–71

haemochromatosis, 309–10
haemoglobinopathies, fructosamine
    monitoring, 71
HbA1c *see* glycosylated haemoglobin
    (HbA1c)
Health-Related Quality of Life, Short
    Form 36 (SF-36), 431

herbal medicine, 234, 412, 483, 495–9,
    496–8
high-density lipoprotein (HDL)
    monitoring, 72
HMG-CoA reductase inhibitors, **150**
HOPE studies, 226
hyperglycaemia, 186–9
aetiology/causes
    alcohol consumption, 96
    corticosteroids, 314
    drug interaction, 115
    enteral nutrition, 282
    exercise, 26
    during insulin therapy, 133
    surgery, 262, 266, 268
associated diseases/disorders
    cancer, 287
    cardiovascular disease, 208
    renal disease, 224
blood glucose level, 186
blood ketone monitoring, 64
brittle diabetes and, 196
documentation, 49
in elderly, **350**
emergency department, 507
fasting, 133
home-based care, 473–4
insulin infusion, 140
maternal, 404–5
overnight, 132
rebound, 304
symptoms, 186
see also ketoacidosis
hyperinsulinaemia, 5
hypernatraemia, 282
hyperosmolar coma, 138, 507
hyperosmolar non-ketotic coma
    (HONK), 197–9
aetiology, 197
embolism, 199
mortality rate, 198
precipitating factors, 198
prevention, 185
surgery complication, 262
treatment, 197–8
hypoglycaemia, 116, 165, 168, 169,
    172, 177, 252, 267, 337, 374–6,
    384–5, 509

hypoglycaemia (*contd.*)
  aetiology/causes, 171
    drug interaction, 115
    enteral nutrition, 283
    exercise, 24
    fasting, 375
    ketoacidosis, 196
    rapid acting insulin, 123
    surgery, 262, 266, 268
  alcohol consumption, 96, 171
  cortisol in, **171**
  glucagon administration, 180–81
  home-based care, 473
  hormonal response, 170–71
  insulin infusions, 139
  investigative procedures, 273
  medicine interactions, 175, **176**
  nocturnal, 173–5
    indicators, 174
    managing, 175
  prolonged, 178
  psychological effects, 179–80
  relative, 175
  risk factors, 178–9
  severe, 507
  signs and symptoms, **169**, 169–70
  unawareness, 172–3
hypoglycaemic agents *see* oral
        hypoglycaemic agents
        (OHAs)
hypokalaemia
  herbal medicine adverse effects, 234
  post ketoacidosis, 196
  thiazide diuretics adverse effects, 213
hypotension
  postprandial, 371
  postural
    autonomic neuropathy, 252
    fall risk, 371
  renal dialysis, 229

impaired fasting glucose (IFG), 3
impaired glucose homeostasis, 3
impaired glucose tolerance (IGT), 3
  corticosteroid related diabetes, 315
  haemochromatosis, 309
impaired insulin response, 304
incretin hormones, 115

infection
  elderly, 369
inflammatory disease, 314
influenza vaccination, 369
insulin(s)
  Actrapid, 123
  allergy, 141
  Apidra, 124, 408
  biphasic, 123–4
  Detemir, 123, 408
  Glargine, 122, 123
  Glulisine, 122
  Humalin, 124
  Humalog, 124
  Humapen Luxura, **129**
  Humulin, 123, 124
  Hypurin, 123
  Hypurin neutral, 123
  infusions, 57, 134, 137–8, 213, 508
    cardiac arrhythmias, 139
    CSII, 133–5
    insulin pumps, 138
  inhaled, 122
  injection technique, 129
  intermediate-acting, 123, 131
  isophane, 122
  Lispro, 122
  long-acting, 123
  Mixtard, 124
  Novorapid, 122
  premixing, 131, 479
  Protophane, 123
  pumps, **129**
  rapid acting, 122–3
  regimens, 131
    basal bolus, 133
    BD, 132
    continuous blood glucose sensors, 135
    continuous subcutaneous insulin
        infusion, 133–5
    daily injection, 131
  resistance syndrome, 10–11, 314
  short-acting, 123, 131
  storage, 124, 478–9
  types of, 122
insulin therapy
  administration, 129–31
  barriers to, 119–21, 120–21

combination therapy
  biguanides, 104
  oral hypoglycaemic agents, 104
  sulphonylureas, 104
continuous ambulatory peritoneal
    dialysis, 230
  instruction sheets, 456–8
insulin delivery devices, **128–9**
  PenMate 3, **128**
  'pens', **128**
  syringes, **128**
investigative procedures, 272
Quality Use of Medicines, 104
renal disease, 227
sliding scales, 135–6
top-up (stat) doses, 136
in Type 2 diabetes, 117–19
visual impairment aids, 221–2
intravenous lines, 285–6
investigative procedures, 271–3
islet cell antibodies (ICA), 73

ketoacidosis (DKA), 189–97, 507
  aetiology, 189
    surgery, 262
  assessment, 191–2
  blood ketone monitoring, 64
  children, 391–2
  complications, 196–7
  consequences, **192**
  differential diagnosis, 190–91
  euglycaemic, 197
  hypothermia, 189
  hypoxia, 189
  initial patient care, 194
  post ketoacidosis, 197
  prevention, 185
  sexual assault, 196
  signs and symptoms, 189–90, **190**
  treatment, 192–3
    insulin infusions, 138, 508
    nursing care, 193, 194–6
    observations, 194–5
  see also blood ketone monitoring;
      hyperglycaemia
ketones, 63, 189
  blood, monitoring *see* blood ketone
    monitoring

urinary, monitoring, 57
ketosis, 64, **187**, 197
  alcoholic, 190
  starvation, 190, 266
kidney disease *see* renal disease
Kussmaul's respirations, ketoacidosis, 189

lactic acidosis, 199–202
  associated with metformin, 201–2
  biguanides adverse effects, 110
  definition, 200
  management, 202
  signs and symptoms, 201
Lantus, 124
latent autoimmune diabetes (LADA), 8–9
leukocyte function, 30
Levemir, 122, 123
lipid
  dietary management, 86
  management guidelines, 150–51
  outpatient stabilisation, 144
  serum, monitoring, 72
lipid lowering agents, 146–50
  adverse effects, 149–50, 339
  cardiovascular prevention trials, 147–8
  classes, **150**
  management strategy, 148–9
liver disease
  aetiology, 307
  caused by CAM medicines, 308
  iron overload, 309
  thiazolidinediones adverse effects, 113
  sulphonylureas adverse effects, 111

macroproteinuria, 224–5
macrovascular disease, 28, 205
maculopathy, 219, 221
magnetic resonance imaging (MRI),
    237–8
malnourishment
  elderly, 360, 362
  nutritional support, 282
malnutrition
  anaemia, 227
  in cancer, 287
  elderly, 360–62
  hypoglycaemia, 375
  renal disease, 227–8

malnutrition-related (tropical)
    diabetes, 13
management (of diabetes mellitus)
    aim, 21–4
    control assessment, **23**
    dietary modification, 85–9
    education *see* education (diabetes)
    exercise *see* exercise
    investigative procedures, 271–8
    model, *25*
    during surgery, 260–71
    team, 20–21
    see also insulin therapy; oral
        hypoglycaemic agents (OHAs)
Mason-type diabetes *see* maturity onset
    diabetes of the young (MODY)
mastopathy, 310
maternal hyperglycaemia
    consequences, 404
    longer term effects, 404–5
maturity onset diabetes of the young
    (MODY), 13–14
medical record, 47
medicine interactions, 209–10,
        372–3, 300
    blood glucose levels, 55
    complementary therapies, 175, 308–9
    food, **94**
    herbal medicine, 495–9
    hypoglycaemia, 175, **176**
    oral hypoglycaemic agents, 115–16
    renal disease, 227
meditation, 483
menopause, 409–10
    complementary approaches, 411–12
    management, 410
    signs and symptoms, 409
metabolic syndrome, 3, 79
meters
    glucose meters, 58–9, 60, 61
    pedometers, 97
metformin, 106, **108**, 111, 201–2, 263
Micral-Test dipstick tests, 67
microalbuminuria
    renal disease, 224–5
    renal failure, 226
    screening, 67–8

microangiopathy, 306
MICROHOPE studies, 226
microvascular disease, 28, 205
Mini Mental State Examination
    (MMSE), 366
monitoring
    beta-hydroxybutyrate, 63
    cholesterol, 72
    continuous ambulatory peritoneal
        dialysis, 73
    C-peptide, 72–3
    creatinine clearance, 73
    education, 69
    fructosamines, 71
    glucose *see* blood glucose monitoring;
        urine ketone monitoring
    glycosylated haemoglobin, 70–71
    islet cell antibodies, 73
    kidney function, 67
    lipids, 72
    lipoproteins, 72
    microalbuminuria, 67
    twice daily, 57
morning surgical procedure, 263,
        267, 269
musculoskeletal diseases, 312–14, **352**
    myocardial infarction, 28, 138, 196,
        208, 209, 507, 509

nasogastric tubes, 283
nausea/vomiting, 110, 111, 273
neonatal hypoglycaemia, 404
nephropathy *see* renal disease
neuropathies, 28, 205, 235, 238, 239,
        309, 351
nicotinamide, 8
nicotine, 292
nocturnal hypoglycaemia, 133,
        173–5, 385
non-alcoholic fatty liver disease
    (NAFLD), 307
non-alcoholic steatohepatitis (NASH), 307
non-insulin-dependent diabetes (NIDDM)
    see Type 2 diabetes mellitus
non-insulin-dependent diabetes of the
    young (NIDDY) *see* maturity onset
    diabetes of the young (MODY)

non-mydriatic fundus photography, 221
non-nutritive sweeteners
  acesulphame-k, 95
  alitame, 95
  aspartame, 95
  cyclamate, 95
  isomalt, 95
  neotame, 95
  saccharin, 95
  sucralose (splenda), 95
nursing care
  aims, 31
  autonomic neuropathy, 252–3
  complementary therapy, 278
  documentation, 47–8
  elderly, 376–7
  emergency department, 507–8
  eye diseases/disorders, 223
  ketoacidosis, 193
  objectives, 31
  outpatient department, 509–10
nursing history, 36–45
nursing responsibilities
  brittle diabetes, 305
  cancer, 289–90
  cardiovascular disease, 213–14
  central lines, 285–6
  children/adolescents, 391
  complementary therapy, 501–2
  documentation, 49
  emergency department, 508
  foot disorders, 243–5
  home-based care, 473
  hospital stabilisation, 142–3
  intravenous lines, 285–6
  monitoring, 69
  nasogastric tubes, 285
  nutrition, 92–3
  nutritional support, 285–6
  outpatient department, 509–10
  percutaneous endoscopic
    techniques, 285
  photocoagulation, 274–5
  renal disease, 231–2
  stabilisation, 142–3
nutrition *see* diet and nutrition
nutritive sweeteners, 95

obesity, 79–80
  definition, 77
  dietary management, 90–91
  food consumption, 81–2
  inadequate protein intake, 85
  measurement, 80–82
  nutritional support, 289
  overview, 77–9
  prevalence, 77
  significance, 79
  and Type 2 diabetes, 82
oral cavity disease (dental) 305–7
oral contraceptives (OC), 397
oral glucose tolerance test (OGTT), 14,
  17
  patient instructions, 18
  patient preparation, 17
  test protocol, 18–19
oral hypoglycaemic agents (OHAs), 104
  blood glucose monitoring, 54, 106
  combination therapy, 116–17
  Diabex, **108**
  Diaformin, **108**
  Diamicron, **107**
  elderly, 371
  enteral nutrition, 284
  Glibenclamide, **107**, 111
  Gliclazide, **107**
  Glimel, **107**
  Glimepiride, **107**
  glipizide, **107**
  glitinides, **108**, 112
  Glucophage, **108**
  investigative procedures, 272
  medicine interactions, 115–16
  Minidiab, **107**
  nataglitinide, **108**
  pioglitazone, **109**, 112
  renal disease, 228
  repaglinide, **108**
  rosiglitazone, **109**, 112
  side effects, 107–9, 110
  sitagliptin, **109**
  vildagliptin, **109**
oral phosphodiesterase type 5 (PDE-5)
  inhibitors, 340
osmotic diuresis, ketoacidosis, 189

osteopenia, 313
osteoporosis, 316–17

pancreas transplants, 141
pancreatic disease, blood glucose levels, 56
Parkinson's disease, 249
PLISSIT model, 344–5
Polycystic Ovarian Syndrome (PCOS),
    387, 395–8, 114
polydipsia, 8, 64, 189
polypharmacy, 154–5
polyuria, 8, 64, 189, 353
'portions', 86
prednisolone, 290, 314
pregnancy, 28, 54, 56, 71, 111, 219,
    398–403, 405
pressure ulcers, 376
professional diabetes associations, 512
psychological issues, 179–80, 418
    and cardiovascular disease, 428–30
    compliance, 428
    'diabetic grief cycle', 420, *420*
    diagnosis, 420–21
    epidemiology, 418
    mental health, 212
    Type 1 diabetes, 419, 426–7
    Type 2 diabetes, 420, 427–8
    see also quality of life

quality of life (QOL), 179, 227, 235–6,
    369–70, 430–32
    Health-Related Quality of Life, Short
        Form 36 (SF-36), 431
    Quality Use of Medicines (QUM), 103–4,
        156, 278, 482, 486

radiocontrast media injection, 275–6
renal disease, 28, 224–35
    anaemia, 227
    aromatherapy, 234
    assessment, 229
    biopsy, 229
    blood glucose levels, 56
    cardiovascular disease, 215
    care objectives, 230–31
    complementary medicine, 234
    damage, herbal medicine adverse
        effects, 234

dialysis
    continuous ambulatory peritoneal
        dialysis (CAPD), 230
    haemodialysis, 229–30
    peritoneal dialysis, 230
    diet, 227–8
    in elderly, 228, **352**
    erythropoietin production, 227
    estimated GFR (e-GFR), 68
    failure, 225–7
    function, urine test, 67
    function monitoring, 67
    glomerular filtration rate (GFR), 67
    insulin therapy, 227
    management, 229
    nursing responsibilities, 231–2
    priorities, 230
    proteinuria, 224
    radiocontrast media injection, 275–6
    retinopathy, 219
    risk factors, 224–5
    threshold, 66
    urinary tract infections, 369, 509
retinopathy *see* eye diseases/disorders

screening (diabetes mellitus), 19, *20*
    nutrition, 85
    pregnancy, 405
    see also diagnosis (of diabetes mellitus)
self-care, 155–7
    in elderly, 367
    during illness, 186
self-management, 154–5, 388
self-monitoring, 52, 53
serum albumin, 286
serum creatinine, 67
serum lipids, 72
serum potassium, 194
serum urea, 286
sexual health, 334, 336, 337, 338,
    340–41, 344–6
    adolescents, 339
    arthritis, 337
    autonomic neuropathy, 338
    blood glucose levels, 338
    causes, 336–8
    complementary medicines, 342
    counsellors, 335, 343–4

elderly, 338, 339
erectile dysfunction, 339–40
  aetiology, 339
  age-associated, 340
  management, 342–3
  partners, 340
infections, 338
investigation, 340
libido decrease, 338
management
  medication, 340–41
  nursing role, 345–6
  PLISSIT model, 344–5
men, 339–40
neuropathy, 337
psychological illness, 337
sexual development, 336
sexual history, 343
vaginal lubrication, 338
vaginal thrush, 339
women, 338–9
sildenafil, 340
sliding scales, insulin therapy, 135–6
smoking cessation, 292–4
  adverse effects, 339
  cardiovascular disease
    management, 215
  interventions, 294
  medications to support, 296–7
  oral glucose tolerance test, 17
  prevalence, 292
  quitting, 293, 295–6
  retinopathy, 219
sodium restriction, 228
Somogyi effect, 174
sorbitol, 95
spiritual healing, 483, 491
stabilisation (of diabetes mellitus), 141–6
starvation ketosis, 190
statins, 146–7
steroids, oral glucose tolerance test, 17
storing insulin, 124
stress, 79–80, **352**
sucralose (splenda), 95
sugar
  dietary management, 86
  hypoglycaemia therapy, 177
sugar-free foods, 93–5

sulphonylureas, **107**, 111
  adverse effects, 111
  in cancer, 289
  drug interactions, 175, **176**
  mode of action, 106
  in pregnancy, 111
  preoperative withdrawal, 263
surgery, 260–71
  afternoon procedure, 267, 269–70
  basal bolus regimes, 269
  complementary therapy, 492–3
  complications, 262
  electrolyte imbalance, 262
  emergency procedures, 270–71
  hormonal effects, **261**
  hypoglycaemia, 267
  insulin infusions, 138
  long-term effects, **261**
  major procedures, 266–7
  management aims, 262–3
  metabolic effects, **261**
  minor procedures, 268–70
  morning procedure, 267, 269
  patient instructions, 269
  postoperative nursing responsibilities,
    267–8
  preoperative nursing care, 263–6

thalassaemia, haemochromatosis, 309
thiazide diuretics
  adverse effects, 213, 339
  oral glucose tolerance test, 17
thiazolidinediones (TZD), **109**, 112–14
  adverse effects, 113–14
  contraindication, 112
  mode of action, 106
thrombolytic agents, 214
total parenteral nutrition (TPN), 57,
  58, 288
transient ischaemic attacks (TIAs), 217
transplantation, 141
  pancreas, 141
triglycerides, 146
  monitoring, 72
tropical diabetes mellitus, 13
Type 1 diabetes mellitus, 2, 7–8, 381,
  383, 384–8, 407–8
  blood ketone monitoring, 64

Type 1 diabetes mellitus (*contd.*)
  causes, 8
  characteristics, **13**
  C-peptide, 72
  idiopathic, 2
  immune-mediated, 2
  instruction sheets, 459–61
  islet cell antibodies, 73
  management, 9
  progression, 8, 9
  psychological issues, 419, 426–7
  sexual problem in women, 338
Type 2 diabetes mellitus, 3, 9–11, 381,
    383, 388, 399, 408
  characteristics, **13**
  complications, 9–10
  C-peptide, 72
  development, 11
  impaired glucose homeostasis, 3
  instruction sheets, 462–4
  insulin therapy, 117–19
  obesity, 79, 82
  prevention, 19–20
  psychological issues, 420, 427–8
  risk factor, 11
  sexual problem in women, 338

ultrasound, 310
United Kingdom Prospective
    Diabetes Study (UKPDS), 28, 104,
    146, 324
urea, 286

urinary tract infections (UTIs)
  autonomic neuropathy, 509
  in elderly, 369
urine glucose testing, 66–8
  indications, 67
  kidney function, 67
  microalbuminuria, 67–8
  stabilisation in hospital, 142
urine ketone monitoring, 57, 63

vardenafil, 340
very low-density lipoprotein (VLDL)
    monitoring, 72
visual impairment *see* eye diseases/
    disorders
vitamin B_{12} absorption, 111
vitamin supplements, **498**

waist-hip ratio (WHR), 81
weight loss, Type 1 diabetes, 8
white cell count, 30
women
  contraception options, 410–11
  gestational diabetes, 405–7
  Type 1 diabetes, 407–8
  Type 2 diabetes, 408
wound healing, 369

xerostomia, 306
xylitol, 95

zinc, **497**

PARK LEARNING CENTRE

The Park Cheltenham
Glouceste·   GL50 2RH
Teleph   ·· ·

UNIVERSITY OF
GLOUCESTERSHIRE
at Cheltenham and Gloucester

Practice